Tarascon Pocket Pharmacopoeia®
2005 Deluxe Lab-coat Pocket Edition

"Desire to take medicines ... distinguishes man from animals."   *Sir William Osler*

CONTENTS

NOTICES 2
INSTRUCTIONS 3
TABLES INDEX 4
ANALGESICS 12
  Antirheumatics 12
  Muscle relaxants 14
  Non-Opioid Combos 16
  NSAIDs 18
  Opioids 22
  Opioid Combos 26
  Other 29
ANESTHESIA 30
  Anesthetics & Sedatives. 30
  Local anesthetics 31
  Neuromuscular blockers. 31
ANTIMICROBIALS 32
  Aminoglycosides 32
  Antifungals 33
  Antimalarials 36
  Antimycobacterials 40
  Antiparasitics 42
  Antivirals 45
  Carbapenems 58
  Cephalosporins 59
  Ketolides 66
  Macrolides 66
  Penicillins 68
  Quinolones 74
  Sulfonamides 77
  Tetracyclines 78
  Other 79
CARDIOVASCULAR 83
  ACE inhibitors 83
  Aldosterone Antagonists 85
  Angiotensin Receptor
    Blockers 86
  Antiadrenergic agents 87
  Antidysrhythmics 88
  Antihyperlipidemics 93
  Antihypertensives 99
  Antiplatelet drugs 104
  Beta blockers 105
  Calcium chan. blockers 108
  Diuretics 110
  Nitrates 113
  Pressors / Inotropes 115
  Thrombolytics 117
  Volume expanders 118
  Other 119
CONTRAST MEDIA 119
DERMATOLOGY 120
  Acne 120

Actinic Keratosis 123
Antibacterials 123
Antifungals 124
Antiparasitics 126
Antipsoriatics 127
Antivirals 128
Atopic Dermatitis 129
Corticosteroids 129
Hemorrhoid care 133
Other 133
ENDOCRINE/METABOLIC
Androgens 137
Bisphosphonates 138
Corticosteroids 139
Diabetes-Related 141
Gout-Related agents ... 146
Minerals 147
Nutritionals 151
Thyroid agents 152
Vitamins 154
Other 158
ENT 162
Antihistamines 162
Antitussives 164
Decongestants 164
Ear preparations 165
ENT combinations 166
Mouth & lip preps 175
Nasal preparations 176
GASTROENTEROLOGY
Antidiarrheals 178
Antiemetics 180
Antiulcer 183
Laxatives 189
Other 192
HEMATOLOGY 196
Anticoagulants 196
Other 201
HERBAL & ALTERNATIVE
  THERAPIES 204
IMMUNIZATIONS 211
Immunizations 211
Immunoglobulins 216
Immunosuppression 218
NEUROLOGY 219
Alzheimer's disease 219
Anticonvulsants 220
Migraine 225
Multiple sclerosis 227
Parkinsonian agents 228
Other 230
OB/GYN 232

Estrogens 232
GnRH Agonists 234
Hormone replacement 235
Labor induction 238
Ovarian stimulants 238
Progestins 239
Selective Estrogen
  Receptor Modulators 240
Tocolytics 240
Uterotonics 241
Vaginal preps 242
Other OB/GYN 244
ONCOLOGY 246
OPHTHALMOLOGY 247
Antibacterials 247
Antihistamines 249
Antivirals 249
Corticosteroids 249
Decongestants 251
Glaucoma 251
Mast cell stabilizers ... 253
Mydriatics/Cycloplegics 254
NSAIDs 255
Other 255
PSYCHIATRY 256
Antidepressants 256
Antimanic agents 261
Antipsychotics 262
Anxiolytics / Hypnotics 265
Drug dependence 268
Stimulants / ADHD /
  Anorexiants 270
Other 272
PULMONARY 273
Beta Agonists 273
Inhaled Steroids 275
Leukotriene inhibitors .. 277
Other 277
TOXICOLOGY 280
UROLOGY 283
BPH 283
Bladder agents 283
Erectile dysfunction 286
Nephrolithiasis 286
Prostate cancer 288
Other 289
INDEX 289
NOTES PAGES 316-317
EMERGENCY DRUGS . 318
CARDIAC DYSRHYTHMIA
  PROTOCOLS 319
ORDERING INFO 320

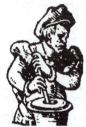

FOR TARASCON BOOKS/SOFTWARE, VISIT: **WWW.TARASCON.COM**

Tarascon Pocket Pharmacopoeia®
- Classic Shirt-Pocket Edition
- Deluxe Labcoat Pocket Edition
- PDA software for Palm OS® or Pocket PC®

Other Tarascon Pocketbooks
- Tarascon Internal Medicine & Critical Care Pocketbook
- Tarascon Adult Emergency Pocketbook
- Tarascon Pocket Orthopaedica®
- Tarascon Primary Care Pocketbook
- Tarascon Pediatric Emergency Pocketbook & software
- How to be a Truly Excellent Junior Medical Student

See faxable order form on page 320

"It's not how much you know, it's how fast you can find the answer."®

Important Caution – Please Read This! The information in the *Pocket Pharmacopoeia* is compiled from sources believed to be reliable, and exhaustive efforts have been put forth to make the book as accurate as possible. The *Pocket Pharmacopoeia* is edited by a panel of drug information experts with extensive peer review and input from more than 50 practicing clinicians of multiple specialties. Our goal is to provide health professionals focused, core prescribing information in a convenient, organized, and concise fashion. We include FDA-approved dosing indications and those off-label uses that have a reasonable basis to support their use. *However the accuracy and completeness of this work cannot be guaranteed.* Despite our best efforts this book may contain typographical errors and omissions. The *Pocket Pharmacopoeia* is intended as a quick and convenient reminder of information you have already learned elsewhere. The contents are to be used as a guide only, and health care professionals should use sound clinical judgment and individualize therapy to each specific patient care situation. This book is not meant to be a replacement for training, experience, continuing medical education, studying the latest drug prescribing literature, raw intelligence, good hair, or common sense. This book is sold without warranties of any kind, express or implied, and the publisher and editors disclaim any liability, loss, or damage caused by the contents. *If you do not wish to be bound by the foregoing cautions and conditions, you may return your undamaged and unexpired book to our office for a full refund.* Tarascon Publishing is independent from and has no affiliation with pharmaceutical companies. Although drug companies purchase and distribute our books as promotional items, the Tarascon editorial staff alone determine all book content.

Tarascon Pocket Pharmacopoeia® 2005 Deluxe Edition

S1

HOW TO USE THE TARASCON POCKET PHARMACOPOEIA

The *Tarascon Pocket Pharmacopoeia* arranges drugs by clinical class with a comprehensive index in the back. Trade names are italicized and capitalized. Drug doses shown in mg/kg are generally intended for children, while fixed doses represent typical adult recommendations. Each drug entry is divided as follows:

WARNING – Black-box warnings, if any, with lower level warnings in the "notes" section.

ADULT – Selected adult FDA-approved indications & doses listed in typical frequency of use.

PEDS – Selected peds FDA-approved indications & doses listed in typical frequency of use.

UNAPPROVED ADULT – Selected adult non-FDA-approved (ie, "off-label") indications and doses listed in typical frequency of use.

UNAPPROVED PEDS – Selected pediatric non-FDA-approved (ie, "off-label") indications and doses listed in typical frequency of use.

FORMS – Formulations available from manufacturers (eg, tabs, caps, liquid, susp, cream, lotion, patches, etc), including specification of trade, generic, and over-the-counter forms. Scored pills are designated as such. Not all pharmacies stock all items, of course.

NOTES – Selected notes, additional warnings, major adverse drug interactions, dosage adjustment in renal/hepatic insufficiency, therapeutic levels, etc.

Each drug entry contains the following codes:

▶ **METABOLISM & EXCRETION:** L = primarily liver, K = primarily kidney, LK = both, but liver>kidney, KL = both, but kidney>liver, LO = liver & onions

♀ **SAFETY IN PREGNANCY:** A = Safety established using human studies, B = Presumed safety based on animal studies, C = Uncertain safety; no human studies and animal studies show an adverse effect, D = Unsafe - evidence of risk that may in certain clinical circumstances be justifiable, X = Highly unsafe - risk of use outweighs any possible benefit. For drugs which have not been assigned a category: +Generally accepted as safe, ?Safety unknown or controversial, -Generally regarded as unsafe.

◗ **SAFETY IN LACTATION:** +Generally accepted as safe, ?Safety unknown or controversial, -Generally regarded as unsafe. Many of our "+" listings are taken from the AAP website, and may differ from those recommended by manufacturers (www.aap.org/policy/0063.html).

© **DEA CONTROLLED SUBSTANCES:** I = High abuse potential, no accepted use (eg, heroin, marijuana), II = High abuse potential and severe dependence liability (eg, morphine, codeine, hydromorphone, cocaine, amphetamines, methylphenidate, secobarbital). Some states require triplicates. III = Moderate dependence liability (eg, *Tylenol #3, Vicodin*), IV = Limited dependence liability (benzodiazepines, propoxyphene, phentermine), V = Limited abuse potential (eg, *Lomotil*).

$ **RELATIVE COST:** Cost codes used are "per month" of maintenance therapy (eg, antihypertensives) or "per course" of short-term therapy (eg, antibiotics). Codes are calculated using average wholesale prices (at press time in US$) for the most common indication & route of each drug at a typical adult dosage. For maintenance therapy, costs are calculated based upon a 30 day supply or the quantity that might typically be used in a given month. For short-term therapy (≤10 days), costs are calculated on a single treatment course. When multiple forms are available (eg,

Code	Cost
$	< $25
$$	$25 to $49
$$$	$50 to $99
$$$$	$100 to $199
$$$$$	≥ $200

generics), these codes reflect the least expensive generally available product. When drugs don't neatly fit into the classification scheme above, we have assigned codes based upon the relative cost of other similar drugs. *These codes should be used as a rough guide only*, as (1) they reflect cost, not charges, (2) pricing often varies substantially from location to location & time to time, and (3) HMOs, Medicaid, and buying groups often negotiate quite different pricing. Your mileage may vary. Check with your local pharmacy if you have any question.

🍁 **CANADIAN TRADE NAMES:** Unique common Canadian trade names not used in the USA are listed after a maple leaf symbol. Trade names used in both nations or only in the USA are displayed without such notation.

PAGE INDEX FOR TABLES

GENERAL
Abbreviations 4
Therapeutic levels 5
Outpt peds drugs............. 6
Peds vitals & IV drugs 7
QT interval drugs............. 7
P450 enzymes 8-9
Conversions.................... 9
Formulas 10
Drug therapy web sites ... 10
Adult emerg drugs 318
Cardiac protocols 319

ANALGESICS
NSAIDs 19
Opioid equivalency 23
Fentanyl transdermal 24

ANTIMICROBIALS
Bacterial pathogens 60
Cephalosporins 61
STDs / Vaginitis 62
Penicillins 70
SBE prophylaxis 72
Quinolones 77

CARDIOVASCULAR
ACE inhibitors 85
LDL goals 94
CAD 10-year risk 95
Statins lipid response 96
HTN risk stratification 112
Cardiac parameters 115
Thrombolysis in MI 117

DERMATOLOGY
Topical steroids 132

ENDOCRINE
Corticosteroids 141
Diabetes numbers 143
Insulin 144
IV solutions 147
Fluoride dose 149
Potassium forms 151
Peds rehydration 152

GASTROENTEROLOGY
H pylori treatment 186

HEMATOLOGY
Heparin dosing 198
Oral anticoagulation 199
Warfarin interactions 200

IMMUNIZATIONS
Adult immunizations 214
Child immunizations 214
Tetanus 216

NEUROLOGY
Nerve roots 219
Lumbosacral spine 219
Glasgow coma scale 220
Dermatomes 225

OB/GYN
Drugs in pregnancy 235
Emerg contraception 236
Oral contraceptives 237
APGAR score 241

OPTHALMOLOGY
Visual acuity screen 256

PSYCHIATRY
Body mass index 270

PULMONARY
Inhaler colors 274
Inhaled steroids 276
Peak flow 277

TOXICOLOGY
Antidotes 282

ABBREVIATIONS IN TEXT

AAP - American Academy of Pediatrics
ac - before meals
ADHD - attention deficit & hyperactivity disorder
AHA - American Heart Association
ANC - absolute neutrophil count
ASA - aspirin
bid - twice per day
BP - blood pressure
BPH - benign prostatic hypertrophy
CAD - coronary artery disease
cap - capsule
CMV - cytomegalovirus
CNS - central nervous system
COPD - chronic obstructive pulmonary disease
CPZ - chlorpromazine
CrCl - creatinine clearance
d - day
D5W - 5% dextrose
DPI - dry powder inhaler
elem - elemental
ET - endotracheal
EPS - extrapyramidal symptoms
g - gram
gtts - drops
GERD - gastroesophageal reflux dz
GU - genitourinary
h - hour
HAART - highly active antiretroviral therapy
HCTZ - hydrochlorothiazide
HRT - hormone replacement therapy
HSV - herpes simplex virus
HTN - hypertension
IM - intramuscular
INR - international normalized ratio
IU - international units
IV - intravenous
JRA - juvenile rheumatoid arthritis
kg - kilogram
LFTs - liver fxn tests
LV - left ventricular
mcg - microgram
MDI - metered dose inhaler
mEq - milliequivalent
mg - milligram
MI - myocardial infarction
min - minute
mL - milliliter
mo - months old
ng - nanogram
NS - normal saline
NYHA - New York Heart Association
N/V -nausea/vomiting
OA - osteoarthritis
pc - after meals
PO - by mouth
PR - by rectum
prn - as needed
q - every
qd - once daily
qhs - at bedtime
qid - four times/day
qod - every other day
q pm - every evening
RA - rheumatoid arthritis
SC - subcutaneous
soln - solution
supp - suppository
susp - suspension
tab - tablet
TB - tuberculosis
TCAs - tricyclic antidepressants
TIA - transient ischemic attack
tid - 3 times/day
TNF - tumor necrosis factor
tiw - 3 times/week
UC - ulcerative colitis
UTI - urinary tract infection
wk - week
yo - years old

THERAPEUTIC DRUG LEVELS

Drug	Level	Optimal Timing
amikacin peak	20-35 mcg/ml	30 minutes after infusion
amikacin trough	<5 mcg/ml	Just prior to next dose
carbamazepine trough	4-12 mcg/ml	Just prior to next dose
cyclosporine trough	50-300 ng/ml	Just prior to next dose
digoxin	0.8-2.0 ng/ml	Just prior to next dose
ethosuximide trough	40-100 mcg/ml	Just prior to next dose
gentamicin peak	5-10 mcg/ml	30 minutes after infusion
gentamicin trough	<2 mcg/ml	Just prior to next dose
lidocaine	1.5-5 mcg/ml	12-24 hours after start of infusion
lithium trough	0.6-1.2 meq/l	Just prior to first morning dose
NAPA	10-30 mcg/ml	Just prior to next procainamide dose
phenobarbital trough	15-40 mcg/ml	Just prior to next dose
phenytoin trough	10-20 mcg/ml	Just prior to next dose
primidone trough	5-12 mcg/ml	Just prior to next dose
procainamide	4-10 mcg/ml	Just prior to next dose
quinidine	2-5 mcg/ml	Just prior to next dose
theophylline	5-15 mcg/ml	8-12 hrs after once daily dose
tobramycin peak	5-10 mcg/ml	30 minutes after infusion
tobramycin trough	<2 mcg/ml	Just prior to next dose
valproic acid trough	50-100 mcg/ml	Just prior to next dose
vancomycin trough	5-10 mcg/ml	Just prior to next dose

Tarascon Pocket Pharmacopoeia® Deluxe PDA Edition

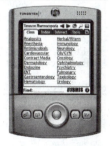

Features
- Palm OS® and Pocket PC® versions
- Meticulously peer-reviewed drug information
- Multiple drug interaction checking
- Continuous internet auto-updates
- Extended memory card support
- Multiple tables & formulas
- Complete customer privacy

Download a FREE 30-day trial version at www.tarascon.com
Subscriptions thereafter priced at $2.29/month

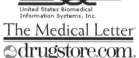

PEDIATRIC DRUGS		*Age*	*2m*	*4m*	*6m*	*9m*	*12m*	*15m*	*2y*	*3y*	*5y*
		Kg	5	6½	8	9	10	11	13	15	19
		Lbs	11	15	17	20	22	24	28	33	42
med	***strength***	***freq***	***teaspoons of liquid per dose*** *(1 tsp= 5 ml)*								
Tylenol (mg)		q4h	80	80	120	120	160	160	200	240	280
Tylenol (tsp)	160/t	q4h	½	½	¾	¾	1	1	1¼	1½	1¾
ibuprofen (mg)		q6h	-	-	75†	75†	100	100	125	150	175
ibuprofen (tsp)	100/t	q6h	-	-	¾†	¾†	1	1	1¼	1½	1¾
amoxicillin or	125/t	bid	1	1¼	1½	1¾	1¾	2	2¼	2¾	3½
Augmentin	200/t	bid	½	¾	1	1	1¼	1¼	1½	1¾	2¼
not otitis media	250/t	bid	½	½	¾	¾	1	1	1¼	1¼	1¾
	400/t	bid	¼	½	½	½	¾	¾	¾	1	1
amoxicillin,	200/t	bid	--	1¼	1¾	2	2	2¼	2¾	3	4
otitis media‡	250/t	bid	--	1¼	1½	1½	1¾	1¾	2¼	2½	3¼
	400/t	bid	--	¾	¾	1	1	1¼	1½	1½	2
Augmentin ES‡	600/t	bid	--	½	½	¾	¾	¾	1	1¼	1½
azithromycin*§	100/t	qd	¼	½†	½	½	½	½	¾	¾	1
(5-day Rx)	200/t	qd	--	¼†	¼	¼	¼	¼	½	½	½
Bactrim/Septra	---	bid	½	¾	1	1	1	1¼	1½	1½	2
cefaclor*	125/t	bid	1	1	1¼	1½	1½	1¾	2	2½	3
"	250/t	bid	½	½	¾	¾	¾	1	1	1¼	1½
cefadroxil	125/t	bid	½	¾	1	1	1¼	1¼	1½	1¾	2¼
"	250/t	bid	¼	½	½	½	¾	¾	¾	1	1
cefdinir	125/t	qd	--	¾†	1	1	1	1¼	1½	1¾	2
cefprozil*	125/t	bid	--	¾†	1	1	1¼	1½	1½	2	2¼
"	250/t	bid	--	½†	½	½	¾	¾	¾	1	1¼
cefuroxime	125/t	bid	½	¾	¾	1	1	1	1½	1¾	2¼
cephalexin	125/t	qid	--	½	¾	¾	1	1	1¼	1½	1¾
"	250/t	qid	--	¼	¼	½	½	½	¾	¾	1
clarithromycin	125/t	bid	--	½†	½	½	¾	¾	¾	1	1¼
"	250/t	bid	--	--	--	¼	½	½	½	½	¾
dicloxacillin	62½/t	qid	½	¾	1	1	1¼	1¼	1½	1¾	2
loracarbef*	100/t	bid	--	1†	1¼	1½	1½	1¾	2	2¼	3
nitrofurantoin	25/t	qid	¼	½	½	½	½	¾	¾	¾	1
Pediazole	---	tid	½	½	¾	¾	1	1	1	1¼	1½
penicillin"	250/t	bid-tid	--	1	1	1	1	1	1	1	1
albuterol	2/t	tid	-	-	-	-	½	½	¾	¾	1
cetirizine	5/t	qd	-	-	-	-	-	-	½	½	½
diphenhydramine	12.5/t	q6h	½	½	¾	¾	1	1	1¼	1½	2
prednisolone	15/t	qd	¼	½	½	¾	¾	¾	1	1	1¼
prednisone	5/t	qd	1	1¼	1½	1¾	2	2¼	2½	3	3¾
Robitussin	---	q4h	-	-	¼†	¼†	½	½	¾	¾	1
Rondec	---	q4h	-	-	-	-	¼†	¼†	½	½	1
Triaminic	---	q4h	-	¼	¼	¼	½	½	1	1	1
Tylenol w/ Codeine		q4h	-	-	-	-	-	-	-	1	1

* Dose shown is for otitis media only; see dosing in text for alternative indications.

† Dosing at this age/weight not recommended by manufacturer.

‡ AAP now recommends high dose (80-90 mg/kg/d) for all otitis media in children; with Augmentin used as ES only.

§Give a double dose of azithromycin the first day.

PEDIATRIC VITAL SIGNS AND INTRAVENOUS DRUGS

Age		Pre- matr	New- born	2m	4m	6m	9m	12m	15m	2y	3y	5y
Weight	(Kg)	2	3½	5	6½	8	9	10	11	13	15	19
	(Lbs)	4½	7½	11	15	17	20	22	24	28	33	42
Maint fluids	(ml/h)	8	14	20	26	32	36	40	42	46	50	58
ET tube	(mm)	2½	3/3½	3½	3½	3½	4	4	4½	4½	4½	5
Defib	(Joules)	4	7	10	13	16	18	20	22	26	30	38
Systolic BP	(high)	70	80	90	100	110	110	120	120	120	120	120
	(low)	50	60	70	70	70	70	70	70	75	75	80
Pulse rate	(high)	145	145	180	180	180	160	160	160	150	150	135
	(low)	100	100	110	110	110	100	100	100	90	90	65
Resp rate	(high)	45	45	45	40	35	35	30	30	30	24	24
	(low)	35	35	35	30	25	25	20	20	20	16	14
adenosine	(mg)	0.2	0.3	0.5	0.6	0.8	0.9	1	1.1	1.3	1.5	1.9
atropine	(mg)	0.1	0.1	0.1	0.13	0.16	0.18	0.2	0.22	0.26	0.30	0.38
Benadryl	(mg)	-	-	5	6½	8	9	10	11	13	15	19
bicarbonate	(meq)	2	3½	5	6½	8	9	10	11	13	15	19
dextrose	(g)	2	3½	5	6½	8	9	10	11	13	15	19
epinephrine	(mg)	.02	.04	.05	.07	.08	.09	0.1	0.11	0.13	0.15	0.19
lidocaine	(mg)	2	3½	5	6½	8	9	10	11	13	15	19
morphine	(mg)	0.2	0.3	0.5	0.6	0.8	0.9	1	1.1	1.3	1.5	1.9
mannitol	(g)	2	3½	5	6½	8	9	10	11	13	15	19
naloxone	(mg)	.02	.04	.05	.07	.08	.09	0.1	0.11	0.13	0.15	0.19
diazepam	(mg)	0.6	1	1.5	2	2.5	2.7	3	3.3	3.9	4.5	5
lorazepam	(mg)	0.1	0.2	0.3	0.35	0.4	0.5	0.5	0.6	0.7	0.8	1.0
phenobarb	(mg)	30	60	75	100	125	125	150	175	200	225	275
ampicillin	(mg)	100	175	250	325	400	450	500	550	650	750	1000
ceftriaxone	(mg)	-	-	250	325	400	450	500	550	650	750	1000
cefotaxime	(mg)	100	175	250	325	400	450	500	550	650	750	1000
gentamicin	(mg)	6	7	10	13	16	18	20	22	26	30	38

SELECTED DRUGS THAT MAY PROLONG THE QT INTERVAL

alfuzosin	dolasetron	isradipine	pentamidine*†	sotalol*†
amiodarone*†	droperidol*	levofloxacin*	phenothiazines‡¶	tacrolimus
arsenic trioxide*	erythromycin*†	levomethadyl*	pimozide*†	tamoxifen
azithromycin*	flecainide	lithium	polyethylene glycol	telithromycin
bepridil*†	foscarnet	mefloquine	(PEG-salt solution)§	tizanidine
chloroquine*	fosphenytoin	methadone*†	procainamide*	vardenafil
cisapride*†	gatifloxacin*	moexipril/HCTZ	quetiapine‡	venlafaxine
clarithromycin*	gemifloxacin	moxifloxacin	quinidine*†	Visicol§
cocaine*	haloperidol*‡	nicardipine	quinine	voriconazole
disopyramide*†	ibutilide*†	octreotide	risperidone‡	ziprasidone‡
dofetilide*	indapamide*	ondansetron	salmeterol	

This table may not include all drugs that prolong the QT interval or cause torsades. Risk of drug-induced QT prolongation may be increased in women, elderly, ↓K, ↓Mg, bradycardia, starvation, & CNS injuries. Hepatorenal dysfunction & drug interactions can ↑ the concentration of QT interval-prolonging drugs. Coadministration of QT interval-prolonging drugs can have additive effects. Avoid these (and other) drugs in congenital prolonged QT syndrome (www.qtdrugs.org). *Torsades reported in product labeling/case reports. †↑Risk in women. ‡QT prolongation: thioridazine>ziprasidone>risperidone, quetiapine, haloperidol. §May be due to electrolyte imbalance. ¶QT prolongation documented for chlorpromazine*, mesoridazine*, thioridazine*.

INHIBITORS, INDUCERS, AND SUBSTRATES OF CYTOCHROME P450 ISOZYMES

Bear in mind that inhibitors and inducers listed on the chart below do not necessarily cause clinically important drug interactions with the substrates listed below. This chart only predicts the *potential* for a drug interaction. Please refer to other resources for more definitive information when a drug interaction is suspected based on the information given in the chart. Many drugs are metabolized by subfamilies of hepatic cytochrome P450. A drug that inhibits the activity of a specific enzyme can block the metabolism of drugs that are substrates of that enzyme. If the body lacks other mechanisms for excreting these drugs, they can accumulate and cause toxicity. A drug that induces the activity of a specific enzyme can stimulate the metabolism of drugs that are substrates of that enzyme. This can lead to decreased levels of these drugs in the body and could reduce their efficacy. Underlined drugs have demonstrated potential for drug interactions in case reports or clinical studies; the contribution of the other drugs to clinically important interactions is unclear. The contents of this table may not be complete since new evidence about drug interactions is continually being identified.

CYP 1A2

Inhibitors: amiodarone, cimetidine, ciprofloxacin, citalopram (weak), clarithromycin, enoxacin, erythromycin, ♦fluvoxamine, ipriflavone, isoniazid, mexiletine, norfloxacin, paroxetine, peginterferon alfa-2a, tacrine, zileuton, ziprasidone.
Inducers: barbiturates, carbamazepine, charcoal-broiled foods, lansoprazole, omeprazole, phenytoin, rifampin, ritonavir, smoking, St Johns wort.
Substrates: acetaminophen, alosetron, amitriptyline, bortezomib, caffeine, clomipramine, clozapine, cyclobenzaprine, duloxetine, estradiol, fluvoxamine, haloperidol, imipramine, levobupivacaine, mexiletine, mirtazapine, naproxen, olanzapine, ondansetron, propranolol, riluzole, ropinirole, ropivacaine, R-warfarin, tacrine, theophylline, verapamil, zileuton, zolmitriptan.

CYP 2C8

Inhibitors: gemfibrozil, trimethoprim.
Inducers: barbiturates, carbamazepine, rifabutin, rifampin.
Substrates: amiodarone, carbamazepine, isotretinoin, paclitaxel, pioglitazone, repaglinide, rosiglitazone, tolbutamide.

CYP 2C9

Inhibitors: amiodarone, cimetidine, cotrimoxazole, delavirdine, disulfiram, fenofibrate, fluconazole, ♦fluvoxamine, gemfibrozil, ginkgo, imatinib, isoniazid, ketoconazole (weak), leflunomide, metronidazole, ticlopidine, voriconazole, zafirlukast.
Inducers: aprepitant, barbiturates, bosentan, carbamazepine, rifampin, rifapentine.
Substrates: alosetron, bortezomib, bosentan, carvedilol, celecoxib, desogestrel, diclofenac, flurbiprofen, fluvastatin, formoterol, glimepiride, ibuprofen, irbesartan, isotretinoin, losartan, mefenamic acid, meloxicam, montelukast, naproxen, nateglinide, phenytoin, piroxicam, rosiglitazone, rosuvastatin, sildenafil, tolbutamide, torsemide, valdecoxib, valsartan, vardenafil, voriconazole, S-warfarin, zafirlukast, zileuton

CYP 2C19

Inhibitors: bortezomib (possible), bosentan (possible), citalopram (weak), clorazepate, delavirdine, esomeprazole, felbamate, fluconazole, fluoxetine, fluvoxamine, isoniazid, letrozole, modafinil, omeprazole, oxcarbazepine, telmisartan, voriconazole.
Inducers: rifampin.
Substrates: amitriptyline, bortezomib, carisoprodol, cilostazol, citalopram, clomipramine, desipramine, diazepam, escitalopram, esomeprazole, formoterol, imipramine, lansoprazole, nelfinavir, omeprazole, pantoprazole, phenytoin, progesterone, proguanil, propranolol, voriconazole, R-warfarin.

CYP 2D6

Inhibitors: amiodarone, bupropion, chloroquine, cimetidine, citalopram (weak), clomipramine, delavirdine, diphenhydramine, duloxetine, escitalopram (weak), fluoxetine, fluphenazine, fluvoxamine, haloperidol, imatinib, paroxetine, perphenazine, pindolol, propafenone, propoxyphene, propranolol, quinacrine, ♦quinidine, ♦ritonavir, sertraline, terbinafine, tolterodine, thioridazine, venlafaxine. **Inducers:** St Johns wort. **Substrates:** almotriptan, amitriptyline, aripiprazole, atomoxetine, bortezomib, carvedilol, cevimeline, chlorpromazine, clomipramine, clozapine, codeine*, delavirdine, desipramine, dextromethorphan, dihydrocodeine*, dolasetron, donepezil, duloxetine, flecainide, fluoxetine, formoterol, galantamine, haloperidol, hydrocodone*, imipramine, loratadine, maprotiline, methadone, methamphetamine, metoprolol, mexiletine, mirtazapine, morphine, nortriptyline, ondansetron, oxycodone, palonosetron, paroxetine, perphenazine, propafenone, propoxyphene, propranolol, risperidone, ritonavir, thioridazine, timolol, tolterodine, tramadol*, trazodone, venlafaxine.

CYP 3A4

Inhibitors: amiodarone, amprenavir, aprepitant, atazanavir, clarithromycin, cyclosporine, danazol, delavirdine, diltiazem, efavirenz, erythromycin, ethinyl estradiol, fluconazole, fluoxetine, fluvoxamine, grapefruit juice, imatinib, indinavir, itraconazole, ketoconazole, miconazole, nefazodone, nelfinavir, quinine, ♦ritonavir, saquinavir, sertraline, *Synercid*, troleandomycin, verapamil, voriconazole, zafirlukast. **Inducers:** barbiturates, bosentan, carbamazepine, dexamethasone, efavirenz, ethosuximide, garlic supplements (suspected inducer), griseofulvin, modafinil, nafcillin, nevirapine, oxcarbazepine, phenytoin, primidone, rifabutin, ♣rifampin, rifapentine, St Johns wort. **Substrates:** acetaminophen, alfentanil, alfuzosin, almotriptan, alosetron, alprazolam, amiodarone, amlodipine, amprenavir, aprepitant, argatroban, aripiprazole, atazanavir, atorvastatin, bepridil, bexarotene, bortezomib, bosentan, budesonide, buspirone, buprenorphine, carbamazepine, carvedilol, cevimeline, cilostazol, cisapride, citalopram, clarithromycin, clomipramine, clonazepam, clopidogrel, clozapine, corticosteroids, cyclophosphamide, cyclosporine, dapsone, delavirdine, desogestrel, dexamethasone, diazepam, dihydroergotamine, diltiazem, disopyramide, docetaxel, dofetilide, dolasetron, donepezil, doxorubicin, dutasteride, efavirenz, eletriptan, eplerenone, ergonovine, ergotamine, erythromycin, esomeprazole, ethinyl estradiol, etoposide, escitalopram, exemestane, felodipine, fentanyl, finasteride, fluticasone, galantamine, gefitinib, glyburide, hydrocodone, ifosfamide, imatinib, imipramine, indinavir, irinotecan, isotretinoin, isradipine, itraconazole, ketoconazole, lansoprazole, letrozole, levobupivacaine, loperamide, lopinavir, loratadine, losartan, lovastatin, methadone, methylergonovine, methylprednisolone, midazolam, mifepristone, mirtazapine, modafinil, mometasone, montelukast, nateglinide, nefazodone, nelfinavir, nicardipine, nifedipine, nimodipine, nisoldipine, ondansetron, oxybutynin, paclitaxel, pantoprazole, pimozide, pioglitazone, praziquantel, quetiapine, quinidine, quinine, repaglinide, rifabutin, ritonavir, saquinavir, sertraline, sibutramine, sildenafil, simvastatin, sirolimus, sufentanil, tacrolimus, tamoxifen, temazepam, testosterone, theophylline, tiagabine, tolterodine, toremifene, tramadol, trazodone, triazolam, trimetrexate, troleandomycin, valdecoxib, vardenafil, venlafaxine, verapamil, vinblastine, vincristine, vinorelbine, voriconazole, R-warfarin, zaleplon, zileuton, ziprasidone, zolpidem, zonisamide.

♦potent inhibitor; rank order of CYP 3A4 inhibition by protease inhibitors: ritonavir >> indinavir = nelfinavir = amprenavir > saquinavir. ♣potent inducer * Metabolism by CYP2D6 required to convert to active analgesic metabolite; analgesia may be impaired by CYP2D6 inhibitors.

CONVERSIONS	Liquid:	Weight:
Temperature:	1 fluid ounce = 30ml	1 kilogram = 2.2 lbs
F = (1.8) C + 32	1 teaspoon = 5ml	1 ounce = 30 g
C = (F - 32)/(1.8)	1 tablespoon = 15ml	1 grain = 65 mg

FORMULAS

Alveolar-arterial oxygen gradient = A-a = 148 - 1.2($PaCO2$) - $PaO2$
  [normal = 10-20 mmHg, breathing room air at sea level]

Calculated osmolality = 2Na + glucose/18 + BUN/2.8
            [norm 280-295 meq/L. Na in meq/L; all others in mg/dL]

Pediatric IV maintenance fluids (see table on page 7)
  4 ml/kg/hr **or** 100 ml/kg/day for first 10 kg, plus
  2 ml/kg/hr **or** 50 ml/kg/day for second 10 kg, plus
  1 ml/kg/hr **or** 20 ml/kg/day for all further kg

$$mcg/kg/min = \frac{16.7 \times \text{Drug Conc [mg/ml]} \times \text{Infusion Rate [ml/h]}}{\text{Weight [kg]}}$$

$$\textit{Infusion rate [ml/h]} = \frac{\text{Desired mcg/kg/min} \times \text{Weight [kg]} \times 60}{\text{Drug concentration [mcg/ml]}}$$

Fractional excretion of sodium =
[Pre-renal, etc <1%; ATN, etc >1%]
$$\left[\frac{\text{urine Na / plasma Na}}{\text{urine creat / plasma creat}} \right] \times 100\%$$

Anion gap = Na – (Cl + HCO3)   [normal = 10-14 meq/L]

Glomerular filtration rate (ml/min/1.73 m^2)
  = 186 x (creatinine)$^{-1.154}$ x (age)$^{-0.203}$ x (0.742 if ♀) x (1.210 if African American)

$$\textit{Creatinine clearance} = \frac{(\text{lean kg})(140 - \text{age})(0.85 \text{ if female})}{(72)(\text{stable creatinine [mg/dL]})}$$
  [normal >80]

Body surface area (BSA) = square root of:
  [in m^2]
$$\left[\frac{\text{height (cm)} \times \text{weight (kg)}}{3600} \right]$$

DRUG THERAPY REFERENCE WEBSITES (selected)

Professional societies or governmental agencies with drug therapy guidelines		
AHRQ	Agency for Healthcare Research and Quality	www.ahcpr.gov
AAP	American Academy of Pediatrics	www.aap.org
ACC	American College of Cardiology	www.acc.org
ACCP	American College of Clinical Pharmacy	www.accp.com
AHA	American Heart Association	www.americanheart.org
ADA	American Diabetes Association	www.diabetes.org
AMA	American Medical Association	www.ama-assn.org
ATS	American Thoracic Society	www.thoracic.org
ASHP	Amer. Society Health-Systems Pharmacists	www.ashp.org
CDC	Centers for Disease Control & Prevention	www.cdc.gov
IDSA	Infectious Diseases Society of America	www.idsociety.org
MHA	Malignant Hyperthermia Association	www.mhaus.org
NHLBI	National Heart, Lung, & Blood Institute	www.nhlbi.nih.gov
Other therapy reference sites		
Cochrane library		www.cochrane.org
Emergency Contraception Website		www.not-2-late.com
Immunization Action Coalition		www.immunize.org
Int'l Registry for Drug-Induced Arrhythmias		www.qtdrugs.org
Managing Contraception		www.managingcontraception.com
Nephrology Pharmacy Associates		www.nephrologypharmacy.com

Pocket Pharmacopoeia Editorial Staff*

*Affiliations are given for information purposes only, and no affiliation sponsorship is claimed.

ANALGESICS: Antirheumatic Agents – Gold Compounds

NOTE: Monitor CBC and urinary protein q 4-12 weeks (oral) or q 1-2 weeks (injectable) due to the risk of myelosuppression and proteinuria.

auranofin (Ridaura) ▶K ♀C ▶+ $$$$
WARNING - Gold toxicity may manifest as marrow suppression, proteinuria, hematuria, pruritus, rash, stomatitis or persistent diarrhea.
ADULT - RA: Initial 3 mg PO bid or 6 mg PO qd. May increase to 3 mg PO tid after 6 months.
PEDS - RA: 0.1-0.15 mg/kg/day PO. Max dose 0.2 mg/kg/day. May be given qd or divided bid.
UNAPPROVED ADULT - Psoriatic arthritis: 3 mg PO bid or 6 mg PO qd.
FORMS - Trade: Caps 3 mg.
NOTES - Contraindicated in patients with a history of any of the following gold-induced disorders: anaphylactic reactions, necrotizing enterocolitis, pulmonary fibrosis, exfoliative dermatitis, bone marrow suppression. Not recommended in pregnancy. Proteinuria has developed in 3%-9% of patients. Diarrhea, rash, stomatitis, chrysiasis (gray-to-blue pigmentation of skin) may occur. Minimize exposure to sunlight or artificial UV light. Auranofin may increase phenytoin levels.

gold sodium thiomalate (Aurolate, ✦Myochrysine) ▶K ♀C ▶+ $$$$$
WARNING - Evaluate patient at each injection for gold toxicity, including marrow suppression, proteinuria, hematuria, pruritus, rash, stomatitis or persistent diarrhea.
ADULT - RA: weekly IM injections: 1st dose, 10 mg. 2nd dose, 25 mg. 3rd & subsequent doses, 25-50 mg. Continue the 25-50 mg dose weekly to a cumulative dose of 0.8-1g. If improvement seen w/o toxicity, 25-50 mg every other week for 2-20 weeks. If stable, increase dosing intervals to q 3-4 weeks.
PEDS - JRA: test dose 10 mg IM, then 1 mg/kg, not to exceed 50 mg for a single injection. Continue this dose weekly to a cumulative dose of 0.8-1g. If improvement seen w/o toxicity, dose every other week for 2-20 weeks. If stable, increase dosing intervals to q 3-4 weeks.
NOTES - Administer only IM, preferably intragluteally. Have patient remain recumbent for approximately 10 minutes after injection. Contraindicated in pregnancy & in patients who have uncontrolled DM, severe debilitation, renal disease, hepatic dysfunction or hepatitis, marked HTN, uncontrolled CHF, SLE, blood dyscrasias, patients recently radiated & those with severe toxicity from previous exposure to gold or other heavy metals, urticaria, eczema & colitis. Arthralgia & dermatitis may occur.

ANALGESICS: Antirheumatic Agents – Immunomodulators

adalimumab (Humira) ▶Serum ♀B ▶- $$$$$
WARNING - Death, sepsis, and serious infections (eg, TB, fungal) have been reported. Do not start if current serious infection, discontinue if serious infection develops, and closely monitor any new infection. Caution in diabetics or others at risk of infections, or those in endemic TB or histoplasmosis regions. Screening for latent TB infection is recommended. Rare CNS disorders (eg, multiple sclerosis, myelitis, optic neuritis) have been reported.
ADULT - RA:. 40 mg SC q2 weeks, alone or in combination w/ methotrexate or other disease-modifying antirheumatic drugs. May increase frequency to q week if not on methotrexate.
PEDS - Not approved in children.
FORMS - Trade: 40 mg pre-filled glass syringes or vials with needles, 2 per pack.
NOTES - Monitor for neutropenia. Refrigerate & protect from light. Avoid live vaccines.

anakinra (Kineret) ▶K ♀B ▶? $$$$$
WARNING - Increased incidence of serious infections. Do not use in active infection or with TNF-blocking drugs such as adalimumab, etanercept or infliximab.
ADULT - RA: 100 mg SC qd, alone or in combination with other disease-modifying antirheumatic drugs (DMARDs) except TNF inhibitors.
PEDS - Not approved in children.
FORMS - Trade: 100 mg pre-filled glass syringes with needles, 7 or 28 per box.
NOTES - Monitor for neutropenia. Refrigerate & protect from light. Avoid live vaccines.

etanercept (Enbrel) ▶Serum ♀B ▶- $$$$$
WARNING - Death, sepsis, and serious infections (eg, TB) have been reported. Do not start if current serious infection, discontinue if serious infection develops, and closely monitor any new infection. Screening for latent TB infection is recommended. Use caution in those with a history of recurring infections or with underlying conditions (eg, DM) that predispose to infec-

tions. Rare nervous system disorders (eg, multiple sclerosis, myelitis, optic neuritis) have been reported.

ADULT - RA, psoriatic arthritis, ankylosing spondylitis: 50 mg SC q week, alone or in combination with methotrexate. Plaque psoriasis: 50 mg SC twice weekly x 3 months, then 50 mg SC q week.

PEDS - JRA 4-17 yo: 0.8 mg/kg SC q week, to max single dose of 50 mg.

FORMS - Supplied in a carton containing four dose trays. Each dose tray contains one 25 mg single-use vial of etanercept, one syringe (1 mL sterile bacteriostatic water for injection, containing 0.9% benzyl alcohol), one plunger, and two alcohol swabs.

NOTES - Max dose per injection site is 25 mg. Appropriate SC injection sites are thigh, abdomen & upper arm. Rotate injection sites. Refrigerate. Avoid live vaccines.

infliximab (*Remicade*) ▶Serum ♀B ▶? $$$$$
WARNING - Death, sepsis, and serious infections (eg, TB, fungal) have been reported. Do not start if current serious infection, discontinue if serious infection develops, and closely monitor any new infection. Screening for latent TB infection is recommended. May worsen heart failure; monitor signs/symptoms of CHF. Hypersensitivity reactions may occur. Rare CNS disorders (eg, multiple sclerosis, myelitis, optic neuritis) have been reported.

ADULT - RA: 3 mg/kg IV in combination with methotrexate at 0, 2 and 6 weeks. Give q8 weeks thereafter. May increase up to 10 mg/kg or q4 weeks if incomplete response. See entry

in GI section for Crohn's disease dosing.
PEDS - Not approved in children.
UNAPPROVED ADULT - Ankylosing spondylitis: 5 mg/kg IV at 0, 2 and 6 weeks.
NOTES - Headache, dyspnea, urticaria, nausea, infections, abdominal pain, & fever. Avoid live vaccines. 3 cases of toxic optic neuropathy reported. Refrigerate.

leflunomide (*Arava*) ▶LK ♀X ▶- $$$$$
WARNING - Hepatotoxicity. Rare reports of lymphoma, pancytopenia, agranulocytosis, thrombocytopenia, Stevens-Johnson Syndrome, & severe HTN. Exclude pregnancy before starting. Women of childbearing potential must use reliable contraception.

ADULT - RA: initial: 100 mg PO qd x 3 days. Maintenance: 10-20 mg PO qd.
PEDS - Not approved in children.
UNAPPROVED ADULT - Psoriatic arthritis: Initial: 100 mg PO qd x 3 days. Maintenance: 10-20 mg PO qd.
FORMS - Trade: Tabs 10, 20, & 100 mg.
NOTES - Avoid in hepatic or renal insufficiency. Monitor LFTs, CBC & creatinine monthly until stable, then q 1-2 months. Avoid in men wishing to father children or with concurrent live vaccines. May increase INR if on warfarin; check INR within 1-2 days of initiation, then weekly for 2-3 weeks & adjust the dose accordingly. Rifampin increases and cholestyramine decreases leflunomide levels. Give charcoal or cholestyramine in case of overdose or drug toxicity. Cholestyramine: 8 g PO tid for up to 11 days. Consecutive days administration not necessary unless rapid level decrease desired.

ANALGESICS: Antirheumatic Agents – Other

azathioprine (*Azasan, Imuran*) ▶LK ♀D ▶- $$$
WARNING - Chronic immunosuppression with azathioprine increases the risk of neoplasia. May cause marrow suppression or GI hypersensitivity reaction characterized by severe N/V.

ADULT - Severe RA: Initial dose 1 mg/kg (50-100 mg) PO qd or divided bid. Increase by 0.5 mg/kg/day at 6-8 weeks and thereafter at 4-week intervals, if no serious toxicity and if initial response is unsatisfactory. Max dose 2.5 mg/kg/day. In patients with clinical response, use the lowest effective dose for maintenance therapy.

PEDS - Not approved in children.
UNAPPROVED ADULT - Crohn's disease: 75-

100 mg PO qd. Myasthenia gravis: 2-3 mg/kg/day PO. Behcet's syndrome, SLE: 2.5 mg/kg/day PO. Vasculitis: 2 mg/kg/day PO.
UNAPPROVED PEDS - JRA: Initial: 1 mg/kg/day PO. Increase by 0.5 mg/kg/day every 4 weeks until response or max dose of 2.5-3 mg/kg/day.
FORMS - Generic/Trade: Tabs 50 mg, scored. Trade (Azasan): 25, 75 & 100 mg, scored.
NOTES - Monitor CBC q 1-2 weeks with dose changes, then q1-3 months. ACE inhibitors, allopurinol & methotrexate may increase activity & toxicity. Azathioprine may decrease the activity of anticoagulants, cyclosporine, & neuromuscular blockers.

hydroxychloroquine (*Plaquenil*) ▶K ♀C ▶+ $$

ADULT - RA: 400-600 mg PO qd to start, taken with food or milk. After clinical response, decrease to 200-400 mg PO qd. If no objective improvement within 6 months, discontinue. SLE: 400 mg PO qd-bid to start. Decrease to 200-400 PO qd for prolonged maintenance.

PEDS - Not approved in children.

UNAPPROVED PEDS - JRA or SLE: 3-5 mg/kg/day, up to a max of 400 mg/day PO qd or divided bid. Max dose 7 mg/kg/day. Take with food or milk.

FORMS - Generic/Trade: Tabs 200 mg, scored.

NOTES - May exacerbate psoriasis or porphyria. Irreversible retinal damage possible with long-term or high dosage (>6.5 mg/kg/day). Baseline & periodic eye exams recommended. Anorexia, nausea & vomiting may occur. May increase digoxin and metoprolol levels.

methotrexate (*Rheumatrex, Trexall*) ▶LK ♀X ▶- $$

WARNING - Deaths have occurred from hepatotoxicity, pulmonary disease, intestinal perforation and marrow suppression. Restrict use to patients with severe, recalcitrant, disabling rheumatic disease unresponsive to other therapy. Use with extreme caution in renal insufficiency. May see diarrhea. Folate deficiency states may increase toxicity. The American College of Rheumatology recommends supplementation with 1 mg/day of folic acid.

ADULT - Severe RA, psoriasis: 7.5 mg/week PO single dose or 2.5 mg PO q12h x 3 doses given as a course once weekly. May be increased gradually to a max weekly dose of 20 mg. After clinical response, reduce to lowest effective dose. Psoriasis: 10-25 mg weekly IV/IM until response, then decrease dose. Supplement with 1 mg/day of folic acid.

PEDS - Severe JRA: 10 mg/meters squared PO q week.

UNAPPROVED ADULT - Severe RA, psoriasis: 25 mg PO q week. After clinical response, reduce to lowest effective dose. Supplement with 1 mg/day of folic acid.

FORMS - Trade: Tabs 5, 7.5, 10 & 15 mg. Generic/Trade: Tabs 2.5 mg, scored.

NOTES - Contraindicated in pregnant & lactating women, alcoholism, liver disease, immunodeficiency, blood dyscrasias. Avoid ethanol. Monitor CBC q month, liver & renal function q 1-3 months.

sulfasalazine (*Azulfidine, Azulfidine EN-tabs*, ✦*Salazopyrin, Salazopyrin EN-Tabs, S.A.S.*) ▶L ♀B ▶- $

WARNING - Beware of hypersensitivity, marrow suppression, renal & liver damage, irreversible neuromuscular & CNS changes, fibrosing alveolitis.

ADULT - RA: 500 mg PO qd-bid after meals to start. Increase to 1g PO bid. Ulcerative colitis: see GI section.

PEDS - JRA: ≥6 yo: 30-50 mg/kg/day (EN-Tabs) PO divided bid to max of 2 g/day. Ulcerative colitis: See GI section.

UNAPPROVED ADULT - Ankylosing spondylitis: 1-1.5g PO bid. Psoriasis: 1.5-2g PO bid. Psoriatic arthritis: 1g PO bid.

FORMS - Generic/Trade: Tabs 500 mg, scored. Enteric coated, Delayed release (EN-Tabs) 500 mg.

NOTES - Contraindicated in children <2 yo. Avoid with hepatic or renal dysfunction, intestinal or urinary obstruction, porphyria, sulfonamide or salicylate sensitivity. Monitor CBC q2-4 weeks for 3 months, then q3 months. Monitor LFTs & renal function. Oligospermia & infertility, and photosensitivity may occur. May decrease folic acid, digoxin, cyclosporine & iron levels. May turn body fluids, contact lenses, or skin orange-yellow. Enteric coated (Azulfidine EN, Salazopyrin EN) tabs may cause fewer GI adverse effects.

ANALGESICS: Muscle Relaxants

NOTE: May cause drowsiness and/or sedation, which may be enhanced by alcohol and other CNS depressants.

baclofen (*Lioresal*) ▶K ♀C ▶+ $$

WARNING - Abrupt discontinuation of intrathecal baclofen has been associated with life-threatening sequelae and/or death.

ADULT - Spasticity related to MS or spinal cord disease/injury: 5 mg PO tid x 3 days, 10 mg PO tid x 3 days, 15 mg PO tid x 3 days, then 20 mg PO tid x 3 days. Max dose: 20 mg PO qid. Spasticity related to spinal cord disease /injury, unresponsive to oral therapy: Specialized dosing via implantable intrathecal pump.

PEDS - Spasticity related to spinal cord disease/injury: Specialized dosing via implantable intrathecal pump.

UNAPPROVED ADULT - Trigeminal neuralgia: 30-80 mg/day PO divided tid-qid. Tardive dyskinesia: 40-60 mg/day PO divided tid-qid. Intractable hiccoughs: 15-45 mg PO divided tid.

UNAPPROVED PEDS - Spasticity: ≥2 yo: 10-15 mg/day PO divided q8h. Max doses 40 mg/day for 2-7 yo, 60 mg/day for ≥8 yo.

FORMS - Generic/Trade: Tabs 10 & 20 mg, trade scored.

NOTES - Hallucinations & seizures with abrupt withdrawal. Administer with caution if impaired renal function. Efficacy not established for typical muscle relaxant indications: rheumatic disorders, stroke, cerebral palsy, Parkinson's disease.

carisoprodol (Soma) ▶LK ♀? ▶- $

ADULT - Musculoskeletal pain: 350 mg PO tid-qid with meals and qhs.

PEDS - Not approved in children.

FORMS - Generic/Trade: Tabs 350 mg.

NOTES - Contraindicated in porphyria, caution in renal or hepatic insufficiency. Abuse potential. Use with caution if addiction-prone.

chlorzoxazone (Parafon Forte DSC) ▶LK ♀C ▶? $$

WARNING - If signs/symptoms of liver dysfunction are observed, discontinue use.

ADULT - Musculoskeletal pain: Start 500 mg PO tid-qid, increase prn to 750 mg tid-qid. After clinical improvement, decrease to 250 mg PO tid-qid.

PEDS - Not approved in children.

UNAPPROVED PEDS - Musculoskeletal pain: 125-500 mg PO tid-qid or 20 mg/kg/day divided tid-qid depending on age & weight.

FORMS - Generic/Trade: Tabs & caplets 250 & 500 mg (Parafon Forte DSC 500 mg tablets scored).

NOTES - Use with caution in patients with history of drug allergies. Discontinue if allergic drug reactions occur or for signs/symptoms of liver dysfunction. May turn urine orange or purple-red.

cyclobenzaprine (Flexeril) ▶LK ♀B ▶? $

ADULT - Musculoskeletal pain: 10 mg PO tid up to max dose of 60 mg/day. Not recommended in elderly or for use >2-3 weeks.

PEDS - Not approved in children.

FORMS - Generic/Trade: Tabs 10 mg. Trade: Tabs 5 mg.

NOTES - Contraindicated with recent or concomitant MAO inhibitor use, immediately post-MI, in patients with arrhythmias, conduction disturbances, CHF, & hyperthyroidism. Not effective for cerebral or spinal cord disease or in children with cerebral palsy. May have similar adverse effects & drug interactions as TCAs. Caution with urinary retention, angle-closure glaucoma, increased intraocular pressure.

dantrolene (Dantrium) ▶LK ♀C ▶- $$$$

WARNING - Hepatotoxicity, monitor LFTs. Use the lowest possible effective dose.

ADULT - Chronic spasticity related to spinal cord injury, stroke, cerebral palsy, MS: 25 mg PO qd to start, increase to 25 mg bid-qid, then by 25 mg up to max of 100 mg bid-qid if necessary. Maintain each dosage level for 4-7 days to determine response. Use the lowest possible effective dose. Malignant hyperthermia: 1 mg/kg rapid IV push q6h continuing until symptoms subside or to a maximum 10 mg/kg/dose. Doses of up to 40 mg/kg have been used. Follow with 4-8 mg/kg/day PO divided tid-qid x 1-3 days to prevent recurrence.

PEDS - Chronic spasticity: 0.5 mg/kg PO bid to start; increase to 0.5 mg/kg tid-qid, then by increments of 0.5 mg/kg up to 3 mg/kg bid-qid. Max dose 100 mg PO qid. Malignant hyperthermia: use adult dose.

UNAPPROVED ADULT - Neuroleptic malignant syndrome, heat stroke: 1-3 mg/kg/day PO/IV divided qid.

FORMS - Trade: Caps 25, 50 & 100 mg.

NOTES - Photosensitization may occur. Warfarin may decrease protein binding of dantrolene & increase dantrolene's effect. The following website may be useful for malignant hyperthermia: www.mhaus.org

diazepam (Valium, Diastat, ♣Vivol, E Pam) ▶LK ♀D ▶- ©IV $

ADULT - Skeletal muscle spasm, spasticity related to cerebral palsy, paraplegia, athetosis, stiff man syndrome: 2-10 mg PO/PR tid-qid. 5-10 mg IM/IV initially, then 5-10 mg q 3-4h prn. Decrease dose in elderly.

PEDS - Skeletal muscle spasm: 0.1-0.8 mg/kg/day PO/PR divided tid-qid. 0.04-0.2 mg/kg/dose IV/IM q2-4h. Max dose 0.6 mg/kg within 8 hours.

FORMS - Generic/Trade: Tabs 2,5,10 mg, trade scored. Generic: Oral drops 2mg/ml, oral soln 1 mg/ml, 5 mg/5 ml & concentrated soln 5 mg/ml, 10 mg/ml. Trade only: Rectal gel: 2.5 mg & 5 mg, 10 mg, 15 mg & 20 mg, in twin packs.

NOTES - Contraindicated in liver disease. Abuse potential. Long half-life may increase the risk of adverse effects in the elderly. Cimetidine, oral contraceptives, disulfiram, fluoxetine, isoniazid, ketoconazole, metoprolol, propoxyphene, propranolol, & valproic acid may increase diazepam concentrations. Diazepam may increase digoxin & phenytoin concentrations. Rifampin may increase the metabolism of diazepam. Avoid combination with protease inhibitors.

metaxalone (*Skelaxin*) ▶LK ♀? ▶? $$$

ADULT - Musculoskeletal pain: 800 mg PO tid-qid.

PEDS - >12 yo: use adult dose.

FORMS - Trade: Tabs 400 & 800 mg, scored.

NOTES - Contraindicated in serious renal or hepatic insufficiency or history of drug-induced hemolytic or other anemia. Beware of hypersensitivity reactions, leukopenia, hemolytic anemia, & jaundice. Monitor LFTs.

methocarbamol (*Robaxin, Robaxin-750*) ▶LK ♀C ▶? $

ADULT - Musculoskeletal pain, acute relief: 1500 mg PO qid or 1000 mg IM/IV tid x 48-72h. Maintenance: 1000 mg PO qid, 750 mg PO q4h, or 1500 mg PO tid. Tetanus: specialized dosing.

PEDS - Tetanus: Specialized dosing.

FORMS - Generic/Trade: Tabs 500 & 750 mg. OTC in Canada.

NOTES - Max IV rate 3 ml/min to avoid syncope, hypotension, & bradycardia. Total parenteral dosage should not exceed 3g/day for >3 consecutive days, except in the treatment of tetanus. Urine may turn brown, black or green.

orphenadrine (*Norflex*) ▶LK ♀C ▶? $$

ADULT - Musculoskeletal pain: 100 mg PO bid. 60 mg IV/IM bid.

PEDS - Not approved in children.

UNAPPROVED ADULT - Leg cramps: 100 mg PO qhs.

FORMS - Generic/Trade: 100 mg extended release. OTC in Canada.

NOTES - Contraindicated in glaucoma, pyloric or duodenal obstruction, BPH, & myasthenia gravis. Some products contain sulfites, which may cause allergic reactions. May increase anticholinergic effects of amantadine & decrease therapeutic effects of phenothiazines. Side effects include dry mouth, difficult urination, constipation, headache & GI upset.

quinine sulfate ▶L ♀X ▶+ $

ADULT - Chloroquine resistant malaria. See Antimicrobial section (Antimalarial Agents).

PEDS - Not approved in children.

UNAPPROVED ADULT - Nocturnal leg cramps: 260-325 mg PO qhs.

FORMS - Rx: Generic: Caps 130,200, 260, 300, 324, 325, 650 mg. Tabs 250, 260, 325 mg.

NOTES - Hemolysis possible in G6PD deficiency. Cinchonism with overdose. Quinine may have quinidine-like activity & may exacerbate cardiac arrhythmias. Beware of hypersensitivity reactions, tinnitus & visual impairment. Do not use with mefloquine. Antacids may decrease quinine absorption; rifampin may increase its metabolism. Cimetidine may reduce quinine clearance & urinary alkalinizers may also increase levels. May increase warfarin, digoxin & neuromuscular blocker activity.

tizanidine (*Zanaflex*) ▶LK ♀C ▶? $$$$

ADULT - Muscle spasticity due to MS or spinal cord injury: 4-8 mg PO q6-8h prn, max dose 36 mg/day.

PEDS - Not approved in children.

FORMS - Generic/Trade: Tabs 2 & 4 mg, scored. Trade 6 mg.

NOTES - Monitor LFTs. Avoid with hepatic or renal insufficiency. Alcohol & oral contraceptives increase tizanidine levels. Concurrent antihypertensives may exacerbate hypotension. Dry mouth, somnolence, sedation, asthenia & dizziness most common side effects.

ANALGESICS: Non-Opioid Analgesic Combinations

NOTE: Refer to individual components for further information. Carisoprodol and butalbital may be habit-forming; butalbital contraindicated with porphyria. May cause drowsiness and/or sedation, which may be enhanced by alcohol & other CNS depressants. Avoid exceeding 4 g/day of acetaminophen in combination products. Caution people who drink ≥3 alcoholic drinks/day to limit acetaminophen use to 2.5 g/day due to additive liver toxicity.

Ascriptin **(aspirin + aluminum hydroxide + magnesium hydroxide + calcium carbonate)** ▶K ♀D ▶? $

WARNING - Multiple strengths; see FORMS.

ADULT - Pain: 1-2 tabs PO q4h.

PEDS - Not approved in children.

FORMS - OTC: Trade: Tabs 325 mg ASA/50 mg magnesium hydroxide/50 mg aluminum hydroxide/calcium carbonate (Ascriptin). 325 mg ASA/75 mg magnesium hydroxide/75 mg aluminum hydroxide/calcium carbonate (Ascriptin A/D). 500 mg ASA/80 mg magnesium hydroxide/80 mg aluminum hydroxide/calcium carbonate (Ascriptin Extra Strength).

NOTES - See NSAIDs - Salicylic Acid subclass warning.

Bufferin **(aspirin + calcium carbonate + magnesium oxide + magnesium carbonate)** ▶K ♀D ▶? $

ADULT - Pain: 2 tabs/caplets PO q4h while symptoms persist. Max 12 in 24 hours.

PEDS - Not approved in children.

FORMS - OTC: Trade: Tabs/caplets 325 mg ASA / 158 mg Ca carbonate / 63 mg Mg oxide / 34 mg Mg carbonate. Bufferin ES: 500 mg ASA / 222.3 mg Ca carbonate / 88.9 mg Mg oxide / 55.6 mg Mg carbonate

NOTES - See NSAIDs - Salicylic Acid subclass warning.

Esgic Plus (acetaminophen + butalbital + caffeine) ▶LK ♀C ▶? $$

ADULT - Tension or muscle contraction headache: 1-2 tabs or caps PO q4h. Max 6 in 24 hours.

PEDS - Not approved in children.

FORMS - Generic/Trade: Tabs/caps acetaminophen 500 mg / butalbital 50 mg / caffeine 40 mg.

Excedrin Migraine (acetaminophen + aspirin + caffeine) ▶LK ♀D ▶? $

ADULT - Migraine headache: 2 tabs/caps/geltabs PO q6h while symptoms persist. Max 8 in 24 hours.

PEDS - ≥12 yo: Use adult dose.

FORMS - Trade: Tabs/caplets/geltabs acetaminophen 250 mg / ASA 250 mg / caffeine 65 mg.

NOTES - See NSAIDs - Salicylates subclass warning.

Fioricet (acetaminophen + butalbital + caffeine) ▶LK ♀C ▶? $$

ADULT - Tension or muscle contraction headache: 1-2 tabs PO q4h. Max 6 in 24 hours.

PEDS - Not approved in children.

FORMS - Generic/Trade: Tabs 325 mg acetaminophen//50 mg butalbital/40 mg caffeine.

Fiorinal (aspirin + butalbital + caffeine, ❤Tecnal) ▶KL ♀D ▶- ©III $$

ADULT - Tension or muscle contraction headache: 1-2 tabs PO q4h. Max 6 tabs in 24 hours.

PEDS - Not approved in children.

FORMS - Generic/Trade: Caps 325 mg aspirin + 50 mg butalbital + 40 mg caffeine.

NOTES - See NSAIDs - Salicylic Acid subclass warning.

Goody's Extra Strength Headache Powder (acetaminophen + aspirin + caffeine) ▶LK ♀D ▶? $

ADULT - Headache: Place one powder on tongue and follow with liquid, or stir powder into a glass of water or other liquid. Repeat in 4-6 hours prn. Max 4 powders in 24 hours.

PEDS - ≥12 yo: Use adult dose.

FORMS - Trade: 260 mg acetaminophen/520 mg ASA/32.5 mg caffeine per powder paper.

NOTES - See NSAIDs - Salicylic Acid subclass warning.

Norgesic (orphenadrine + aspirin + caffeine) ▶KL ♀D ▶? $$$

WARNING - Multiple strengths; see FORMS & write specific product on Rx.

ADULT - Musculoskeletal pain: Norgesic, 1-2 tabs PO tid-qid. Pain: Norgesic Forte, 1 tab PO tid-qid.

PEDS - Not approved in children.

FORMS - Trade: Tabs Norgesic 25 mg orphenadrine/385 mg aspirin/30 mg caffeine. Norgesic Forte 50 mg orphenadrine/770 mg aspirin/60 mg caffeine.

NOTES - See NSAIDs - Salicylic Acid subclass warning.

Phrenilin (acetaminophen + butalbital) ▶LK ♀C ▶? $

ADULT - Tension or muscle contraction headache: 1-2 tabs PO q4h. Max 6 in 24 hours.

PEDS - Not approved in children.

FORMS - Trade: Tabs 325 mg acetaminophen/50 mg butalbital.

Phrenilin Forte (acetaminophen + butalbital) ▶LK ♀C ▶? $

ADULT - Tension or muscle contraction headache: 1 cap PO q4h. Max 6 in 24 hours.

PEDS - Not approved in children.

FORMS - Trade: Tabs 650 mg acetaminophen//50 mg butalbital.

Sedapap (acetaminophen + butalbital) ▶LK ♀C ▶? $

ADULT - Tension or muscle contraction headache: 1-2 tabs PO q4h. Max 6 tabs in 24 hours.

PEDS - Not approved in children.

FORMS - Generic/Trade: Tabs 650 mg acetaminophen//50 mg butalbital.

Soma Compound (carisoprodol + aspirin) ▶LK ♀D ▶- $

ADULT - Musculoskeletal pain: 1-2 tabs PO qid.

PEDS - Not approved in children.

FORMS - Generic/Trade: Tabs 200 mg carisoprodol/325 mg ASA.

NOTES - See NSAIDs - Salicylic Acid subclass warning. Carisoprodol may be habit forming.

Ultracet (tramadol + acetaminophen) ▶KL ♀C ▶- $$

ADULT - Acute pain: 2 tabs PO q4-6h prn, max 8 tabs/day for no more than 5 days. If creatinine clearance <30ml/min, increase the dosing interval to 12 hours. Consider a similar adjustment in elderly patients.

PEDS - Not approved in children.

FORMS - Trade: Tabs 37.5 mg tramadol/325

mg acetaminophen.

NOTES - Do not use with other acetaminophen-containing drugs due to potential for hepatotoxicity. Contraindicated in acute intoxication with alcohol, hypnotics, centrally acting analgesics, opioids or psychotropic drugs. Seizures may occur with concurrent antidepressants or with

seizure disorder. Use with great caution with MAO inhibitors or in combination with SSRIs due to potential for serotonin syndrome; dose adjustment may be needed. Withdrawal symptoms may occur in patients dependent on opioids. The most frequent side effects are somnolence & constipation.

ANALGESICS: Nonsteroidal Anti-Inflammatories – COX-2 Inhibitors

NOTE: Fewer GI side effects than 1st generation NSAIDs & no effect on platelets, but other NSAID-related side effects (renal dysfunction, fluid retention, CNS) are possible. May cause fluid-retention or exacerbate CHF. May elevate BP or blunt effects of antihypertensives & loop diuretics. Not substitutes for aspirin for cardiovascular prophylaxis due to lack of antiplatelet effects. Monitor INR with warfarin. May increase lithium levels. Caution in aspirin-sensitive asthma. Use around the time of conception appears to increase the risk of miscarriage (use acetaminophen instead).

celecoxib (*Celebrex*) ▶L ♀C (D in 3rd trimester) ▶? $$$

ADULT - OA: 200 mg PO qd or 100 mg PO bid. RA: 100-200 mg PO bid. Familial adenomatous polyposis (FAP), as an adjunct to usual care: 400 mg PO bid with food. Acute pain, dysmenorrhea: 400 mg x 1, then 200 mg PO bid. May take an additional 200 mg on day 1.

PEDS - Not approved in children.

FORMS - Trade: Caps 100, 200, & 400 mg.

NOTES - Contraindicated in sulfonamide allergy. See rofecoxib for possible alternative in this situation. Decrease dose by 50% with hepatic dysfunction.

rofecoxib (*Vioxx*) ▶Plasma ♀C (D in 3rd trimester) ▶? $$$

ADULT - OA: 12.5-25 mg PO qd. Acute pain,

primary dysmenorrhea: 50 mg PO qd. RA: 25 mg PO qd. Acute migraine with/without aura: Start 25 mg PO qd at headache onset, max 50 mg PO qd. Avoid chronic daily use.

PEDS - JRA: >12 yo: Use adult dose. 2-11 yo & ≥10 kg: 0.6 mg/kg to max 25 mg.

FORMS - Trade: Tabs 12.5, 25 & 50 mg. Suspension 12.5 mg/5 ml and 25 mg/5 ml.

NOTES - Rifampin decreases rofecoxib levels. Rofecoxib is not related to the sulfonamides and is not contraindicated in pts with such allergies. Use of 50 mg for >5 days for pain management has not been studied. Decrease dose with hepatic dysfunction.

valdecoxib (*Bextra*) ▶Plasma ♀C (D in 3rd trimester) ▶? $$$

WARNING - Cases of Stevens-Johnson syndrome, toxic epidermal necrolysis, exfoliative dermatitis, erythema multiforme & anaphylactoid reactions have been reported.

ADULT - OA, RA: 10 mg PO qd. Primary dysmenorrhea: 20 mg PO bid prn.

PEDS - Not approved in children.

FORMS - Trade: Tabs 10 & 20 mg.

NOTES - Contraindicated in sulfonamide allergy. See rofecoxib for possible alternative in this situation. Can temporarily increase INR in patients on warfarin, monitor for the 1st few weeks. If rash occurs, discontinue immediately. Decrease dose with hepatic dysfunction.

ANALGESICS: Nonsteroidal Anti-Inflammatories – Salicylic Acid Derivatives

NOTE: Avoid in children <17 yo with chickenpox or flu, due to association with Reye's syndrome. May potentiate warfarin, heparin, valproic acid, methotrexate. Unlike aspirin, derivatives may have less GI toxicity & negligible effects on platelet aggregation & renal prostaglandins. Caution in aspirin-sensitive asthma. Ibuprofen and possibly other NSAIDs may antagonize antiplatelet effects of aspirin if given simultaneously. Use around the time of conception appears to increase the risk of miscarriage (use acetaminophen instead).

aspirin (*Ecotrin, Bayer, Anacin, ASA, ♣Asaphen, Entrophen, Novasen*) ▶K ♀D ▶? $

ADULT - Mild to moderate pain, fever: 325-650 mg PO/PR q4h prn. Acute rheumatic fever: 5-8 g/day, initially. RA/OA: 3.2-6g/day in divided doses.

PEDS - Mild to moderate pain, fever: 10-15 mg/kg/dose PO q4-6h not to exceed 60-80 mg/kg/day. JRA: 60-100 mg/kg/day PO divided q6-8h. Acute rheumatic fever: 100 mg/kg/day

PO/PR x 2 weeks, then 75 mg/kg/day x 4-6 weeks. Kawasaki disease 80-100 mg/kg/day divided qid PO/PR until fever resolves, then 3-5 mg/kg/day PO qam x 7 weeks or longer if there is ECG evidence of coronary artery abnormalities.

FORMS - OTC: Tabs 65, 81, 162.5, 300, 320, 324, 325, 486, 500, 640, 650, controlled release tabs 650 (scored). Rx only: 800 mg controlled release tabs & 975 mg enteric coated. OTC: suppositories 120, 125, 300, & 600 mg.

NOTES - Consider discontinuation 1 week prior to surgery because of the possibility of postoperative bleeding. Aspirin intolerance occurs in 4%-19% of asthmatics. Use caution in liver damage, renal insufficiency, peptic ulcer or bleeding tendencies.

choline magnesium trisalicylate (*Trilisate*) ▶K ♀C (D in 3rd trimester) ▶? $

ADULT - RA/OA: 1500 mg PO bid. Mild to moderate pain, fever: 1000-1500 mg PO bid.

PEDS - RA, mild to moderate pain: 50 mg/kg/day (up to 37kg) PO divided bid.

FORMS - Generic/Trade: Tabs 500, 750, & 1000 mg, scored.

NOTES - Contraindicated in patients with ASA allergy.

diflunisal (*Dolobid*) ▶K ♀C (D in 3rd trimester)

▶- $$

ADULT - Mild to moderate pain: Initially: 500 mg-1g PO, then 250-500 mg PO q8-12h. RA/OA: 500 mg-1g PO divided bid. Max dose 1.5g/day.

PEDS - Not approved in children.

FORMS - Generic/Trade: Tabs 250 & 500 mg.

NOTES - Contraindicated in patients with ASA allergy. Do not crush or chew tablets. Increases acetaminophen levels.

salsalate (*Salflex, Disalcid, Amigesic*) ▶K ♀C (D in 3rd trimester) ▶? $

ADULT - RA/OA: 3000 mg/day PO divided q8-12h.

PEDS - Not approved in children.

FORMS - Generic/Trade: Tabs 500 & 750 mg, scored.

NOTES - Contraindicated in ASA allergy.

NSAIDs – If one class fails, consider another. *Salicylic acid derivatives:* aspirin, diflunisal, salsalate, Trilisate. *Propionic acids:* flurbiprofen, ibuprofen, ketoprofen, naproxen, oxaprozin. *Acetic acids:* diclofenac, etodolac, indomethacin, ketorolac, nabumetone, sulindac, tolmetin. *Fenamates:* meclofenamate. *Oxicams:* meloxicam, piroxicam. *COX-2 inhibitors:* celecoxib, rofecoxib, valdecoxib.

ANALGESICS: Nonsteroidal Anti-Inflammatories – Other

NOTE: Chronic use associated with renal insufficiency, gastritis, peptic ulcer disease, GI bleeds. Caution in liver disease. May cause fluid-retention or exacerbate CHF. May elevate BP or blunt effects of antihypertensives & loop diuretics. May increase levels of methotrexate, lithium, phenytoin, digoxin & cyclosporine. May potentiate warfarin. Caution in aspirin-sensitive asthma. Ibuprofen or other NSAIDs may antagonize antiplatelet effects of aspirin if given simultaneously. Use around the time of conception appears to increase the risk of miscarriage (use acetaminophen instead).

***Arthrotec* (diclofenac + misoprostol)** ▶LK ♀X ▶- $$$$

WARNING - Because of the abortifacient property of the misoprostol component, it is contraindicated in women who are pregnant. Caution in women with childbearing potential; effective contraception is essential.

ADULT - OA: one 50/200 PO tid. RA: one 50/200 PO tid-qid. If intolerant, may use 50/200 or 75/200 PO bid.

PEDS - Not approved in children.

FORMS - Trade: Tabs 50 mg/200 mcg & 75 mg/200 mcg diclofenac/misoprostol.

NOTES - Refer to individual components. Abdominal pain & diarrhea may occur. Check LFTs at baseline then periodically. See NSAIDs-Other subclass warning. Do not crush or chew tablets.

diclofenac (*Voltaren, Voltaren XR, Cataflam*, ♥*Voltaren Rapide*) ▶L ♀B (D in 3rd trimester) ▶- $$$

WARNING - Multiple strengths; see FORMS & write specific product on Rx.

ADULT - OA: immediate or delayed release 50 mg PO bid-tid or 75 mg bid. Extended release 100 mg PO qd. RA: immediate or delayed release 50 mg PO tid-qid or 75 mg bid. Extended release 100 mg PO qd-bid. Ankylosing spondylitis: immediate or delayed release 25 mg PO qid & hs. Analgesia & primary dysmenorrhea: immediate or delayed release 50 mg PO tid.

PEDS - Not approved in children.

UNAPPROVED PEDS - JRA: 2-3 mg/kg/day PO.

FORMS - Generic/Trade: Tabs, immediate release (Cataflam) 25, 50 mg. Tabs, delayed release (Voltaren) 25, 50, & 75 mg. Tabs, extended release (Voltaren XR) 100 mg.

NOTES - Check LFTs at baseline then periodically.

etodolac (Lodine, Lodine XL, ✦Ultradol) ▶L ♀C (D in 3rd trimester) ▶- $$

WARNING - Multiple strengths; write specific product on Rx.

ADULT - OA: 400 mg PO bid-tid. 300 mg PO bid-qid. 200 mg tid-qid. Extended release 400-1200 mg PO qd. Mild to moderate pain: 200-400 mg q6-8h. Max dose 1200 mg/day or if ≤60 kg, 20 mg/kg/day.

PEDS - Not approved in children.

UNAPPROVED ADULT - RA, ankylosing spondylitis: 300-400 mg PO bid. Tendinitis, bursitis & acute gout: 300-400 mg PO bid-qid then taper.

FORMS - Generic/Trade: Tabs, immediate release (Lodine) 400 & 500 mg. Caps, immediate release (Lodine) 200 & 300 mg. Generic/Trade: Tabs, extended release (Lodine XL) 400, 500 & 600 mg.

fenoprofen (Nalfon) ▶L ♀C (D in 3rd trimester) ▶- $

ADULT - Other drugs preferred due to nephrotoxicity risk.

PEDS - Not approved in children.

FORMS - Generic/Trade: Caps 200 & 300 mg. Generic only: Tabs 600 mg.

floctafenine (✦Idarac) ▶K ♀C (D in 3rd trimester) ▶- $$

ADULT - Canada only. Acute mild to moderate pain: 200-400 mg PO q6-8h prn. Max 1200 mg/day.

PEDS - Not approved in children.

FORMS - Trade: Tabs 200, 400 mg.

NOTES - Caution in aspirin-sensitive asthma.

flurbiprofen (Ansaid, ✦Froben, Froben SR) ▶L ♀B (D in 3rd trimester) ▶+ $

ADULT - RA/OA: 200-300 mg/day PO divided bid-qid. Max single dose 100 mg.

PEDS - Not approved in children.

UNAPPROVED ADULT - Ankylosing spondylitis: 150-300 mg/day PO divided bid-qid. Mild to moderate pain: 50 mg PO q6h. Primary dysmenorrhea: 50 mg PO qd at onset, d/c when pain subsides. Tendinitis, bursitis, acute gout, acute migraine: 100 mg PO at onset, then 50 mg PO qid, then taper.

UNAPPROVED PEDS - JRA: 4 mg/kg/day PO.

FORMS - Generic/Trade: Tabs immediate release 50 & 100 mg.

ibuprofen (Motrin, Advil, Nuprin, Rufen) ▶L ♀B (D in 3rd trimester) ▶+ $

ADULT - RA/OA: 200-800 mg PO tid-qid. Mild to moderate pain: 400 mg PO q4-6h. Primary dysmenorrhea: 400 mg PO q4h, prn. Fever: 200 mg PO q4-6h prn. Migraine pain: 200-400 mg PO not to exceed 400 mg in 24 hours (OTC dosing). Max dose 3.2g/day.

PEDS - JRA: 30-50 mg/kg/day PO divided q6h. Max dose 2400 mg/24h. 20 mg/kg/day may be adequate for milder disease. Analgesic/antipyretic >6 mo: 5-10 mg/kg PO q6-8h, prn. Max dose 40 mg/kg/day.

FORMS - OTC: Caps, 200 mg. Tabs 100, 200 mg. Chewable tabs 50 mg. Liquid & suspension 50 mg/1.25ml, 100 mg/5 ml, suspension 100 mg/2.5 ml. Infant drops, 50 mg/1.25 ml (calibrated dropper). Rx only: Tabs 400, 600 & 800 mg.

NOTES - May antagonize antiplatelet effects of aspirin if given simultaneously. Take aspirin 2 hours prior to ibuprofen.

indomethacin (Indocin, Indocin SR, ✦Indocid, Rhodacine) ▶L ♀B (D in 3rd trimester) ▶+ $

WARNING - Multiple strengths; see FORMS & write specific product on Rx.

ADULT - RA/OA, ankylosing spondylitis: 25 mg PO bid-tid to start. Increase incrementally to a total daily dose of 150-200 mg. Bursitis/tendinitis: 75-150 mg/day PO/PR divided tid-qid. Acute gout: 50 mg PO/PR tid until pain tolerable, rapidly taper dose to D/C. Sustained release: 75 mg PO qd-bid.

PEDS - Not approved in children.

UNAPPROVED ADULT - Primary dysmenorrhea: 25 mg PO tid-qid. Cluster headache: 75-150 mg SR PO qd. Polyhydramnios: 2.2-3.0 mg/kg/day PO based on maternal weight; premature closure of the ductus arteriosus has been reported.

UNAPPROVED PEDS - JRA: 1-3 mg/kg/day tid-qid to start. Increase prn to max dose of 4 mg/kg/d or 200 mg/d, whichever is less.

FORMS - Generic/Trade: Caps, immediate release 25 & 50 mg. Oral suspension 25 mg/5 ml. Suppositories 50 mg. Caps, sustained release 75 mg.

NOTES - Suppositories contraindicated with history of proctitis or recent rectal bleeding. May aggravate depression or other psychiatric disturbances. Do not crush sustained release capsule.

ketoprofen (Orudis, Orudis KT, Actron, Oruvail, ✦Rhodis, Rhodis EC, Rhodis

SR, Rhovail, Orudis E, Orudis SR) ▶L ♀B (D in 3rd trimester) ▶- $
ADULT - RA/OA: 75 mg PO tid or 50 mg PO qid. Extended release 200 mg PO qd. Mild to moderate pain, primary dysmenorrhea: 25-50 mg PO q6-8h prn.
PEDS - Not approved in children.
UNAPPROVED PEDS - JRA : 100-200 mg/m^2/day PO. Max dose 320 mg/day.
FORMS - OTC: Tabs immediate release, 12.5 mg. Rx: Generic/Trade: Caps, immediate release 25, 50 & 75 mg. Caps, extended release 100, 150 & 200 mg.

ketorolac (*Toradol*) ▶L ♀C (D in 3rd trimester) ▶+ $
WARNING - Indicated for short-term (up to 5 days) therapy only. Ketorolac is a potent NSAID and can cause serious GI and renal adverse effects. It may also increase the risk of bleeding by inhibiting platelet function. Contraindicated in patients with active peptic ulcer disease, recent GI bleeding or perforation, a history of peptic ulcer disease or GI bleeding, and advanced renal impairment.
ADULT - Moderately severe, acute pain, single-dose treatment: 30-60 mg IM or 15-30 mg IV. Multiple-dose treatment: 15-30 mg IV/IM q6h. IV/IM doses are not to exceed 60 mg/day in patients ≥65 yo, <50 kg, & for patients with moderately elevated serum creatinine. Oral continuation therapy: 10 mg PO q4-6h prn, max dose 40 mg/day. Combined duration IV/IM and PO is not to exceed 5 days.
PEDS - Not approved in children.
UNAPPROVED PEDS - Pain: 0.5 mg/kg/dose IM/IV q6h not to exceed 30 mg q6h or 120 mg/day. >50 kg: 10 mg PO q6h prn not to exceed 40 mg/day.
FORMS - Generic/Trade: Tabs 10 mg.

meclofenamate ▶L ♀B (D in 3rd trimester) ▶- $
ADULT - Mild to moderate pain: 50 mg PO q4-6h prn. Max dose 400 mg/day. Menorrhagia & primary dysmenorrhea: 100 mg PO tid for up to 6 days. RA/OA: 200-400 mg/day PO divided tid-qid.
PEDS - Not approved in children.
UNAPPROVED PEDS - JRA: 3-7.5 mg/kg/day PO. Max dose 300 mg/day.
FORMS - Generic: Caps 50 & 100 mg.
NOTES - Reversible autoimmune hemolytic anemia with use for >12 months.

meloxicam (*Mobic*, ♣*Mobicox*) ▶L ♀C (D in 3rd trimester) ▶? $$$
ADULT - RA/OA: 7.5 mg PO qd. Max dose 15 mg/day.

PEDS - Not approved in children.
FORMS - Trade: Tabs 7.5, 15 mg. Suspension 7.5 mg/5 ml.
NOTES - Shake suspension gently before using. This is not a selective COX-2 inhibitor.

nabumetone (*Relafen*) ▶L ♀C (D in 3rd trimester) ▶- $$$
ADULT - RA/OA: Initial: two 500 mg tabs (1000 mg) PO qd. May increase to 1500-2000 mg PO qd or divided bid. Dosages >2000 mg/day have not been studied.
PEDS - Not approved in children.
FORMS - Generic/Trade: Tabs 500 & 750 mg.

naproxen (*Naprosyn, Aleve, Anaprox, EC-Naprosyn, Naprelan*) ▶L ♀B (D in 3rd trimester) ▶+ $$$
WARNING - Multiple strengths; see FORMS & write specific product on Rx.
ADULT - RA/OA, ankylosing spondylitis, pain, dysmenorrhea, acute tendinitis & bursitis, fever: 250-500 mg PO bid. Delayed release: 375-500 mg PO bid (do not crush or chew). Controlled release: 750-1000 mg PO qd. Acute gout: 750 mg PO x 1, then 250 mg PO q8h until the attack subsides. Controlled release: 1000-1500 mg PO x 1, then 1000 mg PO qd until the attack subsides.
PEDS - JRA: 10-20 mg/kg/day PO divided bid. Max dose 1250 mg/24h. Pain >2 yo: 5-7 mg/kg/dose PO q8-12h.
UNAPPROVED ADULT - Acute migraine: 750 mg PO x 1, then 250-500 mg PO prn. Migraine prophylaxis, menstrual migraine: 500 mg PO bid.
FORMS - OTC: Generic/Trade: Tabs immediate release 200 mg. OTC Trade: Capsules & Gelcaps immediate release 200 mg. Rx: Generic/Trade: Tabs immediate release 250, 375 & 500 mg. Delayed release 375 & 500 mg. Rx: Trade: Tabs delayed release enteric coated (EC-Naprosyn), 375 & 500 mg. Tabs, controlled release (Naprelan), 375 & 500 mg. Generic/Trade: Suspension 125 mg/5 ml.
NOTES - All dosing based on naproxen content; 500 mg naproxen = 550 mg naproxen sodium.

oxaprozin (*Daypro, Daypro Alta*) ▶L ♀C (D in 3rd trimester) ▶- $$
ADULT - RA/OA: 1200 mg PO qd. Max 1800 mg/day or 26 mg/kg/day, whichever is lower.
PEDS - Not approved in children.
FORMS - Generic/Trade (Daypro): Caplets, tabs 600 mg, trade scored. Trade (Daypro Alta): Tabs 600 mg.
NOTES - Daypro Alta is the potassium salt of oxaprozin.

piroxicam (*Feldene, Fexicam*) ▶L ♀B (D in 3rd trimester) ▶+ $
ADULT - RA/OA: 20 mg PO qd or divided bid.
PEDS - Not approved in children.
UNAPPROVED ADULT - Primary dysmenorrhea: 20-40 mg PO qd x 3 days.
FORMS - Generic/Trade: Caps 10 & 20 mg.

sulindac (*Clinoril*) ▶L ♀B (D in 3rd trimester) ▶- $
ADULT - RA/OA, ankylosing spondylitis: 150 mg PO bid. Bursitis, tendinitis, acute gout: 200 mg PO bid, decrease after response. Max dose: 400 mg/day.
PEDS - Not approved in children.
UNAPPROVED PEDS - JRA: 4 mg/kg/day PO divided bid.
FORMS - Generic/Trade: Tabs 150 & 200 mg.
NOTES - Sulindac-associated pancreatitis & a potentially fatal hypersensitivity syndrome have occurred.

tiaprofenic acid (✦*Surgam, Surgam SR*) ▶K ♀C (D in 3rd trimester) ▶- $$
ADULT - Canada only. RA or OA: 600 mg PO qd of sustained release, or 300 mg PO bid of regular release. Some OA patients may be maintained on 300 mg/day.
PEDS - Not approved in children.
FORMS - Trade: Caps, sustained release 300 mg. Generic/trade: Tabs 300 mg
NOTES - Caution in renal insufficiency. Cystitis has been reported more frequently than with other NSAIDs.

tolmetin (*Tolectin*) ▶L ♀C (D in 3rd trimester) ▶+ $$$
ADULT - RA/OA: 400 mg PO tid to start. Range 600-1800 mg/day PO divided tid.
PEDS - JRA ≥2 yo: 20 mg/kg/day PO divided tid-qid to start. Range 15-30 mg/kg/day divided tid-qid. Max dose 2g/24h.
UNAPPROVED PEDS - Pain ≥2 yo: 5-7 mg/kg/dose PO q6-8h. Max dose 2g/24h.
FORMS - Generic/Trade: Tabs 200 (trade scored) & 600 mg. Caps 400 mg.
NOTES - Rare anaphylaxis.

ANALGESICS: Opioid Agonist-Antagonists

NOTE: May cause drowsiness and/or sedation, which may be enhanced by alcohol & other CNS depressants. Partial agonist-antagonists may result in withdrawal effects in the opioid-dependent.

buprenorphine (*Buprenex*) ▶L ♀C ▶- ©III $
ADULT - Moderate to severe pain: 0.3-0.6 mg IM or slow IV, q6h prn. Max single dose 0.6 mg. See entry in Psychiatry section for opioid-dependence therapy.
PEDS - Moderate to severe pain: 2-12 yo: 2-6 mcg/kg/dose IM or slow IV q4-6h. Max single dose 6 mcg/kg.
NOTES - May cause bradycardia, hypotension & respiratory depression. Concurrent use with diazepam has resulted in respiratory & cardiovascular collapse.

butorphanol (*Stadol, Stadol NS*) ▶LK ♀C ▶+ ©IV $$$
WARNING - Approved as a nasal spray in 1991 and has been promoted as a safe treatment for migraine headaches. There have been numerous reports of dependence-addiction & major psychological disturbances. These problems have been documented by the FDA. Stadol NS should be used for patients with infrequent but severe migraine attacks for whom all other common ablative treatments have failed. Experts recommend restriction to ≤2 bottles (30 sprays) per month in patients who are appropriate candidates for this medication.
ADULT - Pain, including post-operative pain: 0.5-2 mg IV q3-4h prn. 1-4 mg IM q3-4h prn. Obstetric pain during labor: 1-2 mg IV/IM at full term in early labor, repeat after 4h. Last resort for migraine pain: 1 mg nasal spray (1 spray in one nostril). If no pain relief in 60-90 min, may give a 2nd spray in the other nostril. Additional doses q3-4h prn.
PEDS - Not approved in children.
FORMS - Generic/Trade: Nasal spray 1 mg/spray, 2.5 ml bottle (14-15 doses/bottle).
NOTES - May increase cardiac workload.

nalbuphine (*Nubain*) ▶LK ♀? ▶? $
ADULT - Moderate to severe pain: 10-20 mg SC/IM/IV q3-6h prn. Max dose 160 mg/day.
PEDS - Not approved in children.

pentazocine (*Talwin, Talwin NX*) ▶LK ♀C ▶? ©IV $$$
WARNING - The oral form (Talwin NX) may cause fatal reactions if injected.
ADULT - Moderate to severe pain: Talwin: 30 mg IM/IV q3-4h prn, max dose 360 mg/day. Talwin NX: 1 tab PO q3-4h, max 12 tabs/day.
PEDS - Not approved in children.
FORMS - Generic/Trade: Tabs 50 mg with 0.5 mg naloxone, trade scored.
NOTES - Can cause disorientation, hallucinations, seizures. Rotate injection sites. Use with sibutramine may precip. serotonin syndrome.

OPIOIDS*	Approximate equianalgesic		Recommended starting dose			
			Adults >50kg		Children/Adults 8 to 50 kg	
	IV / SC / IM	PO	IV / SC / IM	PO	IV / SC / IM	PO
Opioid Agonists						
morphine	10 mg q3-4h	†30 mg q3-4h †60 mg q3-4h	10 mg q3-4h	30 mg q3-4h	0.1 mg/kg q3-4h	0.3 mg/kg q3-4h
codeine	75 mg q3-4h	130 mg q3-4h	60 mg q2h	60 mg q3-4h	n/r	1 mg/kg q3-4h
fentanyl	0.1 mg q1h	n/a	0.1 mg q1h	n/a	n/r	n/a
hydromorphone	1.5 mg q3-4h	7.5 mg q3-4h	1.5 mg q3-4h	6 mg q3-4h	0.015 mg/kg q3-4h	0.06 mg/kg q3-4h
hydrocodone	n/a	30 mg q3-4h	n/a	10 mg q3-4h	n/a	0.2 mg/kg q3-4h
levorphanol	2 mg q6-8h	4 mg q6-8h	2 mg q6-8h	4 mg q6-8h	0.02 mg/kg q6-8h	0.04 mg/kg q6-8h
meperidine§	100 mg q3h	300 mg q2-3h	100 mg q3h	n/r	0.75 mg/kg q2-3h	n/r
oxycodone	n/a	30 mg q3-4h	n/a	10 mg q3-4h	n/a	0.2 mg/kg q3-4h
oxymorphone	1 mg q3-4h	n/a	1 mg q3-4h	n/a	n/r	n/a
Opioid Agonist-Antagonist and Partial Agonist						
buprenorphine	0.3-0.4 mg q6-8h	n/a	0.4 mg q6-8h	n/a	0.004 mg/kg q6-8h	n/a
butorphanol	2 mg q3-4h	n/a	2 mg q3-4h	n/a	n/r	n/a
nalbuphine	10 mg q3-4h	n/a	10 mg q3-4h	n/a	0.1 mg/kg q3-4h	n/a
pentazocine	60 mg q3-4h	150 mg q3-4h	n/r	50 mg q4-6h	n/r	n/r

*Approximate dosing, adapted from 1992 AHCPR guidelines, www.ahcpr.gov. All PO dosing is with immediate-release preparations. Individualize all dosing, especially in the elderly, children, and patients with chronic pain, opioid tolerance, or hepatic/renal insufficiency. Many recommend initially using lower than equivalent doses when switching between different opioids. Not available = "n/a". Not recommended = "n/r". Do not exceed 4g/day of acetaminophen or aspirin when using opioid combination formulations. Methadone is excluded due to poor consensus on equivalence.
†30 mg with around the clock dosing, and 60 mg with a single dose or short-term dosing (ie, the opioid-naïve).
§Doses should be limited to <600 mg/24 hrs and total duration of use <48 hrs; not for chronic pain.

ANALGESICS: Opioid Agonists

NOTE: May cause drowsiness and/or sedation, which may be enhanced by alcohol & other CNS depressants. Patients with chronic pain may require more frequent & higher dosing. Opioids commonly create constipation. All opioids are pregnancy class D if used for prolonged periods or in high doses at term.

codeine ▶LK ♀C ▶+ ©II $
  WARNING - Do not use IV in children due to large histamine release and cardiovascular effects.

ADULT - Mild to moderate pain: 15-60 mg PO/IM/IV/SC q4-6h. Max dose 360 mg in 24 hours. Antitussive: 10-20 mg PO q4-6h prn. Max dose 120 mg in 24 hours.
PEDS - Mild to moderate pain in ≥1yo: 0.5-1 mg/kg PO/SC/IM q4-6h, max dose 60 mg/dose. Antitussive: 2-5 yo: 2.5-5 mg PO q4-6h prn, max dose: 30 mg/day. 6-12 yo: 5-10 mg PO q4-6h prn, max dose 60 mg/day.
FORMS - Generic: Tabs 15, 30, & 60 mg. Oral soln: 15 mg/5 ml.

FENTANYL TRANSDERMAL DOSE (based on ongoing morphine requirement)*

Morphine (IV/IM)	Morphine (PO)	Transdermal fentanyl
8-22 mg/day	45-134 mg/day	25 mcg/hr
23-37 mg/day	135-224 mg/day	50 mcg/hr
38-52 mg/day	225-314 mg/day	75 mcg/hr
53-67 mg/day	315-404 mg/day	100 mcg/hr

* For higher morphine doses see product insert for transdermal fentanyl equivalencies.

fentanyl (*Duragesic, Actiq*) ▶L ♀C ▶+ ©II $$$$$

WARNING - Duragesic patches and Actiq are contraindicated in the management of acute or postoperative pain due to potentially life-threatening respiratory depression in opioid non-tolerant patients. Instruct patients and their caregivers that even used patches/lozenges on a stick can be fatal to a child or pet. Dispose via toilet.

ADULT - Duragesic Patches: Chronic pain: 25-100 mcg/hr patch q72 hours. Titrate dose to the needs of the patient. Some patients require q48 hr dosing. May wear more than one patch to achieve the correct analgesic effect. Actiq: Breakthrough cancer pain: 200-1600 mcg sucked over 15 min, max dose 4 lozenges on a stick/day.

PEDS - Transdermal (Duragesic): not approved in children. Actiq: not approved <16yo.

FORMS - Trade: Transdermal patches 25, 50, 75, & 100 mcg/h (Duragesic). Transmucosal forms: lozenges on a stick, raspberry flavored 200, 400, 600, 800, 1,200, & 1,600 mcg (Actiq lozenges on a stick).

NOTES - Do not use patches for acute pain. Oral transmucosal fentanyl doses of 5mcg/kg provide effects similar to 0.75-1.25 mcg/kg of fentanyl IM. Lozenges on a stick should be sucked, not chewed. Flush lozenge remnants (without stick) down the toilet. For transdermal systems: apply patch to non-hairy skin. Clip (not shave) hair if have to apply to hairy area. Fever or external heat sources may increase fentanyl released from patch. Dispose of a used patch by folding with the adhesive side of the patch adhering to itself, then flush it down the toilet immediately upon removal. Do not cut the patch in half. Keep all forms of fentanyl out of the reach of children or pets. For Duragesic patches and Actiq lozenges on a stick: Titrate dose as high as necessary to relieve cancer pain or other types of non-malignant pain where chronic opioids are necessary.

hydromorphone (*Dilaudid, Dilaudid-5, ♥Hydromorph Contin*) ▶L ♀C ▶? ©II $$$

ADULT - Moderate to severe pain: 2-4 mg PO q4-6h. 0.5-2 mg SC/IM or slow IV q4-6h initial dose (opioid naïve). 3 mg PR q6-8h.

PEDS - Not approved in children.

UNAPPROVED PEDS - Pain =<12 yo: 0.03-0.08 mg/kg PO q4-6h prn. 0.015 mg/kg/dose IV q4-6h prn. Pain >12 yo: use adult dose.

FORMS - Generic/Trade: Tabs 2, 4, & 8 mg (8 mg trade scored). Liquid 5 mg/5 ml. Suppositories 3 mg. Trade only: Tabs 1 & 3 mg.

NOTES - In opioid-naïve patients, consider an initial dose of 0.5 mg or less IM/SC/IV. SC/IM/IV doses after initial dose should be individualized. May be given by slow IV injection over 2-5 minutes. Titrate dose as high as necessary to relieve cancer pain or other types of non-malignant pain where chronic opioids are necessary. 1.5 mg IV = 7.5 mg PO.

levorphanol (*Levo-Dromoran*) ▶L ♀C ▶? ©II $$$

ADULT - Moderate to severe pain: 2 mg PO/SC q6-8h prn. Increase to 4 mg, if necessary. May be given by slow IV injection.

PEDS - Not approved in children.

FORMS - Trade: Tabs 2 mg, scored.

meperidine (*Demerol, pethidine*) ▶LK ♀C but + ▶+ ©II $$$

ADULT - Moderate to severe pain: 50-150 mg IM/SC/PO q3-4h prn. OB analgesia: when pains become regular, 50-100 mg IM/SC q1-3h. May also be given slow IV diluted to 10 mg/ml, or by continuous IV infusion diluted to 1 mg/ml.

PEDS - Moderate to severe pain: 1-1.8 mg/kg IM/SC/PO or slow IV (see adult dosing) up to adult dose, q3-4h prn.

FORMS - Generic/Trade: Tabs 50 (trade scored) & 100 mg. Syrup 50 mg/5 ml (trade banana flavored).

NOTES - Avoid in renal insufficiency and in elderly due to risk of metabolite accumulation and increased risk of CNS disturbance / seizures. Multiple drug interactions including MAOIs & SSRIs. Poor oral absorption/efficacy. 75 mg meperidine IV,IM,SC = 300 mg meperidine PO. Take syrup with ½ glass (4 oz) water. Due to the risk of seizures at high doses, meperidine is not a good choice for treatment of chronic pain. Not recommended in children.

methadone (*Dolophine, Methadose, ♥Metadol*) ▶L ♀C ▶+ ©II $

WARNING - High doses (mean ~400 mg/day) have been inconclusively associated with arrhythmia (torsade de pointes), particularly in those with pre-existing risk factors.

ADULT - Severe pain: 2.5-10 mg IM/SC/PO q3-4h prn. Opioid dependence: 20-100 mg PO qd.

PEDS - Not approved in children.

UNAPPROVED PEDS - Pain =<12 yo: 0.7 mg/kg/24h divided q4-6h PO/SC/IM/IV prn. Max 10 mg/dose.

FORMS - Generic/Trade: Tabs 5, 10, various scored. Dispersible tabs 40 mg. Oral concentrate: 10 mg/ml. Generic only: Oral soln 5 & 10 mg/5 ml.

NOTES - Titrate dose as high as necessary to relieve cancer pain or other types of non-malignant pain where chronic opioids are necessary. Treatment for opioid dependence >3 wks is maintenance and only permitted in approved treatment programs. Drug interactions leading to decreased methadone levels with enzyme-inducing HIV drugs (eg, efavirenz, nevirapine). Monitor for opiate withdrawal symptoms and increase methadone if necessary. Rapid metabolizers may require more frequent daily dosing.

morphine (*MS Contin, Kadian, Avinza, Roxanol, Oramorph SR, MSIR, DepoDur, ♣Statex, M-Eslon, M.O.S.*) ▶LK ♀C ▶+ ©II $$$$$

WARNING - Multiple strengths; see FORMS & write specific product on Rx.

ADULT - Moderate to severe pain: 10-30 mg PO q4h (immediate release tabs, caps, or oral soln). Controlled release (MS Contin, Oramorph SR): 30 mg PO q8-12h. (Kadian): 20 mg PO q12-24h. Extended release caps (Avinza): 30 mg PO qd. 10 mg q4h IM/SC. 2.5-15 mg/70kg IV over 4-5 min. 10-20 mg PR q4h. Pain with major surgery (DepoDur): 10-15 mg x 1 epidurally at the lumbar level prior to surgery (max dose 20 mg), or 10 mg epidurally after clamping of the umbilical cord with cesarian section.

PEDS - Moderate to severe pain: 0.1-0.2 mg/kg up to 15 mg IM/SC/IV q2-4h.

UNAPPROVED PEDS - Moderate to severe pain: 0.2-0.5 mg/kg/dose PO (immediate release) q4-6h. 0.3-0.6 mg/kg/dose PO q12h (controlled release).

FORMS - Generic/Trade: Tabs, immediate release: 15 & 30 mg. Trade: Caps 15 & 30 mg. Generic/Trade: Oral soln: 10 mg/5 ml, 10 mg/2.5 ml, 20 mg/5 ml, 20 mg/ml (concentrate) & 100 mg/5 ml (concentrate). Rectal suppositories 5, 10, 20 & 30 mg. Controlled release tabs (MS Contin, Oramorph SR) 15, 30, 60, 100; 200 mg MS Contin only. Controlled release caps (Kadian) 20,30,50,60,100 mg. Extended release caps (Avinza) 30,60,90,120 mg.

NOTES - Titrate dose as high as necessary to relieve cancer pain or other types of non-malignant pain where chronic opioids are necessary. The active metabolite may accumulate in hepatic/renal insufficiency leading to increased analgesic & sedative effects. Do not break, chew, or crush MS Contin or Oramorph SR. Kadian & Avinza caps may be opened & sprinkled on applesauce for easier administration, however the pellets should not be crushed or chewed. Doses >1600 mg/day of Avinza contain a potentially nephrotoxic quantity of fumaric acid. Do not mix DepoDur with other medications; do not administer any other medications into epidural space for at least 48 hours.

oxycodone (*Roxicodone, OxyContin, Percolone, OxyIR, OxyFAST, ♣Endocodone, Supeudol*) ▶L ♀C ▶- ©II $$$

WARNING - Do not Rx Oxycontin tabs on a prn basis. 80 & 160 mg tabs for use in opioid-tolerant patients only. Multiple strengths; see FORMS & write specific product on Rx. Do not break, chew, or crush controlled release preparations.

ADULT - Moderate to severe pain: 5 mg PO q6h prn. Controlled release tabs: 10-40 mg PO q12h. (No supporting data for shorter dosing intervals for controlled release tabs.)

PEDS - Not approved in children.

UNAPPROVED PEDS - Pain =<12 yo: 0.05-0.3 mg/kg/dose q4-6h PO prn to max of 10 mg/dose.

FORMS - Generic/Trade: Immediate release: Tabs (scored) & caps 5 mg. Tabs 15, 30 mg. Oral soln 5 mg/5 ml. Oral concentrate 20 mg/ml. Controlled release tabs (OxyContin): 10, 20, 40, 80 mg.

NOTES - Titrate dose as high as necessary to relieve cancer pain or other types of non-malignant pain where chronic opioids are necessary.

oxymorphone (*Numorphan*) ▶L ♀C ▶? ©II $

ADULT - Moderate to severe pain: 1-1.5 mg IM/SC q4-6h prn. 0.5 mg IV initial dose in healthy patients then q4-6h prn, increase dose until pain adequately controlled. 5 mg PR q4-6h prn.

PEDS - Not approved in children.

FORMS - Trade only: Suppositories 5 mg.

NOTES - Decrease dose in elderly and hepatic dysfunction.

Page 26 ANALGESICS: Opioid Agonists

propoxyphene (Darvon-N, Darvon Pulvules) ▶L ♀C ▶+ ©IV $

ADULT - Mild to moderate pain: 65 mg (Darvon) to 100 mg (Darvon-N) PO q4h prn. Max dose 6 caps/day.

PEDS - Not approved in children.

FORMS - Generic/Trade: Caps 65 mg. Trade only: 100 mg (Darvon-N).

NOTES - Caution in renal & hepatic dysfunction. Avoid in renal insufficiency and in elderly due to risk of metabolite accumulation, and increased risk of CNS disturbance, seizures, and QRS prolongation.

ANALGESICS: Opioid Analgesic Combinations

NOTE: Refer to individual components for further information. May cause drowsiness and/or sedation, which may be enhanced by alcohol & other CNS depressants. Opioids, carisoprodol, and butalbital may be habit-forming. Avoid exceeding 4 g/day of acetaminophen in combination products. Caution people who drink =>3 alcoholic drinks/day to limit acetaminophen use to 2.5 g/day due to additive liver toxicity. Opioids commonly cause constipation. All opioids are pregnancy class D if used for prolonged periods or in high doses at term.

Anexsia (hydrocodone + acetaminophen) ▶LK ♀C ▶- ©III $

WARNING - Multiple strengths; see FORMS & write specific product on Rx.

ADULT - Moderate pain: 1 tab PO q4-6h prn.

PEDS - Not approved in children.

FORMS - Generic/Trade: Tabs 5/500, 7.5/325, 7.5/650, 10/660 mg hydrocodone/mg acetaminophen, scored.

Capital with Codeine suspension (acetaminophen + codeine) ▶LK ♀C ▶? ©V $

ADULT - Moderate pain: 15 ml PO q4h prn.

PEDS - Moderate pain 3-6 yo: 5 ml PO q4-6h prn. 7-12 yo: 10 ml PO q4-6h prn. >12yo use adult dose.

FORMS - Generic = oral soln. Trade = suspension. Both codeine 12 mg/acetaminophen 120 mg/5 ml (trade, fruit punch flavor).

Darvocet (propoxyphene + acetaminophen) ▶L ♀C ▶+ ©IV $

WARNING - Multiple strengths; see Forms below & write specific product on Rx.

ADULT - Moderate pain: 1 tab (100/650 or 100/500) or 2 tabs (50/325) PO q4h prn.

PEDS - Not approved in children.

FORMS - Generic/Trade: Tabs 50/325 (Darvocet N-50), 100/650 (Darvocet N-100), & 100/500 (Darvocet A500), mg propoxyphene/mg acetaminophen.

NOTES - Avoid in renal insufficiency and in elderly due to risk of metabolite accumulation, and increased risk of CNS disturbance, seizures, and QRS prolongation.

Darvon Compound Pulvules (propoxyphene + aspirin + caffeine, ♥Frosst 692) ▶LK ♀D ▶- ©IV $$

WARNING - Multiple strengths; see FORMS & write specific product on Rx.

ADULT - Moderate pain: 1 cap PO q4h prn.

PEDS - Not approved in children.

FORMS - Generic/Trade: Caps, 65 mg propoxyphene/389 mg ASA/32.4 mg caffeine. Trade: 32 mg propoxyphene/389 mg ASA/32.4 mg caffeine.

NOTES - Avoid in renal insufficiency and in elderly due to risk of metabolite accumulation, and increased risk of CNS disturbance, seizures, and QRS prolongation.

Empirin with Codeine (aspirin + codeine, ♥Frosst 292) ▶LK ♀D ▶- ©III $

WARNING - Multiple strengths; see FORMS & write specific product on Rx.

ADULT - Moderate pain: 1-2 tabs PO q4h prn.

PEDS - Not approved in children.

FORMS - Generic/Trade: Tabs 325/30& 325/60 mg ASA/mg codeine. Empirin brand no longer made.

Fioricet with Codeine (acetaminophen + butalbital + caffeine + codeine) ▶LK ♀C ▶- ©III $$$

ADULT - Moderate pain: 1-2 caps PO q4h prn, max dose 6 caps/day.

PEDS - Not approved in children.

FORMS - Generic/Trade: Caps, 325 mg acetaminophen/50 mg butalbital/40 mg caffeine/30 mg codeine.

Fiorinal with Codeine (aspirin + butalbital + caffeine + codeine, ♥Fiorinal C-1/4, Fiorinal C-1/2, Tecnal C-1/4, Tecnal C-1/2) ▶LK ♀D ▶- ©III $$$$

ADULT - Moderate pain: 1-2 caps PO q4h prn, max dose 6 caps/day.

PEDS - Not approved in children.

FORMS - Trade: Caps, 325 mg ASA/50 mg butalbital /40 mg caffeine/30 mg codeine.

Lorcet (hydrocodone + acetaminophen) ▶LK ♀C ▶- ©III $$

WARNING - Multiple strengths; see FORMS & write specific product on Rx.

ADULT - Moderate pain: 1-2 tabs (5/500) PO q4-6h prn, max dose 8 tabs/day. 1 tab PO q4-6h prn (7.5/650 & 10/650).

PEDS - Not approved in children.

FORMS - Generic/Trade: Caps, 2.5/500, 5/500, 7.5/500, 7.5/750, 10/325, 10/500. (Lorcet HD) Tabs, 7.5/650 (Lorcet Plus). Trade: Lorcet - 10/650, mg hydrocodone/mg acetaminophen, scored. Elixir: 7.5/500 (15ml)

Lortab (hydrocodone + acetaminophen) ▶LK ♀C ▶- ©III $

WARNING - Multiple strengths; see FORMS & write specific product on Rx.

ADULT - Moderate pain: 1-2 tabs 2.5/500 & 5/500 PO q4-6h prn, max dose 8 tabs/day. 1 tab 7.5/500 & 10/500 PO q4-6h prn, max dose 5 tabs/day. Elixir 15ml PO q4-6h prn, max 6 doses/day.

PEDS - Not approved in children.

FORMS - Trade: Tabs Lortab 2.5/500. Generic/Trade: Lortab 5/500 (scored), Lortab 7.5/500 (trade scored) & Lortab 10/500 mg hydrocodone/mg acetaminophen. Elixir: 7.5/500 mg hydrocodone/mg acetaminophen/15 ml.

Maxidone (hydrocodone + acetaminophen) ▶LK ♀C ▶- ©III $$$

ADULT - Moderate pain: 1 tab PO q4-6h prn, max dose 5 tabs/day.

PEDS - Not approved in children.

FORMS - Trade: Tabs 10/750 mg hydrocodone/mg acetaminophen.

Mersyndol with Codeine (acetaminophen + codeine + doxylamine) ▶LK ♀C ▶? $

ADULT - Canada only. Headaches, cold symptoms, muscle aches, neuralgia: 1-2 tabs PO q4-6h prn. Maximum 12 tabs/24 hours.

PEDS - Not approved in children.

FORMS - Trade OTC tabs: acetaminophen 325 mg + codeine phos 8 mg + doxylamine 5 mg.

NOTES - May be habit-forming. Hepatotoxicity may be increased with acetaminophen overdose and may be enhanced with concomitant chronic alcohol ingestion.

Norco (hydrocodone + acetaminophen) ▶L ♀C ▶? ©III $$

ADULT - Moderate to severe pain: 1-2 tabs PO q4-6h prn (5/325). 1 tab (7.5/325 & 10/325) PO q4-6h prn up to 6 tabs/day.

PEDS - Not approved in children.

FORMS - Trade: Tabs: 5/325, 7.5/325 & 10/325 mg hydrocodone/mg acetaminophen, scored.

Percocet (oxycodone + acetaminophen, ♥*Percocet-demi, Oxycocet*)▶L♀C ▶- ©II $

WARNING - Multiple strengths; see FORMS & write specific product on Rx.

ADULT - Moderate-severe pain: 1-2 tabs PO q6h prn (2.5/325 & 5/325). 1 tab PO q6 prn (7.5/325, 7.5/500, 10/325 & 10/650).

PEDS - Not approved in children.

FORMS - Trade 2.5/325, 7.5/500, 10/650 oxycodone / acetaminophen. Generic/Trade: Tabs 5/325, 7.5/325, 10/325.

Percodan (oxycodone + aspirin, ♥*Percodan-demi, Oxycodan*) ▶LK ♀D ▶- ©II $

WARNING - Multiple strengths; see FORMS below & write specific product on Rx.

ADULT - Moderate to severe pain: 1 tab (5/325) PO q6h prn. 1-2 tabs (2.5/325) q6h prn.

PEDS - Not approved in children.

UNAPPROVED PEDS - Moderate to severe pain in 6-12 yo: ¼ Demi tab PO q6h prn. >12 yo ½ Demi tab PO q6h prn.

FORMS - Generic/Trade: Tabs Percodan 5/325 (trade scored). Trade only: 2.5/325(Percodan Demi) scored, mg oxycodone/mg ASA.

Propacet (propoxyphene + acetaminophen) ▶L ♀C ▶+ ©IV $$

ADULT - Moderate pain: 1 tab (100/650) PO q4h prn.

PEDS - Not approved in children.

FORMS - Generic/Trade: Tab 100/650 mg propoxyphene/mg acetaminophen.

NOTES - Avoid in renal insufficiency and in elderly due to risk of metabolite accumulation, and increased risk of CNS disturbance, seizures, and QRS prolongation.

Roxicet (oxycodone + acetaminophen) ▶L ♀C ▶- ©II $$

WARNING - Multiple strengths; see FORMS & write specific product on Rx.

ADULT - Moderate to severe pain: 1 tab PO q6h prn. Oral soln: 5 ml PO q6h prn.

PEDS - Not approved in children.

FORMS - Generic/Trade: Tablet Roxicet 5/325, scored. Caplet Roxicet 5/500, scored. Generic: Caps 5/500. Trade only: Roxicet oral soln 5/325 per 5 ml, mg oxycodone/mg acetaminophen.

Soma Compound with Codeine (carisoprodol + aspirin + codeine) ▶L ♀C ▶- ©III $$$

ADULT - Moderate to severe musculoskeletal pain: 1-2 tabs PO qid prn.

PEDS - Not approved in children.

FORMS - Trade: Tabs 200 mg carisoprodol/325 mg ASA/16 mg codeine.

NOTES - Refer to individual components.

Synalgos-DC (dihydrocodeine + aspirin +

caffeine) ▶L ♀C ▶- ©III $

WARNING - Case reports of prolonged erections when taken concomitantly with sildenafil.

ADULT - Moderate-severe pain: 2 caps PO q4h prn.

PEDS - Not approved in children.

FORMS - Trade: Caps, 16 mg dihydrocodeine/356.4 mg ASA/30 mg caffeine. "Painpack"=12 caps.

NOTES - Most common use is dental pain. Refer to individual components.

Talacen (pentazocine + acetaminophen) ▶L ♀C ▶? ©IV $$$

ADULT - Moderate pain: 1 tab PO q4h prn.

PEDS - Not approved in children.

FORMS - Trade: Tabs 25 mg pentazocine/650 mg acetaminophen, scored.

NOTES - Serious skin reactions, including erythema multiforme & Stevens-Johnson syndrome have been reported.

Tylenol with Codeine (codeine + acetaminophen, ✦Lenoltec, Empracet, Emtec) ▶LK ♀C ▶? ©III (Tabs), V(elixir) $

WARNING - Multiple strengths; see FORMS & write specific product on Rx.

ADULT - Moderate pain: 1-2 tabs PO q4h prn.

PEDS - Moderate pain 3-6 yo: 5 ml PO q4-6h prn. 7-12 yo 10 ml PO q4-6h prn.

FORMS - Generic/Trade: Tabs Tylenol #2 (15/300), Tylenol #3 (30/300), Tylenol #4 (60/300). Tylenol with Codeine Elixir 12/120 per 5 ml, mg codeine/mg acetaminophen. Canadian forms come with (Lenoltec, Tylenol) or without (Empracet, Emtec) caffeine.

Tylox (oxycodone + acetaminophen) ▶L ♀C ▶- ©II $

ADULT - Moderate-severe pain: 1 cap PO q6h prn.

PEDS - Not approved in children.

FORMS - Generic/Trade: Caps, 5 mg oxycodone/500 mg acetaminophen.

Vicodin (hydrocodone + acetaminophen) ▶LK ♀C ▶? ©III $

WARNING - Multiple strengths; see FORMS & write specific product on Rx.

ADULT - Moderate pain: 5/500 (max dose 8 tabs/day) & 7.5/750 (max dose of 5 tabs/day): 1-2 tabs PO q4-6h prn. 10/660: 1 tab PO q4-6h prn (max of 6 tabs/day).

PEDS - Not approved in children.

FORMS - Generic/Trade: Tabs Vicodin (5/500), Vicodin ES (7.5/750), Vicodin HP (10/660), scored, mg hydrocodone/mg acetaminophen.

Vicoprofen (hydrocodone + ibuprofen) ▶LK ♀- ▶- ©III $$$

ADULT - Moderate pain: 1 tab PO q4-6h prn, max dose 5 tabs/day.

PEDS - Not approved in children.

FORMS - Generic/Trade: Tabs 7.5 mg hydrocodone/200 mg ibuprofen.

NOTES - See NSAIDs-Other subclass warning.

Wygesic (propoxyphene + acetaminophen) ▶L ♀C ▶? ©IV $$

ADULT - Moderate pain: 1 tab PO q4h prn.

PEDS - Not approved in children.

FORMS - Generic/Trade: Tabs 65 mg propoxyphene/650 mg acetaminophen.

NOTES - Avoid in renal insufficiency and in elderly due to risk of metabolite accumulation, and increased risk of CNS disturbance, seizures, and QRS prolongation.

Zydone (hydrocodone + acetaminophen) ▶LK ♀C ▶? ©III $$

WARNING - Multiple strengths; see FORMS & write specific product on Rx.

ADULT - Moderate pain: 1-2 tabs (5/400) PO q4-6h prn, max dose 8 tabs/day. 1 tab (7.5/400, 10/400) q4-6h prn, max dose 6 tabs/day.

PEDS - Not approved in children.

FORMS - Trade: Tabs (5/400), (7.5/400) & (10/400) mg hydrocodone/mg acetaminophen.

ANALGESICS: Opioid Antagonists

NOTE: May result in withdrawal in the opioid dependent, including life-threatening withdrawal if administered to neonates born to opioid-dependent mothers. Rare pulmonary edema, cardiovascular instability, hypotension, HTN, ventricular tachycardia & ventricular fibrillation have been reported in connection with opioid reversal.

nalmefene (Revex) ▶L ♀B ▶? $$$

ADULT - Opioid overdosage: 0.5 mg/70 kg IV. If needed, this may be followed by a second dose of 1 mg/70 kg, 2-5 minutes later. Max cumulative dose 1.5 mg/70kg. If suspicion of opioid dependency, initially administer a challenge dose of 0.1 mg/70 kg. Post-operative opioid reversal: 0.25 mcg/kg IV followed by 0.25 mcg/kg incremental doses at 2-5 minute intervals, stopping as soon as the desired degree of opioid reversal is obtained. Max cumulative dose 1 mcg/kg.

PEDS - Not approved in children.

FORMS - Trade: Injection 100 mcg/ml nalmefene for postoperative reversal (blue label). 1 mg/ml nalmefene for opioid overdose (green label).

NOTES - Recurrence of respiratory depression is possible, even after an apparently adequate initial response to nalmefene treatment.

naloxone (*Narcan*) ▶LK ♀B ▶? $

ADULT - Management of opioid overdose: 0.4-2 mg IV. May repeat IV at 2-3 minute intervals up to 10 mg. Use IM/SC/ET if IV not available. Intravenous infusion: 2 mg in 500 ml D5W or NS

(0.004 mg/ml); titrate according to response. Partial post-operative opioid reversal: 0.1-0.2 mg IV at 2-3 minute intervals; repeat IM doses may be required at 1-2 hr intervals.

PEDS - Management of opioid overdose: 0.01 mg/kg IV. Give a subsequent dose of 0.1 mg/kg prn. Use IM/SC/ET if IV not available. Partial post-operative opioid reversal: 0.005-0.01 mg IV at 2-3 minute intervals.

NOTES - Watch patients for re-emergence of opioid effects.

ANALGESICS: Other

acetaminophen (*Tylenol, Panadol, Tempra, paracetamol, ♣Abenol, Atasol, Frosst 222 AF*) ▶LK ♀B ▶+ $

ADULT - Analgesic/antipyretic: 325-1000 mg PO q4-6h prn. 650 mg PR q4-6h prn. Max dose 4g/day. OA: ext'd release: 2 caplets PO q8h around the clock. Max dose 6 caplets/ day.

PEDS - Analgesic/antipyretic: 10-15 mg/kg q4-6h PO/PR prn. Max 5 doses/day.

UNAPPROVED ADULT - OA: 1,000 mg PO qid.

FORMS - OTC: Tabs 160, 325, 500, 650 mg. Chewable Tabs 80 mg. Gelcaps 500 mg. Caps 325 & 500 mg. Sprinkle Caps 80 & 160 mg. Extended release caplets 650 mg. Liquid 160 mg/5 ml & 500 mg/15 ml. Drops 80 mg/0.8 ml. Suppositories 80,120,125,300,325, & 650 mg.

NOTES - Risk of hepatotoxicity with chronic use, especially in alcoholics. Chronic use in pts who drink ≥3 drinks/day should be avoided. Rectal administration may produce lower/less reliable plasma levels.

hyaluronate (*Hyalgan, Supartz, ♣Neovisc, Orthovisc*) ▶KL ♀? ▶? $$$$$

WARNING - Do not inject extra-articularly; avoid the synovial tissues & capsule. Do not use disinfectants containing benzalkonium chloride for skin preparation.

ADULT - OA (knee): Hyalgan: 2 mL intra-articular injection q week x 3-5 weeks. Supartz: 2.5 mL intra-articular injection q week x 5 weeks. Orthovisc & Neovisc (Canada): 2 mL intra-articular injection q week x 3 weeks. Inject a local anesthetic SC prior to injections.

PEDS - Not approved in children.

FORMS - Trade: Hyalgan, Neovisc, Orthovisc: 2 ml vials & prefilled syringes. Supartz: 2.5 ml prefilled syringes.

NOTES - For those who have failed conservative therapy. Caution in allergy to eggs, avian proteins or feathers (except Neovisc - synthetic). Remove synovial fluid or effusion be-

fore each injection. Knee pain & swelling most common side effects.

hylan GF-20 (*Synvisc*) ▶KL ♀? ▶? $$$$$

WARNING - Do not inject extra-articularly; avoid the synovial tissues & capsule. Do not use disinfectants containing benzalkonium chloride for skin preparation.

ADULT - OA (knee): 2 mL intra-articular injection q week x 3 weeks.

PEDS - Not approved in children.

FORMS - Trade: 2.25 ml glass syringe w/ 2 mL drug; 3/pack.

NOTES - For those who have failed conservative therapy. Caution in allergy to eggs, avian proteins or feathers. Remove synovial fluid or effusion before each injection. Knee pain & swelling most common side effects.

lidocaine (*Lidoderm, Xylocaine*) ▶LK ♀B ▶+ $$$$

WARNING - Contraindicated in allergy to amide-type anesthetics.

ADULT - Postherpetic neuralgia: apply up to 3 patches to affected area at once for up to 12h within a 24h period.

PEDS - Not approved for use in children.

FORMS - Trade: Patch 5%, box of 30.

NOTES - Apply only to intact skin to cover the most painful area. Patches may be cut into smaller sizes w/scissors prior to removal of the release liner. Store and dispose out of the reach of children & pets to avoid possible toxicity from ingestion.

tramadol (*Ultram*) ▶KL ♀C ▶- $$$

ADULT - Moderate to moderately severe pain: 50-100 mg PO q4-6h prn. Max dose 400 mg/day. If >75 yo, <300 mg/day PO in divided doses. If creatinine clearance <30 ml/min, increase the dosing interval to 12 hours. If cirrhosis, decrease dose to 50 mg PO q12h.

PEDS - Not approved in children <16 yo.

FORMS - Generic/Trade: Tabs immediate release 50 mg.

NOTES - Contraindicated in acute intoxication with alcohol, hypnotics, centrally acting analgesics, opioids or psychotropic drugs. Seizures may occur with concurrent antidepressants or in seizure disorder. Use with great caution with MAO inhibitors or in combination with SSRIs due to potential for serotonin syndrome; dose adjustment may be needed. Withdrawal symptoms may occur in patients dependent on opioids. Carbamazepine decreases tramadol

levels. The most frequent side effects are nausea & constipation.

***Women's Tylenol Menstrual Relief* (acetaminophen + pamabrom)** ▶LK ♀B ▶+ $

ADULT - Menstrual cramps: 2 caplets PO q4-6h.

PEDS - >12 yo: use adult dose.

FORMS - OTC: Caplets 500 mg acetaminophen/25 mg pamabrom (diuretic).

NOTES - Hepatotoxicity with chronic use, especially in alcoholics.

ANESTHESIA: Anesthetics & Sedatives

alfentanil (*Alfenta*) ▶L ♀C ▶? ©II $

ADULT - IV general anesthesia adjunct; specialized dosing.

PEDS - Not approved in children.

dexmedetomidine (*Precedex*) ▶LK ♀C ▶? $$$$

ADULT - ICU sedation <24h: Load 1 mcg/kg over 10 min followed by infusion 0.2-0.7 mcg/kg/h titrated to desired sedation endpoint.

PEDS - Not recommended <18 yo.

NOTES - Alpha 2 adrenergic agonist with sedative properties. Beware of bradycardia and hypotension. Avoid in advanced heart block.

etomidate (*Amidate*) ▶L ♀C ▶? $

ADULT - Anesthesia induction: 0.3 mg/kg IV.

PEDS - Age ≥10 yo: Adult dosing. Age <10 yo: Not approved.

UNAPPROVED PEDS - Anesthesia induction: 0.3 mg/kg IV.

NOTES - Adrenocortical suppression, but rarely of clinical significance.

fentanyl (*Sublimaze*) ▶L ♀C ▶? ©II $

ADULT - IV adjunct to general anesthesia: specialized dosing.

PEDS - IV adjunct to general anesthesia & procedural sedation, specialized dosing.

UNAPPROVED ADULT - Procedural sedation: 50 mcg IV, may repeat q3 min, adjust to desired effect.

UNAPPROVED PEDS - Procedural sedation: 1 mcg/kg/dose IV, may repeat q3 min, adjust to desired effect.

ketamine (*Ketalar*) ▶L ♀? ▶? ©III $

WARNING - Emergence delirium limits value of ketamine in adults; such reactions are rare in children.

ADULT - Dissociative sedation: 1-2 mg/kg IV over 1-2 min or 4-5 mg/kg IM.

PEDS - Dissociative sedation: 1-2 mg/kg IV over 1-2 min or 4-5 mg/kg IM.

NOTES - Raises BP and intracranial pressure;

avoid if coronary artery disease, HTN, head or eye injury. Concurrent atropine minimizes hypersalivation; can be combined in same syringe with ketamine for IM use.

methohexital (*Brevital*) ▶L ♀B ▶? ©IV $

ADULT - Anesthesia induction: 1-1.5 mg/kg IV.

PEDS - Safety in children not established.

UNAPPROVED PEDS - Sedation for diagnostic imaging: 25 mg/kg PR

midazolam (*Versed*) ▶LK ♀D ▶- ©IV $

WARNING - Beware of respiratory depression/apnea. Administer with appropriate monitoring.

ADULT - Sedation/anxiolysis: 0.07-0.08 mg/kg IM (5 mg in average adult); or 1 mg IV slowly q2-3 min up to 5 mg. Anesthesia induction: 0.3-0.35 mg/kg IV over 20-30 seconds.

PEDS - Sedation/anxiolysis: 0.25-1.0 mg/kg to maximum of 20 mg PO, or 0.1-0.15 mg/kg IM. IV route (6 mo to 5 yo): Initial dose 0.05-0.1 mg/kg IV, then titrated to max 0.6 mg/kg. IV route (6-12 yo): Initial dose 0.025-0.05 mg/kg IV, then titrated to max 0.4 mg/kg.

UNAPPROVED PEDS - Sedation/anxiolysis: Intranasal 0.2-0.4 mg/kg. Rectal: 0.25-0.5 mg/kg PR. Higher oral dosing: 0.5-0.75 mg/kg PO, max 20 mg/kg. Status epilepticus: Load 0.15 mg/kg IV followed by infusion 1 mcg/kg/min and titrate dose upward q5 min prn.

FORMS - Oral liquid 2 mg/ml

NOTES - Use lower doses in the elderly, chronically ill, and those receiving concurrent CNS depressants.

pentobarbital (*Nembutal*) ▶LK ♀D ▶? ©II $$

ADULT - Rarely used; other drugs preferred. Hypnotic: 150-200 mg IM or 100 mg IV at a rate of 50 mg/min, maximum dose is 500 mg.

PEDS - FDA approved for active seizing, but other agents preferred.

UNAPPROVED PEDS - Procedural sedation: 1-6 mg/kg IV, adjusted in increments of 1-2 mg/kg to desired effect, or 2-6 mg/kg IM, max

100 mg. Do not exceed 50 mg/min.

propofol (*Diprivan*) ▶L ♀B ▶- $$$
WARNING - Beware of respiratory depression/apnea. Administer with appropriate monitoring.
ADULT - Anesthesia (<55 yo): 40 mg IV q10 sec until induction onset (typical 2-2.5 mg/kg). Follow with maintenance infusion generally 100-200 mcg/kg/min. Lower doses in elderly or for sedation. ICU ventilator sedation: infusion 5-50 mcg/kg/min.
PEDS - Anesthesia (≥3 yo): 2.5-3.5 mg/kg IV over 20-30 seconds, followed with infusion 125-300 mcg/kg/min. Not recommended if <3 yo or for prolonged ICU use.
NOTES - Avoid with egg or soy allergies.

remifentanil (*Ultiva*) ▶L ♀C ▶? ©II $$
ADULT, PEDS - IV general anesthesia adjunct; specialized dosing.

sufentanil (*Sufenta*) ▶L ♀C ▶? ©II $$
ADULT, PEDS - IV anesthesia adjunct: specialized dosing.

thiopental (*Pentothal*) ▶L ♀C ▶? ©III $
ADULT - Anesthesia induction: 3-5 mg/kg IV.
PEDS - Anesthesia induction: 3-5 mg/kg IV.
UNAPPROVED PEDS - Sedation for diagnostic imaging: 25 mg/kg PR
NOTES - Duration 5 minutes. Hypotension, histamine release, tissue necrosis with extravasation.

ANESTHESIA: Local Anesthetics

articaine (*Septocaine*) ▶LK ♀C ▶? ?
ADULT - Dental local anesthesia: 4% injection.
PEDS - Dental local anesthesia and ≥4 yo: 4% injection.
FORMS - 4% (includes epinephrine 1:100,000)
NOTES - Do not exceed 7 mg/kg total dose

bupivacaine (*Marcaine, Sensorcaine*) ▶LK ♀C ▶? $
WARNING - Not for OB anesthesia or children.
ADULT - Local anesthesia, nerve block: 0.25% injection.
PEDS - Not recommended in children <12 yo.
FORMS - 0.25%, 0.5%, 0.75%, all with or without epinephrine.
NOTES - Onset 5 mins, duration 2-4h (longer with epi). Amide group. Max dose 2.5 mg/kg alone, or 3.0 mg/kg with epinephrine.

levobupivacaine (*Chirocaine*) ▶LK ♀B ▶? ?
ADULT - Local & epidural anesthesia, nerve block.
PEDS - Not approved in children.
FORMS - 2.5, 5, 7.5 mg/ml injection.

lidocaine (*Xylocaine*) ▶LK ♀B ▶? $
ADULT - Local anesthesia: 0.5-1% injection.

PEDS - Local anesthesia: 0.5-1% injection.
FORMS - 0.5,1,1.5,2%. With epi: 0.5,1,1.5,2%.
NOTES - Onset <2 mins, duration 30-60 mins (longer with epi). Amide group. Potentially toxic dose 3-5 mg/kg without epinephrine, and 5-7 mg/kg with epinephrine. Use "cardiac lidocaine" (ie, IV formulation) for Bier blocks at maximum dose of 3 mg/kg so that epinephrine and methylparaben are not injected IV.

mepivacaine (*Carbocaine, Polocaine*) ▶LK ♀C ▶? $
ADULT - Nerve block: 1%-2% injection.
PEDS - Nerve block: 1%-2% injection. Use <2% concentration if <3 yo or <30 pounds.
FORMS - 1,1.5,2,3%.
NOTES - Onset 3-5 mins, duration 45-90 mins. Amide group. Max local dose 5 to 6 mg/kg.

Oraquix (lidocaine + prilocaine) ▶LK ♀B ▶? $$
ADULT - Local anesthetic gel applied to periodontal pockets using blunt-tipped applicator: 4% injection.
PEDS - Not approved in children.
FORMS - Gel 2.5% + 2.5% with applicator.

ANESTHESIA: Neuromuscular Blockers

NOTE: Should be administered only by those skilled in airway management and respiratory support.

atracurium (*Tracrium*) ▶Plasma ♀C ▶? $
ADULT - Paralysis: 0.4-0.5 mg/kg IV.
PEDS - Paralysis ≥2yo: 0.4-0.5 mg/kg IV.
NOTES - Duration 15-30 minutes. Hoffman degradation.

cisatracurium (*Nimbex*) ▶Plasma ♀B ▶? $$

ADULT - Paralysis: 0.15-0.2 mg/kg IV.
PEDS - Paralysis: 0.1 mg/kg IV over 5-10 seconds.
NOTES - Duration 30-60 minutes. Hoffman degradation.

doxacurium (*Nuromax*) ▶KL ♀C ▶? $$
ADULT - Paralysis: 0.05 mg/kg IV.
PEDS - Paralysis: 0.03 mg/kg IV.
NOTES - Duration ~100 minutes. Decrease

dose if liver or renal insufficiency.

mivacurium (*Mivacron*) ▶Plasma ♀C ▶? $

ADULT - Paralysis: 0.15 mg/kg IV over 5-15 seconds.

PEDS - Paralysis in children aged 2-12 years: 0.2 mg/kg IV over 5-15 seconds.

NOTES - Duration 20 minutes. Although rapid metabolism by plasma cholinesterase, dose may need to be reduced in renal and liver disease.

pancuronium (*Pavulon*) ▶LK ♀C ▶? $

ADULT - Paralysis: 0.04 to 0.1 mg/kg IV.

PEDS - Paralysis (beyond neonatal age): 0.04 to 0.1 mg/kg IV.

NOTES - Duration 45 minutes. Decrease dose if renal disease.

rocuronium (*Zemuron*) ▶L ♀B ▶? $$

ADULT - Paralysis: 0.6 mg/kg IV. Rapid sequence intubation: 0.6 to 1.2 mg/kg IV. Continuous infusion: 10 to 12 mcg/kg/min; first verify spontaneous recovery from bolus dose.

PEDS - Paralysis (age >3 mo): 0.6 mg/kg IV. Continuous infusion: 12 mcg/kg/min; first verify spontaneous recovery from bolus dose.

NOTES - Duration 30 minutes. Decrease dose if severe liver disease.

succinylcholine (*Anectine, Quelicin*) ▶Plasma ♀C ▶? $

ADULT - Paralysis: 0.6-1.1 mg/kg IV.

PEDS - Paralysis (≥5 yo): 1 mg/kg IV. Paralysis (<5 yo): 2 mg/kg IV; consider pretreatment with atropine 0.02 mg/kg to prevent bradycardia.

NOTES - Avoid in hyperkalemia, myopathies, eye injuries, rhabdomyolysis, subacute burn. If immediate cardiac arrest and ET tube is in correct place & no tension pneumo evident, strongly consider empiric treatment for hyperkalemia.

vecuronium (*Norcuron*) ▶LK ♀C ▶? $

ADULT - Paralysis: 0.08-0.1 mg/kg IV bolus. Continuous infusion: 0.8 to 1.2 mcg/kg/min; first verify spontaneous recovery from bolus dose.

PEDS - Paralysis (age ≥10 yrs): 0.08-0.1 mg/kg IV bolus. Continuous infusion: 0.8 to 1.2 mcg/kg/min; first verify spontaneous recovery from bolus dose. Age 1-10 years: may require a slightly higher initial dose and may also require supplementation slightly more often than older patients. Age 7 weeks to 1 year: moderately more sensitive on a mg/kg dose compared to adults and take 1.5 x longer to recover. Age <7 weeks: Safety has not been established.

NOTES - Duration 15-30 minutes. Decrease dose in severe liver disease.

ANTIMICROBIALS: Aminoglycosides

NOTE: See also dermatology and ophthalmology

amikacin (*Amikin*) ▶K ♀D ▶? $$$$

WARNING - Nephrotoxicity, ototoxicity.

ADULT - Gram negative infections: 15 mg/kg/day up to 1500 mg/day IM/IV divided q8-12h. Peak 20-35 mcg/ml, trough <5 mcg/ml.

PEDS - Gram negative infections: 15 mg/kg/day up to 1500 mg/day IM/IV divided q8-12h. Neonates: 10 mg/kg load, then 7.5 mg/kg IM/IV q12h.

UNAPPROVED ADULT - Once daily dosing: 15 mg/kg IV q24h. TB (2nd-line treatment): 15 mg/kg up to 1 g IM/IV qd. 10 mg/kg up to 750 mg IM/IV qd if >59 yo.

UNAPPROVED PEDS - Severe infections: 15-22.5 mg/kg/day IV divided q8h. Some experts recommend 30 mg/kg/day. Once daily dosing: 15 mg/kg IV q24h. Some experts consider once-daily dosing of aminoglycosides investigational in children. TB (2nd-line treatment): 15-30 mg/kg up to 1 g IM/IV qd.

NOTES - May enhance effects of neuromuscular blockers. Avoid other ototoxic/nephrotoxic drugs. Individualize dose in renal dysfunction, burn patients. Base dose on average of actual and ideal body weight in obesity.

gentamicin (*Garamycin*) ▶K ♀D ▶+ $$

WARNING - Nephrotoxicity, ototoxicity.

ADULT - Gram negative infections: 3-5 mg/kg/day IM/IV divided q8h. Peak 5-10 mcg/ml, trough <2 mcg/ml. Empiric therapy, native valve endocarditis: 1 mg/kg IM/IV q8h plus penicillin/ampicillin and nafcillin/oxacillin. Endocarditis target peak ~3 mcg/ml, trough <1 mcg/ml (no once-daily dosing). See table for prophylaxis of bacterial endocarditis.

PEDS - Gram negative infections: 2-2.5 mg/kg IM/IV q8h. Infants ≥1 week old, >2 kg: 2.5 mg/kg IM/IV q8h. Infants <1 week old, >2 kg: 2.5 mg/kg IM/IV q12h. Cystic fibrosis: 9 mg/kg/day IV in divided doses with target peak of 8-12 mcg/ml.

UNAPPROVED ADULT - Once daily dosing: 5-7 mg/kg IV q24h.

UNAPPROVED PEDS - Once daily dosing: 5-7 mg/kg IV q24h. Age <1 week and full-term: 4 mg/kg IV q24h. Some experts consider once-daily dosing of aminoglycosides investigational

in children.
NOTES - May enhance effects of neuromuscular blockers. Avoid other ototoxic/nephrotoxic drugs. Individualize dose in renal dysfunction, burn dose. Base dose on average of actual and ideal body weight in obesity.

spectinomycin (Trobicin) ▶K ♀B ▶? $$
ADULT - Gonorrhea: 2 g IM single dose.
PEDS - Safety in children not established.
UNAPPROVED ADULT - Disseminated gonorrhea: 2 g IM q12h.
UNAPPROVED PEDS - Gonorrhea: 40 mg/kg IM up to 2 g single dose for <45 kg. Give adult dose for ≥45 kg.
NOTES - Anaphylactoid reactions rarely.

streptomycin ▶K ♀D ▶+ $$$$$
WARNING - Nephrotoxicity, ototoxicity. Monitor audiometry, renal function, and electrolytes.
ADULT - Combined therapy for TB: 15 mg/kg up to 1 g IM/IV qd. 10 mg/kg up to 750 mg IM/IV qd if >59 yo.
PEDS - Combined therapy for TB: 20-40 mg/kg up to 1 g IM qd.
UNAPPROVED ADULT - Same IM dosing can be given IV. Streptococcal endocarditis: 7.5 mg/kg IM bid. Go to www.americanheart.org for further info.
FORMS - Generic: 1 g vials for parenteral use.
NOTES - Contraindicated in pregnancy. Obtain baseline audiogram, vestibular and Romberg testing, and renal function. Monitor renal function and vestibular and auditory sx monthly. May enhance effects of neuromuscular block-

ers. Avoid other ototoxic/nephrotoxic drugs. Individualize dose in renal dysfunction.

tobramycin (Nebcin, TOBI) ▶K ♀D ▶? $$$$
WARNING - Nephrotoxicity, ototoxicity.
ADULT - Gram negative infections: 3-5 mg/kg/day IM/IV divided q8h. Peak 5-10 mcg/ml, trough <2 mcg/ml. Parenteral for cystic fibrosis: 10 mg/kg/day IV divided q6h with target peak of 8-12 mcg/ml. Nebulized for cystic fibrosis (TOBI): 300 mg neb bid 28 days on, then 28 days off.
PEDS - Gram negative infections: 2-2.5 mg/kg IV q8h or 1.5-1.9 mg/kg IV q6h. Premature/full-term neonates ≤1 week old: Up to 4 mg/kg/day divided q12h. Parenteral for cystic fibrosis: 10 mg/kg/day IV divided q6h with target peak of 8-12 mcg/ml. Nebulized for cystic fibrosis (TOBI) ≥6 yo: 300 mg neb bid 28 days on, then 28 days off.
UNAPPROVED ADULT - Once daily dosing: 5-7 mg/kg IV q24h.
UNAPPROVED PEDS - Once daily dosing: 5-7 mg/kg IV q24h. Some experts consider once-daily dosing of aminoglycosides investigational in children.
FORMS - TOBI 300 mg ampules for nebulizer.
NOTES - May enhance effects of neuromuscular blockers. Avoid other ototoxic/nephrotoxic drugs. Individualize dose in renal dysfunction, burn patients. Base dose on average of actual and ideal body weight in obesity. Routine monitoring of tobramycin levels not required with nebulized TOBI.

ANTIMICROBIALS: Antifungal Agents

amphotericin B deoxycholate (Fungizone) ▶Tissues ♀B, C for PO ▶? $$$$
WARNING - IV route not for noninvasive fungal infections (oral thrush, vaginal or esophageal candidiasis) in patients with normal neutrophil counts.
ADULT - Life-threatening systemic fungal infections: Test dose 1 mg slow IV. Wait 2-4 h, and if tolerated start 0.25 mg/kg IV qd. Advance to 0.5-1.5 mg/kg/day depending on fungal type. Maximum dose 1.5 mg/kg/day. Infuse over 2-6 h. Hydrate with 500 ml NS before and after infusion to decrease risk of nephrotoxicity.
PEDS - No remaining FDA approved indications
UNAPPROVED ADULT - Alternative regimen, life-threatening systemic fungal infections: 1 mg test dose as part of 1st infusion (don't need separate IV bag); if tolerated continue infusion, giving target dose of 0.5-1.5 mg/kg on 1st day.

Candidemia, non-neutropenic pts: 0.6-1.0 mg/kg IV qd; or 0.7 mg/kg IV qd + fluconazole 800 mg/day for 4-7 days, then fluconazole 800 mg/day. Treat until 14 days past last + blood culture and signs/sx resolved. Candidemia, neutropenic pts: 0.7-1.0 mg/kg IV qd until 14 days past last + blood culture, signs/sx, and neutropenia resolved. Cryptococcal meningitis in HIV infection: 0.7-1 mg/kg/day IV +/- flucytosine 25 mg/kg PO q6h x 2 wks followed by PO fluconazole. Candidal cystitis: Irrigate bladder with 50 mcg/ml soln periodically/ continuously x 5-10 days.
UNAPPROVED PEDS - Systemic life-threatening fungal infections: Test dose 0.1 mg/kg slow IV. Wait 2-4 h, and if tolerated start 0.25 mg/kg IV qd. Advance to 0.5-1.5 mg/kg/day depending on fungal type. Maximum dose 1.5 mg/kg/day. Infuse over 2-6 h. Hydrate with 10-15 ml/

kg NS before infusion to decrease risk of nephrotoxicity. Alternative dosing regimen: Give 1 mg test dose as part of first infusion (separate IV bag not needed); if tolerated continue infusion, giving target dose of 0.5 to 1.5 mg/kg on first day. Candidemia, non-neutropenic pts: 0.6-1.0 mg/kg IV qd until 14-21 days past signs/sx resolved and neg repeat blood culture.

NOTES - Acute infusion reactions, anaphylaxis, nephrotoxicity, hypokalemia, hypomagnesemia, acidosis, anemia. Monitor renal and hepatic function, CBC, serum electrolytes. Lipid formulations better tolerated, preferred in renal dysfunction..

amphotericin B lipid formulations (*Amphotec, Abelcet, AmBisome*) ▶? ♀B ▶? $$$$$

ADULT - Lipid formulations used primarily in patients refractory/intolerant to amphotericin deoxycholate. Abelcet: Invasive fungal infections: 5 mg/kg/day IV at 2.5 mg/kg/h. Shake infusion bag every 2 h. AmBisome: Infuse IV over 2 h. Empiric therapy of fungal infections in febrile neutropenia: 3 mg/kg/day. Aspergillus, candidal, cryptococcal infections: 3-5 mg/kg/day. Cryptococcal meningitis in HIV infection: 6 mg/kg/day. Amphotec: Test dose of 10 ml over 15-30 minutes, observe for 30 minutes, then 3-4 mg/kg/day IV at 1 mg/kg/h.

PEDS - Lipid formulations used primarily in patients refractory/intolerant to amphotericin deoxycholate. Abelcet: Invasive fungal infections: 5 mg/kg/day IV at 2.5 mg/kg/h. Shake infusion bag every 2 h. AmBisome: Infuse IV over 2 h. Empiric therapy of fungal infections in febrile neutropenia: 3 mg/kg/day. Aspergillus, candidal, cryptococcal infections: 3-5 mg/kg/day. Cryptococcal meningitis in HIV infection: 6 mg/kg/day. Amphotec: Aspergillosis: Test dose of 10 ml over 15-30 minutes, observe for 30 minutes, then 3-4 mg/kg/day IV at 1 mg/kg/h.

NOTES - Acute infusion reactions, anaphylaxis, nephrotoxicity, hypokalemia, hypomagnesemia, acidosis. Lipid formulations better tolerated than amphotericin deoxycholate, preferred in renal dysfunction. Monitor renal and hepatic function, CBC, electrolytes.

caspofungin (*Cancidas*) ▶KL ♀C ▶? $$$$$

ADULT - Infuse IV over 1 h. Invasive aspergillosis refractory / intolerant to other antifungals: 70 mg loading dose on day 1, then 50 mg qd. Candidemia or Candida intra-abdominal abscess, peritonitis, pleural space infections: 70 mg loading dose on day 1, then 50 mg qd. Treat ≥14 days after last positive culture; may

treat longer if persistent neutropenia. Esophageal candidiasis: 50 mg qd. Patients taking rifampin: 70 mg qd. Consider using this dose with other enzyme inducers (such as carbamazepine, dexamethasone, efavirenz, nevirapine, phenytoin).

PEDS - Not approved in children.

NOTES - Administration with cyclosporine increases caspofungin levels & hepatic transaminases; risk of concomitant use unclear. Caspofungin decreases tacrolimus levels. Dosage adjustment in moderate liver dysfunction (Child-Pugh score 7-9): 35 mg IV qd (after 70 mg loading dose in patients with invasive aspergillosis).

clotrimazole (*Mycelex*, ♣*Canesten, Clotrimaderm*) ▶L ♀C ▶? $$$

ADULT - Oropharyngeal candidiasis: 1 troche dissolved slowly in mouth 5x/day x 14 days. Prevention of oropharyngeal candidiasis in immunocompromised patients: 1 troche dissolved slowly in mouth tid until end of chemotherapy/high-dose corticosteroids.

PEDS - Treatment of oropharyngeal candidiasis, ≥3 yo: 1 troche dissolved slowly in mouth 5x/day x 14 days.

FORMS - Trade/generic: Oral troches 10 mg.

fluconazole (*Diflucan*) ▶K ♀C ▶+ $$$$

ADULT - Vaginal candidiasis: 150 mg PO single dose. All other dosing regimens IV/PO. Oropharyngeal/esophageal candidiasis: 200 mg first day, then 100 mg qd for ≥14 days for oropharyngeal, ≥3 weeks & continuing for 2 weeks past symptom resolution for esophageal. Systemic candidiasis: 400 mg qd. Candidal UTI, peritonitis: 50-200 mg qd. Cryptococcal meningitis: 400 mg qd until 10-12 weeks after cerebrospinal fluid is culture negative. Suppression of cryptococcal meningitis relapse in AIDS: 200 mg qd. Prevention of candidiasis after bone marrow transplant: 400 mg qd starting several days before neutropenia and continuing until ANC >1000 cells/mm3 x 7 days.

PEDS - All dosing regimens IV/PO. Oropharyngeal/esophageal candidiasis: 6 mg/kg first day, then 3 mg/kg qd for ≥14 days for oropharyngeal, ≥3 weeks & continuing for 2 weeks past symptom resolution for esophageal. Systemic candidiasis: 6-12 mg/kg qd. Cryptococcal meningitis: 12 mg/kg on first day, then 6 mg/kg qd until 10-12 weeks after cerebrospinal fluid is culture negative. Suppression of cryptococcal meningitis relapse in AIDS: 6 mg/kg qd.

UNAPPROVED ADULT - Onychomycosis, fingernail (2nd line to itraconazole or terbinafine):

150-300 mg PO q week x 3-6 mo. Onychomycosis, toenail (2nd line to itraconazole or terbinafine): 150-300 mg PO q week x 6-12 mo. Recurrent vaginal candidiasis: 150 mg PO x 2 doses 3 days apart, then 100-150 mg PO q week x 6 months. Non-neutropenic candidemia: 400-800 mg/day IV/PO or 800 mg/day + amphotericin B 0.7 mg/kg/day IV for first 4-7 days. Treat until 14 days past last + blood culture and signs/sx resolved. Neutropenic candidemia: 6-12 mg/kg/day IV/PO until 14 days past last + blood culture, signs/sx, and neutropenia resolved. Prevention of candidal infections in high-risk neutropenic pts: 400 mg/day during period of risk for neutropenia.
FORMS - Trade/generic: Tabs 50,100,150,200 mg; susp 10 & 40 mg/ml.
NOTES - Hepatotoxicity. Many drug interactions, including increased levels of cyclosporine, phenytoin, theophylline, and increased INR with warfarin. Do not use with cisapride. Dosing in renal dysfunction: Reduce maintenance dose by 50% for CrCl 11-50 ml/min. Hemodialysis: Give recommended dose after each dialysis.

flucytosine (*Ancobon*) ▶K ♀C ▶- $$$$$
WARNING - Extreme caution in renal or bone marrow impairment. Monitor hematologic, hepatic, renal function in all patients.
ADULT - Candidal/cryptococcal infections: 50-150 mg/kg/day PO divided qid. Initial dose for cryptococcal meningitis: 100 mg/kg/day PO divided qid.
PEDS - Not approved in children.
UNAPPROVED PEDS - Candidal/cryptococcal infections: 50-150 mg/kg/day PO divided qid.
FORMS - Trade: Caps 250, 500 mg.
NOTES - Flucytosine is given with other antifungal agents. Myelosuppression. Reduce nausea by taking caps a few at a time over 15 minutes. Monitor flucytosine levels. Peak 70-80 mg/L, trough 30-40 mg/L. Reduce dose in renal dysfunction.

griseofulvin (*Grisactin 500*) ▶Skin ♀C ▶? $$
ADULT - Tinea: 500 mg PO qd x 4-6 weeks for capitis, 2-4 weeks for corporis, 4-8 weeks for pedis, 4 months for fingernails, 6 months for toenails. Can use 1 g/day for pedis and unguium.
PEDS - Tinea: 11 mg/kg PO qd x 4-6 weeks for capitis, 2-4 weeks for corporis, 4-8 weeks for pedis, 4 months for fingernails, 6 months for toenails.
UNAPPROVED PEDS - Tinea capitis: AAP recommends 15-20 mg/kg (max 1 g) PO qd x 4-6

weeks, continuing for 2 weeks past symptom resolution. Some infections may require 20-25 mg/kg/day or ultramicrosize griseofulvin 5-10 mg/kg (max 750 mg) PO qd.
FORMS - Generic/Trade: Tabs 500 mg. Trade: Tabs 250, susp 125 mg/5 ml.
NOTES - Do not use in liver failure, porphyria. May cause photosensitivity, lupus-like syndrome/ exacerbation of lupus. Decreased INR with warfarin, decreased efficacy of oral contraceptives. Ultramicrosize formulations have greater GI absorption, and are available with different strengths and dosing.

griseofulvin ultramicrosize (*Gris-PEG*) ▶Skin ♀C ▶? $$
ADULT - Tinea: 375 mg PO qd x 4-6 weeks for capitis, 2-4 weeks for corporis, 4-8 weeks for pedis, 4 months for fingernails, 6 months for toenails. Can use 750 mg/day for pedis and unguium. Best absorption when given after meal containing fat.
PEDS - Tinea, >2 yo: 7.3 mg/kg PO qd x 4-6 weeks for capitis, 2-4 weeks for corporis, 4-8 weeks for pedis, 4 months for fingernails, 6 months for toenails. Give 82.5-165 mg PO qd for 13.6-22.6 kg. Tinea capitis: AAP recommends 5-10 mg/ kg (up to 750 mg) PO qd x 4-6 weeks, continuing for 2 weeks past symptom resolution. Best absorption when given after meal containing fat.
FORMS - Generic/trade: Tabs 125,250 mg.
NOTES - Do not use in liver failure, porphyria. May cause photosensitivity, lupus-like syndrome/ exacerbation of lupus. Decreased INR with warfarin, decreased efficacy of oral contraceptives. Microsize formulations, which have lower GI absorption, are available with different strengths and dosing.

itraconazole (*Sporanox*) ▶L ♀C ▶- $$$$$
WARNING - Inhibition of CYP 3A4 metabolism by itraconazole can lead to dangerously high levels of some drugs. High levels of some can prolong QT interval (see QT drugs table). Contraindicated with cisapride, dofetilide, ergot alkaloids, levomethadyl, lovastatin, PO midazolam, pimozide, quinidine, simvastatin, triazolam. Negative inotrope; stop treatment if signs/sx of CHF. Not for onychomycosis if CHF; use for other indications in CHF only if benefit exceeds risk.
ADULT - Caps - Take caps with full meal. Onychomycosis, toenails: 200 mg PO qd x 12 weeks. Onychomycosis "pulse dosing", fingernails: 200 mg PO bid for 1st wk of month x 2

months. Test nail specimen to confirm diagnosis before prescribing. IV/PO - Aspergillosis in patients intolerant/ refractory to amphotericin, blastomycosis, histoplasmosis: 200 mg IV bid x 4 doses, each IV dose over 1 h, then 200 mg IV qd. Can also give 200 mg PO bid or qd. Treat for ≥3 months. For life-threatening infections, load with 200 mg IV bid x 4 doses or 200 mg PO tid x 3 days. Empiric therapy of suspected fungal infection in febrile neutropenia: 200 mg IV bid x 4 doses, then 200 mg IV qd for ≤14 days. Continue oral sol'n 200 mg (20 ml) PO bid until significant neutropenia resolved. Oral soln - Swish & swallow in 10 ml increments on empty stomach. Oropharyngeal candidiasis: 200 mg qd x 1-2 weeks. Oropharyngeal candidiasis unresponsive to fluconazole: 100 mg bid. Esophageal candidiasis: 100-200 mg qd x ≥3 weeks & continuing for 2 weeks past symptom resolution.
PEDS - Not approved in children.
UNAPPROVED ADULT - Caps - Onychomycosis "pulse dosing", toenails: 200 mg PO bid for 1st wk of month x 3-4 months. Confirm diagnosis with nail specimen lab testing before prescribing.
UNAPPROVED PEDS - Caps for systemic fungal infections, 3-16 yo: 100 mg PO qd.
FORMS - Generic/Trade: Cap 100 mg. Trade: Oral soln 10 mg/ml.
NOTES - Hepatotoxicity, even during 1st week of therapy. Monitor LFTs if hepatic history; consider monitoring in all. Decreased absorption of itraconazole with antacids, H2 blockers, proton pump inhibitors, or achlorhydria. Carbamazepine, grapefruit juice (avoid), isoniazid, nevirapine, phenobarbital, phenytoin, rifabutin & rifampin reduce itraconazole levels. Itraconazole inhibits cytochrome P450 3A4 metabolism of many drugs. Not more than 200 mg bid of itraconazole with unboosted indinavir. May increase adverse effects with trazodone; consider reducing trazodone dose. May increase QT interval with disopyramide or halofantrine. Caps and oral soln not interchangeable. Oral sol'n may be preferred in serious infections due to greater absorption. Oral soln may not achieve adequate levels in cystic fibrosis patients; consider alternative if no response. Start therapy for onychomycosis on day 1-2 of menses in women of childbearing potential & advise against pregnancy until 2 months after therapy ends. Do not use IV itraconazole if CrCl <30 ml/min. See package insert for instructions before making/ giving IV soln.

ketoconazole (*Nizoral*) ▶L ♀C ▶?+ $$$$
WARNING - Hepatotoxicity: inform patients of risk & monitor. Do not use with cisapride, midazolam, pimozide, triazolam.
ADULT - Systemic fungal infections: 200-400 mg PO qd.
PEDS - Systemic fungal infections, ≥2 yo: 3.3-6.6 mg/kg PO qd.
UNAPPROVED ADULT - Tinea versicolor: 400 mg PO single dose or 200 mg PO qd x 7 days. Prevention of recurrent mucocutaneous candidiasis in HIV infection: 200 mg PO qd.
UNAPPROVED PEDS - Prevention of recurrent mucocutaneous candidiasis in HIV infection: 5-10 mg/kg/day PO qd or bid; max 400 mg bid.
FORMS - Generic/Trade: Tabs 200 mg.
NOTES - Antacids, H2 blockers, proton pump inhibitors, buffered didanosine, achlorhydria decrease absorption. Isoniazid & rifampin reduce ketoconazole levels. Avoid >200 mg/day of ketoconazole with ritonavir or Kaletra. Ketoconazole inhibits cytochrome P450 3A4 metabolism of many drugs. May increase adverse effects with trazodone; consider reducing trazodone dose.

nystatin (*Mystatin*, ♦*Nilstat, Nyaderm, Candistatin*) ▶Not absorbed ♀B ▶? $
ADULT - Thrush: 4-6 ml PO swish & swallow qid or suck on 1-2 troches 4-5 x daily.
PEDS - Thrush, infants: 2 ml/dose PO with 1 ml in each cheek qid. Premature and low weight infants: 0.5 ml PO in each cheek qid. Thrush, older children: 4-6 ml PO swish & swallow qid or suck on 1-2 troches 4-5 x daily.
FORMS - Generic/Trade: Susp 100,000 units/ml. Trade: Troches 200,000 units.

terbinafine (*Lamisil*) ▶LK ♀B ▶- $$$$$
ADULT - Onychomycosis: 250 mg PO qd x 6 weeks for fingernails, x 12 weeks for toenails.
PEDS - Not approved in children.
UNAPPROVED ADULT - Onychomycosis "pulse dosing": 500 mg PO qd for 1st week of month x 2 months for fingernails, 4 months for toenails.
UNAPPROVED PEDS - Onychomycosis: 67.5 mg PO qd for <20 kg, 125 mg PO qd for 20-40 kg, 250 mg PO qd for >40 kg x 6 weeks for fingernails, x 12 weeks for toenails.
FORMS - Trade: Tabs 250 mg.
NOTES - Hepatotoxicity; monitor AST & ALT at baseline. Neutropenia. May rarely cause or exacerbate lupus. Do not use in liver disease or CrCl ≤50 ml/min. Test nail specimen to confirm diagnosis before prescribing. Inhibitor of CYP 2D6.

voriconazole (*Vfend*) ▸L ♀D ▸? $$$$$

ADULT - IV and PO doses are the same. Invasive aspergillosis, or Scedosporium, Fusarium infections: 6 mg/kg IV q12h x 2 doses, then 4 mg/kg q12h. Dilute to ≤5 mg/mL and infuse at ≤3 mg/kg/h over 1-2 h. When PO tolerated, give 200 mg PO q12h if >40 kg or 100 mg PO q12h if <40 kg. See package insert for dosage adjustments due to poor response/ adverse effects. Esophageal candidiasis: 200 mg PO q12h if ≥40 kg; 100 mg PO q12h if <40 kg for ≥2 weeks and continuing for >1 week past symptom resolution. Take tabs/ susp 1 h before/after meals.

PEDS - Safety & efficacy not established in children <12 yo. Use adult dose if ≥12 yo.

UNAPPROVED ADULT - Serious candidal infections: 3 mg/kg IV q12h.

FORMS - Trade: Tabs 50,200 mg (contains lactose), susp 40 mg/mL.

NOTES - Anaphylactoid reactions (IV only), severe skin reactions & photosensitivity, hepatotoxicity rarely. Transient visual disturbances common; advise against hazardous tasks (if vision impaired); night driving & strong, direct sunlight. Monitor visual (if treated >28 days), liver, and renal function. Many drug interactions. Substrate & inhibitor of CYP 2C9, 2C19, & 3A4. Do not use with carbamazepine, cisapride, efavirenz, ergot alkaloids, phenobarbital, pimozide, quinidine, rifabutin, rifampin, ritonavir 400 mg bid, sirolimus. Dosage adjustments with cyclosporine, omeprazole, phenytoin, tacrolimus in package insert. Increased INR with warfarin. Could inhibit metabolism of benzodiazepines, calcium channel blockers, statins. Vehicle in IV form may accumulate in renal impairment; oral preferred if CrCl <50 mL/minute. Mild/ moderate cirrhosis (Child-Pugh class A/B): Same loading dose & reduce maintenance dose by 50%. Oral susp stable for 14 days at room temperature.

ANTIMICROBIALS: Antimalarials

NOTE: For help treating malaria or getting antimalarials, call the CDC "malaria hotline" (770) 488-7788 Monday-Friday 8 am to 4:30 pm EST. After hours / weekend (404) 639-2888. Information is also available at: http://www.cdc.gov.

chloroquine (*Aralen*) ▸KL ♀C but + ▸+ $

WARNING - Review product labeling for precautions and adverse effects before prescribing.

ADULT - Doses as chloroquine phosphate. Malaria prophylaxis, chloroquine-sensitive areas: 500 mg PO q wk from 1-2 weeks before exposure to 4 weeks after. Malaria: 1 g PO x 1, then 500 mg PO qd x 3 starting 6 h after 1st dose. Total dose is 2.5 g. Extraintestinal amebiasis: 1 g PO qd x 2, then 500 mg PO qd x 2-3 weeks.

PEDS - Doses as chloroquine phosphate. Malaria prophylaxis, chloroquine-sensitive areas: 8.3 mg/kg (up to 500 mg) PO q wk from 1-2 weeks before exposure to 4 weeks after. Malaria: 16.7 mg/kg PO x 1, then 8.3 mg/kg qd x 3 days starting 6 h after 1st dose. Do not exceed adult dose. Chloroquine phosphate 8.3 mg/kg = 5 mg/kg base.

FORMS - Generic: Tabs 250 mg. Generic/ Trade: Tabs 500 mg (500 mg phosphate equivalent to 300 mg base).

NOTES - Retinopathy with chronic/high doses; eye exams required. May cause seizures (caution advised if epilepsy); ototoxicity (caution advised if hearing loss); myopathy (discontinue if muscle weakness develops); bone marrow toxicity (monitor CBC if long-term use); exacerbation of psoriasis; torsades. Concentrates in liver; caution advised if hepatic disease, alcoholism, or hepatotoxic drugs. Antacids reduce absorption; give at least 4h apart. Chloroquine reduces ampicillin absorption; give at least 2h apart. May increase cyclosporine levels. As little as 1 g can cause fatal overdose in a child. Fatal malaria reported after chloroquine used as malaria prophylaxis in areas with chloroquine resistance; use only in areas without resistance. Maternal antimalarial prophylaxis doesn't harm breast-fed infant or protect infant from malaria.

doxycycline (*Adoxa, Vibramycin, Vibra-Tabs, Doryx, Monodox*, ✿*Doxycin*) ▸LK ♀D ▸? $

ADULT - Malaria prophylaxis: 100 mg PO qd starting 1-2 days before exposure until 4 weeks after. Usual dose for other indications: 100 mg PO bid on first day, then 100 mg/day PO divided qd or bid. Severe infections: 100 mg PO bid. Chlamydia, nongonococcal urethritis: 100 mg PO bid x 7 days. Acne vulgaris: Up to 100 mg PO bid. Cholera: 300 mg PO single dose. Syphilis if penicillin-allergic: 100 mg PO bid x 14 days if primary, secondary, early latent, x 4 weeks if late latent or tertiary. Not for neurosyphilis. Periostat for periodontitis: 20 mg PO bid 1 h before breakfast and dinner. IV: 200 mg on first day in 1-2 infusions, then 100-200 mg/day in 1-2 infusions. Bioterrorism anthrax: 100 mg IV x 60 days. Use IV with ≥1 other drug for initial treatment of inhalation or severe cutaneous anthrax. PO monotherapy for less severe cutaneous anthrax or post-exposure prophylaxis. See www.idsociety.org/BT/ToC.htm for more info.

PEDS - Avoid if <8 yo due to teeth staining. Malaria prophylaxis: 2 mg/kg/day up to 100 mg PO qd starting 1-2 days before exposure until 4 weeks after. Usual dose for other indications, children ≤45 kg: 4.4 mg/kg/day PO divided bid on first day, then 2.2-4.4 mg/kg/day PO divided qd or bid. Use adult dose for children >45 kg. Most PO and IV doses are equivalent. Bioterrorism anthrax: 100 mg bid for >8 yo and >45 kg, 2.2 mg/kg bid for >8 yo and ≤45 kg, or ≤8 yo. Treat x 60 days. Use IV with ≥1 other drug for initial treatment of inhalation anthrax, severe cutaneous anthrax, or any case of cutaneous anthrax if <2 yo. PO monotherapy for less-severe cutaneous anthrax in older children or post-exposure prophylaxis. For further info, see http://www.idsociety.org/BT/ToC.htm.

UNAPPROVED ADULT - Malaria treatment: 100 mg PO bid x 7 days with quinine. See table for pelvic inflammatory disease treatment. Lyme disease: 100 mg PO bid x 14-28 days. Prevention of Lyme disease in highly endemic area, with deer tick attachment ≥48h: 200 mg PO single dose with food within 72 h of tick bite. Ehrlichiosis: 100 mg IV/PO bid x 7-14 days.

UNAPPROVED PEDS - Avoid in children <8 yo due to teeth staining. Malaria treatment: 2 mg/kg/day x 7 days with quinine. Lyme disease: 1-2 mg/kg up to 100 mg PO bid x 14-28 days.

FORMS - Generic/Trade: Tabs 75,100 mg, caps 50,100 mg. Trade: Susp 25 mg/5 ml, syrup 50 mg/5 ml. Periostat: Caps 20 mg.

NOTES - Photosensitivity, pseudotumor cerebri, increased BUN, painful IV infusion. May decrease efficacy of oral contraceptives. Increased INR with warfarin. No antacids or calcium supplements within 2 h of doxycycline. Barbiturates, carbamazepine, rifampin, & phenytoin may decrease doxycycline levels. Preferred over tetracycline in renal dysfunction. Maternal antimalarial prophylaxis doesn't harm breast-fed infant or protect infant from malaria. Take with fluids to decrease esophageal irritation; can take with food/milk.

Fansidar (sulfadoxine + pyrimethamine) ▶KL ♀C ▶- $

WARNING - Can cause life-threatening Stevens-Johnson syndrome and toxic epidermal necrolysis. Stop treatment at first sign of rash, bacterial/fungal infection, or change in CBC.

ADULT - Treatment of chloroquine-resistant P falciparum malaria: 2-3 tabs PO single dose.

PEDS - CDC regimen - presumptive treatment: 5-10 kg: ½ tab, 11-20 kg: 1 tab, 21-30 kg: 1½ tab, 31-45 kg: 2 tabs, >45 kg: 3 tabs. Do not use in infants <2 mo; may cause kernicterus.

FORMS - Trade: Tabs sulfadoxine 500 mg + pyrimethamine 25 mg.

NOTES - Do not use in sulfonamide allergy; megaloblastic anemia due to folate deficiency; or for prolonged period in hepatic/renal failure or blood dyscrasia. Can cause hemolytic anemia in G6PD deficiency. Fansidar resistance is common in many malarious regions. Avoid excessive sun exposure.

Malarone (atovaquone + proguanil) ▶Fecal excretion; LK ♀C ▶? $$$$

ADULT - Malaria prophylaxis: 1 adult tab PO qd from 1-2 days before exposure until 7 days after. Malaria treatment: 4 adult tabs PO qd x 3 days. Take with food/milk at same time each day. Repeat dose if vomiting within 1 h. CDC recommends for presumptive self-treatment of malaria (same dose as for treatment, but not for patients taking it for prophylaxis).

PEDS - Safety & efficacy established in children ≥11 kg for prevention, ≥5 kg for treatment. Prevention of malaria: Give PO qd from 1-2 days before exposure until 7 days after: 1 ped tab for 11-20 kg; 2 ped tabs for 21-30 kg; 3 ped tabs for 31-40 kg; 1 adult tab for >40 kg. Treatment of malaria: Give PO qd x 3 days: 2 ped tabs for 5-8 kg; 3 ped tabs for 9-10 kg; 1 adult tab for 11-20 kg; 2 adult tabs for 21-30 kg; 3 adult tabs for 31-40 kg; 4 adult tabs for >40 kg. Take with food or milk at same time each day. Repeat dose if vomiting occurs within 1 h after dose.

FORMS - Trade: Adult tabs atovaquone 250 mg + proguanil 100 mg; pediatric tabs 62.5 mg + 25 mg.

NOTES - Vomiting common with malaria treatment doses. Monitor parasitemia and consider antiemetic in Malarone-treated patients who are vomiting. Plasma levels of atovaquone may be decreased by tetracycline, metoclopramide (use another anti-emetic if possible), and rifampin (avoid).

mefloquine (*Lariam*) ▶L ♀C ▶? $$

ADULT - Malaria prophylaxis, chloroquine-resistant areas: 250 mg PO q week from 1 week before exposure to 4 weeks after. Malaria treatment: 1250 mg PO single dose. Take on full stomach with at least 8 oz water.

PEDS - Malaria treatment: 20-25 mg/kg PO; can divide into 2 doses given 6-8 h apart to reduce risk of vomiting. Repeat full dose if vomiting <30 min after dose; Repeat ½ dose if vomiting <30-60 minutes after dose. Experience limited in infants <3 mo or <5 kg. Malaria prophylaxis: Give PO once weekly starting 1 week before exposure to 4 weeks after: 5-10 kg, 5 mg/kg (prepared by pharmacist); 10-20 kg, ¼ tab; 20-30 kg, ½ tab; 30-45 kg, ¾ tab. Take on full stomach.

UNAPPROVED PEDS - Malaria prophylaxis, chloroquine-resistant areas: CDC recommends these PO doses q week starting 1 week before exposure to 4 weeks after: ≤15 kg, 5 mg/kg, 15-19 kg, ¼ tab; 20-30 kg, ½ tab; 31-45 kg, ¾ tab; >45 kg, 1 tab. Malaria treatment, <45 kg: 15 mg/kg PO, then 10 mg/kg PO given 8-12 h after first dose. Take on full stomach with at least 8 oz water.

FORMS - Generic/trade: Tabs 250 mg.

NOTES - Cardiac conduction disturbances. Do not use with ziprasidone. Do not give until 12 h after the last dose of quinidine, quinine, or chloroquine; may cause ECG changes and seizures. Contraindicated for prophylaxis if depression (active/recent), generalized anxiety disorder, psychosis, schizophrenia, other major psychiatric disorder, or history of seizures. Tell patients to discontinue if psychiatric symptoms occur during prophylaxis. May cause drowsiness (warn about hazardous tasks). Can crush tabs and mix into in small amount of water, milk, or other liquid. Pharmacists can put small doses into caps to mask bitter taste. Decreases valproate levels. Rifampin decreases mefloquine levels. Maternal use of antimalarial prophylaxis doesn't harm or protect breastfed infant from malaria.

primaquine ▶L ♀- ▶- $

WARNING - Review product labeling for precautions and adverse effects before prescribing.

ADULT - Prevention of relapse after leaving malarious region or after P vivax/ ovale treatment: 30 mg base PO qd x 14 days.

PEDS - Not approved in children.

UNAPPROVED ADULT - Pneumocystis in patients intolerant to trimethoprim/sulfamethoxazole: 30 mg primaquine base (2 tabs) PO qd plus clindamycin 600-900 mg IV q8h or 300-450 mg PO q8h x 21 days. Can be used for primary prophylaxis of malaria in special cir-

cumstance; contact CDC at 770-488-7788.

UNAPPROVED PEDS - Prevention of relapse after leaving malarious region or after treatment for P vivax or P ovale: 0.6 mg/kg PO qd x 14 d. Can be used for primary prophylaxis of malaria in special circumstance; contact CDC at 770-488-7788 for info.

FORMS - Generic: Tabs 26.3 mg (equiv to 15 mg base).

NOTES - Causes hemolytic anemia in G6PD deficiency, methemoglobinemia in NADH methemoglobin reductase deficiency. Contraindicated in G6PD deficiency; screen for deficiency before prescribing. Stop if dark urine or anemia. Avoid in patients with rheumatoid arthritis or SLE, recent quinacrine use, or use of other bone marrow suppressants.

quinidine gluconate ▶LK ♀C ▶+ $$$$

ADULT - Life-threatening malaria: Load with 10 mg/kg (max 600 mg) IV over 1-2 h, then 0.02 mg/kg/min. Treat x 72 h, until parasitemia <1%, or PO meds tolerated. Dose given as quinidine gluconate.

PEDS - Safety and efficacy not established in children.

UNAPPROVED PEDS - Life-threatening malaria: Load with 10 mg/kg IV over 1-2h, then 0.02 mg/kg/min. Treat x 72 h, until parasitemia <1%, or PO meds tolerated. Dose given as quinidine gluconate.

NOTES - QRS widening, QT interval prolongation (risk increased by hypokalemia, hypomagnesemia, or bradycardia), hypotension, hypoglycemia. Contraindicated with ziprasidone. Monitor EKG and BP. Drug interactions with some anti-arrhythmics, digoxin, phenytoin, phenobarbital, rifampin, verapamil. For rapid shipment of quinidine gluconate, call Eli Lilly at (800) 821-0538.

quinine ▶L ♀X ▶+? $

ADULT - Malaria: 600-650 mg PO tid x 3-7 days. Also give doxycycline or Fansidar.

PEDS - Not approved in children.

UNAPPROVED PEDS - Malaria: 25-30 mg/kg/ day up to 2 g/day PO divided q8h x 3-7 days. Also give doxycycline or Fansidar.

FORMS - Generic: Tabs 260 mg, caps 200,325 mg.

NOTES - Thrombocytopenia, cinchonism, hemolytic anemia with G6PD deficiency, cardiac conduction disturbances, hearing impairment. Many drug interactions. Rule out G6PD deficiency in breastfed at-risk infant before giving quinine to mother.

ANTIMICROBIALS: Antimycobacterial Agents

NOTE - Two or more drugs are needed for the treatment of active mycobacterial infections. See guidelines at http://www.thoracic.org/statements/. Get baseline LFTs, creatinine, and platelet count before treating TB. Evaluate at least monthly for adverse drug reactions. Routine liver and renal function tests not needed unless baseline dysfunction or increased risk of hepatotoxicity.

clofazimine (*Lamprene*) ▶Fecal excretion ♀C ▶?- $

ADULT - Approved for leprosy therapy.

PEDS - Not approved in children.

UNAPPROVED ADULT - Mycobacterium avium complex in immunocompetent patients: 100-200 mg PO qd until "tan", then 50 mg PO qd or 100 mg PO three times weekly. Use in combination with other antimycobacterial agents. Not for general use in AIDS patients due to increased mortality.

FORMS - Trade: Caps 50 mg. After July 2004, will only be distributed through investigational new drug application by National Hansen's Disease Program (phone 225-578-9861).

NOTES - Abdominal pain common; rare reports of splenic infarction, bowel obstruction, and GI bleeding. Pink to brownish-black skin pigmentation that may persist for months to years after drug is discontinued. Discoloration of urine, body secretions.

dapsone ▶LK ♀C ▶+? $

ADULT - Leprosy: 100 mg PO qd with rifampin +/- clofazimine or ethionamide.

PEDS - Leprosy: 1 mg/kg/day (up to 100 mg) PO qd with other antimycobacterial agents.

UNAPPROVED ADULT - Pneumocystis prophylaxis: 100 mg PO qd. Pneumocystis treatment: 100 mg PO qd with trimethoprim 5 mg/kg PO tid x 21 days.

UNAPPROVED PEDS - Pneumocystis prophylaxis, age ≥1 mo: 2 mg/kg (up to 100 mg) PO qd or 4 mg/kg (up to 200 mg) PO q week.

FORMS - Generic: Tabs 25,100 mg.

NOTES - Blood dyscrasias, severe allergic skin reactions, sulfone syndrome, hemolysis in G6PD deficiency, hepatotoxicity, neuropathy, photosensitivity, leprosy reactional states. Monitor CBC q wk x 4, then monthly x 6, then twice yearly. Monitor LFTs.

ethambutol (*Myambutol*, ✿*Etibi*) ▶LK ♀C but + ▶+ $$$$$

ADULT - TB: ATS and CDC recommend 15-20 mg/kg PO qd. Dose with whole tabs: 800 mg PO qd if 40-55 kg, 1200 mg PO qd if 56-75 kg, 1600 mg PO qd if 76-90 kg. Base dose on estimated lean body weight. Max dose regardless of weight is 1600 mg/day.

PEDS - TB: ATS and CDC recommend 15-20 mg/kg up to 1 g PO qd. Use cautiously if visual acuity cannot be monitored. Manufacturer recommends against use in children <13 yo.

UNAPPROVED ADULT - Treatment or prevention of recurrent Mycobacterium avium complex disease in HIV infection: 15-25 mg/kg up to 1600 mg PO qd with clarithromycin/azithromycin +/- rifabutin.

UNAPPROVED PEDS - Treatment or prevention of recurrent Mycobacterium avium complex disease in HIV infection: 15 mg/kg up to 900 mg PO qd with clarithromycin/azithromycin +/- rifabutin.

FORMS - Generic/Trade: Tabs 100,400 mg.

NOTES - Can cause retrobulbar neuritis. Avoid, if possible, in patients with optic neuritis. Test visual acuity and color discrimination at baseline. Ask about visual disturbances monthly. Monitor visual acuity and color discrimination monthly if dose >15-20 mg/kg, duration >2 months, or renal dysfunction. Advise patients to report any change in vision immediately; do not use in those who cannot report visual sx (eg, children, unconscious). Do not give aluminum hydroxide antacid until >4h after ethambutol dose. Reduce dose in renal impairment.

isoniazid (*INH*, ✿*Isotamine*) ▶LK ♀C but + ▶+ $

WARNING - Hepatotoxicity. Obtain baseline LFTs. Monitor LFTs monthly in high-risk patients (HIV, signs/hx of liver disease, abnormal LFTs at baseline, pregnancy/postpartum, alcoholism/regular alcohol use, some patients >35 yo). Tell all patients to stop isoniazid and call at once if hepatotoxicity sx. Discontinue if AST >3 x upper limit of normal with hepatotoxicity sx or AST >5 x upper limit of normal without hepatotoxicity sx.

ADULT - TB treatment: 5 mg/kg up to 300 mg PO qd or 15 mg/kg up to 900 mg twice weekly. Latent TB: 300 mg PO qd.

PEDS - TB treatment: 10-15 mg/kg up to 300 mg PO qd. Latent TB: 10 mg/kg up to 300 mg PO qd.

UNAPPROVED ADULT - American Thoracic Society regimen, latent tuberculosis: 5 mg/kg up to 300 mg PO qd x 9 months (6 months OK if HIV-negative, but less effective than 9 months).

UNAPPROVED PEDS - American Thoracic Society regimen for latent tuberculosis: 10-20 mg/kg up to 300 mg PO qd for 9 months.

FORMS - Generic: Tabs 100,300 mg, syrup 50 mg/5 ml.

NOTES - To reduce risk of peripheral neuropathy, give pyridoxine 25 mg PO qd if alcoholism, diabetes, HIV, uremia, malnutrition, seizure disorder, pregnant/ breastfeeding woman, breast-fed infant of INH-treated mother. Many drug interactions.

pyrazinamide (PZA, ♥Tebrazid) ▶LK ♀C ▶? $$$

WARNING - The ATS and CDC recommend against general use of 2 mo regimen of rifampin + pyrazinamide for latent TB due to reports of fatal hepatotoxicity.

ADULT - TB: ATS and CDC recommend 20-25 mg/kg up to 2000 mg PO qd. Dose with whole tabs: 1000 mg PO qd if 40-55 kg, 1500 mg PO qd if 56-75 kg, 2000 mg if 76-90 kg. Base dose on estimated lean body weight. Max dose regardless of weight is 2000 mg PO qd.

PEDS - TB: 15-30 mg/kg up to 2000 mg PO qd.

FORMS - Generic: Tabs 500 mg.

NOTES - Hepatotoxicity, hyperuricemia (avoid in acute gout). Obtain LFTs at baseline. Monitor periodically in high-risk patients (HIV infection, alcoholism, pregnancy, signs/history of liver disease, abnormal LFTs at baseline). Discontinue if AST >3 x upper limit of normal with hepatotoxicity sx or AST >5 x upper limit of normal without hepatotoxicity sx. A 2-month regimen of pyrazinamide + rifampin was recommended in the past to treat latent TB. Due to reports of fatal hepatotoxicity, the ATS and CDC now recommend against general use of this regimen. Consider reduced dose in renal dysfunction.

rifabutin (Mycobutin) ▶L ♀B ▶? $$$$$

ADULT - Prevention of disseminated Mycobacterium avium complex disease in AIDS: 300 mg PO qd or 150 mg PO bid. See http://www.cdc.gov/nchstp/tb/TB_HIV_Drugs/TOC.htm for dosage adjustments of rifabutin with antiretroviral regimens.

PEDS - Not approved in children.

UNAPPROVED ADULT - TB or Mycobacterium avium complex disease treatment in AIDS: 300 mg PO qd. See http://www.cdc.gov/nchstp/tb/TB_HIV_Drugs/TOC.htm for dosage adjustments of rifabutin with antiretroviral regimens.

UNAPPROVED PEDS - Mycobacterium avium complex disease prophylaxis: ≥6 yo, 300 mg

PO qd. <6 yo, 5 mg/kg (up to 300 mg) PO qd.

FORMS - Trade: Caps 150 mg.

NOTES - Uveitis (with high doses or if metabolism inhibited by other drugs), hepatotoxicity, thrombocytopenia, neutropenia. Obtain CBC and LFTs at baseline. Monitor periodically in high-risk patients (HIV infection, alcoholism, pregnancy, signs/ history of liver disease, abnormal LFTs at baseline). Do not use alone in patients with active TB. May induce liver metabolism of other drugs including oral contraceptives, protease inhibitors, and azole antifungals. Substrate of CYP 3A4; fluconazole, clarithromycin, and protease inhibitors increase rifabutin levels (see http://www.cdc.gov/nchstp/tb/TB_HIV_Drugs/TOC.htm or www.aidsinfo.nih.gov for dosage adjustments) . Urine, body secretion, soft contact lenses may turn orange-brown. Dosage reduction may be required for hepatic dysfunction.

Rifamate (isoniazid + rifampin) ▶LK ♀C but + ▶+ $$$$

WARNING - Hepatotoxicity.

ADULT - Tuberculosis: 2 caps PO qd on empty stomach.

PEDS - Not approved in children.

FORMS - Trade: Caps isoniazid 150 mg + rifampin 300 mg.

NOTES - See components. Monitor LFTs at baseline and periodically during therapy.

rifampin (Rimactane, Rifadin, ♥Rofact) ▶L ♀C but + ▶+ $$$

WARNING - The ATS and CDC recommend against general use of 2 mo regimen of rifampin + pyrazinamide for latent TB due to reports of fatal hepatotoxicity.

ADULT - Tuberculosis: 10 mg/kg up to 600 mg PO/IV qd. Neisseria meningitidis carriers: 600 mg PO bid x 2 days. Take on empty stomach. IV and PO doses are the same.

PEDS - TB: 10-20 mg/kg up to 600 mg PO/IV qd. Neisseria meningitidis carriers: ≥1 mo, 10 mg/kg up to 600 mg PO bid x 2 days. <1 mo, 5 mg/kg PO bid x 2 days. Take on empty stomach. IV and PO doses are the same.

UNAPPROVED ADULT - Prophylaxis of H influenza type b infection: 20 mg/kg up to 600 mg PO qd x 4 days. Leprosy: 600 mg PO q month with dapsone. American Thoracic Society regimen for latent TB: 10 mg/kg up to 600 mg PO qd x 4 months. Staphylococcal prosthetic valve endocarditis: 300 mg PO q8 hr in combination with gentamicin plus nafcillin, oxacillin, or vancomycin. Take on empty stomach.

UNAPPROVED PEDS - Prophylaxis of H influenza type b infection: ≥1 mo, 20 mg/kg up to 600 mg PO qd x 4 days. <1 mo, 10 mg/kg PO qd x 4 days. Prophylaxis of invasive meningococcal disease: ≥1 mo, 10 mg/kg up to 600 mg PO bid x 2 days. <1 mo, 5 mg/kg PO bid x 2 days. American Thoracic Society regimen for latent tuberculosis: 10-20 mg/kg up to 600 mg PO qd x 4 months. Take on empty stomach.

FORMS - Generic/Trade: Caps 150,300 mg. Pharmacists can make oral suspension.

NOTES - Hepatotoxicity, thrombocytopenia. When treating TB, obtain baseline CBC, LFTs. Monitor periodically in high-risk patients (HIV infection, alcoholism, pregnancy, signs/history of liver disease, abnormal LFTs at baseline). Discontinue if AST >3 x upper limit of normal with hepatotoxicity sx or AST >5 x upper limit of normal without hepatotoxicity sx. A 2-month regimen of pyrazinamide + rifampin was recommended in the past to treat latent TB. Due to reports of fatal hepatotoxicity, the ATS and CDC recommend against general use of this regimen to treat latent TB. Induces hepatic metabolism of many drugs; check other sources for dosage adjustments before prescribing. See http://www.cdc.gov/nchstp/tb/TB_HIV_Drugs/TOC.htm for dosage adjustments of antiretroviral regimens with rifampin. Decreased efficacy of oral contraceptives; use non-hormonal method. Decreased INR with warfarin; monitor daily or as needed. Adjust dose for hepatic impairment. Colors urine, body secretions, soft contact lenses red-orange. IV rifampin is stable for 4h after dilution in dextrose 5%.

rifapentine (Priftin) ▶Esterases, fecal ♀C ▶? $$$

ADULT - TB: 600 mg PO twice weekly x 2 months, then once weekly x 4 months. ATS and CDC recommend use only for continuation therapy in selected HIV-negative patients.

PEDS - Not approved in children <12 yo.

FORMS - Trade: Tabs 150 mg.

NOTES - Hepatotoxicity, thrombocytopenia, exacerbation of porphyria. Obtain CBC and LFTs at baseline. Monitor LFTs periodically in high-risk patients (HIV infection, alcoholism, pregnancy, signs/ history of liver disease, abnormal LFTs at baseline). Do not use in porphyria. Urine, body secretions, contact lenses, and dentures may turn red-orange. May induce liver metabolism of other drugs including oral contraceptives. Avoid with protease inhibitors or NNRTIs.

Rifater (isoniazid + rifampin + pyrazinamide) ▶LK ♀C ▶? $$$$$

WARNING - Hepatotoxicity.

ADULT - TB, initial 2 mo of treatment: 6 tabs PO qd if ≥55 kg, 5 tabs qd if 45-54 kg, 4 tabs qd if ≤44 kg. Additional pyrazinamide tablets required to provide adequate dose in patient >90 kg. Take on empty stomach. Can finish treatment with Rifamate.

PEDS - Ratio of formulation may not be appropriate for children <15 yo.

FORMS - Trade: Tab Isoniazid 50 mg + rifampin 120 mg + pyrazinamide 300 mg.

NOTES - See components. Monitor LFTs at baseline and during therapy. Do not use in patients with renal dysfunction.

ANTIMICROBIALS: Antiparasitics

albendazole (Albenza) ▶L ♀C ▶? $$$

ADULT - Hydatid disease, neurocysticercosis: ≥60 kg - 400 mg PO bid. <60 kg - 15 mg/kg/day (up to 800 mg/day) PO divided bid. Treatment duration varies. Take with food.

PEDS - Hydatid disease, neurocysticercosis: ≥60 kg - 400 mg PO bid. <60 kg: 15 mg/kg/day (up to 800 mg/day) PO divided bid. Treatment duration varies. Take with food.

UNAPPROVED ADULT - Hookworm, whipworm, pinworm, roundworm: 400 mg PO single dose. Repeat in 2 weeks for pinworm. Cutaneous larva migrans: 200 mg PO bid x 3 days. Giardia: 400 mg PO qd x 5 days.

UNAPPROVED PEDS - Roundworm, hookworm, pinworm, whipworm: 400 mg PO single dose. Repeat in 2 weeks for pinworm. Cutane-

ous larva migrans: 200 mg PO bid x 3 days. Giardia: 400 mg PO qd x 5 days.

FORMS - Trade: Tabs 200 mg.

NOTES - Monitor LFTs, WBC. Consider corticosteroids & anticonvulsants in neurocysticercosis. Get negative pregnancy test before treatment & warn against getting pregnant until a month after treatment. Treat close contacts for pinworms.

atovaquone (Mepron) ▶Fecal ♀C ▶? $$$$$

ADULT - Pneumocystis in patients intolerant to trimethoprim/sulfamethoxazole: Treatment 750 mg PO bid x 21 days. Prevention 1500 mg PO qd. Take with meals.

PEDS - Pneumocystis in patients intolerant to trimethoprim/sulfamethoxazole, 13-16 yo: Treatment, 750 mg PO bid x 21 days. Prevention, 1500 mg PO qd. Take with meals. Efficacy & safety not established for <13 yo.

UNAPPROVED PEDS - Prevention of recurrent Pneumocystis in HIV infection: 1-3 mo, 30 mg/kg PO qd. 4-24 mo, 45 mg/kg PO qd. >24 mo, 30 mg/kg PO qd. Take with meals.

FORMS - Trade: Susp 750 mg/5 ml, foil pouch 750 mg/5 ml.

NOTES - Efficacy of atovaquone may be decreased by lopinavir/ ritonavir (Kaletra), rifampin (consider using alternative), rifabutin, rifapentine, and ritonavir.

iodoquinol (*Yodoxin, diiodohydroxyquin,* ♥ *Diodoquin*) ▸Not absorbed ♀? ▸? $$

ADULT - Intestinal amebiasis: 650 mg PO tid after meals x 20 days.

PEDS - Intestinal amebiasis: 40 mg/kg/day PO divided tid x 20 days. Do not exceed adult dose.

FORMS - Generic/Trade: Tabs 650 mg. Trade: Tabs 210 mg.

NOTES - Optic neuritis/atrophy, peripheral neuropathy with prolonged high doses. Interference with some thyroid function tests for up to 6 months after treatment.

ivermectin (*Stromectol*) ▸L ♀C ▸+ $

ADULT - Strongyloidiasis: 200 mcg/kg PO single dose. Onchocerciasis: 150 mcg/kg PO q3-12 months. Take on empty stomach with water.

PEDS - For children ≥15 kg. Strongyloidiasis: 200 mcg/kg PO single dose. Onchocerciasis: 150 mcg/kg PO single dose q 3-12 months. Take on empty stomach with water.

UNAPPROVED ADULT - Scabies: 200 mcg/kg PO single dose. Cutaneous larva migrans: 150-200 mcg/kg PO single dose. Take on empty stomach with water.

UNAPPROVED PEDS - Scabies: 200 mcg/kg PO single dose. Cutaneous larva migrans: 150-200 mcg/kg PO single dose. Take on empty stomach with water. Safety and efficacy not established in children <15 kg.

FORMS - Trade: Tab 3, 6 mg.

NOTES - Mazzotti & ophthalmic reactions with treatment for onchocerciasis. May need repeat/monthly treatment for strongyloidiasis in immunocompromised/HIV-infected patients.

mebendazole (*Vermox*) ▸L ♀C ▸? $

ADULT - Pinworm: 100 mg PO x 1; repeat in 2 weeks. Roundworm, whipworm, hookworm: 100 mg PO bid x 3 days.

PEDS - Pinworm: 100 mg PO x 1; repeat dose in 2 weeks. Roundworm, whipworm, hookworm: 100 mg PO bid x 3 days.

UNAPPROVED ADULT - Roundworm, whip-

worm, hookworm: 500 mg PO single dose.

UNAPPROVED PEDS - Roundworm, whipworm, hookworm: 500 mg PO single dose.

FORMS - Trade/Generic: Chew tab 100 mg.

NOTES - Treat close contacts for pinworms.

metronidazole (*Flagyl,* ♥ *Trikacide, Florazole ER*) ▸KL ♀B ▸?- $

ADULT - Acute amebic dysentery: 750 mg PO tid x 5-10 days. Amebic liver abscess: 500-750 mg PO tid x 5-10 days. Trichomoniasis: Treat patient & sex partners with 2g PO single dose, 250 mg PO tid x 7 days, or 375 mg PO bid x 7 days. Flagyl ER for bacterial vaginosis: 750 mg PO qd x 7 days on empty stomach. H pylori: See table in GI section. Anaerobic bacterial infections: Load 1 g or 15 mg/kg IV, then 500 mg or 7.5 mg/kg IV/PO q6h, each IV dose over 1h (not to exceed 4 g/day). Prophylaxis, colorectal surgery: 15 mg/kg IV completed 1 h preop, then 7.5 mg/kg IV q6h x 2 doses.

PEDS - Amebiasis: 35-50 mg/kg/day PO (max of 750 mg/dose) divided tid x 10 days.

UNAPPROVED ADULT - Giardia: 250 mg PO tid x 5-7 days. Bacterial vaginosis: 500 mg PO bid x 7 days. Bacterial vaginosis in pregnancy: 250 mg PO tid x 7 days. Trichomoniasis (CDC alternative to single dose): 500 mg PO bid x 7 days. Pelvic inflammatory disease: see STD table. Clostridium difficile diarrhea: 250 mg PO qid or 500 mg PO tid x 10 days.

UNAPPROVED PEDS - Giardia: 15 mg/kg/day PO divided tid x 5-7 days. Clostridium difficile diarrhea: 30-50 mg/kg/day PO (not to exceed adult dose) divided tid or qid x 7-10 days. Trichomoniasis: 5 mg/kg PO tid (max 2 g/day) x 7 days. Anaerobic bacterial infections: 30 mg/kg/day IV/PO divided q6h, each IV dose over 1 h (not to exceed 4 g/day).

FORMS - Generic/Trade: Tabs 250,500 mg, ER tabs 750 mg, Caps 375 mg.

NOTES - Peripheral neuropathy (chronic use), seizures. Disulfiram reaction; avoid alcohol until ≥1 day after treatment with tabs, ≥3 days with caps/ Flagyl ER. Do not give within 2 weeks of disulfiram. Interacts with barbiturates, lithium, phenytoin. Increased INR with warfarin. Darkens urine. Give iodoquinol/ paromomycin after treatment for amebic dysentery or liver abscess. Can minimize infant exposure by withholding breastfeeding for 12-24 h after maternal single dose. Decrease dose in liver dysfunction.

nitazoxanide (*Alinia*) ▸L ♀B ▸? $$$

ADULT - Giardiasis: 500 mg PO q12h with food x 3 days.

PEDS - Give PO bid with food x 3 days. Use suspension for <12 yo. Giardiasis dose: 100 mg for 1-3 yo, 200 mg for 4-11 yo, 500 mg for ≥12 yo. Cryptosporidial diarrhea dose: 100 mg for 1-3 yo, 200 mg for 4-11 yo.

FORMS - Trade: Oral susp 100 mg/5 ml 60 ml bottle, tab 500 mg.

NOTES - Contains 1.5 g sucrose/5 ml. Turns urine bright yellow. Store at room temperature for up to 7 days. Can obtain tabs for HIV-positive patients from compassionate access program (813-282-8544 or compassionateaccess@romarklabs.com).

paromomycin (*Humatin*) ▶Not absorbed ♀C ▶- $$$$

ADULT - Intestinal amebiasis: 25-35 mg/kg/day PO divided tid with/after meals x 5-10 days.

PEDS - Intestinal amebiasis: 25-35 mg/kg/day PO divided tid with/after meals x 5-10 days.

UNAPPROVED ADULT - Giardiasis: 500 mg PO tid x 7 days.

UNAPPROVED PEDS - Giardiasis: 25-35 mg/kg /day PO divided tid with/after meals x 7 days.

FORMS - Generic/Trade: Caps 250 mg.

NOTES - Nephrotoxicity possible with systemic absorption in inflammatory bowel disease. Not effective for extra-intestinal amebiasis.

pentamidine (*Pentam, NebuPent, ♣Pentacarinat*) ▶K ♀C ▶- $$$$$

ADULT - Pneumocystis treatment: 4 mg/kg IM/IV qd x 14-21 days. NebuPent for Pneumocystis prevention: 300 mg nebulized q 4 weeks.

PEDS - Pneumocystis treatment: 4 mg/kg IM/IV qd x 14 days. NebuPent not approved in children.

UNAPPROVED PEDS - Pneumocystis prevention: NebuPent, ≥5 yo: 300 mg nebulized q 4 weeks.

FORMS - Trade: Aerosol 300 mg.

NOTES - Contraindicated with ziprasidone. Fatalities due to severe hypotension, hypoglycemia, cardiac arrhythmias with IM/IV. Have patient lie down, check BP, and keep resuscitation equipment handy during IM/IV injection. May cause torsades, hyperglycemia, neutropenia, nephrotoxicity, pancreatitis, and hypocalcemia. Monitor BUN, serum creatinine, blood glucose, CBC, LFTs, serum calcium, and ECG. Bronchospasm with inhalation (consider bronchodilator). Reduce IM/IV dose in renal dysfunction.

praziquantel (*Biltricide*) ▶LK ♀B ▶- $$$

ADULT - Schistosomiasis: 20 mg/kg PO q4-6h x 3 doses. Liver flukes: 25 mg/kg PO q4-6h x 3 doses.

PEDS - Schistosomiasis: 20 mg/kg PO q4-6h x 3 doses. Liver flukes: 25 mg/kg PO q4-6h x 3 doses.

UNAPPROVED ADULT - Neurocysticercosis: 50 mg/kg/day PO divided tid x 15 days. Fish, dog, beef, pork intestinal tapeworms: 10 mg/kg PO single dose.

UNAPPROVED PEDS - Neurocysticercosis: 50-100 mg/kg/day PO divided tid x 15 days. Fish, dog, beef, pork intestinal tapeworms: 10 mg/kg PO single dose.

FORMS - Trade: Tabs 600 mg.

NOTES - Contraindicated in ocular cysticercosis. May cause drowsiness; do not drive or operate machinery for 48 h. Phenytoin, carbamazepine, rifampin (avoid using together), and dexamethasone may lower praziquantel levels enough to cause treatment failure. Take with liquids during a meal. Do not chew tabs. Manufacturer advises against breast feeding until 72 h after treatment.

pyrantel (*Antiminth, Pin-X, Pinworm, ♣Combantrin*) ▶Not absorbed ♀- ▶? $

ADULT - Pinworm, roundworm: 11 mg/kg up to 1 g PO single dose. Repeat in 2 weeks for pinworm.

PEDS - Pinworm, roundworm: 11 mg/kg up to 1 g PO single dose. Repeat in 2 weeks for pinworm.

UNAPPROVED ADULT - Hookworm: 11 mg/kg up to 1 g PO qd x 3 days.

UNAPPROVED PEDS - Hookworm: 11 mg/kg up to 1 g PO qd x 3 days.

FORMS - OTC: Caps 62.5 mg, liquid 50 mg/ml.

NOTES - Purging not necessary. Treat close contacts for pinworms.

pyrimethamine (*Daraprim*) ▶L ♀C ▶+ $$

ADULT - Toxoplasmosis, immunocompetent patients: 50-75 mg PO qd x 1-3 weeks, then reduce dose by 50% for 4-5 more weeks. Give with leucovorin (10-15 mg qd) and sulfadiazine. Reduce initial dose in seizure disorders.

PEDS - Toxoplasmosis: 1 mg/kg/day PO divided bid x 2-4 days, then reduce by 50% x 1 month. Give with sulfadiazine & leucovorin. Reduce initial dose in seizure disorders.

UNAPPROVED ADULT - CNS toxoplasmosis in AIDS: 200 mg PO x 1, then 75-100 mg qd. Secondary prevention after CNS toxoplasmosis in AIDS: 25-50 mg PO qd. Give with leucovorin (10-15 mg qd) and sulfadiazine or clindamycin. Reduce initial dose in seizure disorders.

UNAPPROVED PEDS - AAP regimen for toxoplasmosis: 2 mg/kg/day PO x 3 days, then

1 mg/kg/day (max 25 mg/day) PO (duration of treatment varies). Give with leucovorin (10-25 mg PO with each dose of pyrimethamine) & sulfadiazine. Secondary prevention after CNS toxoplasmosis in HIV infection: 1 mg/kg or 15 mg/m² (max 25 mg/day) PO qd with leucovorin 5 mg PO every 3 days and sulfadiazine. Reduce initial dose in seizure disorders.

FORMS - Trade: Tabs 25 mg.

NOTES - Hemolytic anemia in G6PD deficiency, dose-related folate deficiency, hypersensitivity. Monitor CBC.

thiabendazole (Mintezol) ▶LK ♀C ▶? $

ADULT - Helminths: 22 mg/kg/dose up to 1500 mg PO bid. Treat x 2 days for strongyloidiasis, cutaneous larva migrans. Take after meals.

PEDS - Helminths: 22 mg/kg/dose up to 1500 mg PO bid. Treat x 2 days for strongyloidiasis, cutaneous larva migrans. Limited use in children <13.5 kg. Take after meals.

FORMS - Trade: Chew tab 500 mg, susp 500 mg/5 ml.

NOTES - May cause drowsiness.

tinidazole (Tindamax) ▶KL ♀- ▶?- $?

ADULT - Trichomoniasis or giardiasis: 2 g PO single dose. Amebiasis: 2 g PO qd x 3 days. Take with food.

PEDS - Giardiasis: 50 mg/kg (up to 2 g) PO single dose. Amebiasis: >3 yo: 50 mg/kg (up to 2 g) PO qd x 3 days. Take with food.

FORMS - Trade: Tabs 250,500 mg. Pharma-

cists can compound oral suspension.

NOTES - Give iodoquinol/ paromomycin after treatment for amebic dysentery or liver abscess. Disulfiram reaction; avoid alcohol until ≥3 days after treatment. Can minimize infant exposure by withholding breastfeeding for 12-24 h after maternal single dose. May increase levels of cyclosporine, fluorouracil, lithium, phenytoin, tacrolimus. May increase INR with warfarin. Do not give at same time as cholestyramine. For patients undergoing hemodialysis: Give supplemental ½ dose after dialysis session.

trimetrexate (Neutrexin) ▶LK ♀D ▶- $$$$$

WARNING - Must give leucovorin during therapy & until 72h after last dose of trimetrexate to prevent toxicity.

ADULT - Pneumocystis pneumonia treatment in immunocompromised/ AIDS patients intolerant/unresponsive to trimethoprim/ sulfamethoxazole: 45 mg/m² IV infused over 1h qd x 21 days with leucovorin 20 mg/m² IV/PO q6h x 24 days. Round PO leucovorin dose up to next higher 25 mg increment.

PEDS - Safety and efficacy not established in children. Adult dose has been used in compassionate use.

NOTES - Hematologic, renal, hepatic, mucosal toxicity. Monitor ANC, platelets, renal & hepatic function at least twice weekly. See package insert for dosage adjustments for toxicity.

ANTIMICROBIALS: Antiviral Agents – Anti-CMV

cidofovir (Vistide) ▶K ♀C ▶- $$$$$

WARNING - Nephrotoxicity. Granulocytopenia - monitor neutrophil counts.

ADULT - CMV retinitis: 5 mg/kg IV q wk x 2 wks, then 5 mg/kg every other week. Give probenecid 2 g PO 3h before and 1 g 2h and 8h after infusion. Give normal saline with each infusion.

PEDS - Not approved in children.

NOTES - Fanconi-like syndrome. Stop nephrotoxic drugs ≥1 week before cidofovir. Get serum creatinine, urine protein before each dose. See package insert for dosage adjustments based on renal function. Do not use if creatinine >1.5 mg/dl, CrCl ≤55 ml/min, or urine protein ≥100 mg/dl (≥2+). Hold/ decrease zidovudine by 50% on days cidofovir is given. Tell women not to get pregnant until 1 month after and men to use barrier contraceptive until 3 months after cidofovir. Ocular hypotony - monitor intraocular pressure.

foscarnet (Foscavir) ▶K ♀C ▶? $$$$$

WARNING - Nephrotoxicity; seizures due to mineral/electrolyte imbalance.

ADULT - Hydrate before infusion. CMV retinitis: 60 mg/kg IV (over 1 h) q8h or 90 mg/kg IV (over 1.5-2 h) q12h x 2-3 weeks, then 90-120 mg/kg IV qd over 2h. Acyclovir-resistant HSV infection: 40 mg/kg IV (over 1 h) q8-12h x 2-3 weeks or until healed.

PEDS - Not approved in children. Deposits into teeth & bone of young animals.

UNAPPROVED PEDS - Hydrate before infusion. CMV retinitis: 60 mg/kg IV (over 1 h) q8h or 90 mg/kg IV (over 1.5-2 h) q12h x 2-3 weeks, then 90-120 mg/kg IV qd over 2h. Acyclovir-resistant HSV infection: 40 mg/kg IV (over 1 h) q8h x 2-3 weeks or until healed.

NOTES - Granulocytopenia, anemia, vein irritation, penile ulcers. Decreased ionized serum calcium, especially with IV pentamidine. Must use IV pump to avoid rapid administration. Monitor renal function, serum calcium, magnesium, phosphate, potassium. Reduce dose in renal impairment. Stop foscarnet if CrCl decreases to <0.4 ml/min/kg.

ganciclovir (DHPG, Cytovene) ▶K ♀C ▶- $$$$$
WARNING - Neutropenia, anemia, thrombocytopenia. Do not use if ANC <500/mm3 or platelets <25,000/mm3.
ADULT - CMV retinitis. Induction: 5 mg/kg IV q12h x 14-21 days. Maintenance: 6 mg/kg IV qd x 5 days/week; 5 mg/kg IV qd; 1000 mg PO tid; or 500 mg PO 6 times/day (q3h while awake) with food. Prevention of CMV disease in advanced AIDS: 1000 mg PO tid with food. Prevention of CMV disease after organ transplant: 5 mg/kg IV q12h x 7-14 days, then 6 mg/kg IV qd x 5 days/week or 1000 mg PO tid with food. Give IV infusion over 1 h.
PEDS - Safety and efficacy not established in children; potential carcinogenic or reproductive adverse effects.
UNAPPROVED PEDS - CMV retinitis in immunocompromised patient: Induction 5 mg/kg IV q12h x 14-21 days. Maintenance 5 mg/kg IV qd or 6 mg/kg IV qd x 5 days/week.
FORMS - Trade: Caps 250, 500 mg.
NOTES - Neutropenia (worsened by zidovudine), phlebitis/pain at infusion site, increased seizure risk with imipenem. Monitor CBC, creatinine. Reduce dose if CrCl <70 ml/min. Adequate hydration required. Potential teratogen. Tell women not to get pregnant during & men to use barrier contraceptive until ≥3 months after treatment. Potential carcinogen.

Follow guidelines for handling/ disposal of cytotoxic agents.

valganciclovir (Valcyte) ▶K ♀C ▶- $$$$$
WARNING - Myelosuppression may occur at any time. Monitor CBC frequently. Do not use if ANC <500/mm3, platelets <25,000/mm3, hemoglobin <8 g/dL.
ADULT - CMV retinitis: 900 mg PO bid x 21 days, then 900 mg PO qd. Prevention of CMV disease in high-risk kidney, kidney-pancreas, and heart transplant patients: 900 mg PO qd from within 10 days after transplant until 100 days post-transplant. Give with food. Valganciclovir tabs and ganciclovir caps not interchangeable on mg per mg basis.
PEDS - Safety and efficacy not established in children; potential carcinogenic or reproductive adverse effects.
FORMS - Trade: Tabs 450 mg.
NOTES - Contraindicated in ganciclovir allergy. Not for liver transplant patients due to higher risk of tissue-invasive CMV disease than with ganciclovir. Potential teratogen. Tell women not to get pregnant during and men to use barrier contraceptive until ≥3 months after treatment. CNS toxicity; warn against hazardous tasks. May increase creatinine; monitor renal function. Reduce dose if CrCl <60 ml/min. Use ganciclovir instead in hemodialysis patients. Potential drug interactions with didanosine, mycophenolate. Potential carcinogen. Avoid direct contact with broken/crushed tabs; do not intentionally break/crush tabs. Follow guidelines for handling/ disposal of cytotoxic agents.

ANTIMICROBIALS: Antiviral Agents – Anti-Herpetic

acyclovir (Zovirax, ♥Avirax) ▶K ♀B ▶+ $
ADULT - Genital herpes: 200 mg PO q4h (5x/day) x 10 days for first episode, x 5 days for recurrent episodes. Chronic suppression: 400 mg PO bid. Zoster: 800 mg PO q4h (5x/day) x 7-10 days. Chickenpox: 800 mg PO qid x 5 days. IV: 5-10 mg/kg IV q8h, each dose over 1 h. Zoster in immunocompromised patients: 10 mg/kg IV q8h x 7 days. Herpes simplex encephalitis: 10 mg/kg IV q8h x 10 days. Mucosal/cutaneous herpes simplex in immunocompromised patients: 5 mg/kg IV q8h x 7 days. Treat ASAP after symptom onset.
PEDS - Safety and efficacy of PO acyclovir not established in children <2 yo. Chickenpox: 20 mg/kg PO qid x 5 days. Use adult dose if >40 kg. AAP does not recommend routine treatment of chickenpox with acyclovir. Consider

use if >12 yo, chronic cutaneous or pulmonary disease, or corticosteroid or chronic salicylate use. IV: 250-500 mg/m2 q8h, each dose over 1h. Zoster in immunocompromised patients <12 yo: 20 mg/kg IV q8h x 7 days. Herpes simplex encephalitis: 20 mg/kg IV q8h x 10 days for 3 mo-12 yo, adult dose for ≥12 yo. Neonatal herpes simplex (birth to 3 mo): 10 mg/kg IV q8 h x 10 days. Mucosal/cutaneous herpes simplex in immunocompromised patients: 10 mg/kg IV q8h x 7 days for <12 yo, adult dose for ≥12 yo. Treat ASAP after symptom onset.
UNAPPROVED ADULT - Genital herpes: 400 mg PO tid x 7-10 days for first episode, x 5 days for recurrent episodes, x 5-10 days for current episodes in HIV+ patients. Chronic suppression of genital herpes in HIV+ patients:

400-800 mg PO bid-tid. Orolabial herpes (controversial indication): 400 mg PO 5x/day. Bell's palsy: 400 mg PO 5x/day x 10 days. Treat ASAP after symptom onset.
UNAPPROVED PEDS - Primary herpes gingivostomatitis: 15 mg/kg PO 5x/day x 7 days. First-episode genital herpes: 80 mg/kg/day PO divided tid (max 1.2 g/day) x 7-10 days. Use dose in unapproved adult for adolescents. Treat ASAP after symptom onset.
FORMS - Generic/Trade: Caps 200 mg, tabs 400,800 mg. Trade: Susp 200 mg/5 ml.
NOTES - Need adequate hydration with IV administration. Severe drowsiness with acyclovir plus zidovudine. Reduce dose in renal dysfunction and in elderly. Base IV dose on ideal body weight in obese adults.

famciclovir (*Famvir*) ▶K ♀B ▶? $$$
ADULT - Recurrent genital herpes: 125 mg PO bid x 5 days. Chronic suppression of genital herpes: 250 mg PO bid. Recurrent orolabial/genital herpes in HIV patients: 500 mg PO bid x 7 days. Zoster: 500 mg PO tid x 7 days. Treat ASAP after symptom onset.
PEDS - Not approved in children.
UNAPPROVED ADULT - First-episode genital herpes: 250 mg PO tid x 7-10 days. Chronic suppression of genital herpes in HIV+ patients: 500 mg PO bid. Chickenpox in young adults: 500 mg PO bid x 5 days. Orolabial herpes in immunocompetent patients (controversial indication): 250 mg PO tid. Treat ASAP after symptom onset.
UNAPPROVED PEDS - Chickenpox in adolescents: 500 mg PO tid x 5 days. First-episode genital herpes in adolescents: Use dose in unapproved adult.
FORMS - Trade: Tabs 125,250,500 mg.
NOTES - Reduce dose for CrCl <60 ml/min.

valacyclovir (*Valtrex*) ▶K ♀B ▶? $$$$
ADULT - First-episode genital herpes: 1 g PO bid x 10 days. Recurrent genital herpes: 500 mg PO bid x 3 days. Chronic suppression of genital herpes in immunocompetent patients: 1 g PO qd. Can use 500 mg PO qd if ≤9 recurrences/year; transmission of genital herpes reduced with use of this regimen by source partner, in conjunction with safer sex practices. Chronic suppression of genital herpes in HIV-infected patients: 500 mg PO bid. Herpes labialis: 2 g PO q12h x 2 doses. Zoster: 1 g PO tid x 7 days. Treat ASAP after symptom onset.
PEDS - Herpes labialis, ≥12 yo: 2 g PO q12h x 2 doses. Treat ASAP after symptom onset.
UNAPPROVED ADULT - Recurrent genital herpes: 1 g PO qd x 5 days. Recurrent genital herpes in HIV+ patients: 1 g PO bid x 5-10 days. Orolabial herpes in immunocompromised patients, including HIV-infection: 1 g PO tid x 7 days. Chickenpox in young adults: 1 g PO tid x 5 days. Treat ASAP after symptom onset.
UNAPPROVED PEDS - Chickenpox in adolescents: 1 g PO tid x 5 days. Treat ASAP after symptom onset. First-episode genital herpes in adolescents: Use adult dose.
FORMS - Trade: Tabs 500,1000 mg.
NOTES - Thrombotic thrombocytopenic purpura/hemolytic uremic syndrome at dose of 8 g/day. Reduce dose for CrCl <50 ml/min. Metabolized to acyclovir.

ANTIMICROBIALS: Antiviral Agents – Anti-HIV – Fusion Inhibitors

NOTE: AIDS treatment guidelines available online at www.aidsinfo.nih.gov. Consider monitoring LFTs in patients receiving highly active anti-retroviral therapy (HAART).

enfuvirtide (*Fuzeon, T-20*) ▶Serum ♀B ▶- $$$$$
WARNING - Not for monotherapy.
ADULT - Combination therapy for HIV infection: 90 mg SC bid. Give each injection at new site in upper arm, anterior thigh, or abdomen, avoiding areas with current reaction.
PEDS - Combination therapy for HIV infection, 6-16 yo: 2 mg/kg up to 90 mg SC bid. Give each injection at new site in upper arm, anterior thigh, or abdomen, avoiding areas with current reaction.
FORMS - 30-day kit with vials, diluent, syringes, alcohol wipes. Single-dose vials contain 108 mg to provide 90 mg enfuvirtide.
NOTES - Increased risk of bacterial pneumonia; monitor for signs/sx of pneumonia. Reconstitute with 1.1 ml sterile water for injection. This provides 1.2 ml of solution, of which only 1 ml (90 mg) is injected. Allow vial to stand until powder dissolves completely (up to 45 minutes). Do not shake. 2nd daily dose can be reconstituted ahead of time if stored in refrigerator in original vial and used within 24h. Return to room temp before injecting. Discard unused soln. Patient education on administration available at 1-877-438-9366 or www.fuzeon.com.

ANTIMICROBIALS: Antiviral Agents – Anti-HIV – Non-Nucleoside Reverse Transcriptase Inhibitors

NOTE: AIDS treatment guidelines available at www.aidsinfo.nih.gov. Many serious drug interactions - always check before prescribing! See http://www.cdc.gov/nchstp/tb/TB_HIV_Drugs/TOC.htm for use of rifamycins with NNRTIs. Consider monitoring LFTs in patients receiving highly active anti-retroviral therapy (HAART).

delavirdine (*Rescriptor, DLV*) ▶L ♀C ▶- $$$$$

WARNING - Not for monotherapy.

ADULT - Combination therapy for HIV infection: 400 mg PO tid.

PEDS - Combination therapy for HIV infection, ≥16 yo: 400 mg PO tid. Safety and efficacy not established in younger children.

UNAPPROVED PEDS - Combination therapy for HIV, adolescents <16 yo: 400 mg PO tid.

FORMS - Trade: Tabs 100,200 mg.

NOTES - Rash common in 1st first month of therapy. Can cause Stevens-Johnson syndrome. Many drug interactions. Inhibits cytochrome P450 3A4 & 2C9. Do not use with alprazolam, carbamazepine, cisapride, ergot alkaloids, lovastatin, phenytoin, phenobarbital, pimozide, chronic use of H2 blocker or proton pump inhibitor, simvastatin, St John's wort, triazolam. See http://www.cdc.gov/nchstp/tb/TB_HIV_Drugs/TOC.htm for use of rifamycins with NNRTIs. Midazolam contraindicated in labeling; but can use single dose IV cautiously with monitoring for procedural sedation. Monitor LFTs when delavirdine used with saquinavir. May need to decrease methadone dose. See package insert for clarithromycin dosage reduction if CrCl <60 ml/min. Monitor levels of antiarrhythmics, immunosuppressants. Not more than a single 25 mg dose of sildenafil in 48 hours. Not more than a single 2.5 mg dose of vardenafil in 24 hours. Tadalafil initial dose is 5 mg; not more than 10 mg single dose in 72 hours. Monitor INR with warfarin. Take at least 1 h before/after buffered didanosine or antacids. Can dissolve 100 mg tabs in water. Take with acidic drink if achlorhydria.

efavirenz (*Sustiva, EFV*) ▶L ♀C ▶- $$$$$

WARNING - Not for monotherapy.

ADULT - Combination therapy for HIV infection: 600 mg PO qhs. Avoid with high-fat meal.

PEDS - Consider antihistamine rash prophylaxis before starting. Combination therapy for HIV infection, ≥3 yo: 10-15 kg: 200 mg PO qhs. 15-20 kg: 250 mg qhs. 20 to <25 kg: 300 mg qhs. 25 to <32.5 kg: 350 mg qhs. 32.5 to <40 kg: 400 mg qhs. ≥40 kg: 600 mg qhs. Do not give with high-fat meal.

FORMS - Trade: Caps 50,100,200 mg, tabs 600 mg.

NOTES - Psychiatric/CNS reactions (warn about hazardous tasks), rash (consider antihistamines and/or corticosteroids; stop treatment if severe), increased cholesterol (monitor). To avoid "hangover", give 1st dose at 6-8 pm & start drug over weekend. False-positive with Microgenics cannabinoid screening test. Monitor LFTs if given with ritonavir, hepatotoxic drugs, or to patients with hepatitis B/C. Induces cytochrome P450 3A4. Many drug interactions including decreased levels of anticonvulsants, methadone. Do not give with cisapride, triazolam, ergot derivatives, St John's wort, voriconazole, or with saquinavir as sole protease inhibitor. Midazolam contraindicated in labeling; but can use single dose IV cautiously with monitoring for procedural sedation. See http://www.cdc.gov/nchstp/tb/TB_HIV_Drugs/TOC.htm for use of rifamycins with NNRTIs. High risk of rash when taken with clarithromycin; consider alternative antimicrobial. Potentially teratogenic; get negative pregnancy test before use by women of child-bearing potential and recommend barrier contraceptive.

nevirapine (*Viramune, NVP*) ▶LK ♀C ▶- $$$$$

WARNING - Life-threatening skin reactions, hypersensitivity, and hepatotoxicity. Monitor clinical and lab status intensively during first 18 weeks of therapy (risk of rash and/or hepatotoxicity greatest during first 6 weeks of therapy) and frequently thereafter. Consider LFTs at baseline, before and 2 weeks after dose increase, and at least once monthly. Stop nevirapine and never rechallenge if clinical hepatitis, severe rash, or rash with constitutional sx. Obtain LFTs if rash occurs. Risk of hepatotoxicity with rash high in women or high CD4 count (women with CD4 count >250 especially high risk, including pregnant women). Elevated LFTs or hepatitis B/C infection at baseline increases risk of hepatotoxicity. Not for monotherapy.

ADULT - Combination therapy for HIV infection: 200 mg PO qd x 14 days, then 200 mg PO bid. Dose titration reduces risk of rash. If rash develops, do not increase dose until it resolves. If stopped for >7 days, restart with initial dose.

PEDS - Combination therapy for HIV infection, 2 mo - 8 yo: 4 mg/kg PO qd x 14 days, then 7 mg/kg PO bid. ≥8 yo: 4 mg/kg PO qd x 14 days, then 4 mg/kg PO bid. Max dose 400 mg/day. Dose titration reduces risk of rash. If rash develops, do not increase dose until it resolves. If stopped for >7 days, restart with initial dose.

UNAPPROVED ADULT - Combination therapy for HIV infection: 200 mg PO qd x 14 days, then 400 mg PO qd. Prevention of maternal-fetal HIV transmission, maternal dosing: 200 mg PO single dose at onset of labor.

UNAPPROVED PEDS - Prevention of maternal-fetal HIV transmission, neonatal dosing: 2 mg/kg PO single dose within 3 days of birth.

FORMS - Trade: Tabs 200 mg, susp 50 mg/5ml.

NOTES - Cytochrome P450 3A inducer. May require increased methadone dose. Do not give with ketoconazole, hormonal contraceptives, St John's wort. Do not give with saquinavir unless ritonavir also used.

ANTIMICROBIALS: Antiviral Agents – Anti-HIV – Nucleoside/Nucleotide Reverse Transcriptase Inhibitors

NOTE: AIDS treatment guidelines available online at www.aidsinfo.nih.gov. Consider monitoring LFTs in patients receiving highly active anti-retroviral therapy (HAART). WARNING: Nucleoside reverse transcriptase inhibitors can cause lactic acidosis and hepatic steatosis. Fatalities reported in pregnant women receiving didanosine + stavudine.

abacavir (*Ziagen, ABC*) ▶L ♀C ▶- $$$$$

WARNING - Potentially fatal hypersensitivity (look for fever, rash, GI symptoms, cough, dyspnea, pharyngitis, or other respiratory symptoms). Stop at once & never rechallenge after suspected reaction. Fatal reactions can recur within hours of rechallenge in patients with previously unrecognized reaction.

ADULT - Combination therapy for HIV infection: 300 mg PO bid or 600 mg PO qd. Severe hypersensitivity may be more common with once-daily regimen.

PEDS - Combination therapy for HIV, 3 mo - 16 yo: 8 mg/kg up to 300 mg PO bid.

FORMS - Trade: Tabs 300 mg, oral soln 20 mg/ml.

NOTES - Dosage reduction for mild hepatic dysfunction (Child-Pugh score 5-6): 200 mg (10 mL of oral soln) PO bid.

Combivir **(lamivudine + zidovudine)** ▶LK ♀C ▶- $$$$$

WARNING - Zidovudine: bone marrow suppression, myopathy.

ADULT - Combination therapy for HIV infection: 1 tab PO bid.

PEDS - Combination therapy for HIV infection, ≥12 yo: 1 tab PO bid.

FORMS - Trade: Tabs lamivudine 150 mg + zidovudine 300 mg.

NOTES - See components. Monitor CBC. Not for weight <50 kg, CrCl ≤50 mL/min, hepatic dysfunction, or if dosage adjustment required.

didanosine (*Videx, Videx EC, ddI*) ▶LK ♀B ▶- $$$$$

WARNING - Potentially fatal pancreatitis; avoid use with other drugs that can cause pancreatitis. Avoid didanosine + stavudine in pregnancy due to reports of fatal lactic acidosis with pancreatitis or hepatic steatosis.

ADULT - Combination therapy for HIV infection: Buffered tabs: 200 mg PO bid for ≥60 kg, 125 mg PO bid for <60 kg. Use at least 2 (but not >4) tabs per dose to get adequate buffering. Use qd only when less frequent dosing required (may be less effective): 400 mg PO qd for ≥60 kg, 250 mg PO qd for <60 kg. Buffered powder: 250 mg PO bid for ≥60 kg, 167 mg PO bid for <60 kg. Videx EC: 400 mg PO qd for ≥60 kg, 250 mg PO qd for <60 kg. All formulations usually taken on empty stomach. Dosage reduction of Videx EC with tenofovir: 250 mg if ≥60 kg, 200 mg if <60 kg. Dosage reduction unclear with tenofovir if CrCl <60 mL/min. Give tenofovir + Videx EC on empty stomach or with light meal; give tenofovir + buffered didanosine on empty stomach.

PEDS - Combination therapy for HIV infection: 100 mg/m^2 PO bid for age 2 weeks-8 mo. 120 mg/m^2 PO bid for age >8 mo. Give on empty stomach. Give at least 2 buffered tabs (but not >4) per dose to get adequate buffering. Videx EC not approved for children.

FORMS - Trade: Chew/dispersible buffered tabs 25,50,100,150, 200 mg. Packets of buffered powder for oral soln 100,167,250 mg. Pediatric powder for oral soln 10 mg/ml (buffered with antacid). Delayed-release caps (Videx EC) 125,200,250,400 mg. All forms except Videx

EC are buffered.

NOTES - Peripheral neuropathy (use cautiously with other neurotoxic drugs), retinal changes, optic neuritis, retinal depigmentation in children, hyperuricemia. Risk of lactic acidosis, pancreatitis, and peripheral neuropathy increased by concomitant stavudine. Diarrhea with buffered powder. See package insert for reduced dose if CrCl <60 ml/min. Do not use with allopurinol. Give some medications at least 1 h (amprenavir, delavirdine, indinavir), 2 h (atazanavir, ciprofloxacin, levofloxacin, norfloxacin, ofloxacin, itraconazole, ketoconazole, ritonavir, dapsone, tetracyclines), or 4 h (moxifloxacin, gatifloxacin) before buffered didanosine. Didanosine levels increased by tenofovir or ribavirin; monitor for toxicity and stop if didanosine adverse effect (eg, pancreatitis, neuropathy, hyperlactatemia, lactic acidosis).

emtricitabine (Emtriva, FTC) ▶K ♀B ▶- $$$$$

ADULT - Combination therapy for HIV infection: 200 mg PO qd.

PEDS - Safety and efficacy not established in children.

UNAPPROVED PEDS - Combination therapy for HIV infection, 3 mo-16 yo: 6 mg/kg up to 200 mg PO qd.

FORMS - Trade: Caps 200 mg.

NOTES - Lactic acidosis/hepatic steatosis. Exacerbation of hepatitis B after discontinuation. Dosage reduction in adults with renal dysfunction: 200 mg PO q48h if CrCl 30-49 ml/min; 200 mg PO q72h if CrCl 15-29 ml/min; 200 mg PO q96h if CrCl <15 ml/min or hemodialysis.

Epzicom (abacavir + lamivudine) ▶LK ♀C ▶- $$$$$

WARNING - Abacavir: Potentially fatal hypersensitivity reactions. Abacavir and lamivudine: Lactic acidosis and hepatosteatosis. Lamivudine: Exacerbation of hepatitis B after discontinuation in patients co-infected with HIV and hepatitis B.

ADULT - Combination therapy for HIV infection: 1 tab PO qd.

PEDS - Safety and efficacy not established in children.

FORMS - Trade: Tabs abacavir 600 mg + lamivudine 300 mg.

NOTES - See components. Contraindicated in patients with previous hypersensitivity reaction to abacavir due to risk of fatal rechallenge reaction. Not for patients with CrCl ≤50 mL/min, hepatic dysfunction, or if dosage adjustment required.

lamivudine (Epivir, Epivir-HBV, 3TC, ✦Heptovir) ▶K ♀C ▶- $$$$$

WARNING - Lower dose of lamivudine in Epivir-HBV can cause HIV resistance - test for HIV before prescribing Epivir-HBV.

ADULT - Epivir for combination therapy for HIV infection: 300 mg PO qd or 150 mg PO bid. Epivir-HBV for chronic hepatitis B: 100 mg PO qd.

PEDS - Epivir for HIV infection: 3 mo-16 yo, 4 mg/kg (up to 150 mg) PO bid. Epivir-HBV for chronic hepatitis B, 2-17 yo: 3 mg/kg up to 100 mg PO qd.

UNAPPROVED PEDS - Epivir for HIV infection in adolescents ≥50 kg: 300 mg PO qd.

FORMS - Trade: Epivir, 3TC: Tabs 150, 300 mg, oral soln 10 mg/ml. Epivir-HBV, Heptovir: Tabs 100 mg, oral soln 5 mg/ml.

NOTES - Lamivudine-resistant hepatitis B reported. Exacerbation of hepatitis B reported after discontinuation of lamivudine. Epivir: Pancreatitis in children. Do not use with zalcitabine. See package inserts for dosage adjustments based on renal function.

stavudine (Zerit, d4T) ▶LK ♀C ▶- $$$$$

WARNING - Warn patients to report early signs of lactic acidosis (eg, abdominal pain, N/V, fatigue, dyspnea, weakness). Symptoms can mimic Guillain-Barr? syndrome. Stop stavudine if weakness or lactic acidosis. Potentially fatal pancreatitis & hepatotoxicity with didanosine + stavudine +/- hydroxyurea. Avoid this combo in pregnancy.

ADULT - Combination therapy for HIV infection: 40 mg PO q12h, 30 mg PO q12h if <60 kg. Hold for peripheral neuropathy. If symptoms resolve completely, can restart at 20 mg PO q12h, 15 mg PO q12h if <60 kg. If symptoms recur, consider stopping permanently.

PEDS - Combination therapy for HIV infection: <30 kg and ≥2 weeks old: 1 mg/kg PO bid. 30-59.9 kg: 30 mg bid. ≥60 kg: 40 mg bid.

FORMS - Trade: Caps 15,20,30,40 mg; oral soln 1 mg/ml.

NOTES - Peripheral neuropathy, lactic acidosis, pancreatitis; risk of these adverse reactions increased by concomitant didanosine. Do not use with zidovudine. See package insert for dosage adjustments based on renal function. Oral soln stable in refrigerator for 30 days.

tenofovir (Viread, TDF) ▶K ♀B ▶- $$$$$

WARNING - Stop tenofovir if hepatomegaly or steatosis occur, even if LFTs not abnormal. Exacerbation of hepatitis B after discontinuation in patients co-infected with HIV and hepatitis B.

ADULT - Combination therapy for HIV infection: 300 mg PO qd with a meal. High rate of virologic failure with tenofovir + didanosine + lamivudine; avoid this regimen.

PEDS - Not approved in children. Decreased bone mineral density reported.

FORMS - Trade: Tab 300 mg.

NOTES - Decreased bone mineral density; consider bone monitoring if hx of pathologic fracture or high risk of osteopenia. Consider calcium + vitamin D supplement for HIV-associated osteoporosis/ osteopenia. Exacerbation of hepatitis B after discontinuing tenofovir in patients coinfected with HIV and hepatitis B; monitor liver function for at least several months. Tenofovir increases didanosine levels and possibly serious didanosine adverse effects (eg pancreatitis, lactic acidosis, hyperlactatemia, neuropathy). Reduce Videx EC to 250 mg in patients ≥60 kg or 200 mg if <60 kg. Dosage adjustment of Videx EC unclear if CrCl <60 mL/min. Give tenofovir + Videx EC on empty stomach or with light meal; give tenofovir + buffered didanosine on empty stomach. If atazanavir is used with tenofovir, use 300 mg atazanavir + 100 mg ritonavir. Atazanavir and lopinavir/ritonavir increase tenofovir levels; monitor and discontinue tenofovir if adverse effects. Tenofovir can cause renal impairment including acute renal failure & Fanconi syndrome. Avoid tenofovir if current/ recent nephrotoxic drug use. Drugs that reduce renal function or undergo renal elimination (eg acyclovir, adefovir, ganciclovir) may increase tenofovir levels. Monitor creatinine & phosphate if risk/ history of renal insufficiency or nephrotoxic drug. Dosage reduction if CrCl <50 ml/min: 300 mg q48h if CrCl 30-49 ml/min; 300 mg twice weekly if CrCl 10-29 ml/min, 300 mg once weekly for dialysis patients (given after dialysis).

Trizivir (abacavir + lamivudine + zidovudine) ▶LK ♀C ▶- $$$$$

WARNING - Abacavir: Life-threatening hypersensitivity (see abacavir entry for details). Never restart after a reaction. Zidovudine: Bone marrow suppression, myopathy.

ADULT - HIV infection: 1 tab PO bid.

PEDS - HIV infection in adolescents ≥40 kg: 1 tab PO bid.

FORMS - Trade: Tabs abacavir 300 mg + lamivudine 150 mg + zidovudine 300 mg.

NOTES - See components. Monitor CBC. Not for patients <40 kg, those with CrCl ≤50 mL/

min or those who require dosage adjustment.

Truvada (emtricitabine + tenofovir) ▶K ♀B ▶- $$$$$

WARNING - Emtricitabine and tenofovir: Potentially fatal lactic acidosis and hepatosteatosis; severe acute exacerbation of hepatitis B after discontinuation in patients coinfected with HIV and hepatitis B.

ADULT - Combination therapy for HIV infection: 1 tab PO qd.

PEDS - Safety and efficacy not established in children.

FORMS - Trade: Tabs emtricitabine 200 mg + tenofovir 300 mg.

NOTES - See components. Do not use in a triple nucleoside regimen. Not for patients with CrCl ≤30 mL/min or hemodialysis; hepatic dysfunction; or if dosage adjustment required. Increase dosing interval to q48h if CrCl 30-49 mL/min. Coadminister didanosine and Truvada cautiously; monitor for didanosine adverse effects, and discontinue didanosine if they occur. Reduce didanosine dose to 250 mg in adults >60 kg; dosage adjustment of didanosine unclear if <60 kg. Give Videx EC + Truvada on empty stomach or with light meal. Give buffered didanosine + Truvada on empty stomach. Atazanavir and lopinavir/ ritonavir increase tenofovir levels; monitor and discontinue Truvada if tenofovir adverse effects. Tenofovir decreases atazanavir levels. If atazanavir is used with Truvada, use 300 mg atazanavir + 100 mg ritonavir. Do not use Truvada with lamivudine.

zalcitabine (*Hivid, ddC*) ▶K ♀C ▶- $$$$$

WARNING - Peripheral neuropathy, pancreatitis, hepatotoxicity.

ADULT - Combination therapy for HIV infection: 0.75 mg PO q8h on an empty stomach.

PEDS - Combination therapy for HIV infection, ≥13 yo: 0.75 mg PO q8h on an empty stomach.

UNAPPROVED PEDS - HIV infection, <13 yo: 0.01 mg/kg PO q8h. Take on an empty stomach.

FORMS - Trade: Tabs 0.375, 0.75 mg.

NOTES - Monitor amylase, triglycerides if high risk of pancreatitis. Do not use with lamivudine, didanosine, stavudine, IV pentamidine. Do not give at the same time as magnesium/aluminum antacids. See package insert for dosage adjustments based on renal function or neuropathy symptoms.

zidovudine (*Retrovir, AZT, ZDV*) ▶LK ♀C ▶- $$$$$

WARNING - Bone marrow suppression, myopathy.

ADULT - Combination therapy for HIV infection: 600 mg/day PO divided bid or tid. IV dosing: 1 mg/kg IV over 1 h 5-6 x/day. Prevention of maternal-fetal HIV transmission, maternal dosing (>14 weeks of pregnancy): 200 mg PO tid or 300 mg PO bid until start of labor. During labor, 2 mg/kg IV over 1 h, then 1 mg/kg/h until delivery.

PEDS - Combination therapy for HIV infection. 6 wk -12 yo: 160 mg/m² up to 200 mg PO q8h. Adolescents: Use adult dose. Prevention of maternal-fetal HIV transmission, infant dosing: 2 mg/kg PO q6h from within 12 h of birth until 6 weeks old. Can also give infants 1.5 mg/kg IV over 30 min q6h.

FORMS - Trade: Cap 100 mg, tab 300 mg, syrup 50 mg/5 ml.

NOTES - Do not use with stavudine. Hematologic toxicity; monitor CBC. Increased bone marrow suppression with ganciclovir or valganciclovir. See package insert for dosage adjustments based on renal function or hematologic toxicity.

ANTIMICROBIALS: Antiviral Agents – Anti-HIV – Protease Inhibitors

NOTE: Many serious drug interactions - always check before prescribing! Contraindicated with most antiarrhythmics, cisapride, ergot alkaloids, lovastatin, pimozide, simvastatin, St. John's wort, triazolam. Midazolam contraindicated in labeling; but can use single dose IV cautiously with monitoring for procedural sedation. See http://www.cdc.gov/nchstp/tb/TB_HIV_Drugs/TOC.htm for use of rifamycins with protease inhibitors. Not more than a single 25 mg dose of sildenafil in 48 hours with protease inhibitors. Vardenafil initial dose is 2.5 mg; not more than a single 2.5 mg dose in 72 hours. Sildenafil preferred over vardenafil with unboosted indinavir. Tadalafil initial dose is 5 mg; not more than 10 mg single dose in 72 hours. Adverse effects include spontaneous bleeding in hemophilics, hyperglycemia, hyperlipidemia, and fat redistribution. Coinfection with hepatitis C or other liver disease increases the risk of hepatotoxicity with protease inhibitors; monitor LFTs at least twice in 1st month of therapy, then every 3 months.

amprenavir (*Agenerase, APV***)** ▶L ♀C ▶- $$$$$

WARNING - Oral solution contraindicated in children <4 yo, pregnancy, hepatic/renal failure, therapy with metronidazole/ disulfiram due to potential propylene glycol toxicity.

ADULT - Combination therapy for HIV infection: 1200 mg PO bid. In combination with ritonavir: Give amprenavir 1200 mg PO qd with ritonavir 200 mg PO qd. Or amprenavir 600 mg bid with ritonavir 100 mg bid. Do not take with high-fat meal.

PEDS - Combination therapy for HIV infection. Caps: 13-16 yo, 1200 mg PO bid. 4-12 yo, or 13-16 yo and <50 kg, 20 mg/kg PO bid or 15 mg/kg PO tid. Maximum daily dose of 2400 mg. Oral soln: 4-12 yo, or 13-16 yo and <50 kg, 22.5 mg/kg PO bid or 17 mg/kg PO tid. Max 2800 mg/day. Do not take with high-fat meal.

FORMS - Trade: Caps 50,150 mg, oral soln 15 mg/ml.

NOTES - Life-threatening skin reactions; cross-sensitivity with sulfonamides possible. Monitor lipids. Contains vitamin E; tell patients not to take more. Multivitamin containing minimal vitamin E probably OK. Inhibits cytochrome P450 3A4. Do not give amprenavir plus ritonavir with flecainide or propafenone. Monitor levels of antiarrhythmics, immunosuppressants, tricyclic antidepressants. Monitor INR with warfarin. Avoid using with delavirdine. Using amprenavir with methadone can decrease levels of both drugs. See http://www.cdc.gov/nchstp/tb/TB_HIV_Drugs/TOC.htm for dosage adjustment of rifamycins. Take ≥1 h before/after buffered didanosine/ antacids. Hormonal contraceptives may reduce amprenavir levels; do not use. Oral sol'n and caps not interchangeable on mg per mg basis. Dosage reduction for moderate/ severe hepatic dysfunction: 450 mg bid for Child-Pugh score of 5-8; 300 mg bid for Child-Pugh score of 9-12.

atazanavir (*Reyataz, ATV***)** ▶L ♀B ▶- $$$$$

ADULT - Combination therapy for HIV infection. Therapy-naïve patients: 400 mg PO qd. Efavirenz regimen, therapy-naïve patients: atazanavir 300 mg + ritonavir 100 mg + efavirenz 600 mg all PO qd. Therapy-experienced patients: atazanavir 300 mg PO qd + ritonavir 100 mg PO qd. Tenofovir regimen (must include ritonavir): atazanavir 300 mg + ritonavir 100 mg + tenofovir 300 mg all PO qd with food. Give atazanavir with food; give 2 h before or 1 h after buffered didanosine.

PEDS - Not approved in children. Use adult dose if ≥16 yo. Do not use in infants; may cause kernicterus.

FORMS - Trade: Caps 100,150,200 mg.

NOTES - Does not appear to increase cholesterol or triglycerides. Asymptomatic increases in indirect bilirubin due to inhibition of UDP-glucuronosyl transferase (UGT); may cause jaundice/ scleral icterus. Do not use with indinavir; both may increase bilirubin. Consider other etiology for associated increases in transaminases. May inhibit UGT1A1 metabolism of irinotecan. Do not use with indinavir (also increases bilirubin). Prolongs PR interval and rare cases of second degree AV block reported; caution advised for patients with AV block or on drugs that prolong PR interval. Monitor ECG with calcium channel blockers; consider reducing diltiazem dose by 50%. Reduce clarithromycin dose by 50%; consider alternative therapy for indications other than Mycobacterium avium complex. Acid required for GI absorption. Do not use with proton pump inhibitors; separate dose from H2 blockers by ≥12h. Give 2 h before or 1 h after antacids or buffered didanosine. Inhibits cytochrome P450 1A2, 2C9, and 3A4. See http://www.cdc.gov/nchstp/tb/TB_HIV_Drugs/TOC.htm for dosage adjustment of rifamycins. Monitor levels of antiarrhythmics, immunosuppressants, tricyclic antidepressants. Monitor INR with warfarin. Increases levels of ethinyl estradiol and norethindrone; use lowest dose of both in oral contraceptives. In mild to moderate hepatic impairment (Child-Pugh class B), consider dosage reduction to 300 mg PO qd with food. Do not use in Child-Pugh Class C.

fosamprenavir (Lexiva, 908) ▶L ♀C ▶- $$$$$
ADULT - Combination therapy for HIV infection. Therapy-naïve patients: 1400 mg PO bid (without ritonavir). OR fosamprenavir 1400 mg + ritonavir 200 mg both PO qd. OR 700 mg fosamprenavir + 100 mg ritonavir both PO bid. Protease inhibitor-experienced patients: 700 mg fosamprenavir + 100 mg ritonavir both PO bid. Do not use once-daily regimen. If once-daily ritonavir-boosted regimen given with efavirenz, increase ritonavir to 300 mg/day; no increase of ritonavir dose needed for bid regimen with efavirenz. No meal restrictions.
PEDS - Not approved in children. Use adult dose if ≥16 yo. Do not use in infants; may cause kernicterus.
FORMS - Trade: 700 mg (equivalent to amprenavir 600 mg).
NOTES - Lower pill burden than amprenavir. Life-threatening skin reactions possible (reported with amprenavir). Cross-sensitivity with sulfonamides possible; use caution in sulfona-mide-allergic patients. Hypertriglyceridemia; monitor lipids. Fosamprenavir is inhibitor & substrate of cytochrome P450 3A4. Do not use fosamprenavir + ritonavir with flecainide or propafenone. Do not use fosamprenavir with delavirdine. See http://www.cdc.gov/nchstp/tb/TB_HIV_Drugs/TOC.htm for dosage adjustment of rifamycins. Monitor levels of antiarrhythmics, immunosuppressants, tricyclic antidepressants. May need to increase dose of methadone. Monitor INR with warfarin. Not >200 mg/day ketoconazole/ itraconazole with fosamprenavir + ritonavir; may need to reduce antifungal dose if >400 mg/day itraconazole/ketoconazole with unboosted fosamprenavir. Not >20 mg/day of atorvastatin. Not >2.5 mg vardenafil q24h with unboosted fosamprenavir or q72h for fosamprenavir + ritonavir. Do not use hormonal contraceptives. More adverse reactions when fosamprenavir given with Kaletra; appropriate dose for combination therapy unclear. Mild to moderate hepatic dysfunction (Child-Pugh score 5-8): 700 mg PO bid for unboosted fosamprenavir; no data for ritonavir-boosted regimen.

indinavir (Crixivan, IDV) ▶LK ♀C ▶- $$$$$
ADULT - Combination therapy for HIV infection: 800 mg PO q8h between meals with water (at least 48 oz/day).
PEDS - Not approved in children. Do not use in infants; may cause kernicterus.
UNAPPROVED ADULT - Combination therapy for HIV infection: 800 mg PO bid with ritonavir 100-200 mg PO bid. Or 400 mg bid with ritonavir 400 mg bid. Can be given without regard to meals when given with ritonavir.
UNAPPROVED PEDS - Combination therapy for HIV infection, adolescents: 800 mg PO q8h between meals with water (at least 48 oz/day). Children: 350-500 mg/m²/dose (max of 800 mg/dose) PO q8h.
FORMS - Trade: Caps 100,200,333,400 mg.
NOTES - Nephrolithiasis (may be more common in children), hemolytic anemia, indirect hyperbilirubinemia, possible hepatitis, interstitial nephritis with asymptomatic pyuria. Do not use with atazanavir; both may increase bilirubin. Inhibits cytochrome P450 3A4. Avoid using with carbamazepine if possible. Give indinavir and buffered didanosine 1 h apart on empty stomach. http://www.cdc.gov/nchstp/tb/TB_HIV_Drugs/TOC.htm for dosage adjustment of rifamycins and indinavir. Reduce indinavir dose to 600 mg PO q8h when given with ketoconazole, itraconazole 200 mg bid, or delavirdine

400 mg tid. Increase indinavir dose to 1000 mg PO q8h when given with efavirenz, nevirapine. For mild to moderate hepatic cirrhosis, give 600 mg PO q8h.

lopinavir-ritonavir (*Kaletra, LPV/r*) ►L ♀C ▶- $$$$$

ADULT - Combination therapy for HIV infection: 3 caps or 5 ml PO bid. Give 4 caps or 6.5 ml PO bid w/ efavirenz/nevirapine. Take with food.

PEDS - Combination therapy for HIV infection, 6 mo-12 yo: lopinavir 12 mg/kg PO bid for 7 to <15 kg, 10 mg/kg PO bid for 15-40 kg. Do not exceed adult dose. Use adult dose for >12 yo or >40 kg. With efavirenz/nevirapine, increase to 13 mg/kg PO bid for 7 to <15 kg, 11 mg/kg PO bid for 15-45 kg. Do not exceed adult dose. Use adult dose for >12 yo or >45 kg. Take with food.

FORMS - Trade: Caps 133.3 mg lopinavir + 33.3 mg ritonavir. Oral soln 80 mg lopinavir + 20 mg ritonavir/ml.

NOTES - Medication errors can occur if Keppra (levetiracetam) confused with Kaletra. May cause pancreatitis. Ritonavir (inhibits cytochrome P450 3A4 & 2D6) included in formulation to inhibit metabolism and boost levels of lopinavir. Many other drug interactions including decreased efficacy of oral contraceptives. See http://www.cdc.gov/nchstp/tb/TB_HIV_Drugs/TOC.htm for dosage adjustment of rifamycins. May require higher methadone dose. Give buffered didanosine 1 h before/ 2 h after Kaletra. Monitor INR with warfarin. Oral soln contains alcohol. Use caps/oral soln within 2 months if patient stores at room temperature.

nelfinavir (*Viracept, NFV*) ►L ♀B ▶- $$$$$

ADULT - Combination therapy for HIV infection: 750 mg PO tid or 1250 mg PO bid with meals. Absorption improved when meal contains ≥500 calories with 11-28 g of fat.

PEDS - Combination therapy for HIV infection, ≥2 yo: 45-55 mg/kg PO bid or 25-35 mg/kg PO tid to max of 2500 mg/day. Take with meals. Use powder or 250 mg tabs.

UNAPPROVED PEDS - Combination therapy for HIV infection: Up to 45 mg/kg/dose PO tid with meals. Absorption improved when meal contains ≥500 calories with 11-28 g of fat.

FORMS - Trade: Tab 250,625 mg, powder 50 mg/g.

NOTES - Diarrhea common. Inhibits cytochrome P450 3A4. Decreases efficacy of oral contraceptives. May require higher methadone dose. See http://www.cdc.gov/nchstp/tb/TB_HIV_Drugs/TOC.htm for dosage adjustment of rifa-

mycins and nelfinavir. Give nelfinavir 2 h before/1 h after buffered didanosine. Oral powder stable for 6 h after mixing if refrigerated.

ritonavir (*Norvir, RTV*) ►L ♀B ▶- $$$$$

WARNING - Contraindicated with many drugs due to risk of drug interactions.

ADULT - Full-dose regimen (600 mg PO bid) poorly tolerated. Lower doses of 100 mg PO qd to 400 mg PO bid used to boost levels of other protease inhibitors. Best tolerated regimen with saquinavir may be ritonavir 400 mg bid with Invirase 400 mg bid. Saquinavir 1000 mg bid (Invirase) with ritonavir 100 mg bid also used. In combination with amprenavir: Give amprenavir 1200 mg PO qd with ritonavir 200 mg qd. Or amprenavir 600 mg bid with ritonavir 100 bid.

PEDS - Combination therapy for HIV infection: 250 mg/m² PO q12h, increasing by 50 mg/m²/dose every 2-3 days to 400 mg/m² PO q12h. Max dose 600 mg PO bid. Give with meals.

UNAPPROVED ADULT - Combination therapy for HIV infection: 100-200 mg PO bid with indinavir 800 mg PO bid.

UNAPPROVED PEDS - Used at lower than labeled doses to boost levels of other protease inhibitors.

FORMS - Trade: Cap 100 mg. Oral soln 80 mg/ml.

NOTES - Nausea & vomiting, pancreatitis, alterations in AST, ALT, GGT, CPK, uric acid. Inhibits hepatic cytochrome P450 3A & 2D6. Do not use ritonavir 400 mg BID with voriconazole. Not >200 mg/day of ketoconazole with ritonavir. See http://www.cdc.gov/nchstp/tb/TB_HIV_Drugs/TOC.htm for dosage adjustment of rifamycins. Not more than a single dose of vardenafil 2.5 mg or tadalafil 10 mg in 72 h with ritonavir. Decreases efficacy of oral contraceptives. Increases methadone requirements. May cause serotonin syndrome with fluoxetine. May increase adverse effects with trazodone; consider reducing trazodone dose. Give ritonavir 2.5h before/after buffered didanosine. Contains alcohol. Do not refrigerate oral soln. Try to refrigerate caps, but stable for 30 days at <77 degrees F.

saquinavir (*Fortovase, Invirase, SQV, FTV*) ►L ♀B ▶? $$$$$

ADULT - Combination therapy for HIV infection. Fortovase: 1200 mg PO tid with/after meals. Ritonavir-boosted regimens: Saquinavir 400 mg PO bid with ritonavir 400 mg PO bid. Or saquinavir 1000 mg PO bid with ritonavir 100 mg PO bid. In ritonavir-boosted regimens, Invirase has better GI tolerance than Fortovase and no meal restrictions.

PEDS - Combination therapy for HIV, ≥16 yo. Fortovase: 1200 mg PO tid with/after meals. Invirase: 600 mg PO tid within 2 h after meals. Do not use saquinavir as sole protease inhibitor in children; boost with ritonavir or nelfinavir.

UNAPPROVED ADULT - Combination therapy for HIV infection: Saquinavir 1000 mg PO bid with standard doses of Kaletra.

UNAPPROVED PEDS - Fortovase, combination therapy for HIV infection: 33 mg/kg PO q8h with/after meals. Use adult dose in adolescents. Do not use saquinavir as sole protease inhibitor in children; boost with ritonavir or nelfinavir.

FORMS - Trade: Fortovase (soft gel), Invirase (hard gel) caps 200 mg.

NOTES - Do not give Invirase without ritonavir. Do not use saquinavir with garlic supplements. Delavirdine or ketoconazole increases saquinavir levels. Monitor LFTs if given with delavirdine. See http://www.cdc.gov/nchstp/tb/TB_HIV_Drugs/TOC.htm for dosage adjustment of rifamycins. Nevirapine and efavirenz lower levels of saquinavir; avoid combo therapy unless ritonavir also used. Use Fortovase caps within 3 months when stored at room temp.

ANTIMICROBIALS: Antiviral Agents – Anti-Influenza

NOTE: Whenever possible, immunization is the preferred method of prophylaxis. Consider chemoprophylaxis in high-risk patients vaccinated after influenza activity has begun, care-givers for high-risk patients, patients with immunodeficiency (including HIV infection), and those who request it. Provide chemoprophylaxis to all residents during institutional outbreaks of influenza, continuing for ≥2 weeks or until 1 week after end of outbreak.

amantadine (*Symmetrel*, ✚*Endantadine*) ▶K ♀C ▶? $

ADULT - Influenza A: 100 mg PO bid. ≥65 yo: 100 mg PO qd.

PEDS - Safety and efficacy not established in infants <1 yo. Influenza A, treatment or prophylaxis, ≥10 yo: 100 mg PO bid. 1-9 yo and any child <40 kg: 5 mg/kg/day up to 150 mg/day PO divided bid.

FORMS - Generic: Cap 100 mg. Generic/Trade: Tab 100 mg, syrup 50 mg/5 ml.

NOTES - CNS toxicity, suicide attempts, neuroleptic malignant syndrome with dosage reduction/withdrawal, anticholinergic effects, orthostatic hypotension. For prophylaxis after influenza exposure, start ASAP and continue for ≥10 days. Continue amantadine for 2-4 weeks after influenza vaccination while antibodies develop. For treatment, start within 48 h of symptom onset, continue for 3-5 days or until 24-48 h after signs/sx resolve. Do not stop abruptly in Parkinson's disease. Dosage reduction in adults with renal dysfunction: 200 mg PO 1st day, then 100 mg PO qd for CrCl 30-50 ml/min. 200 mg PO 1st day, then 100 mg PO qod for CrCl 15-29 ml/min. 200 mg PO q week for CrCl <15 ml/min or hemodialysis.

oseltamivir (*Tamiflu*) ▶LK ♀C ▶? $$$

ADULT - Influenza A/B, treatment: 75 mg PO bid x 5 days starting within 2 days of symptom onset. Prophylaxis: 75 mg PO qd. Start within 2 days of exposure and continue for ≥7 days. Take with food to improve tolerability.

PEDS - Influenza A/B treatment ≥1 yo: 30 mg PO bid for ≤15 kg, 45 mg PO bid for 16-23 kg, 60 mg PO bid for 24-40 kg, 75 mg PO bid for >40 kg or ≥13 yo. Treat for 5 days starting within 2 days of symptom onset. Prophylaxis ≥13 yo: 75 mg PO qd. Start within 2 days of exposure and continue for ≥7 days. Suspension comes with graduated syringe calibrated to 30, 45, and 60 mg; use 30 mg plus 45 mg to measure 75 mg dose. Take with food to improve tolerability.

FORMS - Trade: Caps 75 mg, susp 12 mg/ml.

NOTES - Not for infants <1 yo; immature blood brain barrier could lead to high oseltamivir levels in CNS. Patients with suspected influenza may have primary/ concomitant bacterial pneumonia. Antibiotics may be indicated. Dosage adjustment for CrCl 10-30 ml/min: 75 mg PO qd x 5 days for treatment, 75 mg PO qod for prophylaxis. Susp stable for 10 days at room temperature.

rimantadine (*Flumadine*) ▶LK ♀C ▶- $$

ADULT - Prophylaxis/treatment of influenza A: 100 mg PO bid. Start treatment ≤48 h of symptom onset and continue x 7 days. Reduce to 100 mg/day if side effects in patients ≥65 yo, severe hepatic dysfunction, CrCl ≤10 ml/min, elderly nursing home patient.

PEDS - Prophylaxis of influenza A, ≥10 yo: 100 mg PO bid. 1-9 yo or any child <40 kg: 5 mg/kg/day up to 150 mg/day PO divided qd or bid.

FORMS - Trade: Tabs 100 mg, syrup 50 mg/5

ml.

NOTES - CDC recommends treatment for 3-5 days or until 24-48 h after signs/sx resolve.

zanamivir (*Relenza*) ▶K ♀C ▶? $$

ADULT - Influenza A/B, treatment: 2 puffs bid x 5 days. Take 2 doses on day 1 at least 2 h apart. Start within 2 days of symptom onset.

PEDS - Influenza A/B, treatment, ≥7 yo: 2 puffs bid x 5 days. Take 2 doses on day 1 at least 2 h apart. Start within 2 days of symptom onset. Not approved in children <7 yo.

UNAPPROVED ADULT - Influenza A/B, prophylaxis: 2 puffs qd.

FORMS - Trade: Rotadisk inhaler 5 mg/puff (20 puffs).

NOTES - May cause bronchospasm & worsen pulmonary function in asthma or COPD. Avoid if underlying airway disease, stop if bronchospasm/decline in respiratory function. Patients with suspected influenza may have primary/concomitant bacterial pneumonia; consider antibiotics. Show patient how to use inhaler.

ANTIMICROBIALS: Antiviral Agents – Other

adefovir (*Hepsera*) ▶K ♀C ▶- $$$$$

WARNING - Nephrotoxic; monitor renal function. HIV resistance in untreated HIV infection; test for HIV before prescribing. Lactic acidosis with hepatic steatosis. Discontinuation may exacerbate hepatitis B; monitor liver function.

ADULT - Chronic hepatitis B: 10 mg PO qd.

PEDS - Not approved in children.

FORMS - Trade: Tabs 10 mg.

NOTES - Monitor renal function. See package insert for dosage reduction if CrCl <50 mL/minute. Other nephrotoxic drugs may increase risk of nephrotoxicity.

interferon alfa-2b (*Intron A*) ▶K? ♀C ▶?+ $$$$$

WARNING - May cause or worsen serious neuropsychiatric, autoimmune, ischemic, & infectious diseases. Frequent clinical & lab monitoring required. Stop interferon if signs/sx of these conditions are persistently severe or worsen.

ADULT - Chronic hepatitis B: 5 million units/day or 10 million units 3 times/week SC/IM x 16 weeks. Chronic hepatitis C: 3 million units SC/IM 3 times/week x 16 weeks. Continue for 18-24 mo if ALT normalized. Other indications: condylomata acuminata, AIDS-related Kaposi's sarcoma.

PEDS - Not approved in children.

UNAPPROVED ADULT - Prevention of chronic hepatitis C in acute hepatitis C: 5 million units SC qd x 4 weeks then 5 million units SC 3 times/week x 20 weeks.

FORMS - Trade: Powder/soln for injection 3,5, 10 million units/vial. Soln for injection 18,25 million units/multidose vial. Multidose injection pens 3,5,10 million units/dose (6 doses/pen).

NOTES - Monitor for depression, suicidal behavior, other severe neuropsychiatric effects. Thyroid abnormalities, hepatotoxicity, flu-like sx, pulmonary & cardiovascular reactions, retinal damage, neutropenia, thrombocytopenia,

hypertriglyceridemia (consider monitoring). Increases theophylline levels. Monitor CBC, TSH, LFTs, electrolytes. Dosage adjustments for hematologic toxicity in package insert.

interferon alfacon-1 (*Infergen*) ▶Plasma ♀C ▶? $$$$$

WARNING - May cause or worsen serious neuropsychiatric, autoimmune, ischemic, & infectious diseases. Frequent clinical & lab monitoring required. Stop interferon if signs/sx of these conditions are persistently severe or worsen.

ADULT - Chronic hepatitis C: 9 mcg SC 3 times/week x 24 weeks. Increase to 15 mcg SC 3 times/week x 24 weeks if relapse/no response. Reduce to 7.5 mcg SC 3 times/week if intolerable adverse effects.

PEDS - Not approved in children.

FORMS - Trade: Vials injectable soln 9,15 mcg.

NOTES - Monitor for depression, suicidal behavior, other severe neuropsychiatric effects. Thyroid dysfunction, cardiovascular reactions, retinal damage, flu-like symptoms, thrombocytopenia, neutropenia, exacerbation of autoimmune disorders, hypertriglyceridemia (consider monitoring). Monitor CBC, thyroid function. Refrigerate injectable soln.

palivizumab (*Synagis*) ▶L ♀C ▶? $$$$$

PEDS - Prevention of respiratory syncytial virus pulmonary disease in high-risk patients: 15 mg/kg IM q month during RSV season with first injection before season starts (November to April in northern hemisphere). Consider for children <2 yo treated for chronic lung disease in last 6 mo or with hemodynamically significant congenital heart disease; infants born <28 wk gestation who are now <12 mo; infants born 29-32 wk gestation who are now <6 mo. Give a dose ASAP after cardiopulmonary bypass (due to decreased palivizumab levels) even if <1 month after last dose.

NOTES – Use preservative-free <6h of reconstitution. Not more than 1 ml per injection site.

peginterferon alfa-2a (*Pegasys*) ▶LK ♀C ▶- $$$$$

WARNING - May cause or worsen serious neuropsychiatric, autoimmune, ischemic, & infectious diseases. Frequent clinical & lab monitoring recommended. Discontinue if signs/sx of these conditions are persistently severe or worsen.

ADULT - Chronic hepatitis C not previously treated with alfa interferon: 180 mcg SC in abdomen or thigh once weekly for 48 weeks.

PEDS - Not approved in children.

FORMS - Trade: 180 mcg/1 mL solution in single-use vial, 180 mcg/0.5 mL prefilled syringe.

NOTES - Monitor for depression, suicidal behavior, other severe neuropsychiatric events. Thrombocytopenia, neutropenia, thyroid dysfunction, hyperglycemia, hypoglycemia, cardiovascular events, colitis, pancreatitis, hypersensitivity, flu-like sx, pulmonary & ophthalmologic disorders. Cytochrome P450 1A2 inhibitor; may increase theophylline levels (monitor). Use cautiously if CrCl <50 ml/min. Monitor CBC, blood chemistry. Dosage adjustments for adverse effects, hepatic dysfunction, or hemodialysis in package insert. Store in refrigerator.

peginterferon alfa-2b (*PEG-Intron*) ▶K? ♀C ▶- $$$$$

WARNING - May cause or worsen serious neuropsychiatric, autoimmune, ischemic, & infectious diseases. Frequent clinical & lab monitoring recommended. Discontinue if signs/sx of these conditions are persistently severe or worsen.

ADULT - Chronic hepatitis C not previously treated with alfa interferon. Give SC once weekly for 1 year. Dose and vial strength based on weight. Monotherapy: 1 mcg/kg/week. ≤45 kg: 40 mcg (0.4 ml, 50 mcg/0.5 ml vial). 46-56 kg: 50 mcg (0.5 ml, 50 mcg/0.5 ml vial). 57-72 kg: 64 mcg (0.4 ml, 80 mcg/0.5 ml vial). 73-88 kg: 80 mcg (0.5 ml, 80 mcg/0.5 ml vial). 89-106 kg: 96 mcg (0.4 ml, 120 mcg/0.5 ml vial). 107-136 kg: 120 mcg (0.5 ml, 120 mcg/0.5 ml vial). 137-160 kg: 150 mcg (0.5 ml, 150 mcg/0.5 ml vial). In combo with oral ribavirin (see Rebetol entry): 1.5 mcg/kg/week. <40 kg: 50 mcg (0.5 ml, 50 mcg/0.5 ml vial). 40-50 kg: 64 mcg (0.4 ml, 80 mcg/0.5 ml vial). 51-60 kg: 80 mcg (0.5 ml, 80 mcg/0.5 ml vial). 61-75 kg: 96 mcg (0.4 ml, 120 mcg/0.5 ml vial). 76-85 kg: 120 mcg (0.5 ml, 120 mcg/0.5 ml vial). >95 kg: 150 mcg (0.5 ml, 150 mcg/0.5 ml vial). Give at bedtime or with antipyretic to minimize flu-like sx. Consider stopping if HCV RNA is not below limit of detection after 24 weeks of therapy.

PEDS - Not approved in children.

FORMS - Trade: 50,80,120,150 mcg/0.5 ml single-use vials with diluent, 2 syringes, and alcohol swabs. Disposable single-dose Redipen 50,80,120,150 mcg.

NOTES - Due to limited supply, patients must enroll in access program (888-437-2608). Monitor for depression, suicidal behavior, other severe neuropsychiatric effects. Thrombocytopenia, neutropenia, thyroid dysfunction, hyperglycemia, cardiovascular events, colitis, pancreatitis, hypersensitivity, flu-like sx, pulmonary damage. Use cautiously if CrCl <50 ml/min. Monitor CBC, blood chemistry. Dosage adjustments for adverse effects in package insert. Peginterferon should be used immediately after reconstitution, but can be refrigerated for up to 24 h.

***Rebetron* (interferon alfa-2b + ribavirin)** ▶K ♀X ▶- $$$$$

WARNING - Ribavirin is contraindicated if pregnancy possible in patient/ partner because it is teratogenic. Female patients and female partners of male patients must avoid pregnancy by using 2 forms of birth control during and for 6 months after stopping ribavirin. Obtain pregnancy test at baseline and monthly. See interferon alfa-2b entry for warnings.

ADULT - Chronic hepatitis C: Interferon alfa-2b 3 million units SC 3 times/week and ribavirin (Rebetol) 600 mg PO bid if >75 kg; 400 mg q am and 600 q pm if ≤75 kg. Get CBC at baseline, weeks 2 & 4, then as needed. See package insert for dosage reductions if hemoglobin declines. Duration of therapy is 24-48 weeks depending on HCV RNA levels and genotype.

PEDS - Efficacy for chronic hepatitis C not established. Dosing in children ≥25 kg: Interferon alfa-2b 3 million units/m^2 SC 3 times/week and PO ribavirin according to weight. Ribavirin: 200 mg bid for 25-36 kg; 200 mg qam and 400 mg q pm for 37-49 kg; 400 mg bid for 50-61 kg. Use adult dose for >61 kg.

FORMS - Trade: Each kit contains a 2-week supply of interferon alfa-2b, ribavirin caps 200 mg. Rebetol oral soln also available.

NOTES - Interferon alfa-2b: Depression, suicidal behavior, thyroid dysfunction, flu-like symptoms, pulmonary reactions, retinal damage, hypersensitivity, hypertriglyceridemia (consider monitoring). Suicidal ideation/ attempts more frequent in children/ adolescents. Give SC for platelets <50,000/mm3. Ribavirin: Hemolytic anemia. Do not use ribavirin in significant/unstable heart disease. Decreased INR with warfarin; monitor INR weekly for 4 weeks after ribavirin started/ stopped. May increase risk of lactic acidosis with nucleoside reverse transcriptase inhibitors. Do not use with didanosine. Do not use ribavirin if CrCl <50 ml/minute.

ribavirin - inhaled (*Virazole*) ▶Lung ♀X ▶- $$$$$
WARNING - Beware of sudden pulmonary deterioration with ribavirin. Drug precipitation may cause ventilator dysfunction.
PEDS - Severe respiratory syncytial virus infection: Aerosol 12-18 hours/day x 3-7 days.
NOTES - Minimize exposure to health care workers, especially pregnant women.

ribavirin - oral (*Rebetol, Copegus*) ▶Cellular, K ♀X ▶- $$$$$
WARNING - Teratogen; contraindicated if pregnancy possible in patient/ partner. Female patients and female partners of male patients must avoid pregnancy by using 2 forms of birth control during and for 6 months after stopping ribavirin. Obtain pregnancy test at baseline and monthly. Hemolytic anemia that may worsen cardiac disease. Do not use in significant/ unstable heart disease. Baseline ECG if preexisting cardiac dysfunction.
ADULT - Chronic hepatitis C. Rebetol: In combo with interferon alfa-2b: 600 mg PO bid if >75 kg; 400 mg q am and 600 mg q pm if ≤75 kg. Take without regard to meals, but consistently

the same. In combo with peginterferon alfa 2b: 400 mg PO bid with food. Copegus: In combo with peginterferon alfa 2a (Pegasys): For genotype 1 or 4, treat x 48 wks with 1200 mg/day if ≥75 kg; 1000 mg/day if <75 kg. For genotype 2 or 3, treat x 24 wks with 800 mg/day PO. Take bid with food. See package inserts for dosage reductions if Hb declines.
PEDS - Rebetol in combo with interferon alfa-2b: For patients ≤25 kg or who cannot swallow caps: 15 mg/kg/day of soln PO divided bid. Caps: 200 mg PO bid for 25-36 kg; 200 mg qam and 400 mg q pm for 37-49 kg; 400 mg bid for 50-61 kg. Use adult dose for >61 kg. Take without regard to meals, but consistently the same.
UNAPPROVED PEDS - Combination therapy with interferon alfa for chronic hepatitis C. 200 mg bid for 25-36 kg; 200 mg qam and 400 mg q pm for 37-49 kg; 400 mg bid for 50-61 kg. Use adult dosing for >61 kg.
FORMS - Trade: Caps 200 mg (Rebetol), tabs 200 mg (Copegus). Generic: Caps 200 mg (Ribasphere, others). Trade: Rebetol oral soln 40 mg/ml.
NOTES - Contraindicated in hemoglobinopathies. Get CBC at baseline, weeks 2 & 4, and prn. Do not use if CrCl <50 ml/min. Decreased INR with warfarin; monitor INR weekly for 4 weeks after ribavirin started/ stopped. May increase risk of lactic acidosis with nucleoside reverse transcriptase inhibitors. Avoid didanosine, stavudine, zidovudine.

ANTIMICROBIALS: Carbapenems

ertapenem (*Invanz*) ▶K ♀B ▶? $$$$$
ADULT - Community-acquired pneumonia, complicated intra-abdominal, skin, urinary tract, acute pelvic infections: 1g IM/IV over 30 minutes q24h x ≤14 days for IV, x ≤7 days for IM.
PEDS - Not approved in children.
NOTES - Possible cross-sensitivity with other beta-lactams; pseudomembranous colitis; superinfection; seizures (especially if renal dysfunction or CNS disorder). Not active against Pseudomonas and Acinetobacter species. IM diluted with lidocaine; contraindicated if allergic to amide-type local anesthetics. For adults with renal dysfunction: 500 mg q24h for CrCl ≤30 ml/min or hemodialysis. Give 150 mg supplemental dose if daily dose given within 6 h before hemodialysis. Do not dilute in dextrose.

imipenem-cilastatin (*Primaxin*) ▶K ♀C ▶? $$$$$

ADULT - Pneumonia, sepsis, endocarditis, polymicrobic, intra-abdominal, gynecologic, bone & joint, skin infections. Normal renal function, ≥70 kg - Mild infection: 250-500 mg IV q6h. Moderate infection: 500 mg IV q6-8h or 1 g IV q8h. Severe infection: 500 mg IV q6h to 1 g IV q6-8h. Complicated UTI: 500 mg IV q6h. See product labeling for doses in adults <70 kg. Can give up to 1.5 g/day IM for mild/moderate infections.
PEDS - Pneumonia, sepsis, endocarditis, polymicrobic, intra-abdominal, bone & joint, skin infections. Age >3 mo: 15-25 mg/kg IV q6h. 1-3 mo: 25 mg/kg IV q6h. 1-4 weeks old: 25 mg/kg IV q8h. <1 week old: 25 mg/kg IV q12h. Not for children with CNS infections, or <30 kg with renal dysfunction.
UNAPPROVED ADULT - Malignant otitis externa, empiric therapy for neutropenic fever:

500 mg IV q6h.

NOTES - Possible cross-sensitivity with other beta-lactams, pseudomembranous colitis, superinfection, seizures (especially if given with ganciclovir, elderly with renal dysfunction, or cerebrovascular or seizure disorder). See product labeling for dose if CrCl <70 ml/min. Not for CrCl <5 ml/min unless dialysis started within 48 h.

meropenem (Merrem IV) ▶K ♀B ▶? $$$$$

ADULT - Intra-abdominal infections: 1 g IV q8h.

PEDS - Meningitis: age ≥3 mo, 40 mg/kg/dose IV q8h. >50 kg, 2 g IV q8h. Intra-abdominal infection: age ≥3 mo, 20 mg/kg/dose IV q8h. >50 kg, 1 g IV q8h.

UNAPPROVED ADULT - Meningitis: 40 mg/kg (max 2 g) IV q 8h. Hospital-acquired pneumonia, complicated UTI, malignant otitis externa: 1 g IV q8h.

UNAPPROVED PEDS - Infant >2 kg: 20 mg/kg IV q12h for ≤1 week old, q8h for 1-4 wks old.

NOTES - Possible cross-sensitivity with other beta-lactams; pseudomembranous colitis; superinfection; seizures; thrombocytopenia in renal dysfunction. Reduces valproic acid levels. For adults with renal dysfunction: 1 g IV q12h for CrCl 26-50 ml/min, 500 mg IV q12h for CrCl 10-25 ml/min, 500 mg IV q24h for CrCl <10 ml/min.

ANTIMICROBIALS: Cephalosporins – 1st Generation

NOTE: Cephalosporins are 2nd-line to penicillin for group A strep pharyngitis, can be cross-sensitive with penicillin, and can cause pseudomembranous colitis.

cefadroxil (Duricef) ▶K ♀B ▶+ $$$

ADULT - Simple UTI: 1-2 g/day PO divided qd-bid. Other UTIs: 1 g PO bid. Skin infections: 1 g/day PO divided qd-bid. Group A strep pharyngitis: 1 g/day PO divided qd-bid x 10 days. See bacterial endocarditis prophylaxis table.

PEDS - UTIs, skin infections: 30 mg/kg/day PO divided bid. Group A streptococcal pharyngitis/tonsillitis, impetigo: 30 mg/kg/day PO divided qd-bid. Treat pharyngitis for 10 days.

FORMS - Generic/Trade: Tabs 1 g, caps 500 mg. Trade: Susp 125,250, & 500 mg/5 ml.

NOTES - Renal dysfunction in adults: 1 g load, then 500 mg PO q12h for CrCl 25-50 ml/min, 500 mg PO q24h for CrCl 10-25 ml/min, 500 mg PO q36h for CrCl <10 ml/min.

cefazolin (Ancef, Kefzol) ▶K ♀B ▶+ $$$

ADULT - Pneumonia, sepsis, endocarditis, skin, bone & joint, genital infections. Mild infections due to gram-positive cocci: 250-500 mg IM/IV q8h. Moderate/severe infections: 0.5-1 g IM/IV q6-8h. Life-threatening infections: 1-1.5 g IV q6h. Simple UTI: 1 g IM/IV q12h. Pneumococcal pneumonia: 500 mg IM/IV q12h. Surgical prophylaxis: 1 g IM/IV 30-60 min preop, additional 0.5-1 g during surgery >2h, and 0.5-1 g q6-8h x 24h postop. See table for prophylaxis of bacterial endocarditis.

PEDS - Pneumonia, sepsis, endocarditis, skin, bone & joint infections. Mild/moderate infections, age ≥1 mo: 25-50 mg/kg/day IM/IV divided q6-8h. Severe infections, age ≥1 mo:

100 mg/kg/day IV divided q6-8h. See table for prophylaxis of bacterial endocarditis.

NOTES - Renal dysfunction in adults: Usual 1st dose, then usual dose q8h for CrCl 35-54 ml/min, 50% of usual dose q12h for CrCl 11-34 ml/min, 50% of usual dose q18-24h for CrCl <10 ml/min. Renal dysfunction in children: Usual 1st dose, then 60% of usual dose q12h for CrCl 40-70 ml/min, 25% of usual dose q12h for 20-40 ml/min, 10% of usual dose q24h for CrCl 5-20 ml/min.

cephalexin (Keflex, Keftab) ▶K ♀B ▶? $$

ADULT - Pneumonia, bone, GU infections. Usual dose: 250-500 mg PO qid. Max: 4g/day. Group A strep pharyngitis, skin infections, simple UTI: 500 mg PO bid. Treat pharyngitis for 10 days. See table for prophylaxis of bacterial endocarditis.

PEDS - Pneumonia, GU, bone, skin infections, group A strep pharyngitis. Usual dose: 25-50 mg/kg/day PO in divided doses. Max dose: 100 mg/kg/day. Can give bid for strep pharyngitis in children >1 yo, skin infections. Group A strep pharyngitis, skin infections, simple UTI in patients >15 yo: 500 mg PO bid. Treat pharyngitis x 10 days. Not for otitis media, sinusitis.

FORMS - Generic/Trade: Caps 250,500 mg, tabs 500 mg, susp 125 & 250 mg/5 ml. Generic: Tabs 250 mg. Keftab: 500 mg. Panixine DisperDose 125,250 mg scored tabs for oral susp.

NOTES - Mix Panixine tab with 2 tsp water and drink mixture, then rinse container with a little water and drink that. Do not chew or swallow tab whole. Use only for doses that can be delivered by half or whole tabs.

OVERVIEW OF BACTERIAL PATHOGENS (selected)

Gram Positive Aerobic Cocci: *Staph epidermidis* (coagulase negative), *Staph aureus* (coagulase positive), Streptococci: *S pneumoniae* (pneumococcus), *S pyogenes* (Group A), *S agalactiae* (Group B), enterococcus

Gram Positive Aerobic / Facultatively Anaerobic Bacilli: *Bacillus, Corynebacterium diphtheriae, Erysipelothrix rhusiopathiae, Listeria monocytogenes, Nocardia*

Gram Negative Aerobic Diplococci: *Moraxella catarrhalis, Neisseria gonorrhoeae & meningitidis*

Gram Negative Aerobic Coccobacilli: *Haemophilus ducreyi, Haemoph. influenzae*

Gram Negative Aerobic Bacilli: *Acinetobacter, Bartonella* species, *Bordetella pertussis, Brucella, Burkholderia cepacia, Campylobacter, Francisella tularensis, Helicobacter pylori, Legionella pneumophila, Pseudomonas aeruginosa, Stenotrophomonas maltophilia, Vibrio cholerae, Yersinia*

Gram Neg Facultatively Anaerobic Bacilli: *Aeromonas hydrophila, Eikenella corrodens, Pasteurella multocida, Enterobacteriaceae: E coli, Citrobacter, Shigella, Salmonella, Klebsiella, Enterobacter, Hafnia, Serratia, Proteus, Providencia*

Anaerobes: *Actinomyces, Bacteroides fragilis, Clostridium botulinum, Clostridium difficile, Clostridium perfringens, Clostridium tetani, Fusobacterium, Lactobacillus, Peptostreptococcus*

Defective Cell Wall Bacteria: *Chlamydia pneumoniae, Chlamydia psittaci, Chlamydia trachomatis, Coxiella burnetii, Myocoplasma pneumoniae, Rickettsia prowazekii, Rickettsia rickettsii, Rickettsia typhi, Ureaplasma urealyticum*

Spirochetes: *Borrelia burgdorferi, Leptospira, Treponema pallidum*

Mycobacteria: *M avium complex, M kansasii, M leprae, M tuberculosis*

ANTIMICROBIALS: Cephalosporins: 2nd Generation

NOTE: Cephalosporins are 2nd-line to penicillin for group A strep pharyngitis, can be cross-sensitive with penicillin, and can cause pseudomembranous colitis.

cefaclor (*Ceclor, Raniclor*) ▶K 9B ▶? $$$
ADULT - Otitis media, pneumonia, group A strep pharyngitis, UTI, skin infections: 250-500 mg PO tid. Ceclor CD: Acute exacerbation of chronic bronchitis, secondary bacterial infection of acute bronchitis: 500 mg PO bid with food. Group A streptococcal pharyngitis, skin infections: 375 mg PO bid with food. Treat pharyngitis for 10 days.
PEDS - Pneumonia, group A strep pharyngitis, UTI, skin infections: 20-40 mg/kg/ day up to 1 g/day PO divided bid for pharyngitis, tid for other infections. Treat pharyngitis x 10d. Otitis media: 40 mg/kg/day PO divided bid.
FORMS - Generic/Trade: Caps 250,500 mg, susp 125,187,250, 375 mg/5 ml. Generic/Trade: Extended release (Ceclor CD): 375,500 mg. Generic: Chew tabs 125,187,250,375 mg.
NOTES - Serum sickness-like reactions with repeated use.

cefotetan (*Cefotan*) ▶K/Bile 9B ▶? $$$$$
ADULT - Usual dose: 1-2 g IM/IV q12h. UTI: 0.5-2 g IM/IV q12h or 1-2 g IM/IV q24h. Pneumonia, gynecologic, intra-abdominal, bone & joint infections: 1-3 g IM/IV q12h. Skin infec-

tions: 1-2 g IM/IV q12h or 2 g IV q24h. Surgical prophylaxis: 1-2 g IV 30-60 min preop. Give after cord clamp for C-section.
PEDS - Not approved in children.
UNAPPROVED PEDS - Usual dose: 40-80 mg/kg/day IV divided q12h.
NOTES - Hemolytic anemia (higher risk than other cephalosporins), clotting impairment rarely. Disulfiram-like reaction with alcohol. Dosing reduction in adults with renal dysfunction: Usual dose q24h for CrCl 10-30 ml/min, usual dose q48h for CrCl <10 ml/min.

cefoxitin (*Mefoxin*) ▶K 9B ▶+ $$$$$
ADULT - Pneumonia, UTI, sepsis, intra-abdominal, gynecologic, skin, bone & joint infections: Uncomplicated, 1 g IV q6-8h. Moderate to severe, 1 g IV q4h or 2 g IV q6-8h. Infections requiring high doses, 2 g IV q4h or 3 g IV q6h. Uncontaminated gastrointestinal surgery, vaginal/abdominal hysterectomy: 2 g IV 30-60 min preop, then 2 g IV q6h x 24h. C-section: 2 g IV after cord clamped or 2 g IV q4h x 3 doses with 1st dose given after cord clamped.
PEDS - Pneumonia, UTI, sepsis, intra-abdominal, skin, bone & joint infections, age ≥3 mo: 80-160 mg/kg/day IV divided into 4-6 doses, max 12 g/day. Mild-moderate infections: 80-100 mg/kg/day IV divided into 3-4 doses. Surgical prophylaxis: 30-40 mg/kg IV 30-60 min preop and for not more than 24h postop.

NOTES - Eosinophilia & increased AST with high doses in children. Dosing reduction in adults with renal dysfunction: Load with 1-2 g IV; then 1-2 g IV q8-12h for CrCl 30-50 ml/min, 1-2 g IV q12-24h for CrCl 10-29 ml/min, 0.5-1 g IV q12-24h for CrCl 5-9 ml/min, 0.5 g IV q24-48h for CrCl <5 ml/min. Give 1-2 g loading dose after each hemodialysis.

cefprozil (*Cefzil*) ▶K ♀B ▶+ $$$$
ADULT - Group A strep pharyngitis: 500 mg PO qd x 10 days. Sinusitis: 250-500 mg PO bid. Acute exacerbation of chronic/secondary infection of acute bronchitis: 500 mg PO bid. Skin infections: 250-500 mg PO bid or 500 mg qd.
PEDS - Otitis media: 15 mg/kg/dose PO bid. Group A strep pharyngitis: 7.5 mg/kg/dose PO bid x 10 days. Sinusitis: 7.5-15 mg/kg/dose PO bid. Skin infections: 20 mg/kg PO qd. Use adult dose for ≥13 yo.
FORMS - Trade: Tabs 250,500 mg, susp 125 & 250 mg/5 ml.
NOTES - Give 50% of usual dose at usual interval for CrCl <30 ml/min.

cefuroxime (*Zinacef, Ceftin, Kefurox*) ▶K ♀B ▶? $$$$
ADULT - IM/IV cefuroxime. Uncomplicated pneumonia, simple UTI, skin infections, disseminated gonorrhea: 750 mg IM/IV q8h. Bone & joint, or severe/complicated infections: 1.5 g IV q8h. Sepsis: 1.5 g IV q6-8h or 3 g IV q8h. Gonorrhea: 1.5 g IM single dose split into 2 injections, given with probenecid 1 g PO. Surgical prophylaxis: 1.5 g IV 30-60 min preop, then 750 mg IM/IV q8h for prolonged procedures. Open heart surgery: 1.5 g IV q12h x 4 with 1st dose at induction of anesthesia. Cefuroxime axetil tabs. Group A strep pharyngitis, acute sinusitis: 250 mg PO bid x 10 days. Acute exacerbation of chronic/secondary infection of acute bronchitis, skin infections: 250-500 mg PO bid. Early Lyme disease: 500 mg PO bid x 20 days. Simple UTI: 125-250 mg PO bid. Gonorrhea: 1 g PO single dose.
PEDS - IM/IV cefuroxime. Most infections: 50-100 mg/kg/day IM/IV divided q6-8h. Bone & joint infections: 150 mg/kg/day IM/IV divided q8h not to exceed maximum adult dose. Cefu-

roxime axetil tabs: Group A strep pharyngitis: 125 mg PO bid x 10 days. Otitis media, sinusitis: 250 mg PO bid x 10 days. Cefuroxime axetil oral susp. Group A strep pharyngitis: 20 mg/kg/day (up to 500 mg/day) PO divided bid x 10 days. Otitis media, sinusitis, impetigo: 30 mg/kg/day (up to 1 g/day) PO divided bid x 10 days. Use adult dose for ≥13 yo.
UNAPPROVED PEDS - Early Lyme disease: 30 mg/kg/day PO divided bid (max 500 mg/dose). Community-acquired pneumonia: 150 mg/kg/day IV divided q8h.
FORMS - Generic/trade: Tabs 250,500 mg. Trade: Susp 125 & 250 mg/5 ml.
NOTES - AAP recommends 5-7 days of therapy for older (≥6 yo) children with non-severe otitis media, and 10 days for younger children and those with severe disease. Dosage adjustment for renal dysfunction in adults: 750 mg IM/IV q12h for CrCl 10-20 ml/min, 750 mg IM/IV q24h for CrCl <10 ml/min. Give supplemental dose after hemodialysis. Tabs & susp not bioequivalent on mg/mg basis. Do not crush tabs.

loracarbef (*Lorabid*) ▶K ♀B ▶? $$$$
ADULT - Acute exacerbation of chronic bronchitis, pneumonia, sinusitis, uncomplicated pyelonephritis: 400 mg PO bid. Secondary infection of acute bronchitis: 200-400 mg PO bid. Group A strep pharyngitis: 200 mg PO bid x 10 days. Skin infections: 200 mg PO bid. Simple UTI: 200 mg PO qd. Take on empty stomach.
PEDS - Otitis media (use suspension), sinusitis: 30 mg/kg/day PO divided bid. Use susp for otitis media. Group A strep pharyngitis, impetigo: 15 mg/kg/day up to 500 mg/day PO divided bid. Treat pharyngitis for 10 days. Use adult dose for ≥13 yo. Take on empty stomach.
FORMS - Trade: Caps 200,400 mg, susp 100 & 200 mg/5 ml.
NOTES - Poor activity against penicillin-nonsusceptible pneumococci. Dosing in renal dysfunction: 50% of recommended dose at usual interval or full recommended dose at twice the usual interval for CrCl 10-49 ml/min, give recommended dose q3-5 days for CrCl <10 ml/min. Give supplemental dose following hemodialysis.

CEPHALOSPORINS – GENERAL ANTIMICROBIAL SPECTRUM

1st generation: gram positive (including Staph aureus); basic gram neg. coverage
2nd generation: diminished Staph aureus, improved gram negative coverage compared to 1st generation; some with anaerobic coverage
3rd generation: further diminished Staph aureus, further improved gram negative coverage compared to 1st & 2nd generation; some with Pseudomonal coverage & diminished gram positive coverage
4th generation: same as 3rd generation plus coverage against Pseudomonas

SEXUALLY TRANSMITTED DISEASES & VAGINITIS*

Bacterial vaginosis: 1) metronidazole 5 g of 0.75% gel intravaginally qd for 5 days. 2) metronidazole 500 mg PO bid for 7 days. 3) clindamycin 5 g of 2% cream intravaginally qhs for 7 days. In pregnancy: 1) metronidazole 250 mg PO tid for 7 days. 2) clindamycin 300 mg PO bid for 7 days.

Candidal vaginitis: 1) intravaginal clotrimazole, miconazole, terconazole, nystatin, tioconazole, or butoconazole. 2) fluconazole 150 mg PO single dose.

Chancroid: 1) azithromycin 1 g PO single dose. 2) ceftriaxone 250 mg IM single dose.

Chlamydia: 1) azithromycin 1 g PO single dose. 2) doxycycline 100 mg PO bid for 7 days. 3) ofloxacin 300 mg PO bid for 7 days. 4) levofloxacin 500 mg PO qd for 7 days. 5) erythromycin base 500 mg PO qid for 7 days.

Chlamydia (in pregnancy): 1) erythromycin base 500 mg PO qid for 7 days or 250 mg PO qid for 14 days. 2) amoxicillin 500 mg PO tid for 7 days. 3) azithromycin 1 g PO single dose.

Epididymitis: 1) ceftriaxone 250 mg IM single dose + doxycycline 100 mg PO bid x 10 days. 2) ofloxacin 300 mg PO bid or levofloxacin 500 mg PO qd for 10 days if enteric organisms suspected, cephalosporin/doxycycline allergic, or >35 yo.

Gonorrhea: Single dose of: 1) ceftriaxone 125 mg IM 2) cefixime 400 mg PO single dose 3) ciprofloxacin 500 mg PO 4) ofloxacin 400 mg PO or 5) levofloxacin 250 mg PO. Treat chlamydia empirically. Due to high resistance rates, quinolones not recommended for infections acquired in Hawaii, California, Asia, or Pacific islands, or in men who have sex with men.

Gonorrhea, disseminated: Initially treat with ceftriaxone 1 g IM/IV q24h until 24-48 h after improvement. Alternatives: 1) ciprofloxacin 400 mg IV q12h. 2) ofloxacin 400 mg IV q12h. 3) levofloxacin 250 mg IV qd. 4) spectinomycin 2 g IV q12h. Complete 1 week of treatment with 1) ciprofloxacin 500 mg PO bid. 2) ofloxacin 400 mg PO bid. 3) levofloxacin 500 mg PO qd. Due to high resistance rates, quinolones not recommended for infections acquired in Hawaii, California, Asia or Pacific islands, or in men who have sex with men.

Gonorrhea, meningitis: ceftriaxone 1-2 g IV q12h for 10-14 days.

Gonorrhea, endocarditis: ceftriaxone 1-2 g IV q12h for at least 4 weeks.

Granuloma inguinale: 1) trimethoprim-sulfamethoxazole 1 double-strength tab PO bid for at least 3 weeks. 2) doxycycline 100 mg PO bid for at least 3 weeks.

Herpes simplex (genital, first episode): 1) acyclovir 400 mg PO tid for 7-10 days. 2) famciclovir 250 PO tid for 7-10 days. 3) valacyclovir 1 g PO bid for 7-10 days.

Herpes simplex (genital, recurrent): 1) acyclovir 400 mg PO tid for 5 days. 2) famciclovir 125 mg PO bid for 5 days. 3) valacyclovir 500 mg PO bid for 3-5 days. 4) valacyclovir 1 g PO qd for 5 days.

Herpes simplex (suppressive therapy): 1) acyclovir 400mg PO bid. 2) famciclovir 250 mg PO bid. 3) valacyclovir 500-1000 mg PO qd.

Herpes simplex (genital, recurrent in HIV infection): 1) Acyclovir 400 mg PO tid for 5-10 days. 2) famciclovir 500 mg PO bid for 5-10 days. 3) Valacyclovir 1 g PO bid for 5-10 days.

Herpes simplex (suppressive therapy in HIV infection): 1) Acyclovir 400-800 mg PO bid-tid. 2) Famciclovir 500 mg PO bid. 3) Valacyclovir 500 mg PO bid.

Herpes simplex (prevention of transmission in immunocompetent patients with <=9 recurrences/year): Valacyclovir 500 mg PO qd by source partner, in conjunction with safer sex practices.†

Lymphogranuloma venereum: 1) doxycycline 100 mg PO bid for 21 days. 2) erythromycin base 500 mg PO qid for 21 days.

Pelvic inflammatory disease (PID), inpatient regimens: 1) cefotetan 2 g IV q12h/ cefoxitin 2 g IV q6h + doxycycline 100 mg IV/PO q12h. 2) clindamycin 900 mg IV q8h + gentamicin 2 mg/kg IM/IV loading dose, then 1.5 mg/kg IM/IV q8h (See gentamicin entry for alternative qd dosing). Can switch to PO therapy within 24 h of improvement.

Pelvic inflammatory disease (PID), outpatient treatment: 1) ceftriaxone 250 mg IM single dose + doxycycline 100 mg PO bid +/- metronidazole 500 mg PO bid for 14 days. 2) ofloxacin 400 mg PO bid/ levofloxacin 500 mg PO qd +/- metronidazole 500 mg PO bid for 14 days.

Proctitis, proctocolitis, enteritis: ceftriaxone 125 mg IM single dose + doxycycline 100 mg PO bid x7d.

Sexual assault prophylaxis: ceftriaxone 125 mg IM single dose + metronidazole 2 g PO single dose + azithromycin 1 g PO single dose/doxycycline 100 mg PO bid for 7 days. Consider giving antiemetic.

Syphilis (primary and secondary): 1) benzathine penicillin 2.4 million units IM single dose. 2) doxycycline 100 mg PO bid for 2 weeks if penicillin allergic.

SEXUALLY TRANSMITTED DISEASES & VAGINITIS, continued*

Syphilis (early latent, i.e. duration <1 y): 1) benzathine penicillin 2.4 million units IM single dose. 2) doxycycline 100 mg PO bid for 2 weeks if penicillin allergic.

Syphilis (late latent or unknown duration): 1) benzathine penicillin 2.4 million units IM q week for 3 doses. 2) doxycycline 100 mg PO bid for 4 weeks if penicillin allergic.

Syphilis (tertiary): 1) benzathine penicillin 2.4 million units IM q week for 3 doses. 2) doxycycline 100 mg PO bid for 4 weeks if penicillin allergic.

Syphilis (neuro): 1) penicillin G 18-24 million units/day continuous IV infusion or 3-4 million units IV q4h for 10-14 days. 2) procaine penicillin 2.4 million units IM qd + probenecid 500 mg PO qid, both for 10-14 days.

Syphilis in pregnancy: Treat only with penicillin regimen for stage of syphilis as noted above. Use penicillin desensitization protocol if penicillin-allergic.

Trichomonal vaginitis: metronidazole 2 g PO single dose or 500 mg bid for 7 days. Can use 2 g single dose in pregnant women.

Urethritis, Cervicitis: Test for chlamydia and gonorrhea. Treat based on test results or treat for both if testing not available or if patient unlikely to return for follow-up.

Urethritis (persistent/recurrent): 1) metronidazole 2 g PO single dose + erythromycin base 500 mg PO qid for 7 days.

* MMWR 2002;51:RR-6 or http://www.cdc.gov/std/.   †NEJM 2004;350:11.
Treat sexual partners for all except herpes, candida, and bacterial vaginosis.

ANTIMICROBIALS: Cephalosporins – 3rd Generation

NOTE: Cephalosporins are 2nd-line to penicillin for group A strep pharyngitis, can be cross-sensitive with penicillin, and can cause pseudomembranous colitis.

cefdinir (_Omnicef_) ▶K ♀B ▶? $$$
ADULT - Community-acquired pneumonia, skin infections: 300 mg PO bid x 10 days. Sinusitis: 600 mg PO qd or 300 mg PO bid x 10 days. Group A strep pharyngitis, acute exacerbation of chronic bronchitis: 600 mg PO qd x 10 days or 300 mg PO bid x 5-10 days.
PEDS - Group A strep pharyngitis, otitis media: 14 mg/kg/day PO divided bid x 5-10 days or qd x 10 days. Sinusitis: 14 mg/kg/day PO divided qd-bid x 10 days. Skin infections: 14 mg/kg/day PO divided bid x 10 days. Use adult dose for ≥13 yo.
FORMS - Trade: Cap 300 mg, susp 125 mg/5 ml.
NOTES - AAP recommends 5-7 days of therapy for older (≥6 yo) children with non-severe otitis media, and 10 days for younger children and those with severe disease. Complexation with iron may turn stools red. Dosage reduction for renal dysfunction: 300 mg PO qd for adults with CrCl <30 ml/min. 7 mg/kg/day PO qd up to 300 mg/day for children with CrCl <30 ml/min. Hemodialysis: 300 mg or 7 mg/kg PO after hemodialysis, then 300 mg or 7 mg/kg PO qod.

cefditoren (_Spectracef_) ▶K ♀B ▶? $$
ADULT - Skin infections, group A strep pharyn-

gitis: 200 mg PO bid x 10 days. Give 400 mg bid x 10 days for acute exacerbation of chronic bronchitis, x 14 days for community-acquired pneumonia. Take with food.
PEDS - Not approved for <12 yo. Skin infections, group A strep pharyngitis, adolescents ≥12 yo: 200 mg PO bid with food x 10 days.
FORMS - Trade: Tabs 200 mg.
NOTES - Contraindicated if milk protein allergy or carnitine deficiency. Not for long-term use due to potential risk of carnitine deficiency. Do not take with drugs that reduce gastric acid (antacids, H2 blockers, etc). Dosage adjustment for renal dysfunction: Not more than 200 mg bid if CrCl 30-49 ml/min, not more than 200 mg qd if CrCl <30 ml/min.

cefixime (_Suprax_) ▶K/Bile ♀B ▶? ?
ADULT - Simple UTI, pharyngitis, acute bacterial bronchitis, acute exacerbation of chronic bronchitis: 400 mg PO qd or 200 mg PO bid. Gonorrhea: 400 mg PO single dose.
PEDS - Otitis media: 8 mg/kg/day susp PO divided qd-bid. Pharyngitis: 8 mg/kg/day PO divided qd-bid x 10 days. Use adult dose for >50 kg or ≥13 yo.
UNAPPROVED PEDS - Febrile UTI (3-24 mo): 16 mg/kg PO on first day, then 8 mg/kg PO qd to complete 14 days. Gonorrhea: 8 mg/kg (max 400 mg) PO single dose for <45 kg, 400 mg PO single dose for ≥45 kg.
FORMS - Generic: Tabs 200,400 mg, susp 100

mg/5 ml.

NOTES - Generic cefixime, marketed under Suprax brand name, approved by FDA in February 2004; Suprax had been discontinued by manufacturer in 2002. Cross-sensitivity with penicillins possible, pseudomembranous colitis. Poor activity against S aureus. Increased INR with warfarin. May increase carbamazepine levels. Susp stable at room temp or refrigerated x 14 days. Dosing in renal dysfunction: 75% of usual dose at usual interval for CrCl 21-60 ml/min or hemodialysis. 50% of usual dose at usual interval for CrCl <20 ml/min or continuous peritoneal dialysis.

cefoperazone (*Cefobid*) ▶Bile/K ♀B ▶? $$$$$

ADULT - Peritonitis, sepsis, respiratory, intra-abdominal, skin infections, endometritis, pelvic inflammatory disease & other gynecologic infections: Usual dose 2-4 g/day IV divided q12h. Infections with less sensitive organisms/severe infections: 6-12 g/day IV divided q6-12h. Use q6h for Pseudomonas infections. 1-2 g doses can be given IM.

PEDS - Not approved in children.

UNAPPROVED PEDS - Mild to moderate infections, age ≥1 mo: 100-150 mg/kg/day IM/IV divided q8-12h.

NOTES - Possible clotting impairment. Disulfiram-like reaction w/ alcohol. Not for meningitis.

cefotaxime (*Claforan*) ▶KL ♀B ▶+ $$$$$

ADULT - Pneumonia, sepsis, GU & gynecologic, skin, intra-abdominal, bone & joint infections: Uncomplicated, 1 g IM/IV q12h. Moderate/severe, 1-2 g IM/IV q8h. Infections usually requiring high doses, 2 g IV q6-8h. Life-threatening, 2 g IV q4h. Meningitis: 2g IV q4-6h. Gonorrhea: 0.5-1 g IM single dose.

PEDS - Neonates, ≤1 week old: 50 mg/kg/dose IV q12h. 1-4 weeks old: 50 mg/kg/dose IV q8h. Labeled dose for pneumonia, sepsis, GU, skin, intra-abdominal, bone/joint, CNS infections, 1 mo-12 yo: 50-180 mg/kg/day IM/IV divided q4-6h. AAP recommendations: 225-300 mg/kg/day IV divided q6-8h for S pneumoniae meningitis. Mild to moderate infections: 75-100 mg/kg/day IV/IM divided q6-8h. Severe infections: 150-200 mg/kg/day IV/IM divided q6-8h.

NOTES - Bolus injection through central venous catheter can cause arrhythmias. Decrease dose by 50% for CrCl <20 ml/min.

cefpodoxime (*Vantin*) ▶K ♀B ▶? $$$$

ADULT - Acute exacerbation of chronic bronchitis, acute sinusitis: 200 mg PO bid x 10 days. Community-acquired pneumonia: 200 mg PO bid x 14 days. Group A strep pharyngitis: 100

mg PO bid x 5-10 days. Skin infections: 400 mg PO bid x 7-14 days. Simple UTI: 100 mg PO bid x 7 days. Gonorrhea: 200 mg PO single dose. Give tabs with food.

PEDS - 5 mg/kg PO bid x 5 days for otitis media, x 5-10 days for group A strep pharyngitis, x 10 days for sinusitis. Use adult dose if ≥12 yo.

FORMS - Trade: Tabs 100,200 mg, susp 50 & 100 mg/5 ml.

NOTES - AAP recommends 5-7 days of therapy for older (≥6 yo) children with non-severe otitis media, and 10 days for younger children and those with severe disease. Do not give antacids within 2 h before/after cefpodoxime. Dosing in renal dysfunction: Increase dosing interval to q24h for CrCl <30 ml/min. Give 3 times/week after dialysis for hemodialysis patients. Susp stable for 14 days refrigerated.

ceftazidime (*Ceptaz, Fortaz, Tazidime, Tazicef*) ▶K ♀B ▶+ $$$$$

ADULT - Simple UTI: 250 mg IM/IV q12h. Complicated UTI: 500 mg IM/IV q8-12h. Uncomplicated pneumonia, mild skin infections: 500 mg - 1g IM/IV q8h. Serious gynecologic, intra-abdominal, bone & joint, life-threatening infections, meningitis, empiric therapy of neutropenic fever: 2 g IV q8h. Pseudomonas lung infections in cystic fibrosis: 30-50 mg/kg IV q8h to max of 6 g/day.

PEDS - Use sodium formulations in children (Fortaz, Tazidime, Tazicef). UTIs, pneumonia, skin, intra-abdominal, bone & joint infections, 1 mo - 12 yo: 100-150 mg/kg/day IV divided q8h to max of 6 g/day. Meningitis, 1 mo - 12 yo: 150 mg/kg/day IV divided q8h to max of 6 g/day. Infants up to 4 weeks old: 30 mg/kg IV q12h. Use adult dose & formulations if ≥12 yo.

UNAPPROVED ADULT - P aeruginosa osteomyelitis of the foot from nail puncture: 2 g IV q8h.

UNAPPROVED PEDS - AAP dosing for infants >2 kg: 50 mg/kg IV q8-12h for <1 week old, q8h for ≥1 week old.

NOTES - High levels in renal dysfunction can cause CNS toxicity. Dosing in adults with renal dysfunction: 1 g IV q12h for CrCl 31-50 ml/min; 1 g q24h for CrCl 16-30 ml/min; load with 1 g, then 500 mg q24h for CrCl 6-15 ml/min; load with 1 g, then 500 mg q48h for CrCl <5 ml/min. 1 g IV load in hemodialysis patients, then 1 g IV after hemodialysis sessions.

ceftibuten (*Cedax*) ▶K ♀B ▶? $$$

ADULT - Group A strep pharyngitis, acute exacerbation of chronic bronchitis, otitis media not due to S pneumoniae: 400 mg PO qd x 10 days.

PEDS - Group A strep pharyngitis, otitis media not due to S pneumoniae, age >6 mo: 9 mg/kg up to 400 mg PO qd. Give susp on empty stomach.

FORMS - Trade: Cap 400 mg, susp 90 mg/5 ml.

NOTES - Poor activity against S aureus and S pneumoniae. Dosing in adults with renal dysfunction: 200 mg PO qd for CrCl 30-49 ml/min, 100 mg PO qd for CrCl 5-29 ml/min. Dosing in children with renal dysfunction: 4.5 mg/kg PO qd for CrCl 30-49 ml/min, 2.25 mg/kg PO qd for CrCl 5-29 ml/min. Hemodialysis: adults 400 mg PO & children 9 mg/kg PO after each dialysis session. Susp stable for 14 days refrigerated.

ceftizoxime (Cefizox) ▶K ♀B ▶? $$$$$

ADULT - Simple UTI: 500 mg IM/IV q12h. Pneumonia, sepsis, intra-abdominal, skin, bone & joint infections: 1-2 g IM/IV q8-12h. Pelvic inflammatory disease: 2 g IV q8h. Life-threatening infections: 3-4 g IV q8h. Gonorrhea: 1 g IM single dose. Split 2 g IM dose into 2 injections.

PEDS - Pneumonia, sepsis, intra-abdominal, skin, bone & joint infections, age ≥6 mo: 50 mg/kg/dose IV q6-8h. Up to 200 mg/kg/day for serious infections, not to exceed max adult dose.

NOTES - Can cause transient rise in eosinophils, ALT, AST, CPK in children. Not for meningitis. Dosing in adults with renal dysfunction: For less severe infection load with 500 mg - 1 g IM/IV, then 500 mg q8h for CrCl 50-79 ml/min, 250-500 mg q12h for CrCl 5-49 ml/min, 500 mg q48h or 250 mg q24h for hemodialysis. For life-threatening infection, give loading dose, then 750 mg - 1.5 g IV q8h for CrCl 50-79 ml/min, 500 mg - 1 g q12h for CrCl 5-49 ml/min, 500 mg - 1 g q48h or 500 mg q24h for hemodialysis. For hemodialysis patients, give dose at end of dialysis.

ceftriaxone (Rocephin) ▶K/Bile ♀B ▶+ $$$$$

ADULT - Pneumonia, UTI, pelvic inflammatory disease (hospitalized), sepsis, meningitis, skin, bone & joint, intra-abdominal infections: Usual dose 1-2 g IM/IV q24h (max 4 g/day divided q12h). Gonorrhea: single dose 125 mg IM (250 mg if ambulatory treatment of PID).

PEDS - Meningitis: 100 mg/kg/day (max 4 g/day) IV divided q12-24h. Skin, pneumonia, other serious infections: 50-75 mg/kg/day (max 2 g/day) IM/IV divided q12-24h. Otitis media: 50 mg/kg (max 1 g) IM single dose.

UNAPPROVED ADULT - Lyme disease carditis, arthritis, meningitis: 2 g IV qd. Chancroid: 250 mg IM single dose. Disseminated gonorrhea: 1 g IM/IV q24h. Prophylaxis, invasive meningococcal disease: 250 mg IM single dose.

UNAPPROVED PEDS - Refractory otitis media (no response after 3 days of antibiotics): 50 mg/kg IM q24h x 3 doses. Lyme disease carditis, arthritis, meningitis: 75-100 mg/kg IM/IV qd (max 2 g/day). Prophylaxis, invasive meningococcal disease: Single IM dose of 125 mg for ≤15 yo, 250 mg for >15 yo. Gonorrhea: 125 mg IM single dose; use adult regimens in STD table if ≥45 kg. Gonococcal bacteremia/arthritis: 50 mg/kg (max 1 g if <45 kg) IM/IV qd x 7 days. Gonococcal ophthalmia neonatorum/ gonorrhea prophylaxis in newborn: 25-50 mg/kg up to 125 mg IM/IV single dose at birth. Disseminated gonorrhea, infants: 25-50 mg/kg/day IM/IV qd x 7 days. Typhoid fever: 50-75 mg/kg IM/IV qd x 14 days.

NOTES - Can cause prolonged prothrombin time (due to vitamin K deficiency), biliary sludging/symptoms of gallbladder disease. Do not give to neonates with hyperbilirubinemia. Dilute in 1% lidocaine for IM use. Do not exceed 2 g/day in patients with both hepatic & renal dysfunction.

ANTIMICROBIALS: Cephalosporins – 4th Generation

NOTE: Cross-sensitivity with penicillins possible. May can cause pseudomembranous colitis.

cefepime (Maxipime) ▶K ♀B ▶? $$$$$

ADULT - Mild, moderate UTI: 0.5-1 g IM/IV q12h. Severe UTI, complicated intra-abdominal, skin infections: 2 g IV q12h. Pneumonia: 1-2 g IV q12h. Empiric therapy of febrile neutropenia: 2 g IV q8h.

PEDS - UTI, skin infections, pneumonia, ≤40 kg: 50 mg/kg IV q12h. Empiric therapy for febrile neutropenia, ≤40 kg: 50 mg/kg IV q8h. Do not exceed adult dose.

UNAPPROVED ADULT - P aeruginosa osteomyelitis of the foot from nail puncture: 2 g IV q12h.

NOTES - High levels in renal dysfunction can cause CNS toxicity; dosing for CrCl <60 ml/min in package insert.

ANTIMICROBIALS: Ketolides

telithromycin (*Ketek*) ▶LK ♀C ▶? $$$$
ADULT - 800 mg PO qd x 5 days for acute exacerbation of chronic bronchitis, acute sinusitis, x 7 days for community-acquired pneumonia.
PEDS – Safety and efficacy not established.
FORMS - Trade: 400 mg tabs. Ketek Pak: #10, 400 mg tabs.
NOTES - May prolong QT interval. Avoid using in proarrhythmic conditions or with drugs that prolong QT interval. Cytochrome P450 3A4

substrate and inhibitor. Contraindicated with cisapride, pimozide, rifampin, ergot alkaloids. Withhold simvastatin, lovastatin, or atorvastatin during course of telithromycin. Give telithromycin and theophylline at least 1 h apart. Monitor for increased toxicity of digoxin, midazolam, metoprolol. Cytochrome P450 3A4 inducers (ie phenytoin, carbamazepine) could reduce telithromycin levels. Dosage adjustment for CrCl <30 ml/min not established.

ANTIMICROBIALS: Macrolides

azithromycin (*Zithromax*) ▶L ♀B ▶? $$
ADULT - Community-acquired pneumonia: 500 mg IV over 1 h qd x ≥2 days, then 500 mg PO qd x 7-10 days total. Pelvic inflammatory disease: 500 mg IV qd x 1-2 days, then 250 mg PO qd to complete 7 days. Oral for acute exacerbation of chronic bronchitis, community-acquired pneumonia, group A streptococcal pharyngitis (second-line to penicillin), skin infections: 500 mg PO on 1st day, then 250 mg PO qd to complete 5 days. Acute sinusitis, alternative for acute exacerbation of chronic bronchitis: 500 mg PO qd x 3 days. Chlamydia, chancroid: 1 g PO single dose. Gonorrhea: 2 g PO single dose. Observe patient for ≥30 minutes for poor GI tolerability. Prevention of disseminated Mycobacterium avium complex disease: 1200 mg PO q week.
PEDS - Oral for otitis media, community-acquired pneumonia: 10 mg/kg up to 500 mg PO on 1st day, then 5 mg/kg up to 250 mg PO qd to complete 5 days. Acute sinusitis: 10 mg/kg PO qd x 3 days. Short regimens for otitis media: 30 mg/kg PO single dose or 10 mg/kg PO qd x 3 days. Group A streptococcal pharyngitis (second-line to penicillin): 12 mg/kg up to 500 mg PO qd x 5 days. Take susp on empty stomach.
UNAPPROVED ADULT - See table for prophylaxis of bacterial endocarditis. Nongonococcal urethritis: 1 g PO single dose. Campylobacter gastroenteritis: 500 mg PO qd x 3 days. Traveler's diarrhea: 500 mg PO on 1st day, then 250 mg PO qd to complete 5 days; or 1 g PO single dose. Mycobacterium avium complex disease treatment in AIDS: 500 mg PO qd (use ≥2 drugs for active infection). Pertussis: 500 mg PO qd x 5-7 days.
UNAPPROVED PEDS - Prevention of disseminated Mycobacterium avium complex disease:

20 mg/kg PO q week not to exceed adult dose. Mycobacterium avium complex disease treatment: 5 mg/kg PO qd (use ≥2 drugs for active infection). Cystic fibrosis & colonized with P aeruginosa (≥6 yo): 250 mg (<40 kg) or 500 mg (≥40 kg) PO three times weekly x 24 weeks. Chlamydia trachomatis (≥8 yo, or <8 yo & ≥45 kg): 1 g PO single dose. Pertussis: 10-12 mg/kg PO qd x 5-7 days. See table for bacterial endocarditis prophylaxis. Traveler's diarrhea: 5-10 mg/kg PO single dose. Cholera: 20 mg/kg up to 1 g PO single dose.
FORMS - Trade: Tab 250,600 mg, packet 1000 mg, susp 100 & 200 mg/5 ml. Z-Pak: #6, 250 mg tab. Tri-Pak: #3, 500 mg tab.
NOTES - Severe allergic/skin reactions rarely, IV site reactions, hearing loss with prolonged use. Potential for QT interval prolongation and torsades cannot be excluded in patients at risk for prolonged cardiac repolarization. Does not inhibit cytochrome P450 enzymes. Do not take at the same time as Al/Mg antacids. Contraindicated with pimozide. Single dose and 3-day regimens cause more vomiting than 5-day regimen for otitis media. Mechanism of action in cystic fibrosis is unknown; macrolides may inhibit P aeruginosa virulence factors or reduce inflammation.

clarithromycin (*Biaxin, Biaxin XL*) ▶KL ♀C ▶? $$$
ADULT - Group A streptococcal pharyngitis (second-line to penicillin): 250 mg PO bid x 10 days. Acute sinusitis: 500 mg PO bid x 14 days. Acute exacerbation of chronic bronchitis (S pneumoniae/M catarrhalis), community-acquired pneumonia, skin infections: 250 mg PO bid x 7-14 days. Acute exacerbation of chronic bronchitis (H influenzae): 500 mg PO bid x 7-14 days. H pylori: See table in GI sec-

tion. Mycobacterium avium complex disease prevention/ treatment: 500 mg PO bid. Two or more drugs are needed for the treatment of active mycobacterial infections. Biaxin XL: Acute sinusitis: 1000 mg PO qd x 14 days. Acute exacerbation of chronic bronchitis, community-acquired pneumonia: 1000 mg PO qd x 7 days. Take Biaxin XL with food.

PEDS - Group A streptococcal pharyngitis (second-line to penicillin), community-acquired pneumonia, sinusitis, otitis media, skin infections: 7.5 mg/kg PO bid x 10 days. Mycobacterium avium complex prevention/treatment: 7.5 mg/kg up to 500 mg PO bid. Two or more drugs are needed for the treatment of active mycobacterial infections.

UNAPPROVED ADULT - See table for prophylaxis of bacterial endocarditis. Pertussis: 500 mg PO bid x 14 days. Community-acquired pneumonia: 500 mg PO bid.

UNAPPROVED PEDS - See table for prophylaxis of bacterial endocarditis. Pertussis: 7.5 mg/kg PO bid x 14 days. Prophylaxis of pertussis in household contacts: 7.5 mg/kg PO bid x 14 days.

FORMS - Trade: Tab 250,500 mg, susp 125, 187.5 & 250 mg/5 ml. Extended release tabs (Biaxin XL) 500 mg. Biaxin XL-Pak: #14, 500 mg tabs.

NOTES - Rare arrhythmias in patients with prolonged QT. Cytochrome P450 3A4 & 1A2 inhibitor. Contraindicated with cisapride, pimozide. Many drug interactions including increased levels of carbamazepine, cyclosporine, digoxin, disopyramide, lovastatin, rifabutin, simvastatin (avoid), tacrolimus, theophylline. Toxicity with ergotamine/ dihydroergotamine. Monitor INR with warfarin. Clarithromycin levels decreased by efavirenz (avoid concomitant use) and nevirapine enough to impair efficacy in Mycobacterium avium complex disease. AAP recommends 5-7 days of therapy for older (≥6 yo) children with non-severe otitis media, and 10 days for younger children and those with severe disease. Dosage reduction for renal insufficiency patients taking ritonavir or lopinavir/ ritonavir (Kaletra): Decrease by 50% for CrCl 30-60 ml/min, decrease by 75% for CrCl <30 ml/min. Reduce clarithromycin dose by 50% if given with atazanavir; consider alternative for indications other than Mycobacterium avium complex. Do not refrigerate susp.

dirithromycin (Dynabac) ▶L ♀C ▶? $$$
ADULT - 500 mg PO qd x 5-7 days for acute exacerbation of chronic bronchitis and skin in-

fections, x 7 days for secondary infection of acute bronchitis, x 10 days for group A streptococcal pharyngitis (second-line to penicillin), and x 14 days for community-acquired pneumonia. Take with food or within 1 h of eating.

PEDS - Not approved in children <12 yo.

FORMS - Trade: Tab 250 mg. Dynabac D5-Pak: #10, 250 mg tabs.

NOTES - Serum levels too low to treat bacteremia.

erythromycin base (Eryc, E-mycin, Ery-Tab, ✤Erybid, Erythromid) ▶L ♀B ▶+ $
ADULT - Respiratory, skin infections: 250-500 mg PO qid or 333 mg PO tid. Mycoplasma pneumonia, pertussis: 500 mg PO q6h. S aureus skin infections: 250 mg PO q6h or 500 mg PO q12h. Secondary prevention of rheumatic fever: 250 mg PO bid. Chlamydia in pregnancy, nongonococcal urethritis: 500 mg PO qid x 7 days. Alternative for chlamydia in pregnancy if high dose not tolerated: 250 mg PO qid x 14 days. Erythrasma: 250 mg PO tid x 21 days. Legionnaires' disease: 2 g/day PO in divided doses x 14-21 days.

PEDS - Usual dose: 30-50 mg/kg/day PO divided qid x 10 days. Can double dose for severe infections. Pertussis: 40-50 mg/kg/day PO divided qid x 14 days. Chlamydia, newborn - <45 kg: 50 mg/kg/day PO divided qid x 14 days.

UNAPPROVED ADULT - Chancroid: 500 mg PO tid x 7 days. Campylobacter gastroenteritis: 500 mg PO bid x 5 days.

FORMS - Generic/Trade: Tab 250, 333, 500 mg, delayed-release cap 250.

NOTES - Rare arrhythmias in patients with prolonged QT. May aggravate myasthenia gravis. Hypertrophic pyloric stenosis in infants primarily ≤2 weeks of age. Cytochrome P450 3A4 & 1A2 inhibitor. Many drug interactions including increased levels of carbamazepine, cyclosporine, digoxin, disopyramide, tacrolimus, theophylline, some benzodiazepines and statins (avoid simvastatin). Monitor INR with warfarin. Contraindicated with cisapride, pimozide.

erythromycin estolate ▶L ♀B ▶+ $
WARNING - Hepatotoxicity, primarily in adults.
ADULT - Other erythromycin forms preferred in adults.

PEDS - Usual dose: 30-50 mg/kg/day PO divided bid-qid. Can double dose for severe infections. Group A streptococcal pharyngitis: 20-40 mg/kg/day (up to 1 g/day) PO divided bid to qid x 10d. Secondary prevention of rheumatic fever: 250 mg PO bid. Pertussis: 40-50 mg/kg/day PO divided qid x 14 days.

FORMS - Generic: Caps 250 mg, susp 125 & 250 mg/5 ml.

NOTES - Contraindicated in liver disease. Rare arrhythmias in patients with prolonged QT. May aggravate myasthenia gravis. Hypertrophic pyloric stenosis in infants primarily ≤2 weeks of age. Cytochrome 450 3A4 & 1A2 inhibitor. Many drug interactions including increased levels of carbamazepine, cyclosporine, digoxin, disopyramide, tacrolimus, theophylline, some benzodiazepines and statins. Monitor INR with warfarin. Contraindicated with cisapride, pimozide.

erythromycin ethyl succinate (EES, Eryped) ▶L ♀B ▶+ $

ADULT - Usual dose: 400 mg PO qid. Nongonococcal urethritis: 800 mg PO qid x 7 days. Chlamydia in pregnancy: 800 mg PO qid x 7 days or 400 mg PO qid x 14 days if high dose not tolerated. Secondary prevention of rheumatic fever: 400 mg PO bid. Legionnaires' disease: 3.2 g/day in divided doses x 14-21 days.

PEDS - Usual dose: 30-50 mg/kg/day PO divided qid. Maximum dose: 100 mg/kg/day. Group A streptococcal pharyngitis: 40 mg/kg/day (up to 1 g/day) PO divided bid to qid x 10 days. Secondary prevention of rheumatic fever: 400 mg PO bid. Pertussis: 40-50 mg/kg/day up to 2 g/day PO divided qid x 14 days.

FORMS - Generic/Trade: Tab 400 tab, susp 200 & 400 mg/5 ml. Trade: Chew tab 200 tab.

NOTES - Rare arrhythmias in patients with prolonged QT. May aggravate myasthenia gravis. Hypertrophic pyloric stenosis in infants primarily ≤2 weeks of age. Cytochrome P450 3A4 & 1A2 inhibitor. Many drug interactions including increased levels of carbamazepine, cyclosporine, digoxin, disopyramide, tacrolimus, theophylline, some benzodiazepines and statins (avoid simvastatin). Monitor INR with warfarin. Contraindicated with cisapride, pimozide.

erythromycin lactobionate (✦Erythrocin IV) ▶L ♀B ▶+ $$$$

ADULT - For severe infections/PO not possible: 15-20 mg/kg/day (max 4g) IV divided q6h. Legionnaires' disease: 4 g/day IV divided q6h.

PEDS - For severe infections/PO not possible: 15-20 mg/kg/day (max 4g) IV divided q6h.

UNAPPROVED PEDS - 20-50 mg/kg/day IV divided q6h.

NOTES - Dilute and give slowly to minimize venous irritation. Reversible hearing loss (increased risk in elderly given ≥4 g/day), allergic reactions, arrhythmias in patients with prolonged QT, exacerbation of myasthenia gravis. Hypertrophic pyloric stenosis in infants primarily ≤2 weeks of age. Cytochrome P450 3A4 & 1A2 inhibitor. Many drug interactions including increased levels of carbamazepine, cyclosporine, digoxin, disopyramide, tacrolimus, theophylline, some benzodiazepines and statins (avoid simvastatin). Monitor INR with warfarin. Contraindicated with cisapride, pimozide.

Pediazole (erythromycin ethyl succinate + sulfisoxazole) ▶KL ♀C ▶- $

PEDS - Otitis media, age >2 mo: 50 mg/kg/day (based on EES dose) PO divided tid-qid.

FORMS - Generic/Trade: Susp, erythromycin ethyl succinate 200 mg + sulfisoxazole 600 mg/5 ml.

NOTES - Sulfisoxazole: Stevens-Johnson syndrome, toxic epidermal necrolysis, hepatotoxicity, blood dyscrasia, hemolysis in G6PD deficiency. Increased INR with warfarin. Erythromycin: Rare arrhythmias in patients with prolonged QT. May aggravate myasthenia gravis. Cytochrome P450 3A4 & 1A2 inhibitor. Many drug interactions including increased levels of carbamazepine, cyclosporine, digoxin, disopyramide, tacrolimus, theophylline, some benzodiazepines and statins. Monitor INR with warfarin. Contraindicated with cisapride, pimozide. AAP recommends 5-7 days of therapy for older (≥6 yo) children with non-severe otitis media, and 10 days for younger children and those with severe disease.

ANTIMICROBIALS: Penicillins – 1st Generation – Natural

NOTE: Anaphylaxis occurs rarely with penicillins; cross-sensitivity with cephalosporins is possible.

benzathine penicillin (Bicillin L-A, ✦Megacillin) ▶K ♀B ▶? $

ADULT - Group A streptococcal pharyngitis: 1.2 million units IM single dose. Secondary prevention of rheumatic fever: 1.2 million units IM q month (q 3 weeks for high-risk patients) or 600,000 units IM q 2 weeks. Primary, secondary, early latent syphilis: 2.4 million units IM single dose. Tertiary, late latent syphilis: 2.4 million units IM q week x 3 doses.

PEDS - Group A streptococcal pharyngitis (AHA regimen): 600,000 units IM for ≤27 kg, 1.2 million units IM for >27 kg. Secondary prevention of rheumatic fever: 1.2 million units IM q month (q 3 weeks for high-risk patients) or 600,000 units IM q 2 weeks. Primary, secondary, early latent syphilis: 50,000 units/kg (up to 2.4 million units) IM single dose. Late latent syphilis: 50,000 units/ kg (up to 2.4 million units) IM x 3 weekly doses.

UNAPPROVED ADULT - Prophylaxis of diphtheria/treatment of carriers: 1.2 million units IM single dose.

UNAPPROVED PEDS - Prophylaxis of diphtheria/treatment of carriers: 1.2 million units IM single dose for ≥30 kg or ≥6 yo. 600,000 units IM single dose for <30 kg or <6 yo.

FORMS - 600,000 units/ml; 1, 2, 4 ml syringes.

NOTES - Do not give IV. Doses last 2-4 wks. Not for neurosyphilis.

benzylpenicilloyl polylysine (Pre-Pen) ▶K ♀? ▶? $

ADULT - Skin testing for penicillin allergy: 1 drop in needle scratch, then 0.01-0.02 ml intradermally if no reaction.

PEDS - Not approved in children.

NOTES - Systemic allergic reactions; do not test if known to be highly sensitive to penicillin. See CDC 2002 STD guideline for penicillin allergy skin testing protocols.

Bicillin C-R (procaine penicillin + benzathine penicillin) ▶K ♀B ▶? $

ADULT - Scarlet fever, erysipelas, upper-respiratory, skin and soft-tissue infections due to Group A strep: 2.4 million units IM single dose. Pneumococcal infections other than meningitis: 1.2 million units IM q2-3 days until temperature normal x 48 h.

PEDS - Scarlet fever, erysipelas, upper-respiratory, skin & soft-tissue infections due to Group A strep: 2.4 million units IM for >27 kg, 900,000-1.2 million units IM for 13.6-27 kg, 600,000 units IM for <13.6 kg. Pneumococcal infections other than meningitis: 600,000 units IM q2-3 days until temperature normal x 48 h.

FORMS - Trade: for IM use in mixes of 1.2/1.2 million, 300/300, 600/600, 300/900 thousand units procaine/benzathine penicillin.

NOTES - Contraindicated if allergic to procaine. Do not give IV.

penicillin G ▶K ♀B ▶? $$$

ADULT - Penicillin-sensitive pneumococcal pneumonia: 8-12 million units/day IV divided q4-6h. Penicillin-sensitive pneumococcal meningitis: 24 million units/day IV divided q2-4h. Empiric therapy, native valve endocarditis: 20 million units/day IV continuous infusion or divided q4h plus nafcillin/oxacillin and gentamicin. Neurosyphilis: 18-24 million units/day continuous IV infusion or 3-4 million units IV q4h x 10-14 d. Bioterrorism anthrax: See www.

idsociety.org/BT/ToC.htm.

PEDS - Mild to moderate infections: 25,000-50,000 units/kg/day IV divided q6h. Severe infections including pneumococcal and meningococcal meningitis: 250,000-400,000 units/day IV divided q4-6h. Neonates <1 week, >2 kg: 25,000 units/kg IV q8h. Neonates ≥1 week, >2 kg: 25,000 units/kg IV q6h. Group B streptococcal meningitis: ≤7 days old, 250,000-450,000 units/kg/d IV divided q8h. >7 days old, 450,000-500,000 units/kg/d IV divided q4-6h. Congenital syphilis: 50,000 units/kg/dose IV q12h during first 7 days of life, then q8h thereafter to complete 10d. Congenital syphilis or neurosyphilis in children >1 month old: 50,000 units/kg IV q4-6 h x 10 days.

UNAPPROVED ADULT - Prevention of perinatal group B streptococcal disease: Give to mother 5 million units IV at onset of labor/after membrane rupture, then 2.5 million units IV q4h until delivery. Diphtheria: 100,000-150,000 units/kg/day IV divided q6h x 14 days.

UNAPPROVED PEDS - Diphtheria: 100,000-150,000 units/kg/day IV divided q6h x 14 days.

NOTES - Decrease dose by 50% if CrCl <10 ml/min.

penicillin V (Pen-Vee K, Veetids, ✚PVF) ▶K ♀B ▶? $

ADULT - Usual dose: 250-500 mg PO qid. AHA dosing for group A streptococcal pharyngitis: 500 mg PO bid or tid x 10 days. Secondary prevention of rheumatic fever: 250 mg PO bid. Vincent's infection: 250 mg PO q6-8h.

PEDS - Usual dose: 25-50 mg/kg/day PO divided tid or qid. Use adult dose for ≥12 yo. AHA dosing for group A streptococcal pharyngitis: 250 mg PO bid or tid x 10 days. Secondary prevention of rheumatic fever: 250 mg PO bid.

UNAPPROVED PEDS - Prevention of pneumococcal infections in functional/anatomic asplenia: 125 mg PO bid for <3 yo, 250 mg PO bid for ≥3 yo.

FORMS - Generic/Trade: Tabs 250,500 mg, oral soln 125 & 250 mg/5 ml.

NOTES - Oral soln stable in refrigerator for 14 days.

procaine penicillin (Wycillin) ▶K ♀B ▶? $$$

ADULT - Pneumococcal & streptococcal infections, Vincent's infection, erysipeloid: 0.6-1.0 million units IM qd. Neurosyphilis: 2.4 million units IM qd plus probenecid 500 mg PO q6h, both x 10-14 days.

PEDS - Pneumococcal & streptococcal infections, Vincent's infection, erysipeloid, <27 kg: 300,000 units IM qd. AAP dose for mild-tomoderate infections, >1 mo: 25,000-50,000 units/kg/day IM divided qd-bid. Congenital syphilis: 50,000 units/kg IM qd x 10 days.

NOTES - Peak 4h, lasts 24h. Contraindicated if procaine allergy; skin test if allergy suspected. Transient CNS reactions with high doses.

ANTIMICROBIALS: Penicillins – 2nd Generation – Penicillinase-Resistant

NOTE: Anaphylaxis occurs rarely with penicillins; cross-sensitivity with cephalosporins is possible.

cloxacillin (♥*Orbenin*) ▶KL ♀B ▶? $$
ADULT - Staph infections: 250-500 mg PO qid on empty stomach. Severe infections: 1-2 g IV/IM q4h. Staph osteomyelitis: 2 g IV/IM q6h. IV/IM not available in US.
PEDS - Staph infections: 50-100 mg/kg/day PO divided q6h on empty stomach. Use adult dose for ≥20 kg.
FORMS - Generic: Caps 250,500 mg, oral soln 125 mg/5 ml. Parenteral not available in US.
NOTES - Oral soln stable in refrigerator x 14 d.

dicloxacillin (*Dynapen*) ▶KL ♀B ▶? $$
ADULT - Usual dose: 250-500 mg PO qid. Take on empty stomach.
PEDS - Mild to moderate upper respiratory, skin & soft-tissue infections, age >1 mo: 12.5 mg/kg/day PO divided qid. Pneumonia, disseminated infections, age >1 mo: 25 mg/kg/day PO divided qid. Follow-up therapy after IV antibiotics for Staph osteomyelitis: 50-100 mg/kg/day PO divided qid. Use adult dose for ≥40 kg. Give on empty stomach.
FORMS - Generic: Caps 250,500 mg. Trade: Susp 62.5 mg/5 ml.
NOTES - Oral susp stable at room temperature for 7d, in refrigerator 14d.

nafcillin (*Nallpen*) ▶L ♀B ▶? $$$$$
ADULT - Staph infections, usual dose: 500 mg IM q4-6h or 500-2000 mg IV q4h. Osteomyelitis: 1-2 g IV q4h. Empiric therapy, native valve endocarditis: 2 g IV q4h plus penicillin/ampicillin and gentamicin.
PEDS - Staph infections, usual dose: Neonates, 10 mg/kg IM q12h. <40 kg, 25 mg/kg IM q12h.
UNAPPROVED PEDS - Mild to moderate infections: 50-100 mg/kg/day IM/IV divided q6h. Severe infections: 100-200 mg/kg/day IM/IV divided q4-6h. Neonates <1 week, >2 kg: 25 mg/kg IM/IV q8h. Neonates ≥1 week, >2 kg: 25-35 mg/kg IM/IV q6h.
NOTES - Reversible neutropenia with prolonged use. Decreased INR with warfarin. Decreased cyclosporine levels.

oxacillin (*Bactocill*) ▶KL ♀B ▶? $
ADULT - Staph infections: 250 mg-2g IM/IV q4-6h. Osteomyelitis: 1.5-2 g IV q4h. Empiric therapy, native valve endocarditis: 2 g IV q4h with penicillin/ampicillin and gentamicin.
PEDS - Mild to moderate infections: 100-150 mg/kg/day IM/IV divided q6h. Severe infections: 150-200 mg/kg/day IM/IV divided q4-6h. Use adult dose for ≥40 kg. AAP regimens for newborns >2 kg: <1 week, 25-50 mg/kg IM/IV q8h. ≥1 week, 25-50 mg/kg IM/IV q6h.
NOTES - Hepatic dysfunction possible with doses >12 g/day; monitor LFTs. Oral soln stable for 3 days at room temperature, 14 days refrigerated.

PENICILLINS - GENERAL ANTIMICROBIAL SPECTRUM

1st generation: Most streptococci; oral anaerobic coverage
2nd generation: Most streptococci; Staph aureus
3rd generation: Most streptococci; basic gram negative coverage
4th generation: Pseudomonas

ANTIMICROBIALS: Penicillins – 3rd Generation – Aminopenicillins

NOTE: Anaphylaxis occurs rarely with penicillins; cross-sensitivity with cephalosporins is possible.

amoxicillin (*Amoxil, DisperMox, Polymox, Trimox*) ▶K ♀B ▶+ $
ADULT - ENT, skin, GU infections: 250-500 mg PO tid or 500-875 mg PO bid. Pneumonia: 500 mg PO tid or 875 mg PO bid. H pylori: See table in GI section. See table for prophylaxis of bacterial endocarditis.
PEDS - ENT, skin, GU infections: 20-40 mg/kg/day PO divided tid or 25-45 mg/kg/day PO divided bid. See "unapproved" for AAP acute otitis media dosing. Pneumonia: 40 mg/kg/day PO divided tid or 45 mg/kg/day PO divided bid. In-

fants <3 mo: 30 mg/kg/day PO divided q12h. See bacterial endocarditis prophylaxis table.

UNAPPROVED ADULT - Acute sinusitis with antibiotic use in past month &/or drug-resistant S pneumoniae rate >30%: 3-3.5 g/day PO. High-dose for community-acquired pneumonia: 1 g PO tid. Early Lyme disease: 500 mg PO tid x 3 weeks. Chlamydia in pregnancy: 500 mg PO tid x 7 days. Bioterrorism anthrax: See www.idsociety.org/BT/ToC.htm.

UNAPPROVED PEDS - Otitis media (AAP high-dose): 80-90 mg/kg/day PO divided bid-tid. Community-acquired pneumonia, 4 mo-4 yo: 80-100 mg/kg/day PO divided tid-qid. Lyme disease: 25-50 mg/kg/day (up to 1-2 g/day) PO divided tid x 21 days. Bioterrorism anthrax: See www.idsociety.org/BT/ToC.htm.

FORMS - Generic/Trade: Caps 250,500 mg, tabs 500,875 mg, chews 125,250 mg, susp 125, 250 mg/5 ml, susp 200 & 400 mg/5 ml. Trade: chews 200,400 mg, infant drops 50 mg/ml. DisperMox 200,400,600 mg tabs for oral susp.

NOTES - Rash in patients with mononucleosis. AAP recommends 5-7 days of therapy for older (≥6 yo) children with non-severe otitis media, and 10 days for younger children and those with severe disease. Dosing in adults with renal dysfunction: Do not use 875 mg tab for CrCl <30 ml/min. Use 250-500 mg PO bid for CrCl 10-30 ml/min, 250-500 mg PO qd for CrCl <10 ml/min or hemodialysis. Give additional dose both during & at end of dialysis. Oral susp & infant drops stable for 14 days at room temperature or in the refrigerator. Mix DisperMox tab with 2 tsp water and drink mixture, then rinse container with a little water and drink that. Do not chew or swallow tab whole. Use only for doses that can be delivered by whole tabs.

amoxicillin-clavulanate (*Augmentin, Augmentin ES-600, Augmentin XR, ♣Clavulin*) ▶K ♀B ▶? $$$

ADULT - Pneumonia, otitis media, sinusitis, skin infections, UTIs: Usual dose - 500 mg PO bid or 250 mg PO tid. More severe infections: 875 mg PO bid or 500 mg PO tid. Augmentin XR: 2 tabs PO q12h with meals x 10 days for acute sinusitis, x 7-10 days for community-acquired pneumonia.

PEDS - 200,400 chewables & 200,400/5 ml susp for bid administration: Pneumonia, otitis media, sinusitis: 45 mg/kg/day PO divided bid. (See "unapproved" for AAP high-dose for otitis media.) Less severe infections such as skin, UTIs: 25 mg/kg/day PO divided bid. 125,250

chewables & 125,250/5 ml susp for tid administration: Pneumonia, otitis media, sinusitis: 40 mg/kg/day PO divided tid. Less severe infections such as skin, UTIs: 20 mg/kg/day PO divided tid. Age <3 months: Use 125 mg/5 ml susp and give 30 mg/kg PO q12 hr. Use adult dose for ≥40 kg. Augmentin ES-600 susp for ≥3 mo and <40 kg. Recurrent/ persistent otitis media with risk factors (antibiotics for otitis media in past 3 months and either age ≤2 yo or daycare): 90 mg/kg/day PO divided bid with food x 10 days.

UNAPPROVED ADULT - Prevention of infection after dog/cat bite: 875 mg PO bid or 500 mg PO tid x 3-5 days. Treatment of infected dog/cat bite: 875 mg PO bid or 500 mg PO tid, duration of treatment based on response.

UNAPPROVED PEDS - AAP otitis media: Augmentin ES 90 mg/kg/day divided bid. Group A streptococcal pharyngitis, repeated culture-positive episodes: 45 mg/kg/day PO divided bid x 10 days.

FORMS - Trade: (amoxicillin + clavulanate) tabs 250+125, 500+125, 875+125 mg, chewables and susp 125+31.25, 200+28.5, 250+62.5, 400 +57 mg per tab or 5 mL. Augmentin ES-600 susp 600+42.9 mg/5 mL. Extended-release tabs (Augmentin XR) 1000+62.5 mg. Generic: Tabs 500+125, 875+125, susp 200+28.5, 400+ 57/5 ml, chewables 200+28.5, 400+ 57.

NOTES - Rash in patients with mononucleosis; diarrhea common (less diarrhea with bid dosing). AAP recommends 5-7 days of therapy for older (≥6 yo) children with non-severe otitis media, and 10 days for younger children and those with severe disease. Do not interchange Augmentin products with different clavulanate content. 250 mg tab contains too much clavulanate for children <40 kg. Suspensions stable in refrigerator for 10 days. See package insert for dosage reduction of Augmentin tabs if CrCl <30 ml/min. Augmentin XR contraindicated if CrCl <30 ml/min.

ampicillin (*Principen*) ▶K ♀B ▶? $$$

ADULT - Usual dose: 1-2 g IV q4-6h or 250-500 mg PO qid. Sepsis, meningitis: 150-200 mg/kg/day IV divided q3-4h. Empiric therapy, native valve endocarditis: 12 g/day IV continuous infusion or divided q4h plus nafcillin/oxacillin and gentamicin. See table for prophylaxis of bacterial endocarditis. Take oral ampicillin on an empty stomach.

PEDS - AAP recommendations: Mild to moderate infections: 100-150 mg/kg/day IM/IV divided q6h or 50-100 mg/kg/day PO divided qid.

Severe infections: 200-400 mg/kg/day IM/IV divided q6h. Infants >2 kg: 25-50 mg/kg IV q8h if <1 week old and q6h if ≥1 week old. Use adult doses for ≥40 kg. Give oral ampicillin on an empty stomach. Group B streptococcal meningitis: ≤1 week old, 200-300 mg/kg/day IV divided q8h. ≥1 week old, 300 mg/kg/day IV divided q4-6h. Give with gentamicin initially. See table for prophylaxis of bacterial endocarditis.
UNAPPROVED ADULT - Prevention of neonatal group B strep disease: Give to mother 2 g IV during labor, then 1-2 g IV q4-6h until delivery.
FORMS - Generic/Trade: Caps 250,500 mg, susp 125 & 250 mg/5 ml.
NOTES - Rash in patients with mononucleosis or taking allopurinol; pseudomembranous colitis. Susp stable for 7 days at room temperature, 14 days in the refrigerator. Reduce dosing interval to q12-24h for CrCl <10 ml/min. Give dose after hemodialysis.

ampicillin-sulbactam (*Unasyn*) ▶K ♀B ▶? $$$$$
ADULT - Skin, intra-abdominal, gynecologic infections: 1.5-3 g IM/IV q6h.
PEDS - Skin infections, ≥1 yo: <40 kg, 300 mg/kg/day IV divided q6h. ≥40 kg: adult dose.
UNAPPROVED ADULT - Community-acquired pneumonia: 1.5-3 g IM/IV q6h with a macrolide or doxycycline.
UNAPPROVED PEDS - AAP regimens. Mild to moderate infections: 100-150 mg/kg/day of ampicillin IM/IV divided q6h. Severe infections:

200-400 mg/kg/day of ampicillin IM/IV divided q6h.
NOTES - Rash in patients with mononucleosis or taking allopurinol; pseudomembranous colitis. Dosing in renal impairment: Give usual dose q6-8h for adults with CrCl ≥30 ml/min, q12h for CrCl 15-29 ml/min, q24 h for CrCl 5-14 ml/min.

pivampicillin (*Pondocillin*) ▶K ♀? ▶? $
ADULT - Canada only. Respiratory tract, ENT, gynecologic, urinary tract infections: Usual dose is 500 mg PO bid; 1000 mg PO bid for severe infections. Treat pharyngitis x 10 d.
PEDS - Canada only. Not recommended for severe infections. Avoid in infants <3 mo. Susp, 3-12 mo: 40-60 mg/kg/day PO divided bid. Susp, ≤10 yo: 25-35 mg/kg/day up to 525 mg PO bid. 5 ml PO bid for 1-3 yo, 7.5 ml PO bid for 4-6 yo, 10 ml PO bid for 7-10 yo. Treat pharyngitis x 10 d.
FORMS - Trade: Tabs 500 mg (377 mg ampicillin), # 20, oral susp 35 mg/ml (26 mg ampicillin), 100,150,200 ml bottles.
NOTES - Long-term therapy or repeated courses may increase carnitine excretion; avoid with valproate or in carnitine deficiency. Avoid with lymphocytic leukemia or infectious mononucleosis due to high risk of rash; allopurinol can also increase risk of rash. Pseudomembranous colitis. Susp stable for 7 days at room temperature, 14 days in the refrigerator. Reduce dose in severe renal dysfunction.

PROPHYLAXIS FOR BACTERIAL ENDOCARDITIS*

For dental, oral, respiratory tract, or esophageal procedures	
Standard regimen	amoxicillin[1] 2 g PO 1h before procedure
Unable to take oral meds	ampicillin[1] 2 g IM/IV within 30 minutes before procedure
Allergic to penicillin	clindamycin[2] 600 mg PO; or cephalexin[1] or cefadroxil[1] 2 g PO; or azithromycin[3] or clarithromycin[3] 500 mg PO 1h before procedure
Allergic to penicillin and unable to take oral meds	clindamycin[2] 600 mg IV; or cefazolin[4] 1 g IM/IV within 30 minutes before procedure
For genitourinary and gastrointestinal (excluding esophageal) procedures	
High-risk patients	ampicillin[1] 2 g IM/IV plus gentamicin 1.5 mg/kg (max 120 mg) within 30 min of starting procedure; 6h later ampicillin[4] 1 g IM/IV or amoxicillin[4] 1 g PO.
High-risk patients allergic to ampicillin	vancomycin[2] 1 g IV over 1-2h plus gentamicin 1.5 mg/kg IV/IM (max 120 mg) complete within 30 minutes of starting procedure
Moderate-risk patients	amoxicillin[1] 2 g PO or ampicillin[1] 2 g IM/IV within 30 minutes of starting procedure
Moderate-risk patients allergic to ampicillin	vancomycin[2] 1 g IV over 1-2h complete within 30 minutes of starting procedure

*JAMA 1997; 277:1794-1801 or http://www.americanheart.org
Footnotes for pediatric doses: 1 = 50 mg/kg; 2 = 20 mg/kg; 3 = 15 mg/kg; 4 = 25 mg/kg. Total pediatric dose should not exceed adult dose.

ANTIMICROBIALS: Penicillins – 4th Generation – Extended Spectrum

NOTE: Anaphylaxis occurs rarely with penicillins; cross-sensitivity with cephalosporins is possible.

piperacillin (*Pipracil*) ▶K/Bile ♀B ▶? $$$$$

ADULT - Canada only: Simple UTI, community-acquired pneumonia: 6-8 g/day IM/IV divided q6-12h. Complicated UTI: 8-16 g/day IV divided q6-8h. Serious infections: 12-18 g/day IV divided q4-6h. Max dose: 24 g/day.

PEDS - Canada only: Safety and efficacy not established in children <12 yo. Use adult dose for ≥12 yo.

UNAPPROVED ADULT - Empiric therapy of neutropenic fever: 3 g IV q4h or 4 g IV q6h with an aminoglycoside.

UNAPPROVED PEDS - Mild to moderate infections: 100-150 mg/kg/day IV divided q6h. Severe infections: 200-300 mg/kg/day IV divided q4-6h.

NOTES - Hypokalemia; bleeding & coagulation abnormalities possible especially with renal impairment. May prolong neuromuscular blockade with non-depolarizing muscle relaxants. Adult dosing with renal dysfunction: Serious infections: 4 g IV q8h for CrCl 20-40 ml/min, 4 g IV q12h for CrCl <20 ml/min. Complicated UTI: 3 g IV q8h for CrCl 20-40 ml/min, 3 g IV q12h for CrCl <20 ml/min. Simple UTI: 3 g IV q12h for CrCl <20 ml/min.

piperacillin-tazobactam (*Zosyn*, ✚*Tazocin*) ▶K ♀B ▶? $$$$$

ADULT - Appendicitis, peritonitis, skin infections, postpartum endometritis, pelvic inflammatory disease, moderate community-acquired pneumonia: 3.375 g IV q6h. Nosocomial pneumonia: 4.5 g IV q6h (with aminoglycoside initially and if P. aeruginosa is cultured).

PEDS - Not approved in children <12 yo.

UNAPPROVED ADULT - Serious infections: 4.5 g IV q6h.

UNAPPROVED PEDS - 240 mg/kg/day of piperacillin IV divided q8h.

NOTES - Hypokalemia; bleeding & coagulation abnormalities possible especially with renal impairment. May reduce renal excretion of methotrexate; monitor methotrexate levels and toxicity. Dosing in renal impairment: 2.25 g IV q6h for CrCl 20-40 ml/min, 2.25 g IV q8h for CrCl <20 ml/min. Hemodialysis: Maximum dose of 2.25 g IV q8h plus 0.75 g after each dialysis.

ticarcillin (*Ticar*) ▶K ♀B ▶+ $$$$$

ADULT - Sepsis, pneumonia, skin & soft tissue, intra-abdominal, female GU infections: 3 g IV q4h or 4 g IV q6h. Simple UTI: 1 g IM/IV q6h. Complicated UTI: 3 g IV q6h.

PEDS - Sepsis, pneumonia, skin & soft tissue, intra-abdominal infections, <40 kg: 200-300 mg/kg/day IV divided q4-6h. Simple UTI, <40 kg: 50-100 mg/kg/day IM/IV divided q6-8h. Complicated UTI, <40 kg: 150-200 mg/kg/day IV divided q4-6h. Use adult dose for ≥40 kg. Severe infections, neonates ≥2 kg: <1 week, 75 mg/kg IV q8h. >1 week, 100 mg/kg IV q8h or 75 mg/kg IV q6h.

NOTES - Hypokalemia; bleeding & coagulation abnormalities possible with renal impairment. Not more than 2 g/IM injection site. Up to 6.5 mEq sodium/g ticarcillin. Adult dosing with renal dysfunction: 3 g IV load, then 2 g IV q4h for CrCl 30-60 ml/min, 2 g IV q8h for CrCl 10-30 ml/min, 2 g IV q12h or 1 g IM q6h for CrCl <10 ml/min. Liver dysfunction and CrCl <10 ml/min: 2 g IV q24h or 1 g IM q12h. Peritoneal dialysis: 3 g IV q12h. Hemodialysis: 2 g IV q12h and 3 g IV after each dialysis session.

ticarcillin-clavulanate (*Timentin*) ▶K ♀B ▶? $$$$$

ADULT - Systemic infections or UTIs: 3.1 g IV q4-6h. Gynecologic infections: Moderate, 200 mg/kg/day IV divided q6h. Severe, 300 mg/kg/day IV divided q4h. Adults <60 kg: 200-300 mg/kg/day (based on ticarcillin content) IV divided q4h. Use q4h dosing interval for Pseudomonas infections.

PEDS - Mild to moderate infections: ≥60 kg, 3.1 g IV q6h. Age ≥3 mo and <60 kg, 200 mg/kg/day (based on ticarcillin content) IV divided q6h. Severe infections: ≥60 kg, 3.1 g IV q4h. Age ≥3 mo and <60 kg, 300 mg/kg/day (based on ticarcillin content) IV divided q4h.

NOTES - Timentin 3.1 g = 3 g ticarcillin + 0.1 g clavulanate. Hypokalemia; bleeding & coagulation abnormalities possible especially in patients with renal impairment. 4.75 mEq sodium/g Timentin. IV dosing in adults with renal dysfunction: Load with 3.1 g, then 2 g q4h for CrCl 30-60 ml/min, 2 g q8h for CrCl 10-30 ml/min, 2 g q12h for CrCl <10 ml/min, 2 g q24h for CrCl <10 ml/min and liver dysfunction. Peritoneal dialysis: 3.1 g q12h. Hemodialysis: 3.1 g load, then 2 g q12h & 3.1 g after each dialysis.

ANTIMICROBIALS: Quinolones – 1st Generation

NOTE: Important quinolone drug interactions with warfarin, antacids, iron, zinc, magnesium, sucralfate, cimetidine, caffeine, cyclosporine, hydantoins, theophylline, etc.

nalidixic acid (*NegGram*) ▶KL ♀C ▶? $$$$
ADULT - UTI: 1 g PO qid for 1-2 weeks, may reduce to 2 g/day thereafter.
PEDS - UTI, age ≥3 mo: 55 mg/kg/day PO divi-
ded qid, may then reduce to 33 mg/kg/day.
FORMS - Trade: Tabs 0.25,0.5,1 g, susp 250 mg/5 ml.
NOTES - CNS toxicity; photosensitivity; hemolytic anemia in G6PD deficiency. Contraindicated if seizure history. Arthropathy in animal studies - use cautiously in prepubertal children. Monitor CBC and LFTs if used for >2 weeks.

ANTIMICROBIALS: Quinolones – 2nd Generation

NOTE: Avoid in children unless absolutely necessary due to potential cartilage toxicity. Can cause tendon rupture (rare; risk increased by corticosteroids, especially in elderly), phototoxicity (risk varies among agents), QT interval prolongation (risk varies among agents; see QT drugs table), exacerbation of myasthenia gravis, CNS toxicity, and hypersensitivity. Important quinolone drug interactions with antacids, iron, zinc, magnesium, sucralfate, buffered didanosine, cimetidine, caffeine, cyclosporine, phenytoin, anticoagulants, theophylline, etc.

ciprofloxacin (*Cipro, Cipro XR*) ▶LK ♀C but teratogenicity unlikely ▶?+ $$$$
ADULT - UTI: 250-500 mg PO bid or 200-400 mg IV q12h. Simple UTI: 100 mg PO bid x 3 days or Cipro XR 500 mg PO qd x 3 days. Cipro XR for complicated UTI, uncomplicated pyelonephritis: 1000 mg PO qd x 7-14 days. Pneumonia, skin, bone/joint infections: 400 mg IV q8-12h or 500-750 mg PO bid. Treat bone/joint infections x 4-6 weeks. Acute sinusitis: 500 mg PO bid x 10 days. Chronic bacterial prostatitis: 500 mg PO bid x 28 days. Infectious diarrhea: 500 mg PO bid x 5-7 days. Typhoid fever: 500 mg PO bid x 10 days. Gonorrhea, CDC regimen: 500 mg PO single dose (not for infections acquired in California, Hawaii, Asia or Pacific islands, or in men who have sex with men). Nosocomial pneumonia: 400 mg IV q8h. Complicated intra-abdominal infection (with metronidazole): 400 mg IV q12 h, then 500 mg PO bid. Empiric therapy of febrile neutropenia: 400 mg IV q8h with piperacillin. Bioterrorism anthrax. Inhalation or severe cutaneous anthrax treatment: 400 mg IV q12h with ≥1 other drug initially, then monotherapy with 500 mg PO bid to complete 60 days. Monotherapy for post-exposure prophylaxis or treatment of less severe cutaneous anthrax: 500 mg PO bid x 60 days. See www.idsociety.org/BT/ToC.htm for
more info.
PEDS - Safety and efficacy not established for most indications in children; arthropathy in juvenile animals. Still limited data, but case series of treated children show no evidence of arthropathy other than transient large-joint arthralgias. Musculoskeletal adverse events reported with ciprofloxacin treatment of complicated UTI in peds patients were mild to moderate in severity and resolved within 1 month after treatment. Complicated UTI, pyelonephritis, 1-17 yo: 6-10 mg/kg IV q8h, then 10-20 mg/kg PO q12h. Max dose is 400 mg IV or 750 mg PO even for peds patients >51 kg. Bioterrorism anthrax. Treatment of inhalation anthrax, severe cutaneous anthrax, or cutaneous anthrax in any case <2 yo: 10-15 mg/kg IV q12h with ≥1 other drug initially, then monotherapy with 10-15 mg/kg up to 500 mg PO bid to complete 60 days. Monotherapy for post-exposure prophylaxis or less severe cutaneous anthrax treatment: 10-15 mg/kg up to 500 mg PO bid x 60 days. See www.idsociety.org/BT/ToC.htm for more info.
UNAPPROVED ADULT - Acute uncomplicated pyelonephritis: 500 mg PO bid x 7 days. See STD table for disseminated gonorrhea. Chancroid: 500 mg PO bid x 3 days. Prophylaxis, high-risk GU surgery: 500 mg PO or 400 mg IV. Prophylaxis, invasive meningococcal disease: 500 mg PO single dose. Traveler's diarrhea (treatment preferred over prophylaxis): Treatment - 500 mg PO bid x 1-3 days or 750 mg PO single dose. Prophylaxis - 500 mg PO qd x ≤3 weeks. Infectious diarrhea: 500 mg PO bid x 1-3 days for shigella, x 5-7 days for nontyphi salmonella (usually not treated). Malignant otitis externa: 400 mg IV or 750 mg PO q12h. TB (2nd-line treatment): 750-1500 mg/day IV/PO. Sanford's has 750 mg PO qd x 5 days/week.

UNAPPROVED PEDS - Acute pulmonary exacerbation of cystic fibrosis: 10 mg/kg/dose IV q8h x 7 days, then 20 mg/kg/dose PO q12h to complete 10-21 days of treatment.

FORMS - Generic/trade: Susp 250 & 500 mg/5 ml. Tabs 100,250,500,750 mg. Trade: Extended release tabs (Cipro XR) 500, 1000 mg.

NOTES - Crystalluria if alkaline urine. May cause peripheral neuropathy rarely. Ciprofloxacin inhibits cytochrome P450 1A2, an enzyme that metabolizes caffeine, clozapine, tacrine, theophylline, and warfarin. Give 2 h before or 6 h after antacids, iron, sucralfate, calcium, zinc, buffered didanosine. Can give with meals containing dairy products, but not with yogurt, milk, or calcium-fortified fruit juice alone. Do not give Cipro XR within 2h of calcium doses >800 mg. Watch for hypoglycemia with glyburide. Do not give oral susp in feeding tube. Cipro XR and immediate-release tabs are not interchangeable. Do not split, crush, or chew Cipro XR. Dosing in adults with renal dysfunction: 250-500 mg PO q12h for CrCl 30-50 ml/min; 250-500 mg PO q18h or 200-400 mg IV q18-24h for CrCl 5-29 ml/min; 250-500 mg PO q24h given after dialysis for hemodialysis/peritoneal dialysis.

enoxacin (*Penetrex*) ▶LK ♀C ▶? $$$

ADULT - Gonorrhea: 400 mg PO single dose (not for infections acquired in California, Hawaii, Asia, or Pacific islands, or in men who have sex with men). Simple UTI: 200 mg PO bid x 7 days. Complicated UTI: 400 mg PO bid x 14 days. Take on empty stomach.

PEDS - Safety and efficacy not established in children; arthropathy in juvenile animals.

FORMS - Trade: Tabs 200,400 mg.

NOTES - Enoxacin inhibits cytochrome P450 1A2, an enzyme that metabolizes caffeine, clozapine, tacrine, theophylline, and warfarin. May increase digoxin levels. Give ranitidine, antacids, iron, zinc, bismuth subsalicylate, sucralfate, buffered didanosine 8 h before or 2 h after enoxacin. Give 50% of usual dose q12h for CrCl ≤30 ml/min.

lomefloxacin (*Maxaquin*) ▶LK ♀C ▶? $$$

ADULT - Acute exacerbation of chronic bronchitis not due to S pneumoniae, simple UTI due to K pneumoniae, P mirabilis, S saprophyticus: 400 mg PO qd x 10 days. Simple E coli UTI: 400 mg PO qd x 3 days. Complicated UTI: 400 mg PO qd x 14 days. Take in the evening to decrease risk of phototoxicity.

PEDS - Safety and efficacy not established in children; arthropathy in juvenile animals.

FORMS - Trade: Tabs 400 mg.

NOTES - High risk of phototoxicity. Avoid sunlight during and for several days after treatment. Give Al/Mg antacids, sucralfate 4 h before or 2 h after lomefloxacin. Dosing in renal dysfunction: 400 mg PO load, then 200 mg PO qd for CrCl 11-39 ml/min or hemodialysis.

norfloxacin (*Noroxin*) ▶LK ♀C ▶? $$$

ADULT - Simple UTI due to E coli, K pneumoniae, P mirabilis: 400 mg PO bid x 3 days. UTI due to other organisms: 400 mg PO bid x 7-10 days. Complicated UTI: 400 mg PO bid x 10-21 days. Gonorrhea: 800 mg PO single dose (not for infections acquired in California, Hawaii, Asia, or Pacific islands, or in men who have sex with men). Acute/chronic prostatitis: 400 mg PO bid x 28 days. Take on empty stomach.

PEDS - Safety and efficacy not established in children; arthropathy in juvenile animals.

UNAPPROVED ADULT - Traveler's diarrhea (treatment preferred over prophylaxis): Treatment - 400 mg PO bid x 1-3 days. Prophylaxis - 400 mg PO qd for up to 3 weeks. Infectious diarrhea: 400 mg PO bid x 5-7 days for nontyphi salmonella (usually not treated), x 1-3 days for shigella. Take on an empty stomach.

FORMS - Trade: Tabs 400 mg.

NOTES - Crystalluria with high doses. Maintain adequate hydration. May cause peripheral neuropathy rarely. Norfloxacin inhibits cytochrome P450 1A2, an enzyme that metabolizes caffeine, clozapine, tacrine, theophylline, and warfarin. Increased INR with warfarin. Do not take with dairy products. Give antacids, zinc, iron, sucralfate, multivitamins, or buffered didanosine 2 h before/after norfloxacin. Dosing for CrCl <30 ml/min: single dose 400 mg PO qd.

ofloxacin (*Floxin*) ▶LK ♀C ▶?+ $$$$

ADULT - IV & PO doses are the same. Acute exacerbation of chronic bronchitis, community-acquired pneumonia, skin infections: 400 mg bid x 10 days. Gonorrhea: 400 mg PO single dose (not for infections acquired in California, Hawaii, Asia, or Pacific islands, or in men who have sex with men). Chlamydia: 300 mg bid x 7 days. Pelvic inflammatory disease: See table. Simple UTI due to E coli, K pneumoniae: 200 mg bid x 3 days. Simple UTI due to other organisms: 200 mg bid x 7 days. Complicated UTI: 200 mg bid x 10 days. Chronic bacterial prostatitis: 300 mg PO bid x 6 weeks.

PEDS - Safety and efficacy not established in children; arthropathy in juvenile animals.

UNAPPROVED ADULT - Epididymitis: 300 mg PO bid x 10 days. Traveler's diarrhea, treatment: 300 mg PO bid x 1-3 days. Infectious diarrhea: 300 mg PO bid x 1-3 days for shigella, 5-7 days for non-typhi salmonella (usually not treated). TB (2nd-line treatment): 600-800 mg PO qd.

FORMS - Generic/trade: Tabs 200,300,400 mg.

NOTES - Give antacids, iron, sucralfate, multivitamins containing zinc, buffered didanosine 2h before or after ofloxacin. May decrease metabolism of theophylline, increase INR with warfarin. Monitor glucose with antidiabetic agents. Dosing in renal dysfunction: Usual dose given q24h for CrCl 20-50 ml/min, 50% of usual dose q24h for CrCl <20 ml/min.

ANTIMICROBIALS: Quinolones – 3rd Generation

NOTE: Avoid in children unless absolutely necessary due to potential cartilage toxicity. Can cause tendon rupture (rare; risk increased by corticosteroids, especially in elderly), phototoxicity (risk varies among agents), QT interval prolongation (risk varies among agents), CNS toxicity, and hypersensitivity. Important quinolone drug interactions with antacids, iron, zinc, magnesium, sucralfate, cimetidine, caffeine, cyclosporine, phenytoin, anticoagulants, theophylline, etc.

levofloxacin (*Levaquin*) ▶KL ♀C ▶? $$$
ADULT - IV & PO doses are the same. Community-acquired pneumonia: 500 mg qd x 7-14 days or 750 mg qd x 5 days. Nosocomial pneumonia or complicated skin infections: 750 mg qd x 7-14 days. Other: 500 mg qd x 7 days for acute exacerbation of chronic bronchitis, x 7-10 days for uncomplicated skin infections, x 10-14 days for acute sinusitis, x 28 days for chronic bacterial prostatitis. 250 mg PO qd x 3 days for simple UTI, x 10 days for complicated UTI or acute pyelonephritis. Infuse IV doses over 60 minutes (250-500 mg) to 90 minutes (750 mg).

PEDS - Safety and efficacy not established in children; arthropathy in juvenile animals.

UNAPPROVED ADULT - Legionnaires' disease: 1 g IV/PO on 1st day, then 500 mg IV/PO qd. Chlamydia, epididymitis, gonorrhea, pelvic inflammatory disease: See STD table. TB (2nd-line treatment): 500-1000 mg/day IV/PO. Traveler's diarrhea, treatment: 500 mg PO qd x 1-3 days. Infectious diarrhea: 500 mg PO qd x 1-3 days for shigella, x 5-7 days for salmonella.

FORMS - Trade: Tabs 250,500,750 mg. Leva-Pak: #5, 750 mg tabs.

NOTES - May prolong QT interval. Give Mg/Al antacids, iron, sucralfate, multivitamins containing zinc, buffered didanosine 2 h before/after PO levofloxacin. Increased INR with warfarin. Monitor glucose with antidiabetic agents. Dosing in renal dysfunction: For most indications and CrCl <50 ml/min, load with 500 mg, then 250 mg qd for CrCl 20-49 ml/min, 250 mg qod CrCl 10-19 ml/min, hemodialysis, peritoneal dialysis. For complicated UTI/pyelonephritis and CrCl 10-19 ml/min, give 250 mg qod.

ANTIMICROBIALS: Quinolones – 4th Generation

NOTE: Avoid in children unless absolutely necessary due to potential cartilage toxicity. Can cause tendon rupture (rare; risk increased by corticosteroids, especially in elderly), phototoxicity (risk varies among agents), QT interval prolongation (risk varies among agents), CNS toxicity, and hypersensitivity. Important quinolone drug interactions with antacids, iron, zinc, magnesium, sucralfate, cimetidine, caffeine, cyclosporine, phenytoin, anticoagulants, theophylline, etc.

gatifloxacin (*Tequin*) ▶K ♀C ▶- $$$
ADULT - IV & PO doses are the same. Community-acquired pneumonia: 400 mg qd x 7-14 days. Acute exacerbation of chronic bronchitis: 400 mg qd x 5 days. Complicated UTI, acute pyelonephritis, uncomplicated skin infections: 400 mg qd x 7-10 days. Acute sinusitis: 400 mg qd x 10 days. Simple UTI: 400 mg single

dose or 200 mg qd x 3 days. Gonorrhea: 400 mg single dose (not for infections acquired in California, Hawaii, Asia, or Pacific islands, or in men who have sex with men).

PEDS - Safety and efficacy not established in children; arthropathy in juvenile animals.

UNAPPROVED ADULT - IV & PO doses are the same. Acute uncomplicated pyelonephritis: 400 mg qd x 7 days. TB (2nd-line treatment): 400 mg IV/PO qd.

FORMS - Trade: Tabs 200,400 mg. Teq-Paq: #5, 400 mg tabs.

NOTES - May prolong QT interval. Avoid using in proarrhythmic conditions or with drugs that prolong QT interval. Contraindicated with ziprasidone. Do not exceed recommended IV dose or infusion rate; high concentrations of gatifloxacin might increase risk of QT interval prolongation. Monitor blood glucose in diabetics; expect hypoglycemia in first 2 days of therapy; hyperglycemia after 3rd day. Give PO gatifloxacin 4 h before or with Al/Mg antacids, iron, multivitamins with zinc, buffered didanosine. May increase digoxin levels. Dosing for renal dysfunction in adults: 400 mg loading dose on day 1. On day 2, reduce dose to 200 mg PO qd for CrCl <40 ml/min, hemodialysis, continuous peritoneal dialysis.

gemifloxacin (*Factive*) ▶Feces, K ♀C ▶- $$$
ADULT - Acute exacerbation of chronic bronchitis: 320 mg PO qd x 5 days. Community-acquired pneumonia (including multi-drug resistant S pneumoniae): 320 mg PO qd x 7 days.
PEDS - Safety and efficacy not established in children; arthropathy in juvenile animals.
FORMS - Trade: Tabs 320 mg.
NOTES - May prolong QT interval. Avoid using in proarrhythmic conditions or with drugs that prolong QT interval, including Class 1A and Class III antiarrhythmics. Maintain fluid intake to prevent crystalluria. Give 2 h before or 3 h after Al/Mg antacids, iron, multivitamins with zinc, buffered didanosine. Give ≥2 h before sucralfate. Discontinue if rash develops. Dosage reduction for CrCl ≤40 ml/min, hemodialy-

sis, or CAPD: 160 mg PO qd.
moxifloxacin (*Avelox*) ▶LK ♀C ▶- $$$
ADULT - 400 mg PO/IV qd x 5 days (chronic bronchitis exacerbation), 7 days (skin infections), 10 days (acute sinusitis), or 7-14 days (community acquired pneumonia, including penicillin-resistant S pneumoniae). IV infused over 60 minutes.
PEDS - Safety and efficacy not established in children; arthropathy in juvenile animals.
UNAPPROVED ADULT - TB (2nd-line treatment): 400 mg IV/PO qd.
FORMS - Trade: Tabs 400 mg.
NOTES - Prolonged QT interval. Avoid using in proarrhythmic conditions or with drugs that prolong QT interval, including Class 1A and Class III antiarrhythmics. Do not exceed recommended IV dose or infusion rate; high concentrations of moxifloxacin might increase risk of QT interval prolongation. Contraindicated with ziprasidone. May cause peripheral neuropathy rarely. Give tabs ≥4 h before or 8 h after Mg/Al antacids, iron, multivitamins with zinc, sucralfate, buffered didanosine. Monitor INR with warfarin. Avoid in moderate or severe hepatic insufficiency.

QUINOLONES- GENERAL ANTIMICROBIAL SPECTRUM

1st generation: gram negative (excluding Pseudomonas), urinary tract only, no atypicals
2nd generation: gram negative (including Pseudomonas); Staph aureus but not pneumococcus; some atypicals
3rd generation: gram negative (including Pseudomonas); gram positive (including Staph aureus and pneumococcus); expanded atypical coverage
4th generation: same as 3rd generation plus enhanced coverage of pneumococcus, decreased activity vs. Pseudomonas.

ANTIMICROBIALS: Sulfonamides

NOTE: Sulfonamides can cause Stevens-Johnson syndrome; toxic epidermal necrolysis; hepatotoxicity; blood dyscrasias; hemolysis in G6PD deficiency. Avoid maternal sulfonamides when the breastfed infant is ill, stressed, premature, has hyperbilirubinemia, or has glucose-6-phosphate dehydrogenase deficiency.

Pediazole (erythromycin ethyl succinate + sulfisoxazole) ▶KL ♀C ▶- $
PEDS - Otitis media, age >2 mo: 50 mg/kg/day (based on EES dose) PO divided tid-qid.
FORMS - Generic/Trade: Susp, eryth ethyl succinate 200 mg, sulfisoxazole 600 mg/5 ml.
NOTES - Sulfisoxazole: Significantly increased

INR with warfarin; avoid concomitant use if possible. Erythromycin: Rare arrhythmias in patients with prolonged QT. May aggravate myasthenia gravis. Cytochrome P450 3A4 & 1A2 inhibitor. Many drug interactions including increased levels of carbamazepine, cyclosporine, digoxin, disopyramide, tacrolimus, theophylline, some benzodiazepines and statins. Monitor INR with warfarin. Contraindicated with cisapride, pimozide. AAP recommends 5-7 days of therapy for older (≥6 yo) children with non-severe otitis media, and 10 days for younger children and those with severe disease.
sulfadiazine ▶K ♀C ▶+ $$$$$

ADULT - Usual dose: 2-4 g PO initially, then 2-4 g/day divided into 3-6 doses. Secondary prevention of rheumatic fever: 1 g PO qd. Toxoplasmosis treatment: 1-1.5 g PO qid with pyrimethamine and leucovorin.

PEDS - Not for infants <2 mo, except as adjunct to pyrimethamine for congenital toxoplasmosis. Usual dose: Give 75 mg/kg PO initially, then 150 mg/kg/day up to 6 g/day divided into 4-6 doses. Secondary prevention of rheumatic fever, <27 kg: 500 mg PO qd. Use adult dose for >27 kg.

UNAPPROVED ADULT - Secondary prevention after CNS toxoplasmosis in AIDS: 0.5-1 g PO qid with pyrimethamine and leucovorin.

UNAPPROVED PEDS - Not for infants <2 mo, except as adjunct to pyrimethamine for congenital toxoplasmosis. AAP regimen for toxoplasmosis: 100-200 mg/kg/day PO with pyrimethamine and leucovorin (duration varies). Secondary prevention after CNS toxoplasmosis in HIV-infection: 85-120 mg/kg/day PO divided in 2-4 doses with pyrimethamine and leucovorin.

FORMS - Generic: Tab 500 mg.

NOTES - Not effective for streptococcal pharyngitis. Maintain fluid intake to prevent crystalluria & stone formation. Reduce dose in renal insufficiency. May increase INR with warfarin. May increase levels of methotrexate, phenytoin.

sulfisoxazole (Gantrisin) ▶KL ♀C ▶+ $
PEDS - Usual dose: 75 mg/kg PO load, then 150 mg/kg/day PO divided q4-6h (max 6 g/day). Not for infants <2 mo, except as adjunct to pyrimethamine for congenital toxoplasmosis.

UNAPPROVED PEDS - Prophylaxis for recurrent otitis media: 50 mg/kg PO qhs.

FORMS - Trade: susp 500 mg/5 ml. Generic: Tabs 500 mg.

NOTES - May increase levels of methotrexate, phenytoin. Significantly increased INR with warfarin; avoid concomitant use if possible. Reduce dose in renal failure. Maintain fluid intake to prevent crystalluria/stone formation.

trimethoprim-sulfamethoxazole (Bactrim, Septra, Sulfatrim, cotrimoxazole) ▶K ♀C ▶+ $

ADULT - UTI, shigellosis, acute exacerbation of chronic bronchitis: 1 tab PO bid, double strength (DS, 160 TMP/800 SMX). Travelers' diarrhea: 1 DS tab PO bid x 5 days. Pneumocystis treatment: 15-20 mg/kg/day (based on TMP) IV divided q6-8h or PO divided q6h x 21 days total. Pneumocystis prophylaxis: 1 DS tab qd.

PEDS - UTI, shigellosis, otitis media: 5 ml susp/ 10 kg (up to 20 ml)/dose PO bid. Pneumocystis treatment: 15-20 mg/kg/day (based on TMP) IV divided q6-8h or 5 ml susp/8 kg/dose PO q6h. Pneumocystis prophylaxis: 150 mg/m²/day (based on TMP) PO divided bid on 3 consecutive days each week. Do not use in infants <2 mo; may cause kernicterus.

UNAPPROVED ADULT - Bacterial prostatitis: 1 DS tab PO bid x 10-14 days for acute, x 1-3 months for chronic. Sinusitis: 1 DS tab PO bid x 10 days. Burkholderia cepacia pulmonary infection in cystic fibrosis: 5 mg/kg (based on TMP) IV q6h. Pneumocystis prophylaxis: 1 SS tab PO qd. Primary prevention of toxoplasmosis in AIDS: 1 DS PO qd. Pertussis: 1 DS tab bid x 14 days (second-line to erythromycin).

UNAPPROVED PEDS - Head lice unresponsive to usual therapy: 10 mg/kg/day (based on TMP) PO divided bid x 10 days in combo with standard doses of permethrin 1%. Pertussis: 8 mg/kg/day (based on TMP) PO divided bid x 14 days (second-line to erythromycin).

FORMS - Generic/Trade: Tabs 80 mg TMP/400 mg SMX (single strength), 160 mg TMP/800 mg SMX (double strength; DS), susp 40 mg TMP/200 mg SMX per 5 ml. 20 ml susp = 2 SS tabs = 1 DS tab.

NOTES - Not effective for streptococcal pharyngitis. No activity against penicillin-nonsusceptible pneumococci. Bone marrow depression with high IV doses. Significantly increased INR with warfarin; avoid concomitant use if possible. Increases levels of methotrexate, phenytoin. AAP recommends 5-7 days of therapy for older (≥6 yo) children with non-severe otitis media, and 10 days for younger children and those with severe disease. Dosing in renal dysfunction: Use 50% of usual dose for CrCl 15-30 ml/min. Don't use for CrCl <15 ml/min.

ANTIMICROBIALS: Tetracyclines

NOTE: Tetracyclines can cause photosensitivity and pseudotumor cerebri. May decrease efficacy of oral contraceptives. Increased INR w/ warfarin.

doxycycline (Adoxa, Vibramycin, Doryx, Monodox, ✚Doxycin) ▶LK ♀D ▶?+ $
ADULT - Usual dose: 100 mg PO bid on first day, then 100 mg/day PO divided qd or bid.

Severe infections: 100 mg PO bid. Chlamydia, nongonococcal urethritis: 100 mg PO bid x 7 days. Acne vulgaris: Up to 100 mg PO bid. Periostat for periodontitis: 20 mg PO bid 1 h before breakfast and dinner. Cholera: 300 mg PO single dose. Primary, secondary, early latent syphilis if penicillin-allergic: 100 mg PO bid x 14 days. Late latent or tertiary syphilis if penicillin allergic: 100 mg PO bid x 4 weeks. Not for neurosyphilis. Malaria prophylaxis: 100 mg PO qd starting 1-2d before exposure until 4 wks after. Intravenous: 200 mg on first day in 1-2 infusions, then 100-200 mg/day in 1-2 infusions. Bioterrorism anthrax: 100 mg bid x 60 days. Use IV with ≥1 other drug for initial treatment of inhalation or severe cutaneous anthrax. PO monotherapy for less severe cutaneous anthrax or post-exposure prophylaxis. See www.idsociety.org/BT/ToC.htm for more info.

PEDS - Avoid in children <8 yo due to teeth staining. Usual dose, children ≤45 kg: 4.4 mg/kg/day PO divided bid on first day, then 2.2-4.4 mg/kg/day PO divided qd or bid. Use adult dose for children >45 kg. Malaria prophylaxis: 2 mg/kg/day up to 100 mg PO qd starting 1-2 days before exposure until 4 weeks after. Most PO and IV doses are equivalent. Bioterrorism anthrax: 100 mg bid for >8 yo and >45 kg, 2.2 mg/kg bid for >8 yo and ≤45 kg, or ≤8 yo. Treat x 60 days. Use IV with ≥1 other drug for initial treatment of inhalation anthrax, severe cutaneous anthrax, or cutaneous anthrax in any case <2 yo. PO monotherapy for less severe cutaneous anthrax and post-exposure prophylaxis. See www.idsociety.org/BT/ToC.htm for more info.

UNAPPROVED ADULT - See sexually-transmitted diseases table for pelvic inflammatory disease treatment. Lyme disease: 100 mg PO bid x 14-28 days. Prevention of Lyme disease in highly endemic area, with deer tick attachment ≥48h: 200 mg PO single dose with food within 72 h of tick bite. Ehrlichiosis: 100 mg IV/PO bid x 7-14 days. Malaria treatment: 100 mg PO bid x 7 days with quinine.

UNAPPROVED PEDS - Avoid in children <8 yo due to teeth staining. Lyme disease: 1-2 mg/kg PO up to 100 mg bid x 14-28 days. Malaria treatment: 2 mg/kg/day PO x 7d with quinine.

FORMS - Generic/Trade: Tabs 75,100 mg, caps 50,100 mg. Trade: Susp 25 mg/5 ml, syrup 50 mg/5 ml, Periostat: Caps 20 mg.

NOTES - Increased BUN, pain with IV infusion. Do not give antacids or calcium supplements within 2 h of doxycycline. Barbiturates, carbamazepine, rifampin, and phenytoin may decrease doxycycline levels. Preferred over tetracycline in renal dysfunction. Take with fluids to decrease esophageal irritation; can take with food/ milk.

minocycline (*Minocin, Dynacin*) ▶LK ♀D ▶?+ $

ADULT - Usual dose: 200 mg IV/PO 1st dose, then 100 mg q12h. IV and PO doses are the same. Not more than 400 mg/day IV.

PEDS - Avoid in children <8 yo due to teeth staining. Usual dose: 4 mg/kg PO 1st dose, then 2 mg/kg bid. IV and PO doses are the same.

UNAPPROVED ADULT - Acne vulgaris: 50 mg PO bid.

FORMS - Generic/Trade: Caps, tabs 50,75,100 mg. Trade: Susp 50 mg/5 ml.

NOTES - Dizziness, hepatotoxicity, lupus. Do not give antacids or calcium supplements within 2h of minocycline. May cause drowsiness. Take with fluids (not milk) to decrease esophageal irritation. Use with caution in renal dysfunction; doxycycline preferred.

tetracycline (*Sumycin*) ▶LK ♀D ▶?+ $

ADULT - Usual dose: 250-500 mg PO qid on empty stomach. H pylori: See table in GI section. Primary, secondary, early latent syphilis if penicillin-allergic: 500 mg PO qid x 14 days. Late latent syphilis if penicillin allergic: 500 mg PO qid x 28 days.

PEDS - Avoid in children <8 yo due to teeth staining. Usual dose: 25-50 mg/kg/day PO divided bid-qid on empty stomach.

FORMS - Generic/Trade: Caps 250,500 mg. Trade: Tabs 250, 500 mg, susp 125 mg/5 ml.

NOTES - Increased BUN/hepatotoxicity in patients with renal dysfunction. Increased INR with warfarin. Do not give antacids or calcium supplements within 2 h of tetracycline. Use with caution in renal dysfunction; doxycycline preferred. Take with fluids (not milk) to decrease esophageal irritation.

ANTIMICROBIALS: Other

aztreonam (*Azactam*) ▶K ♀B ▶+ $$$$$

ADULT - UTI: 500 mg-1 g IM/IV q8-12h. Pneumonia, sepsis, skin, intra-abdominal, gynecological infections: Moderate, 1-2 g IM/IV q8-12h. Severe or P aeruginosa infections, 2 g IV q6-8h. Use IV route for doses >1 g.

PEDS - Serious gram-negative infections, usual dose: 30 mg/kg/dose IV q6-8h.

UNAPPROVED PEDS - P aeruginosa pulmonary infection in cystic fibrosis: 50 mg/kg/dose IV q6-8h.

NOTES - Dosing in adults with renal dysfunction: 1-2 g IV load, then 50% of usual dose for CrCl 10-30 ml/min. 0.5-2 g IV load, then 25% of usual dose for CrCl <10 ml/min. For life-threatening infections, also give 12.5% of initial dose after each hemodialysis.

chloramphenicol (*Chloromycetin*) ▶LK ♀C ▶- $$$$$

WARNING - Serious & fatal blood dyscrasias. Dose-dependent bone marrow suppression common.

ADULT - Typhoid fever, rickettsial infections: 50 mg/kg/day IV divided q6h. Up to 75-100 mg/kg/day IV for serious infections untreatable with other agents.

PEDS - Severe infections including meningitis: 50-100 mg/kg/day IV divided q6h. AAP recommends 75-100 mg/kg/day for invasive pneumococcal infections only in patients with life-threatening beta-lactam allergy.

NOTES - Monitor CBC every 2 days. Monitor serum levels. Therapeutic peak: 10-20 mcg/ml. Trough: 5-10 mcg/ml. Use cautiously in acute intermittent porphyria/G6PD deficiency. Gray baby syndrome in preemies and newborns. Barbiturates, rifampin decrease chloramphenicol levels. Chloramphenicol increases barbiturate, phenytoin levels and may increase INR with warfarin. Dosing in adults with hepatic dysfunction: 1 g IV load, then 500 mg q6h.

clindamycin (*Cleocin*, ✦*Dalacin C*) ▶L ♀B ▶?+ $$$

WARNING - Pseudomembranous colitis.

ADULT - Serious anaerobic, Staph, streptococcal, infections: 600-900 mg IV q8h or 150-450 mg PO qid. See tables for prophylaxis of bacterial endocarditis, treatment of sexually transmitted diseases (pelvic inflammatory disease).

PEDS - Serious anaerobic, streptococcal, Staph infections: 20-40 mg/kg/day IV divided q6-8h or 8-20 mg/kg/day (as Caps) PO divided tid-qid or 8-25 mg/kg/day (as palmitate oral soln) PO divided tid-qid. Do not give <37.5 mg of oral soln PO tid for ≤10 kg. Infants <1 mo: 15-20 mg/kg/day IV divided tid-qid. See table for prophylaxis of bacterial endocarditis.

UNAPPROVED ADULT - Bacterial vaginosis: 300 mg PO bid x 7 days. Oral/dental infection: 300 mg PO qid. Prevention of perinatal group B streptococcal disease: 900 mg IV to mother

q8h until delivery. CNS toxoplasmosis, AIDS (with leucovorin, pyrimethamine): treatment 600 mg PO/IV q6h; secondary prevention 300-450 mg PO q6-8h. Group A streptococcal pharyngitis, repeated culture-positive episodes: 600 mg/day PO in 2-4 divided doses x 10 days.

UNAPPROVED PEDS - Group A streptococcal pharyngitis, repeated culture-positive episodes: 20-30 mg/kg/day PO divided q8h x 10 days. Otitis media: 30-40 mg/kg/day PO divided tid.

FORMS - Generic/Trade: Cap 150,300 mg. Trade: Cap 75 mg, oral soln 75 mg/5 ml.

NOTES - Not for meningitis. Do not give orally at the same time as kaolin-pectin antidiarrheals. Not more than 600 mg/IM injection site. Avoid if lincomycin hypersensitivity.

daptomycin (*Cubicin, Cidecin*) ▶K ♀B ▶? $$$$$

ADULT - Complicated skin infections: 4 mg/kg IV qd infused over 30 min x 7-14 days.

PEDS - Not approved in children.

NOTES - May cause myopathy; monitor CK levels weekly. Stop if myopathy symptoms and CK >5 x upper limit of normal, or no symptoms and CK ≥10 x upper limit of normal. Consider withholding statins during daptomycin treatment. May cause neuropathy. Not effective for community-acquired pneumonia. Dosage reduction in adults with CrCl <30 ml/min: 4 mg/kg IV q48h. Reconstituted soln stable for up to 12 h at room temp or 48 h in refrigerator (combined time in vial + IV bag).

drotrecogin (*Xigris*) ▶Plasma ♀C ▶? $$$$$

ADULT - To reduce mortality in sepsis: 24 mcg/kg/h IV x 96 h. Reduced mortality only in patients with APACHE II score ≥25.

PEDS - Not approved in children.

NOTES - Can cause severe bleeding. Contraindicated with conditions and drugs that increase risk of bleeding; see package insert for details. Criteria for use include systemic inflammatory response plus acute organ dysfunction. Stop infusion 2 h before invasive procedure, or if bleeding occurs. May prolong APTT. Complete IV infusion within 12 h of reconstitution. Do not expose IV solution to heat or direct sunlight.

fosfomycin (*Monurol*) ▶K ♀B ▶? $$

ADULT - Simple UTI in women: One 3 g packet PO single dose. Dissolve granules in 1/2 cup of water.

PEDS - Not approved in children <12 yo.

FORMS - Trade: 3 g packet of granules.

NOTES - Metoclopramide decreases urinary excretion of fosfomycin. No benefit with multiple dosing. Single dose less effective than ciprofloxacin or TMP/SMX; equivalent to nitrofurantoin.

lincomycin (*Lincocin*) ▶LK ♀C ▶- $$$$$
WARNING - Pseudomembranous colitis.
ADULT - Serious gram-positive infections: 600 mg IM q12-24h. 600-1000 mg IV q8-12h. Max IV daily dose is 8 g. Dilute to 1 g/100 mL or less, and infuse over at least 1 h. Reserve for patients who are allergic or do not respond to penicillins.
PEDS - Serious gram-positive infections, >1 mo: 10-20 mg/kg/day IV divided q8-12h. Dilute to 1 g/100 mL or less, and infuse over at least 1 h. Reserve for patients who are allergic or do not respond to penicillins.
NOTES - Do not use in patients with clindamycin hypersensitivity. Monitor hepatic and renal function and CBC during prolonged therapy. Do not coadminister with erythromycin due to potential antagonism. May enhance effects of neuromuscular blockers. Reduce dose by 25% to 30% in patients with severe renal dysfunction and consider monitoring levels.

linezolid (*Zyvox*, ✚*Zyvoxam*) ▶Oxidation/K ♀C ▶? $$$$$
ADULT - IV & PO doses are the same. Vancomycin-resistant E. faecium infections: 600 mg IV/PO q12h x 14-28 days. Pneumonia, complicated skin infections (including diabetic foot): 600 mg IV/PO q12h x 10-14 days. Uncomplicated skin infections: 400 mg PO q12h x 10-14 days. Infuse over 30-120 minutes.
PEDS - Pneumonia, complicated skin infections, ≤11 yo: 10 mg/kg IV/PO q8h x 10-14 days. Vancomycin-resistant E. faecium infections, ≤11 yo: 10 mg/kg IV/PO q8h x 14-28 days. Uncomplicated skin infections: 10 mg/kg PO q8h if <5 yo, q12h if 5-11 yo x 10-14 days.
FORMS - Trade: Tabs 600 mg, susp 100 mg/5 ml. 400 mg tab approved, but not marketed.
NOTES - Myelosuppression. Monitor CBC weekly, esp. if >2 weeks of therapy, preexisting myelosuppression, other myelosuppressive drugs, or chronic infection treated with other antibiotics. Consider stopping if myelosuppression occurs or worsens. Inhibits MAO; may interact with adrenergic and serotonergic drugs, high tyramine foods. Limit tyramine to <100 mg/meal. Reduce initial dose of dopamine/epinephrine. Store susp at room temperature; stable for 21 days. Gently turn bottle over 3-5 times before giving a dose; do not shake.

methenamine hippurate (*Hiprex, Urex*) ▶KL ♀C ▶? $$$
ADULT - Long-term suppression of UTI: 1 g PO bid.
PEDS - Long-term suppression of UTI: 0.5-1 g PO bid for 6-12 yo, 1 g PO bid for >12 yo.
FORMS - Trade: Tabs 1g.
NOTES - Not for UTI treatment. Contraindicated if renal or severe hepatic impairment, severe dehydration. Acidify urine if Proteus, Pseudomonas infections. Give 1-2 g vitamin C PO q4h if urine pH >5. Avoid sulfonamides, alkalinizing foods & medications.

methenamine mandelate (*Mandelamine*) ▶KL ♀C ▶? $$$
ADULT - Long-term suppression of UTI: 1 g PO qid after meals and qhs.
PEDS - Long-term suppression of UTI: 18.4 mg/kg PO qid for <6 yo, 500 mg PO qid for 6-12 yo. Give after meals and qhs.
FORMS - Generic/Trade: Tabs 0.5,1 g. Generic: Susp 0.5 g/5 ml.
NOTES - Not for UTI treatment. Contraindicated with renal or severe hepatic impairment, severe dehydration. Acidify urine for Proteus, Pseudomonas infections. If urine pH >5, give 1-2 g vitamin C PO q4h. Avoid alkalinizing foods/medications, avoid sulfonamides.

metronidazole (*Flagyl*, ✚*Florazole ER, Trikacide*) ▶KL ♀B ▶?- $
ADULT - Trichomoniasis: Treat patient & sex partners with 2 g PO single dose, 250 mg PO tid x 7 days, or 375 mg PO bid x 7 days. Flagyl ER for bacterial vaginosis: 750 mg PO qd x 7 days on empty stomach. H pylori: See table in GI section. Anaerobic bacterial infections: Load 1 g or 15 mg/kg IV, then 500 mg or 7.5 mg/kg IV/PO q6h, each IV dose over 1h (not to exceed 4 g/day). Prophylaxis, colorectal surgery: 15 mg/kg IV completed 1 h preop, then 7.5 mg/kg IV q6h x 2 doses. Acute amebic dysentery: 750 mg PO tid x 5-10 days. Amebic liver abscess: 500-750 mg PO tid x 5-10 days.
PEDS - Amebiasis: 35-50 mg/kg/day PO (max of 750 mg/dose) divided tid x 10 days.
UNAPPROVED ADULT - Bacterial vaginosis: 500 mg PO bid x 7 days. Bacterial vaginosis in pregnancy: 250 mg PO tid x 7 days. Trichomoniasis (CDC alternative to single dose): 500 mg PO bid x 7 days. Pelvic inflammatory disease & recurrent/persistent urethritis: see STD table. Clostridium difficile diarrhea: 250 mg PO qid or 500 mg PO tid x 10 days. Giardia: 250 mg PO tid x 5-7 days.
UNAPPROVED PEDS - Clostridium difficile diarrhea: 30-50 mg/kg/day PO divided tid or qid x 7-10 days (not to exceed adult dose). Trichomoniasis: 5 mg/kg PO tid (max 2 g/day) x 7

days. Giardia: 15 mg/kg/day PO divided tid x 5-7 days. Anaerobic bacterial infections: 30 mg/kg/day IV/PO divided q6h, each IV dose over 1h (not to exceed 4 g/day).

FORMS - Generic/Trade: Tabs 250,500 mg, ER tabs 750 mg, Caps 375 mg.

NOTES - Peripheral neuropathy (chronic use), seizures. Disulfiram reaction; avoid alcohol until ≥1 day after treatment with tabs, ≥3 days with caps/ Flagyl ER. Do not give within 2 weeks of disulfiram. Interacts with barbiturates, lithium, phenytoin. Increased INR with warfarin. Darkens urine. Give iodoquinol/ paromomycin after treatment for amebic dysentery or liver abscess. Can minimize infant exposure by withholding breastfeeding for 12-24 h after maternal single dose. Decrease dose in liver dysfunction.

nitrofurantoin (*Furadantin, Macrodantin, Macrobid*) ▶KL ♀B ▶+? $$

WARNING - Pulmonary fibrosis with prolonged use.

ADULT - Acute uncomplicated cystitis: 50-100 mg PO qid with food/milk x 7 days or x 3 days after sterile urine. Long-term suppressive therapy: 50-100 mg PO qhs. Sustained release Macrobid: 100 mg bid with food/milk x 7 days.

PEDS - UTI: 5-7 mg/kg/day PO divided qid x 7 days or x 3 days after sterile urine. Long-term suppressive therapy: Doses as low as 1 mg/kg/day PO divided qd-bid. Give with food/milk. Macrobid, >12 yo: 100 mg PO bid with food/milk x 7 days.

FORMS - Macrodantin: Caps 25,50,100 mg. Generic: Caps 50,100 mg. Furadantin: Susp 25 mg/5 ml. Macrobid: Caps 100 mg.

NOTES - Contraindicated if CrCl <60 ml/min, pregnancy ≥38 weeks, infant <1 mo. Hemolytic anemia in G6PD deficiency (including susceptible infants exposed through breast milk), hepatotoxicity, peripheral neuropathy. May turn urine brown. Do not use for complicated UTI or pyelonephritis.

rifampin (*Rimactane, Rifadin, ♣Rofact*) ▶L ♀C ▶+ $$$

WARNING - See anti-mycobacterial subsection for TB regimens.

ADULT - Neisseria meningitidis carriers: 600 mg PO bid x 2 days. Take on empty stomach. IV & PO doses are the same.

PEDS - Neisseria meningitidis carriers: age ≥1 mo, 10 mg/kg up to 600 mg PO bid x 2 days. Age <1 mo, 5 mg/kg PO bid x 2 days. Take on empty stomach.

UNAPPROVED ADULT - Prophylaxis of H influenza type b infection: 20 mg/kg up to 600 mg PO qd x 4 days. Staphylococcal prosthetic valve endocarditis: 300 mg PO q8 hr in combination with gentamicin plus nafcillin, oxacillin, or vancomycin. IV & PO doses are the same.

UNAPPROVED PEDS - Prophylaxis of H influenza type b infection: age ≥1 mo, 20 mg/kg up to 600 mg PO qd x 4 days. Age <1 mo, 10 mg/kg PO qd x 4 days. Prophylaxis of invasive meningococcal disease: age ≥1 mo, 10 mg/kg up to 600 mg PO bid x 2 days. Age <1 mo, 5 mg/kg PO bid x 2 days. IV & PO doses are the same.

FORMS - Generic/Trade: Caps 150,300 mg. Pharmacists can make oral suspension.

NOTES - Hepatotoxicity, thrombocytopenia. Induces hepatic metabolism of many drugs. Induces hepatic metabolism of many drugs; check other sources for dosage adjustments before prescribing. See http://www.cdc.gov/nchstp/tb/TB_HIV_Drugs/TOC.htm for dosage adjustments of antiretroviral regimens with rifampin. Decreased efficacy of oral contraceptives; use non-hormonal method. Decreased INR with warfarin; monitor daily or as needed. Adjust dose for hepatic impairment. Colors urine, body secretions, contact lenses red-orange. IV rifampin is stable for 4h after dilution in dextrose 5%.

rifaximin (*Xifaxan*) ▶Feces, no GI absorption ♀C ▶? ?

ADULT - Travelers diarrhea: 200 mg PO tid x 3 days.

PEDS - Not approved in children <12 yo.

FORMS - Trade: Tab 200 mg.

NOTES - Not effective for diarrhea complicated by fever/blood in stool or caused by pathogens other than E coli. Consider switching to another agent if diarrhea persists for 24-48 h or worsens.

Synercid (*quinupristin + dalfopristin*) ▶Bile ♀B ▶? $$$$$

ADULT - Vancomycin-resistant E faecium infections (Not active against E. faecalis): 7.5 mg/kg IV q8h. Complicated staphylococcal/ streptococcal skin infections: 7.5 mg/kg IV q12h. Infuse over 1 h.

PEDS - Safety and efficacy not established.

UNAPPROVED PEDS - Vancomycin-resistant E faecium infections (Not active against E. faecalis): 7.5 mg/kg IV q8h. Complicated staphylococcal/streptococcal skin infections: 7.5 mg/kg IV q12h. Infuse over 1 h.

NOTES - Venous irritation - flush with D5W (not normal saline/heparin) after peripheral infusion, arthralgias/myalgias, hyperbilirubinemia. Cytochrome P450 3A4 inhibitor. Increases levels of cyclosporine, midazolam, nifedipine, others.

trimethoprim *(Primsol*, ♣*Proloprim)* ▶K ♀C ▶- $

ADULT - Uncomplicated UTI: 100 mg PO bid or 200 mg PO qd.

PEDS - Safety not established in infants <2 mo; Otitis media, age ≥6 mo (not for M catarrhalis): 10 mg/kg/day PO divided bid x 10 days.

UNAPPROVED ADULT - Prophylaxis of recurrent UTI: 100 mg qhs. Pneumocystis treatment: 5 mg/kg PO tid with dapsone 100 mg PO qd x 21 days.

FORMS - Generic/Trade: Tabs 100,200 mg. Primsol: Oral soln 50 mg/5 ml.

NOTES - Contraindicated in megaloblastic anemia due to folate deficiency. Blood dyscrasias. Trimethoprim alone not first-line for otitis media. Inhibits metabolism of phenytoin and procainamide. Dosing in adults with renal dysfunction: 50 mg PO q12h for CrCl 15-30 ml/min. Do not use if CrCl <15 ml/min.

vancomycin *(Vancocin)* ▶K ♀C ▶? $$$$

ADULT - Severe Staph infections, endocarditis: 1g IV q12h, each dose over 1h or 30 mg/kg/day IV divided q12h. Empiric therapy, native valve endocarditis: 15 mg/kg (max 2 g/day unless levels monitored) IV q12h with gentamicin. Clostridium difficile diarrhea: 125

mg PO qid x 7-10 days. IV administration ineffective for this indication. See table for prophylaxis of bacterial endocarditis.

PEDS - Severe Staph infections, endocarditis: 10 mg/kg IV q6h. Infants <1 week old: 15 mg/kg IV load, then 10 mg/kg q12h. Infants 1 week - 1 mo: 15 mg/kg IV load, then 10 mg/kg q8h. Clostridium difficile diarrhea: 40-50 mg/kg/ day up to 500 mg/day PO divided qid x 7-10 days. IV administration ineffective for this indication.

UNAPPROVED PEDS - AAP dosing for infants: 10-15 mg/kg IV q8-12h for infants <1 week. 10-15 mg/kg IV q6-8h for infants ≥1 week. Bacterial meningitis: 60 mg/kg/day IV divided q6h. Nonmeningeal pneumococcal infections: 40-45 mg/kg/day IV divided q6h.

FORMS - Generic/Trade: oral soln 1 g/20 ml bottle. Trade: Caps 125,250 mg; oral soln 500 mg/6 ml.

NOTES - "Red Neck" (or "Red Man") syndrome with rapid IV administration, vein irritation with IV extravasation, reversible neutropenia, ototoxicity or nephrotoxicity rarely. Enhanced effects of neuromuscular blockers. Use caution with other ototoxic/nephrotoxic drugs. Peak 30-40 mcg/ml 1.5-2.5 h after 1-h infusion, trough 5-10 mcg/ml. Individualize dose if renal dysfunction. Oral vancomycin poorly absorbed; do not use for extraluminal infections.

CARDIOVASCULAR: ACE Inhibitors

NOTE: See also antihypertensive combinations. Renoprotection and decreased cardiovascular morbidity/mortality seen with some ACE inhibitors are most likely a class effect. To minimize the risk of hypotension in diuretic-treated patients who are elderly, volume depleted, hyponatremic or have heart failure exacerbation, hold diuretic dose (if possible) for 2-3 days before starting an ACE inhibitor and use a low ACE inhibitor dose. If diuretics cannot be held, then reduce the dose (if possible). Use with caution in volume depleted or hyponatremic patients. Hyperkalemia possible, especially if used concomitantly with other drugs that increase K+ and in patients with CHF or renal impairment. ACE inhibitor use during pregnancy may cause injury or death to the developing fetus: use reliable form of contraception in women of child-bearing age; discontinue as soon as pregnancy is detected. Avoid with a history of angioedema. Consider intestinal angioedema if abdominal pain (with or without N/V). African Americans may be at higher risk for angioedema.

benazepril *(Lotensin)* ▶LK ♀C (1st trimester) D (2nd & 3rd) ▶? $$

ADULT - HTN: Start 10 mg PO qd, usual maintenance dose 20-40 mg PO qd or divided bid, max 80 mg/day, but added effect not apparent above 40 mg/day. Elderly, renal impairment, or concomitant diuretics: Start 5 mg PO qd.

PEDS - HTN: Start 0.2 mg/kg/day (max 10 mg/ day) as monotherapy; doses >0.6 mg/kg/day (or >40 mg/day) have not been studied. Do not use if age <6 years or if glomerular filtration rate <30 mL/min.

UNAPPROVED ADULT - Renoprotective dosing: 10 mg PO qd. CHF: Start 5 mg PO qd, usual 5-20 mg/day, max 40 mg/day (in 1-2 doses).

FORMS - Generic/Trade: Tabs, non-scored 5, 10,20,40 mg.

NOTES - BID dosing may be required for 24-hour BP control.

captopril *(Capoten)* ▶LK ♀C (1st trimester) D (2nd & 3rd) ▶+ $

ADULT - HTN: Start 25 mg PO bid-tid, usual maintenance dose 25-150 mg PO bid-tid, max 450 mg/day (max 150 mg/day typical). Elderly, renal impairment, or concomitant diuretic therapy: Start 6.25-12.5 mg PO bid-tid. CHF: Start 6.25-12.5 mg PO tid, usual 50-100 mg PO tid, max 450 mg/day (max 150 mg/day typical). Diabetic nephropathy: Titrate to 25 mg PO tid.
PEDS - Not approved in children.
UNAPPROVED ADULT - Hypertensive urgency: 12.5-25 mg PO, repeated once or twice if necessary at intervals of ≥30-60 minutes.
UNAPPROVED PEDS - HTN: Neonates: initial dose 0.1-0.4 mg/kg/day PO divided q6-8h. Infants: initial dose 0.15-0.3 mg/kg/dose, titrate to effective dose, max dose 6 mg/kg/day divided qd-qid. Children: initial dose 0.5-1 mg/kg/day PO divided tid. Titrate to effective dose, maximum dose 6 mg/kg/day.
FORMS - Generic/Trade: Tabs, scored 12.5,25, 50,100 mg.
NOTES - A captopril solution or suspension (1 mg/mL) can be made by dissolving Tabs in distilled water or flavored syrup. The solution is stable for 7days at room temperature.

cilazapril (❤*Inhibace*) ▶LK ♀C (1st trimester) D (2nd & 3rd) ▶? $
ADULT - Canada only. HTN: Initial dose 2.5 mg PO qd, usual maintenance dose 2.5-5 mg qd, max 10 mg qd. Elderly or concomitant diuretic therapy: initiate 1.25 mg PO qd. CHF adjunct: Initially 0.5 mg PO qd, increase to usual maintenance of 1-2.5 mg qd. Renal Impairment with CrCl 10-40 ml/min, initiate 0.5 mg qd, max 2.5mg/day. CrCl <10 ml/min 0.25-0.5 mg once or twice per week, according to BP response.
PEDS - Not approved in children.
FORMS - Trade: Scored tabs 1, 2.5, 5 mg.
NOTES - Reduce dose in hepatic / renal impairment

enalapril (*enalaprilat, Vasotec*) ▶LK ♀C (1st trimester) D (2nd & 3rd) ▶+ $
ADULT - HTN: Start 5 mg PO qd, usual maintenance dose 10-40 mg PO qd or divided bid, max 40 mg/day. If oral therapy not possible, can use 1.25 mg IV q6h over 5 minutes, and increase up to 5 mg IV q6h if needed. Renal impairment or concomitant diuretic therapy: Start 2.5 mg PO qd. CHF: Start 2.5 mg PO bid, usual 10-20 mg PO bid, max 40 mg/day.
PEDS - Not approved in children.
UNAPPROVED ADULT - Hypertensive crisis: 1.25-5 mg IV q6h. Renoprotective dosing: 10-20 mg PO qd.
UNAPPROVED PEDS - HTN: Start 0.1

mg/kg/day PO qd or divided bid, titrate to effective dose, maximum dose 0.5 mg/kg/day; 0.005-0.01 mg/kg/dose IV q8-24 hours.
FORMS - Generic/Trade: Tabs, scored 2.5,5, non-scored 10, 20 mg.
NOTES - BID dosing may be required for 24-hour BP control. An enalapril oral susp (0.2 mg/ml) can be made by dissolving one 2.5 mg tab in 12.5 ml sterile water, use immediately.

fosinopril (*Monopril*) ▶LK ♀C (1st trimester) D (2nd & 3rd) ▶? $$
ADULT - HTN: Start 10 mg PO qd, usual maintenance dose 20-40 mg PO qd or divided bid, max 80 mg/day, but added effect not apparent above 40 mg/day. Elderly, renal impairment, or concomitant diuretic therapy: Start 5 mg PO qd. CHF: Start 5-10 mg PO qd, usual 20-40 mg PO qd, max 40 mg/day.
PEDS - HTN: 6-16 years & weight >50 kg: 5-10 mg PO qd.
UNAPPROVED ADULT - Renoprotective dosing: 10-20 mg PO qd.
FORMS - Generic/Trade: Tabs, scored 10, non-scored 20,40 mg.
NOTES - Elimination 50% renal, 50% hepatic. Accumulation of drug negligible with impaired renal function.

lisinopril (*Prinivil, Zestril*) ▶K ♀C (1st trimester) D (2nd & 3rd) ▶? $$
ADULT - HTN: Start 10 mg PO qd, usual maintenance dose 20-40 mg PO qd, max 80 mg/day, but added effect not apparent above 40 mg/day. Renal impairment or concomitant diuretic therapy: Start 2.5-5 mg PO qd. CHF, acute MI: start 2.5-5 mg PO qd, usual 5-20 mg PO qd, max 40 mg/day.
PEDS - HTN ≥6 yo: 0.07 mg/kg PO qd; 5 mg/day max. Not recommended <6 yo or with glomerular filtration rate <30 mL/min/1.73 meters squared.
UNAPPROVED ADULT - Renoprotective dosing: 10-20 mg PO qd.
FORMS - Generic/Trade: Tabs, non-scored 2.5,10,20,30,40, scored 5 mg.

moexipril (*Univasc*) ▶LK ♀C (1st trimester) D (2nd & 3rd) ▶? $
ADULT - HTN: Start 7.5 mg PO qd, usual maintenance dose 7.5-30 mg PO qd or divided bid, max 30 mg/day. Renal impairment or concomitant diuretic therapy: Start 3.75 mg PO qd.
PEDS - Not approved in children.
FORMS - Generic/trade: Tabs, scored 7.5, 15 mg.
NOTES - BID dosing may be required for 24-hour BP control.

perindopril (*Aceon*, ♣ *Coversyl*) ▶K ♀C (1st trimester) D (2nd & 3rd) ▶? $$
ADULT - HTN: Start 4 mg PO qd, usual maintenance dose 4-8 mg PO qd or divided bid, max 16 mg/day. Renal impairment or concomitant diuretics: Start 2 mg PO qd or divided bid.
PEDS - Not approved in children.
UNAPPROVED ADULT - CHF: Start 2 mg PO qd, usual dose 4 mg qd, max dose 8 mg qd. Reduction of cardiovascular events in stable coronary heart disease: Start 4 mg PO qd x 2 weeks, max dose 8 mg qd; Elderly (≥70 years): 2 mg PO qd x 1 week, 4 mg PO qd x 1 week, max dose 8 mg qd. Recurrent stroke prevention: 4 mg PO qd with indapamide.
FORMS - Trade: Tabs, scored 2,4,8 mg.
NOTES - BID dosing does not provide clinically significant BP lowering compared to once daily dosing.

quinapril (*Accupril*) ▶LK ♀C (1st trimester) D (2nd & 3rd) ▶? $$
ADULT - HTN: Start 10-20 mg PO qd, usual maintenance dose 20-80 mg PO qd or divided bid, max 80 mg/day, but added effect not apparent above 40 mg/day. Renal impairment or concomitant diuretic therapy: Start 2.5-5 mg PO qd. CHF: Start 5 mg PO bid, usual maintenance dose 20-40 mg/day divided bid.
PEDS - Not approved in children.
FORMS - Trade: Tabs, scored 5, non-scored 10,20,40 mg.
NOTES - BID dosing may be required for 24-hour BP control.

ramipril (*Altace*) ▶LK ♀C (1st trimester) D (2nd & 3rd) ▶? $$
ADULT - HTN: Start 2.5 mg PO qd, usual maintenance dose 2.5-20 mg PO qd or divided bid, max 20 mg/day. Renal impairment or concomitant diuretic therapy: Start 1.25 mg PO qd. CHF post-MI: Start 2.5 mg PO bid, usual maintenance dose 5 mg PO bid. Reduce risk of MI, stroke, death from cardiovascular causes: Start 2.5 mg PO qd for 1 week, then 5 mg PO qd for 3 weeks, increase as tolerated to maintenance dose 10 mg qd.
PEDS - Not approved in children.
UNAPPROVED ADULT - Renoprotective dosing: Titrate to 10 mg PO qd.
FORMS - Trade: Caps, 1.25,2.5,5,10 mg.
NOTES - BID dosing may be required for 24-hour BP control. cap contents can be sprinkled on applesauce and eaten or mixed with 120 mL of water or apple juice and swallowed. Mixtures are stable for 24 hr at room temperature or 48 hr refrigerated.

trandolapril (*Mavik*) ▶LK ♀C (1st trimester) D (2nd & 3rd) ▶? $$
ADULT - HTN: Start 1 mg PO qd in non-black patients or 2 mg PO qd in black patients, usual maintenance dose 2-4 mg PO qd or divided bid, max 8 mg/day, but added effect not apparent above 4 mg/day. Renal impairment or concomitant diuretic therapy: Start 0.5 mg PO qd. CHF/post-MI: Start 0.5-1 mg PO qd, titrate to target dose 4 mg PO qd.
PEDS - Not approved in children.
FORMS - Trade: Tabs, scored 1, non-scored 2,4 mg.

ACE INHIBITOR DOSING	Hypertension		Heart Failure		
	Initial	*Max/day*	*Initial*	*Target*	*Max*
benazepril (*Lotensin*)	10 mg qd*	80 mg	-	-	-
captopril (*Capoten*)	25 mg bid/tid	450 mg	6.25-12.5 mg tid	50 mg tid	150 mg tid
enalapril (*Vasotec*)	5 mg qd*	40 mg	2.5 mg bid	10 mg bid	20 mg bid
fosinopril (*Monopril*)	10 mg qd*	80 mg	10 mg qd	20 mg qd	40 mg qd
lisinopril (*Zestril/Prinivil*)	10 mg qd	80 mg	5 mg qd	20 mg qd	40 mg qd
moexipril (*Univasc*)	7.5 mg qd*	30-60 mg	-	-	-
perindopril (*Aceon*)	4 mg qd*	16 mg	-	-	-
quinapril (*Accupril*)	10-20 mg qd*	80 mg	5 mg bid	10 mg bid	20 mg bid
ramipril (*Altace*)	2.5 mg qd*	20 mg	2.5 mg bid	5 mg bid	10 mg bid
trandolapril (*Mavik*)	1-2 mg qd*	8 mg	1 mg qd	4 mg qd	4 mg qd

Data taken from prescribing information.   *May require bid dosing for 24-hour BP control.

CARDIOVASCULAR: Aldosterone Antagonists

NOTE: Beware of hyperkalemia. Use cautiously with other agents that may cause hyperkalemia (ie. ACEIs, ARBs).

eplerenone (*Inspra*) ▶L ♀B ▶? $$$$
ADULT - HTN: Start 50 mg PO qd, increase after 4 weeks if needed to max dose 50 mg bid.

Start 25 mg qd if concomitant drugs that mildly inhibit CYP 3A4 isoenzyme (eg, erythromycin, verapamil, fluconazole, saquinavir). Improve survival of stable patients with left ventricular systolic dysfunction (EF ≤40%) and CHF post-MI: Start 25 mg PO qd; titrate to target dose 50 mg PO qd within 4 weeks, if tolerated.

PEDS - Not approved in children.

FORMS - Trade: Tabs non-scored 25, 50 mg

NOTES - Contraindicated in all patients with potassium >5.5 mEq/L; CrCl ≤30 mL/min; strong CYP 3A4 inhibitors (ketoconazole, itraconazole, nefazodone, troleandomycin, clarithromycin, ritonavir, nelfinavir). For treatment of HTN, contraindications include Type 2 DM with microalbuminuria; serum creat >2 mg/dL in males or >1.8 mg/dL in females; CrCl <50 mL/min; concomitant therapy with K+ supplements, K-sparing diuretics. Hyperkalemia more common with concomitant ACE inhibitors/ARBs. Measure serum K+ before initiating, within 1st week , at 1 month after starting treatment or dose adjustment, then prn. Monitor lithium levels. Monitor BP if used with NSAIDs.

spironolactone (*Aldactone*) ▶LK ♀D ▶+ $

ADULT - Edema (CHF, cirrhosis, nephrotic syndrome): Start 100 mg PO qd or divided bid, maintain for 5 days, increase as needed to achieve diuretic response, usual dose range 25-200 mg/day. Other diuretics may be needed. HTN: 50-100 mg PO qd or divided bid, generally used in combination with a thiazide diuretic to maintain serum potassium, increase dose as needed based on serum potassium and BP. Diuretic-induced hypokalemia: 25-100 mg PO qd when potassium supplements/sparing regimens inappropriate.

PEDS - Edema: 3.3 mg/kg PO qd or divided bid.

UNAPPROVED ADULT - Severe CHF: Start 12.5-25 mg PO qd, usual maintenance dose 25 mg qd, max dose 50 mg qd.

UNAPPROVED PEDS - Edema/HTN: 1-3.3 mg/kg/day, PO qd or divided bid, max 200 mg/day.

FORMS - Generic/Trade: Tabs, non-scored 25; scored 50,100 mg.

NOTES - Gynecomastia, impotence in males. Dosing more frequently than BID not necessary. Hyperkalemia more likely with ≥50 mg/day and with concomitant ACE inhibitors or K+ supplements.

CARDIOVASCULAR: Angiotensin Receptor Blockers (ARBs)

NOTE: See also antihypertensive combinations. To minimize the risk of hypotension in diuretic treated patients who are elderly, volume depleted, hyponatremic or have heart failure exacerbation, hold diuretic dose (if possible) for 2-3 days before starting an ARB and use a low ARB dose. If diuretics cannot be held, reduce the dose (if possible). Use with caution in volume-depleted or hyponatremic patients. ARB use during pregnancy may cause injury or death to the developing fetus: use reliable form of contraception in women of child-bearing age; discontinue as soon as pregnancy is detected. Use with caution in patients with a history of ACE inhibitor-induced angioedema. African Americans may be at higher risk for angioedema. Rare cases of rhabdomyolysis have been reported with ARBs.

candesartan (*Atacand*) ▶K ♀C (1st trimester) D (2nd & 3rd) ▶? $$

ADULT - HTN: Start 16 mg PO qd, max 32 mg/day. Volume-depleted patients: Start 8 mg PO qd.

PEDS - Not approved in children.

UNAPPROVED ADULT - Reduce cardiovascular death or CHF hospitalizations in chronic CHF and ejection fraction ≤40%, with or without ACE inhibitors; reduce CHF hospitalizations in chronic CHF & ejection fraction >40%: Start 4 mg PO qd, double dose q 2 weeks; target dose 32 mg/day.

FORMS - Trade: Tabs, non-scored 4,8,16,32 mg.

NOTES - May increase lithium levels.

eprosartan (*Teveten*) ▶Fecal excretion ♀C (1st trimester) D (2nd & 3rd) ▶? $$

ADULT - HTN: Start 600 mg PO qd, maximum 800 mg/day given qd or divided bid.

PEDS - Not approved in children.

FORMS - Trade: tabs non-scored 400, 600 mg.

irbesartan (*Avapro*) ▶L ♀C (1st trimester) D (2nd & 3rd) ▶? $$

ADULT - HTN: Start 150 mg PO qd, max 300 mg/day. Volume depleted patients: Start 75 mg PO qd. Type 2 diabetic nephropathy: Start 150 mg PO qd, target dose 300 mg qd.

PEDS - Not approved in children.

FORMS - Trade: Tabs, non-scored 75,150,300 mg.

losartan (*Cozaar*) ▶L ♀C (1st trimester) D (2nd & 3rd) ▶? $$

ADULT - HTN: Start 50 mg PO qd, max 100 mg/day given qd or divided bid. Volume-depleted patients or history of hepatic impairment: Start 25 mg PO qd. Stroke risk reduction in patients with HTN & left ventricular hypertrophy: Start 50 mg PO qd. Max 100 mg/day and/or add HCTZ. Type 2 diabetic nephropathy: Start 50 mg PO qd, target dose 100 mg qd.

PEDS - HTN: Start 0.7 mg/kg/day (up to 50 mg), doses >1.4 mg/kg/day (or >100 mg) have not been studied. Do not use if age <6 years or if glomerular filtration rate <30 mL/min.

UNAPPROVED ADULT - CHF: Start 12.5 mg PO qd, target dose 50 mg qd. Renoprotective dosing: Start 50 mg PO qd, increase to 100 mg qd as needed for BP control.

FORMS - Trade: Tabs, non-scored 25,50,100 mg.

NOTES - Black patients with HTN & left ventricular hypertrophy may have less stroke risk reduction than non-Blacks. Monitor BP control when adding or discontinuing rifampin, fluconazole, or erythromycin.

olmesartan (*Benicar*) ▶K ♀C (1st trimester) D (2nd & 3rd) ▶? $$

ADULT - HTN: Start 20 mg PO qd, maximum 40 mg/day.

PEDS - Not approved in children.

FORMS - Trade: Tabs, non-scored 5,20,40 mg.

telmisartan (*Micardis*) ▶L ♀C (1st trimester) D (2nd & 3rd) ▶? $$

ADULT - HTN: Start 40 mg PO qd, max 80 mg/day.

PEDS - Not approved in children.

FORMS - Trade: Tabs, non-scored 20,40,80 mg.

NOTES - Swallow tabs whole, do not break or crush. Caution in hepatic insufficiency. May need to monitor digoxin levels when initiating, adjusting dose, or discontinuing.

valsartan (*Diovan*) ▶L ♀C (1st trimester) D (2nd & 3rd) ▶? $$$

ADULT - HTN: Start 80-160 mg PO qd, max 320 mg/d. CHF: Start 40 mg PO bid, target dose 160 mg bid.

PEDS - Not approved in children.

UNAPPROVED ADULT - Renoprotective dosing: 80-160 mg PO qd. Reduce mortality/morbidity post-MI with left ventricular systolic dysfunction (EF ≤35%) and/or CHF: Start 20 mg PO bid, target dose 160 mg bid.

FORMS - Trade: Tabs, nonscored 80, 160, 320 mg.

CARDIOVASCULAR: Antiadrenergic Agents

clonidine (*Catapres*) ▶LK ♀C ▶? $

ADULT - HTN: Start 0.1 mg PO bid, usual maintenance dose 0.2-1.2 mg/day divided bid-tid, max 2.4 mg/day. Transdermal (Catapres-TTS): Start 0.1 mg/24 hour patch q week, titrate to desired effect, max effective dose 0.6 mg/24 hour (two, 0.3 mg/24 hour patches).

PEDS - HTN: Start 5-7 mcg/kg/day PO divided q6-12 hr, titrate at 5-7 day intervals to 5-25 mcg/kg/day divided q6h; max 0.9 mg/day. Transdermal therapy not recommended in children.

UNAPPROVED ADULT - HTN urgency: Initially, 0.1-0.2 mg PO, followed by 0.1 mg q1h as needed up to a total dose of 0.5-0.7 mg.

FORMS - Generic/Trade: Tabs, non-scored 0.1, 0.2, 0.3 mg. Trade only: transdermal weekly patch 0.1 mg/day (TTS-1), 0.2 mg/day (TTS-2), 0.3 mg/day (TTS-3).

NOTES - Sedation. Bradycardia. Can get rebound HTN with abrupt discontinuation of tabs, especially at doses ≥0.8 mg/d. Taper therapy over 4-7 days to avoid rebound HTN. Dispose of used patches carefully, keep away from children.

doxazosin (*Cardura*) ▶L ♀C ▶? $

WARNING - Not first line agent for hyperten-

sion. Increased risk of CHF in patients who used doxazosin compared to diuretic in treating HTN.

ADULT - HTN: Start 1 mg PO qhs, max 16 mg/day. BPH: see urology section. Avoid use of doxazosin alone to treat combined HTN and BPH.

PEDS - Not approved in children.

FORMS - Generic/Trade: Tabs, scored 1,2,4,8 mg.

NOTES - Dizziness, drowsiness, lightheadedness, syncope. Bedtime dosing may minimize side effects. Initial 1 mg dose is used to decrease postural hypotension that may occur after the first few doses. If therapy is interrupted for several days, restart at the 1 mg dose. Monitor BP after first dose, after each dose adjustment, and periodically thereafter. Contraindicated with vardenafil or tadalafil; increases risk of hypotension.

guanabenz (*Wytensin*) ▶LK ♀C ▶- $$

WARNING - Sedation, rebound HTN with abrupt discontinuation especially with high doses.

ADULT - HTN: Start 2-4 mg PO bid, max 32 mg bid.

PEDS - Children >12 years of age: initial dose 0.5-2 mg/day divided bid, usual maintenance dose 4-24 mg/day divided bid.

FORMS - Generic/Trade: Tabs, non-scored 4, scored 8 mg.

NOTES - Sedation. Can get rebound HTN with abrupt discontinuation, especially at higher doses (32 mg/day). Taper therapy over 4-7 days to avoid rebound HTN.

guanfacine (Tenex) ▶K ♀B ▶? $

ADULT - HTN: Start 1 mg PO qhs, increase to 2-3 mg qhs if needed after 3-4 weeks, max 3 mg/day.

PEDS - HTN: ≥12 years of age, same as adult.

FORMS - Generic/Trade: Tabs, non-scored 1,2 mg.

NOTES - Sedation. Most of the drug's therapeutic effect is seen at 1 mg/day. Rebound HTN with abrupt discontinuation, but generally BP returns to pretreatment measurements slowly without ill effects.

methyldopa (Aldomet) ▶LK ♀B ▶ı $

ADULT - HTN: Start 250 mg PO bid-tid, usual maintenance dose 500-3000 mg/day divided bid-qid, max 3000 mg/day. Hypertensive crisis: 250-500 mg IV q6h, maximum 1gm IV q6h.

PEDS - HTN: 10 mg/kg/day PO divided bid-qid, titrate dose to a max dose 65 mg/kg/day.

FORMS - Generic/Trade: Tabs, non-scored 125,250,500 mg.

NOTES - Drug of choice for pregnancy-induced HTN, except near term or during labor. Otherwise, reserved as a 2nd or 3rd line agent for HTN. IV form has a slow onset of effect and other agents preferred for rapid reduction of BP. Hemolytic anemia possible.

prazosin (Minipress) ▶L ♀C ▶? $

WARNING - Not first line agent for hypertension. Increased risk of CHF in patients who used doxazosin compared to diuretic in treating HTN.

ADULT - HTN: Start 1 mg PO bid-tid, usual maintenance dose 20 mg/day divided bid-tid, max 40 mg/day, but doses >20 mg/day usually

do not increase efficacy.

PEDS - Not approved in children.

UNAPPROVED PEDS - HTN: Start 0.005 mg/kg PO single dose; increase slowly as needed up to maintenance dose 0.025-0.150 mg/kg/day divided q6 hours; max dose 0.4 mg/kg/day.

FORMS - Generic/Trade: Caps 1,2,5 mg.

NOTES - To avoid syncope, start with 1 mg qhs, and increase dose gradually. Contraindicated with vardenafil or tadalafil; increases risk of hypotension.

reserpine (Serpasil) ▶LK ♀C ▶- $

ADULT - HTN: Start 0.05-0.1 mg PO qd or 0.1 mg PO qod, max dose 0.25 mg/day.

PEDS - Not approved in children.

FORMS - Generic: Tabs, scored, 0.1,0.25 mg.

NOTES - Usually used in combination with a diuretic to counteract side effects and augment BP control. Drowsiness, fatigue, lethargy. May cause depression at higher doses, avoid use in patients with depression.

terazosin (Hytrin) ▶LK ♀C ▶? $$

WARNING - Not first line agent for hypertension. Increased risk of CHF in patients who used doxazosin compared to diuretic in treating HTN.

ADULT - HTN: Start 1 mg PO qhs, usual effective dose 1-5 mg PO qd or divided bid, max 20 mg/day. BPH: see urology section.

PEDS - Not approved in children.

FORMS - Generic (Caps, Tabs)/Trade (Caps): 1,2,5,10 mg.

NOTES - Dizziness, drowsiness, lightheadedness, syncope. Bedtime dosing may minimize side effects. Initial 1 mg dose is used to decrease postural hypotension that may occur after the first few doses. If therapy is interrupted for several days, restart at the 1 mg dose. Monitor BP after first dose, after each dose adjustment, and periodically thereafter. Contraindicated with vardenafil or tadalafil; increases risk of hypotension.

CARDIOVASCULAR: Anti-Dysrhythmics / Cardiac Arrest

adenosine (Adenocard) ▶Plasma ♀C ▶? $$$

ADULT - PSVT conversion (not A-fib): 6 mg rapid IV & flush, preferably through a central line. If no response after 1-2 mins then 12 mg. A third dose of 12 mg may be given prn.

PEDS - PSVT conversion <50 kg: initial dose 50-100 mcg/kg IV, give subsequent doses q1-2 min prn by increasing 50-100 mcg/kg each time, up to a max single dose of 300 mcg/kg or 12 mg. ≥50 kg: Same as adult.

UNAPPROVED PEDS - PSVT conversion: Initial dose 0.1-0.2 mg/kg IV bolus.

NOTES - Half-life is <10 seconds. Give doses by rapid IV push followed by normal saline flush. Need higher dose if on theophylline or caffeine, lower dose if on dipyridamole or carbamazepine. May cause respiratory collapse in patients with asthma, COPD. Use in setting with cardiac resuscitation readily available. Do not confuse with adenosine phosphate used for the symptomatic relief of varicose vein complications.

amiodarone *(Cordarone, Pacerone)* ▶L ♀D ▶- $$$$

WARNING - Life-threatening pulmonary and hepatoxicity. Proarrhythmic. Contraindicated with marked sinus bradycardia and 2nd/3rd degree heart block if no pacemaker. Loading doses for inpatients only.

ADULT - Life-threatening ventricular arrhythmia: Load 150 mg IV over 10 min, then 1 mg/min x 6 hrs, then 0.5 mg/min x 18h. Mix in D5W. Oral loading dose 800-1600 mg PO qd for 1-3 weeks, reduce dose to 400-800 mg qd for 1 month when arrhythmia is controlled or adverse effects are prominent, then reduce to lowest effective dose, usually 200-400 mg qd.

PEDS - Not approved in children.

UNAPPROVED ADULT - Refractory atrial fibrillation: loading dose 600-800 mg PO qd for 7-10 days, then 200-400 mg qd. Shock-refractory VF/pulseless VT: 300 mg or 5 mg/kg IV over 10 min followed by unsynchronized shock, additional 150 mg bolus over 10 min may be given if serious arrhythmias recur. Stable monomorphic ventricular tachycardia: 150 mg IV over 10 min, repeat q10-15 min prn.

UNAPPROVED PEDS - May cause death or other serious side effects in children (see NOTES); do not use in infants <30 days of age and use only if medically warranted if >30 days of age. Ventricular arrhythmia: Loading dose 10-15 mg/kg/day PO for 4-14 days and/or until arrhythmia is controlled or adverse effects are prominent, then reduce to 5 mg/kg/d for several weeks. Reduce to lowest effective dose. IV therapy limited data; 5 mg/kg IV over 30 minutes; followed by 5 mcg/kg/min infusion; increase infusion as needed up to max 10 mcg/kg/min. Give loading dose in 1 mg/kg aliquots with each aliquot given over 5-10 min; do not exceed 30 mg/min.

FORMS - Generic: Tabs, scored 300 mg. Generic/Trade: Tabs, scored 200; unscored 100, 400 mg.

NOTES - Photosensitivity with oral therapy. Hypo/hyperthyroidism possible. Monitor LFTs, TFTs, and PFTs. Prompt eye exam needed with changes in visual acuity or decreased peripheral vision. Long elimination half-life, approximately 25-50 days. Drug interactions may persist after discontinuance due to long half-life. May increase digoxin levels up to 70% and INRs with warfarin therapy up to 100%. A dosage reduction in warfarin of 33-50% is recommended. Increased myopathy risk with simvastatin or lovastatin. Caution with simvastatin >20 mg/day or lovastatin >40 mg/day, unless clinical benefit outweighs risk of myopathy. Give bid if intolerable GI effects occur with qd dosing. IV therapy may cause hypotension & bradycardia in adults. Administer IV infusion using a nonevacuated glass bottle and in-line IV filter. Use central line when concentration >2 mg/ml. May cause congenital hypothyroidism and hyperthyroidism if given during pregnancy. Avoid use in children <1 month of age: IV form contains benzyl alcohol, which may cause gasping syndrome (gasping respirations, hypotension, bradycardia, and cardiovascular collapse). In children 1 month to 15 years of age may cause life-threatening hypotension, bradycardia, and AV block. May adversely affect male reproductive tract development in infants & toddlers from plasticizer exposure from IV tubing; use IV bolus doses instead of IV tubing to administer doses to infants and toddlers.

atropine ▶K ♀C ▶- $

ADULT - Bradyarrhythmia/CPR: 0.5-1.0 mg IV q3-5 mins, max 0.04 mg/kg (2 mg).

PEDS - CPR: 0.02 mg/kg/dose IV q5 mins for 2-3 doses prn (max single dose 0.5 mg); minimum single dose, 0.1 mg; max cumulative dose 1 mg.

UNAPPROVED ADULT - ET administration prior to IV access: 2-2.5 x the recommended IV dose in 10 ml of NS or distilled water.

bicarbonate ▶K ♀C ▶? $

ADULT - Cardiac arrest: 1 mEq/kg/dose IV initially, followed by repeat doses up to 0.5 mg/kg at 10 minute intervals during continued arrest. Severe acidosis: 2-5 mEq/kg dose IV administered as a 4-8 hour infusion. Repeat dosing based on lab values. Prevention of contrast-induced nephropathy: Administer sodium bicarbonate 154 mEq/L soln at 3 ml/kg/hr IV x 1h before contrast, followed by infusion of 1 ml/kg/hr x 6 hrs post-procedure. If >110 kg dose based on 110 kg weight.

PEDS - Cardiac arrest: Neonates or infants <2 years of age, 1 mEq/kg dose IV slow injection initially, followed by repeat doses up to 1 mEq/kg at 10 minute intervals during continued arrest. To avoid intracranial hemorrhage due to hypertonicity, use a 1:1 dilution of 8.4% (1 mEq/mL) sodium bicarbonate and dextrose 5% or use the 4.2% (0.5 mEq/mL) product.

NOTES - Full correction of bicarb deficit should not be attempted during the first 24h. May paradoxically exacerbate intracellular acidosis.

bretylium (*Bretylol*) ▸K ♀C ▸? $

ADULT - Ventricular arrhythmia: Initial 5 mg/kg IV bolus over 1 minute, then 10 mg/kg if needed at 5-30 minute intervals up to a total 30-35 mg/kg. Infusion 500 mg in 50 ml D5W (10 mg/mL) at 1-3 mg/min (6-18 mL/h).

PEDS - Not approved in children.

UNAPPROVED PEDS - Ventricular fibrillation: Initial dose 5 mg/kg IV, followed by 10 mg/kg IV if ventricular fibrillation persists.

NOTES - Hyperthermia; considered 2nd line agent due to delayed onset of antiarrhythmic action, hypotension (occurs commonly), and increased ventricular irritability.

digoxin (*Lanoxin, Lanoxicaps, Digitek, digitalis*) ▸KL ♀C ▸+ $

ADULT - Atrial fibrillation/CHF: 0.125-0.25 mg PO qd. Rapid A-fib: Load 0.5 mg IV, then 0.25 mg IV q6h x 2 doses, maintenance 0.125-0.375 mg IV/PO qd. Other agents (ie, beta blockers, calcium channel blockers) generally more effective in controlling rate in A-fib.

PEDS - Arrhythmia: Oral loading dose with tabs or elixir: premature neonate, 20-30 mcg/kg; full-term neonate, 25-35 mcg/kg; 1-24 months, 35-60 mcg/kg; 2-5 years, 30-40 mcg/kg; 5-10 years, 20-35 mcg/kg; >10 years, 10-15 mcg/kg. Use 25-35% of oral loading dose for maintenance dose. Caution - pediatric doses are in mcg, elixir product is labeled in mg/ml.

UNAPPROVED ADULT - Reentrant PSVT associated w/ ST-elevation MI (after carotid massage, IV adenosine, IV beta blocker, IV diltiazem): 8-15 mcg/kg IV, give 50% of total dose initially with additional increment in 4 hours.

FORMS - Generic/Trade: Tabs, scored (Lanoxin, Digitek) 0.125,0.25 mg; elixir 0.05 mg/mL. Trade only: Caps (Lanoxicaps)0.05,0.1,0.2 mg.

NOTES - Adjust dose based on response and therapeutic serum levels (range from 0.8-2.0 ng/mL). CHF may respond at lower levels (≥0.5 ng/ml) while A-fib may need higher. Serum digoxin concentration of 0.5-0.8 ng/mL is associated with decreased mortality in men with CHF and ejection fraction ≤45%. Toxicity exacerbated by hypokalemia. 100 mcg Lanoxicaps = 125 mcg tabs or elixir. Avoid administering IM due to severe local irritation. Elimination prolonged with renal impairment, monitor levels carefully. Many drug and herb interactions.

digoxin immune Fab (*Digibind, Digifab*) ▸K ♀C ▸? $$$$$

ADULT - Digoxin toxicity: 2-20 vials IV, one formula is: Number vials = (serum dig level in ng/mL) x (kg) / 100.

PEDS - Same as adult.

UNAPPROVED ADULT - Reentrant PSVT associated w/ ST-elevation MI (after carotid massage, IV adenosine, beta blocker, diltiazem): 8-15 mcg/kg IV.

NOTES - Do not draw serum digoxin concentrations after administering digoxin-immune Fab; levels will be falsely elevated for several days. One vial binds approximately 0.5 mg digoxin.

disopyramide (*Norpace, Norpace CR, ♥Rythmodan-LA*) ▸KL ♀C ▸+ $$$$

WARNING - Proarrhythmic. Increased mortality in patients with non-life threatening ventricular arrhythmias and structural heart disease (i.e. MI, LV dysfunction).

ADULT - Rarely indicated, consult cardiologist. Ventricular arrhythmia: 400-800 mg PO daily in divided doses (immediate-release, q6h or extended-release, q12h).

PEDS - Ventricular arrhythmia: Divide dose q6h. <1 yr, 10-30 mg/kg/day; 1-4 yrs, 10-20 mg/kg/day; 4-12 yrs, 10-15 mg/kg/day; 12-18 yrs, 6-15 mg/kg/day.

FORMS - Generic/Trade: Caps, immediate-release, 100,150 mg; extended-release 150 mg. Trade only: extended-release 100 mg.

NOTES - Anticholinergic side effects (dry mouth, constipation, blurred vision, urinary hesitancy) commonly occur. Reduce dose in patients with CrCl <40 mL/min. Initiate as an outpatient with extreme caution.

dofetilide (*Tikosyn*) ▸KL ♀C ▸- $$$$

WARNING - Consult cardiologist before using. Tikosyn is available only to hospitals and prescribers who have received appropriate dosing and treatment initiation education. Contraindicated if CrCl is <20 ml/min or QTc interval >440 msec, or >500 msec in patients with ventricular conduction abnormalities. Tikosyn must be initiated or re-initiated in a facility that can provide CrCl calculation, ECG monitoring, and cardiac resuscitation. Monitor in this setting for ≥3 days. Do not discharge if ≤12 h since electrical or pharmacological conversion to normal sinus rhythm.

ADULT - Conversion of A-fib/flutter: Specialized dosing based on CrCl and QTc interval.

PEDS - Not approved in children.

FORMS - Trade: Caps, 0.125,0.25,0.5 mg.

NOTES - Use when heart rate <50 bpm has not been studied. Monitor K+ and Mg+ (low levels increase risk of arrhythmias). Assess CrCl and QTc prior to first dose. Continuously monitor ECG during hospital initiation and adjust dose based on QTc interval. Effects may be increased by known cytochrome P450 3A4 inhibitors and drugs that inhibit renal elimination. Contraindicated with HCTZ, SMZ-TMP, verapamil, cimetidine, prochlorperazine, megestrol, and ketoconazole.

epinephrine (*EpiPen, EpiPen Jr*, adrenalin) ▶Plasma ♀C ▶- $
ADULT - Cardiac arrest: 1 mg (1:10,000 solution) IV, repeat every 3-5 minutes if needed; infusion 1 mg in 250 mL D5W (4 mcg/mL) at 1-4 mcg/min (15-60 mL/h). Anaphylaxis: 0.1-0.5 mg SC/IM (1:1,000 solution), may repeat SC dose every 10-15 minutes for anaphylactic shock.
PEDS - Cardiac arrest: 0.01 mg/kg IV/intraosseous or 0.1 mg/kg ET, repeat 0.1-0.2 mg/kg IV/IO/ET every 3-5 minutes if needed. Neonates: 0.01-0.03 mg/kg IV/ET, repeat every 3-5 minutes if needed; IV infusion start 0.1 mcg/kg/min, increase in increments of 0.1 mcg/kg/min if needed, max 1 mcg/kg/min. Anaphylaxis: 0.01 mg/kg SC, may repeat SC dose at 20 min to 4h intervals depending on severity of condition.
UNAPPROVED ADULT - Symptomatic bradycardia unresponsive to atropine: 2-10 mcg/min IV infusion. ET administration prior to IV access: 2-2.5 x the recommended IV dose in 10 ml of NS or distilled water.
FORMS - Adults: EpiPen Auto-injector delivers 0.3 mg (1:1,000 soln) IM dose. Children: EpiPen Jr. Autoinjector delivers 0.15 mg (1:2,000 solution) IM dose.
NOTES - Use the 1:10,000 injectable solution for IV use in cardiac arrest (10 mL = 1 mg). For pediatric patients, use 1:10,000 for initial IV dose, then 1:1,000 for subsequent dosing or ET doses. Use the 1:1,000 injectable solution for SC/IM use in anaphylaxis (0.1 mL = 0.1 mg).

flecainide (*Tambocor*) ▶K ♀C ▶- $$$$
WARNING - Proarrhythmic. Increased mortality in patients with non-life threatening ventricular arrhythmias, structural heart disease (i.e. MI, LV dysfunction), and chronic atrial fibrillation.
ADULT - Prevention of paroxysmal atrial fib/flutter or PSVT, with symptoms & no structural heart disease: Start 50 mg PO q12h, may increase by 50 mg bid q4 days, max 300 mg/day. Life-threatening ventricular arrhythmias without structural heart disease: Start 100 mg PO q12h, may increase by 50 mg bid q 4 days, max 400 mg/day. With severe renal impairment (CrCl<35 mL/min): Start 50 mg PO bid.

PEDS - Consult pediatric cardiologist.
UNAPPROVED ADULT - Cardioversion of recent-onset atrial fib: 300 mg PO single dose.
FORMS - Generic/Trade: Tabs, non-scored 50, scored 100,150 mg.
NOTES - Consider inpatient rhythm monitoring during initiation of therapy, especially when treating life-threatening arrhythmias. Do not use with structural heart disease. Reduce dose if QRS widening >20% from baseline or if 2nd/3rd degree AV block. Correct hypo/hyperkalemia before giving. Increases digoxin level 13-19%. Consult cardiologist before using with other antiarrhythmic agents. Reduce dose of flecainide 50% when used with amiodarone. Quinidine, cimetidine may increase levels. Use cautiously with disopyramide, verapamil, or impaired hepatic function. Use cautiously with impaired renal function; will take >4 days to reach new steady state level. Target trough level 0.2-1 mcg/mL.

ibutilide (*Corvert*) ▶K ♀C ▶? $$$$$
WARNING - Proarrhythmic; use only by trained personnel with continuous ECG monitoring.
ADULT - Recent onset A-fib/flutter: Patients >60 kg: 1 mg (10 mL) IV over 10 mins, may repeat if no response after 10 additional minutes. Patients <60 kg: 0.01 mg/kg over 10 min, may repeat if no response after 10 additional minutes. Useful in combination with DC cardioversion if cardioversion alone is unsuccessful.
PEDS - Not approved in children.
NOTES - Keep on cardiac monitor ≥4 hours. Use with caution, if at all, when QT interval is >500 ms, severe LV dysfunction, or in patients already using class Ia or III antiarrhythmics. Stop infusion when arrhythmia is terminated.

isoproterenol (*Isuprel*) ▶LK ♀C ▶? $$
ADULT - Refractory bradycardia or third degree AV block: 0.02-0.06 mg (1-3 mL of a 1:50,000 dilution) IV bolus or IV infusion (2 mg in 250 mL D5W = 8 mcg/mL) at 5 mcg/min; 5 mcg/min = 37 mL/h. General dose range 2-20 mcg/min.
PEDS - Refractory bradycardia or third degree AV block: Start IV infusion 0.05 mcg/kg/min, increase every 5-10 min by 0.1 mcg/kg/min until desired effect or onset of toxicity, max 2 mcg/kg/min. 10 kg: 0.1 mcg/kg/min = 8 mL/h.

lidocaine (*Xylocaine, Xylocard*) ▶LK ♀B▶? $
ADULT - Ventricular arrhythmia: Load 1 mg/kg IV, then 0.5 mg/kg IV q8-10min as needed to max 3 mg/kg. IV infusion: 4 gm in 500 mL D5W (8 mg/ml) at 1-4 mg/min.
PEDS - Ventricular arrhythmia: Loading dose 1 mg/kg IV/intraosseous slowly; may repeat for 2

doses 10-15 minutes apart; max 3-5 mg/kg in 1 hour. ET tube: Use 2-2.5 times IV dose. IV infusion: 4 gm in 500 ml D5W (8 mg/ml) at 20-50 mcg/kg/min. 10 kg: 40 mcg/kg/min=3 mL/h.

UNAPPROVED ADULT - ET administration prior to IV access: 2-2.5 x the recommended IV dose in 10 ml of NS or distilled water. Shock refractory VF/pulseless VT: 1 mg/kg q3-5min as needed to max 3 mg/kg.

NOTES - Reduce infusion in CHF, liver disease, elderly. Not for routine use after acute MI. Monitor for CNS side effects with prolonged infusions.

mexiletine (*Mexitil*) ▶L ♀C ▶- $$$

WARNING - Proarrhythmic. Increased mortality in patients with non-life threatening ventricular arrhythmias and structural heart disease (i.e. MI, LV dysfunction).

ADULT - Rarely indicated, consult cardiologist. Ventricular arrhythmia: Start 200 mg PO q8h with food or antacid, max dose 1,200 mg/day. Patients responding to q8h dosing may be converted to q12h dosing with careful monitoring, max dose 450 mg q12h.

PEDS - Not approved in children.

FORMS - Generic/Trade: Caps 150, 200, 250 mg.

NOTES - Patients may require decreased dose with severe liver disease. CNS side effects may limit dose titration. Monitor level when given with phenytoin, rifampin, phenobarbital, cimetidine, fluvoxamine. May increase theophylline level.

moricizine (*Ethmozine*) ▶L ♀B ▶? $$$$

WARNING - Proarrhythmic. Increased mortality in patients with non-life threatening ventricular arrhythmias and structural heart disease (i.e. MI, LV dysfunction).

ADULT - Rarely indicated, consult cardiologist. Ventricular arrhythmia: Start 200 mg PO q8h, max dose 900 mg/day. Patients responding to q8h dosing may be converted to q12h dosing with careful monitoring.

PEDS - Not approved in children.

FORMS - Trade: Tabs, non-scored 200,250,300 mg.

procainamide (*Procanbid, Pronestyl*) ▶LK ♀C ▶? $

WARNING - Proarrhythmic. Increased mortality in patients with non-life threatening ventricular arrhythmias and structural heart disease (i.e. MI, LV dysfunction). Positive ANA titer, blood dyscrasias, and lupus erythematosus-like syndrome.

ADULT - Ventricular arrhythmia: 50 mg/kg/day PO; 250-625 mg PO q3h (immediate-release products), 500-1250 mg PO q6h (SR products), 500-1000 mg PO q12h (Procanbid product). IV dosing: Load 100 mg IV q10 min or 20 mg/min (150 mL/h) until: 1) QRS widens >50%, 2) dysrhythmia suppressed, 3) hypotension, or 4) total of 17 mg/kg or 1000 mg. Infusion 2g in 250 ml D5W (8 mg/ml) at 2-6 mg/min (15-45 mL/h). If rhythm unresponsive, guide therapy by serum procainamide/NAPA levels.

PEDS - Not approved in children.

UNAPPROVED ADULT - Shock responsive VF/pulseless VT: up to 50 mg/min until: 1) QRS widens >50%, 2) dysrhythmia suppressed, 3) hypotension, or 4) total of 17 mg/kg or 1000 mg.

UNAPPROVED PEDS - Arrhythmia: 15-50 mg/kg/day PO immediate-release products divided q 3-6 h; 2-6 mg/kg IV over 5 min, max loading dose 100 mg, repeat loading dose every 5-10 min as needed up to max 15 mg/kg; 20-80 mcg/kg/min IV infusion, max dose 2 g/day. Consult peds cardiologist or intensivist.

FORMS - Generic/Trade: Caps, immediate release 250 mg; tabs, sustained-release, non-scored (Pronestyl SR). Generic only: tabs, sustained-release, non-scored (generic procainamide SR, q6h dosing) 750,1000 mg; caps, immediate release 500 mg. Trade only: Tabs, immediate-release, non-scored (Pronestyl) 250, 375, 500 mg, extended-release, non-scored (Procanbid, q12h dosing) 500,1000 mg.

NOTES - Do not break or crush SR or XR products. Swallow Tabs whole.

propafenone (*Rythmol, Rythmol SR*) ▶L ♀C ▶? $$$$

WARNING - Proarrhythmic. Increased mortality in patients with non-life threatening ventricular arrhythmias and structural heart disease (ie, MI, LV dysfunction).

ADULT - Prevention of paroxysmal atrial fib/flutter or PSVT, with symptoms & no structural heart disease; or life-threatening ventricular arrhythmias: Start (immediate release) 150 mg PO q8h; may increase after 3-4 days to 225 mg PO q8h; max 900 mg/day. Prolong time to recurrence of symptomatic atrial fib without structural heart disease: 225 mg SR PO q12h, may increase >=5 days to 325 mg PO q12h, max 425 mg q12h.

PEDS - Not approved in children.

UNAPPROVED ADULT - Cardioversion of recent onset atrial fib: 600 mg PO single dose.

FORMS - Generic/Trade: Tabs (immediate release), scored 150,225,300 mg; Trade: SR, capsules 225,325,425 mg.

NOTES - Consider inpatient rhythm monitoring during initiation of therapy, especially when treating life-threatening arrhythmias. Do not use with structural heart disease or for ventricular rate control during atrial fib. Reduce dose if QRS widening >20% from baseline or if 2nd/3rd degree AV block. Correct hypo/hyperkalemia before giving. Consult cardiologist before using with other antiarrhythmic agents. May increase digoxin level 35-85%. May increase beta blocker, cyclosporine, desipramine, theophylline levels. Increases warfarin activity; monitor INR. Cimetidine may increase level. Instruct patient to report any changes in OTC, prescription, supplement use and symptoms that may be associated with altered electrolytes (prolonged/excessive diarrhea, sweating, vomiting, thirst, appetite loss). Reduce dose 70-80% with impaired hepatic function. Use cautiously with impaired renal function. Bioavailability of 325 mg SR bid = 150 mg immediate release tid. Poorly metabolized by 10% population; reduce dose & monitor for toxicity.

quinidine ▶LK ♀C ▶? $$-gluconate, $-sulfate

WARNING - Proarrhythmic. Increased mortality in patients with non-life threatening ventricular arrhythmias and structural heart disease (i.e. MI, LV dysfunction).

ADULT - Arrhythmia: gluconate, extended-release: 324-648 mg PO q8-12h; sulfate, immediate-release: 200-400 mg PO 6-8h; sulfate, extended-release: 300-600 mg PO q8-12h. Consider inpatient rhythm and QT monitoring during initiation of therapy.

PEDS - Not approved in children.

UNAPPROVED PEDS - Arrhythmia: Test dose (oral sulfate or IM/IV gluconate) 2 mg/kg (max 200 mg). Sulfate: 15-60 mg/kg/day PO divided q6h. Gluconate IV: 2-10 mg/kg/dose q3-8h prn.

FORMS - Generic gluconate: Tabs, extended-release non-scored 324 mg; Generic sulfate: Tabs, scored immediate-release 200,300 mg.

Generic sulfate: Tabs, ext'd-release 300 mg.

NOTES - Do not chew, break, or crush extended-release tabs.

sotalol (*Betapace, Betapace AF, ✦Rylosol, Sotacor*) ▶K ♀B ▶- $$$$

WARNING - Patients should be in a facility for ≥3 days with ECG monitoring, cardiac resuscitation available, and CrCl calculated when initiating or re-initiating Betapace AF. Do not substitute Betapace for Betapace AF.

ADULT - Ventricular arrhythmia (Betapace), symptomatic A-fib/A-flutter (Betapace AF): Start 80 mg PO bid, usual maintenance dose 160-320 mg/day divided bid, max 640 mg/day.

PEDS - Not approved in children.

FORMS - Generic/Trade: Tabs, scored 80,120, 160,240 mg. Trade only: 80,120,160 mg (Betapace AF).

NOTES - Proarrhythmic. Caution, higher incidence of torsades de pointes with doses >320 mg/day, use in women, or CHF. Adjust dose if CrCl <60 mL/min.

tocainide (*Tonocard*) ▶L ♀C ▶? $$$

WARNING - Blood dyscrasias, pulmonary fibrosis. Proarrhythmic. Increased mortality in patients with non-life threatening ventricular arrhythmias and structural heart disease (i.e. MI, LV dysfunction).

ADULT - Rarely indicated, consult cardiologist. Ventricular arrhythmia: Start 400 mg PO q8h, max dose 2400 mg/day. Patients responding to q8h dosing may be converted to q12h dosing with careful monitoring.

PEDS - Not approved in children.

FORMS - Trade: Tabs, scored 400,600 mg.

vasopressin (*Pitressin, ADH, ✦Pressyn AR*) ▶LK ♀C ▶? $

ADULT - See endocrine section.

PEDS - Not approved in children.

UNAPPROVED ADULT - Cardiac arrest: 40 units IV; may repeat if no response after 3 minutes. Septic shock: 0.01-0.1 units/min IV infusion, usual dose <0.04 units/min.

CARDIOVASCULAR: Anti-Hyperlipidemic Agents – Bile Acid Sequestrants

cholestyramine (*Questran, Questran Light, Prevalite, LoCHOLEST, LoCHOLEST Light*) ▶Not absorbed ♀C ▶+ $

ADULT - Elevated LDL cholesterol: Start 4 g PO qd-bid before meals, usual maintenance 12-24 g/day in divided doses bid-qid before meals, max 24 g/day.

PEDS - Not approved in children.

UNAPPROVED ADULT - Cholestasis-associated pruritus: 4-8 g bid-tid.

UNAPPROVED PEDS - Elevated LDL cholesterol: Start 240 mg/kg/day PO divided tid before meals, usual maintenance 8-16 g/day divided tid.

FORMS - Generic/Trade: Powder for oral suspension, 4 g cholestyramine resin / 9 g powder (Questran, LoCHOLEST), 4 g cholestyramine resin / 5 g powder (Questran Light), 4 g cholestyramine resin / 5.5 g powder (Prevalite, LoCHOLEST Light).

NOTES - BID dosing recommended, but may divide up to 6x/day. Mix powder with 60-180 mL of water, milk, fruit juice, or drink (avoid carbonated liquids). GI problems common, eg, constipation. Administer other drugs at least 1 hour before or 4-6 h after cholestyramine to avoid decreased absorption of the other agent. May cause elevation of HDL cholesterol and no change or elevated triglycerides.

colesevelam (*Welchol*) ▶Not absorbed ♀B ▶+ $$$$

ADULT - Elevated LDL cholesterol: 3 Tabs bid with meals or 6 Tabs once daily with a meal, max dose 7 Tabs/day. Same dose when used in combination with other agents (eg, statin).
PEDS - Not approved in children.
FORMS - Trade: Tabs, non-scored, 625 mg.
NOTES - Take with a full glass of water or other non-carbonated liquid. GI problems common, mainly constipation. May cause elevation of HDL cholesterol and triglycerides.

colestipol (*Colestid, Colestid Flavored*)
▶Not absorbed ♀B ▶+ $$$

ADULT - Elevated LDL cholesterol: Tabs: Start 2 g PO qd-bid, max 16 g/day. Granules: Start 5 g PO qd-bid, increase by 5 g increments as tolerated at 1-2 month intervals, max 30 g/day.
PEDS - Not approved in children.
UNAPPROVED PEDS - 125-250 mg/kg/day PO in divided doses bid-qid, dosing range 10-20 g/day.
FORMS - Trade: Tab 1 g. Granules for oral suspension, 5 g / 7.5 g powder.
NOTES - Mix granules in at least 90 mL of water, milk, fruit juice, or drink. Avoid carbonated liquids for mixing. Swallow tabs whole with a full glass of liquid to avoid tab disintegration in the esophagus. GI problems common, mainly constipation. Administer other drugs at least 1 hour before or 4-6 h after colestipol to avoid decreased absorption of the other agent. May cause elevation of HDL cholesterol and no change or elevated triglycerides .

LDL CHOLESTEROL GOALS[1]

Risk Category	LDL Goal (mg/dL)	Lifestyle Changes at LDL (mg/dL)[2]	Also Consider Meds at LDL (mg/dL)[3]
High risk: CHD or equivalent risk[4] 10-year risk >20%	<100 (optional goal < 70)*	≥100**	≥100 (<100: consider Rx options)#
Moderately high risk: 2+ risk factors[5] 10-year risk 10-20%	<130	≥130**	≥130 (100-129: consider Rx options)##
Moderate risk: 2+ risk factors[5] 10-year risk <10%	<130	≥130	≥160
Lower risk: 0 to 1 risk factor[5]	<160	≥160	≥190 (160-189: Rx optional)

1. CHD=coronary heart disease. LDL=low density lipoprotein. Adapted from NCEP: *JAMA* 2001; 285:2486; NCEP Report: Circulation 2004;110:227-239. All 10-year risks based upon Framingham stratification. **2.** Dietary modification, weight reduction, exercise. **3.** When using LDL lowering therapy, achieve at least 30-40% LDL reduction. **4.** Equivalent risk defined as diabetes, other atherosclerotic disease (peripheral artery disease, abdominal aortic aneurysm, symptomatic carotid artery disease), or ≥ 2 risk factors such that 10 year risk >20%. **5.** Risk factors: Cigarette smoking, HTN (BP≥140/90 mmHg or on antihypertensive meds), low HDL (<40 mg/dL), family hx of CHD (1° relative: ♂ <55 yo, ♀ <65 yo), age (♂ ≥45 yo, ♀ ≥55 yo). * With very high risk factors (hospitalized with acute coronary syndrome; CVD with: multiple risk factors, severe/poorly controlled risk factors, or metabolic syndrome), LDL goal <70 & non-HDL <100 (with ↑TG). ** Regardless of LDL, lifestyle changes are indicated when lifestyle-related risk factors (obesity, physical inactivity, ↑TG, ↓ HDL, or metabolic syndrome) are present. # If baseline LDL <100, starting LDL lowering therapy is an option based on clinical trials. With ↑TG or ↓HDL, consider combining fibrate or nicotinic acid with LDL lowering drug. ## At baseline or after lifestyle changes - initiating LDL lowering therapy to achieve LDL <100 is an option based on clinical trials.

CORONARY ARTERY DISEASE 10-YEAR RISK

Framingham model for calculating 10-year risk for coronary artery disease (CAD) in patients without diabetes or clinically evident CAD. Diabetes is considered a CAD risk "equivalent", i.e., the prospective risk of CAD in diabetics is similar to those with established CAD.   (NCEP, *JAMA* 2001; 285:2497)

MEN

Age	Points	Age	Points
20-34	-9	55-59	8
35-39	-4	60-64	10
40-44	0	65-69	11
45-49	3	70-74	12
50-54	6	75-79	13

Choles-	Age (years)				
terol*	20-39	40-49	50-59	60-69	70-79
<160	0	0	0	0	0
160-199	4	3	2	1	0
200-239	7	5	3	1	0
240-279	9	6	4	2	1
280+	11	8	5	3	1

*Total in mg/dL

Age (years)	20-39	40-49	50-59	60-69	70-79
Nonsmoker	0	0	0	0	0
Smoker	8	5	3	1	1

HDL mg/dL	Points	HDL mg/dL	Points
60+	-1	40-49	1
50-59	0	<40	2

Systolic BP	If Untreated	If Treated
<120 mmHg	0	0
120-129 mmHg	0	1
130-139 mmHg	1	2
140-159 mmHg	1	2
160+ mmHg	2	3

Point Total	10-Year Risk	Point Total	10-Year Risk
0	1%	9	5%
1	1%	10	6%
2	1%	11	8%
3	1%	12	10%
4	1%	13	12%
5	2%	14	16%
6	2%	15	20%
7	3%	16	25%
8	4%	17+	30+%

WOMEN

Age	Points	Age	Points
20-34	-7	55-59	8
35-39	-3	60-64	10
40-44	0	65-69	12
45-49	3	70-74	14
50-54	6	75-79	16

Choles-	Age (years)				
terol*	20-39	40-49	50-59	60-69	70-79
<160	0	0	0	0	0
160-199	4	3	2	1	1
200-239	8	6	4	2	1
240-279	11	8	5	3	2
280+	13	10	7	4	2

Age (years)	20-39	40-49	50-59	60-69	70-79
Nonsmoker	0	0	0	0	0
Smoker	9	7	4	2	1

HDL mg/dL	Points	HDL mg/dL	Points
60+	-1	40-49	1
50-59	0	<40	2

Systolic BP	If Untreated	If Treated
<120 mmHg	0	0
120-129 mmHg	1	3
130-139 mmHg	2	4
140-159 mmHg	3	5
160+ mmHg	4	6

Point Total	10-Year Risk	Point Total	10-Year Risk
< 9	< 1%	17	5%
9	1%	18	6%
10	1%	19	8%
11	1%	20	11%
12	1%	21	14%
13	2%	22	17%
14	2%	23	22%
15	3%	24	27%
16	4%	25+	30+%

STATINS*

Minimum Dose for 30-40% LDL Reduction	LDL	LFT Monitoring**
atorvastatin 10 mg	-39%	B, 12 wk, semiannually
fluvastatin 40 mg bid	-36%	B, 8 wk
fluvastatin XL 80 mg	-35%	B, 8 wk
lovastatin 40 mg	-31%	B, 6 & 12 wk, semiannually
pravastatin 40mg	-34%	B, prior to dose increase
rosuvastatin 5 mg	-45%	B, 12 wk, semiannually
simvastatin 20 mg	-38%	B, ***

*Adapted from *Circulation* 2004;110:227-239. Data taken from prescribing information for primary hypercholesterolemia. B=baseline, LDL=low-density lipoprotein, LFT=liver function tests. Will get ~6% decrease in LDL with every doubling of dose. **ACC/AHA/NHLBI schedule for LFT monitoring: baseline, ~12 weeks after starting therapy, annually, when clinically indicated. Stop statin therapy if LFTs are >3 times upper limit of normal. ***Get LFTs prior to & 3 months after dose increase to 80 mg, then semiannually for first year.

CARDIOVASCULAR: Anti-Hyperlipidemic Agents – HMG-CoA Reductase Inhibitors ("Statins") and Combinations

NOTE: Hepatotoxicity - monitor LFTs initially, approximately 12 weeks after starting therapy, then annually or more frequently if indicated. Evaluate muscle symptoms & creatine kinase before starting therapy. Evaluate muscle symptoms 6-12 weeks after starting therapy & at each follow-up visit. Obtain creatine kinase when patient complains of muscle soreness, tenderness, or pain. These factors increase risk of myopathy: advanced age (especially >80, women >men); multisystem disease (eg, chronic renal insufficiency, especially due to diabetes); multiple medications; perioperative periods; alcohol abuse; grapefruit juice (>1 quart/day); specific concomitant medications: fibrates (especially gemfibrozil), nicotinic acid (rare), cyclosporine, erythromycin, clarithromycin, itraconazole, ketoconazole, protease inhibitors, nefazodone, verapamil, amiodarone. Weigh potential risk of combination therapy against potential benefit

Advicor (lovastatin + niacin) ▶LK ♀X ▶- $$$
ADULT - Hyperlipidemia: 1 tab PO qhs with a low-fat snack. Establish dose using extended-release niacin first, or if already on lovastatin substitute combo product with lowest niacin dose.
PEDS - Not approved in children.
FORMS - Trade: Tabs, non-scored ext'd release niacin/lovastatin 500/20, 750/20, 1000/20 mg.
NOTES - Do not break, chew, or crush. Swallow whole. Aspirin or ibuprofen 30 min prior may decrease niacin flushing reaction. Niacin may worsen glucose control, peptic ulcer disease, gout, headaches, and menopausal flushing. Significantly lowers LDL-cholesterol and triglyc-

erides, raises HDL-cholesterol. Increased risk of myopathy and rhabdomyolysis when used with a fibric acid agent or known inhibitors of cytochrome P450 3A4 enzyme system (erythromycin, clarithromycin, cyclosporine, ketoconazole, itraconazole, HIV protease inhibitors, nefazodone, grapefruit juice), increasing risk of myopathy. Do not exceed >2000/40 mg.

atorvastatin (Lipitor) ▶L ♀X ▶- $$$
ADULT - Prevention of cardiovascular disease/hyperlipidemia: Start 10 mg PO qd, 40 mg qd for LDL-C reduction >45%, increase at ≥4-week intervals to a max of 80 mg/day.
PEDS - Hyperlipidemia, ≥10 years: Same as adult.
UNAPPROVED ADULT - Prevention of cardiovascular events & death post-acute coronary syndrome: 80 mg PO qd.
FORMS - Trade: Tabs, non-scored 10,20,40,80 mg.
NOTES - Metabolism may be decreased by known inhibitors of cytochrome P450 3A4 enzyme system (erythromycin, clarithromycin, cyclosporine, ketoconazole, itraconazole, HIV protease inhibitors, nefazodone, grapefruit and grapefruit juice), increasing risk of myopathy. Increased risk of myopathy and rhabdomyolysis when used with a fibric acid agent or niacin. Give either 1 hour before or 4 hours after bile acid resins.

Caduet (amlodipine + atorvastatin) ▶L ♀X ▶- $$$$
ADULT - Simultaneous treatment of HTN and hypercholesterolemia: Establish dose using component drugs first. Dosing interval: qd

PEDS - Not approved in children.
FORMS - Trade: Tabs, 5/10,5/20,5/40,5/80, 10/10,10/20,10/40,10/80 mg.

fluvastatin (Lescol, Lescol XL) ▶L ♀X ▶- $$$

ADULT - Hyperlipidemia: Start 20 mg PO qhs for LDL-C reduction to a goal of <25%, 40-80 mg qhs for goal of ≥25%, max 80 mg/day, give 80 mg/day qd (Lescol XL) or 40 mg bid. Prevention of cardiac events post percutaneous coronary intervention: 80 mg of extended release PO qhs, max 80 mg qd.
PEDS - Not approved in children.
FORMS - Trade: Caps, 20,40 mg; tab, extended-release, non-scored 80 mg.
NOTES - Not metabolized substantially by the cytochrome P450 isoenzyme 3A4, so less potential for drug interactions. Increased risk of myopathy and rhabdomyolysis when used with a fibric acid agent or niacin. Give either 1 hour before or 4 hours after bile acid resins.

lovastatin (Mevacor, Altocor, Altoprev) ▶L ♀X ▶- $$$

ADULT - Reduced cardiovascular morbidity, hyperlipidemia: Start 20 mg PO qd with the evening meal, increase at ≥4 week intervals to max 80 mg/day (qd or divided bid). Altocor dosed qd with max dose 60 mg/day.
PEDS - Hyperlipidemia, ≥10 years: Same as adult.
FORMS - Generic/Trade: Tabs, non-scored 10, 20,40 mg. Trade only: Tabs, extended-release (Altocor, Altoprev) 20,40,60 mg.
NOTES - Metabolism significantly decreased by known inhibitors of cyt P450 3A4 enzyme system (erythromycin, clarithromycin, cyclosporine, ketoconazole, itraconazole, HIV protease inhibitors, nefazodone, grapefruit juice >1 quart/day), increasing risk of myopathy. Do not use with itraconazole, ketoconazole, erythromycin, clarithromycin, HIV protease inhibitors, nefazodone, grapefruit juice >1 quart/day. Do not exceed 20 mg/day when used with a cyclosporine, fibric acid agent, or niacin ≥1 g/day; do not exceed 40 mg/day when used with amiodarone or verapamil. Give either 1 hour before or 4 hours after bile acid resins.

pravastatin (Pravachol) ▶L ♀X ▶- $$$

ADULT - Primary/secondary prevention of coronary events, hyperlipidemia: Start 40 mg PO qd, increase at ≥4-week intervals to max 80 mg/day. Renal or hepatic impairment: Start 10 mg PO qd.
PEDS - Hyperlipidemia, 8-13 yo: 20 mg PO qd. 14-18 yo: 40 mg PO qd.

FORMS - Trade: Tabs, non-scored 10,20,40,80 mg.
NOTES - Not metabolized substantially by the cytochrome P450 isoenzyme 3A4, less potential for drug interactions. Increased risk of myopathy and rhabdomyolysis when used with a fibric acid agent. Give either 1 hour before or 4 hours after bile acid resins.

Pravigard PAC (pravastatin + aspirin) ▶L ♀X ▶- $$$$

ADULT - Reduce cardiovascular events in cardiovascular and/or cerebrovascular disease: Start 40 mg pravastatin with 81 or 325 mg aspirin PO qd; max pravastatin 80 mg/day.
PEDS - Not approved in children.
FORMS - Trade: co-packaged pravastatin/buffered ASA 20/81, 40/81, 80/81, 20/325, 40/325, 80/325 mg.

rosuvastatin (Crestor) ▶L ♀X ▶- $$$

ADULT - Hyperlipidemia: Start 10 mg qd, may adjust dose after 2-4 weeks. Use 40 mg only with severe hypercholesterolemia when treatment goal not achieved with 20 mg qd. Severe renal impairment: Start 5 mg PO qd, max 10 mg/day. With predisposing factors for myopathy (renal impairment, advanced age, hypothyroidism): Start 5 mg PO qd.
PEDS - Canada only: May use with age >8 yrs with homozygous familial hypercholesterolemia. Specialist should supervise use.
FORMS - Trade: tabs non-scored 5, 10, 20, 40 mg.
NOTES - Do not exceed 10 mg/day with severe renal impairment or gemfibrozil. Do not exceed 5 mg/day with cyclosporine. Give aluminum & magnesium containing antacids >2 hours after rosuvastatin. May potentiate effects of warfarin; monitor INR. Proteinuria, with unknown clinical significance, reported with 40 mg/day; consider dose reduction when using 40 mg/day with unexplained persistent proteinuria. May increase levels of ethinyl estradiol & norgestrel. Use cautiously with other drugs that may decrease levels/activity of endogenous steroid hormones (ketoconazole, spironolactone, cimetidine).

simvastatin (Zocor) ▶L ♀X ▶- $$$$

ADULT - Hyperlipidemia: Start 20-40 mg PO q pm. High risk for coronary heart disease event (existing coronary heart disease, DM, peripheral vascular disease, history of stroke or cerebrovascular disease): 40 mg q pm. Increase prn at ≥4 week intervals to max 80 mg/day.
PEDS - Hyperlipidemia, ≥10 years: Start 10 mg PO q pm, max 40 mg/day.
FORMS - Trade: Tabs, non-scored 5,10,20,40,

80 mg.

NOTES - Metabolism significantly decreased by known inhibitors of cytochrome P450 3A4 enzyme system (erythromycin, clarithromycin, cyclosporine, ketoconazole, itraconazole, HIV protease inhibitors, nefazodone, grapefruit juice >1 quart/day), increasing risk of myopathy. Do not exceed 10 mg/day when used with gemfibrozil, cyclosporine; or 20 mg/day when used with amiodarone or verapamil; increased risk of myopathy. Use caution with other fibrates, niacin ≥1 g/day; may cause myopathy. Give either 1 hour before or 4 hours after bile acid resins.

***Vytorin* (simvastatin + ezetimibe)** ▶L ♀X ▶- $$$

ADULT - Hyperlipidemia: Start 10/20 mg PO q pm, max 10/80 mg/day. Start 10/40 if need >55% LDL reduction.

PEDS - Not approved in children.

FORMS - Trade: Tabs, non-scored ezetimibe/ simvastatin 10/10, 10/20, 10/40, 10/80 mg.

CARDIOVASCULAR: Anti-Hyperlipidemic Agents – Other

bezafibrate (✖*Bezalip*) ▶K ♀D ▶- $$$

ADULT - Canada only. Hyperlipidemia/hypertriglyceridemia: 200 mg of immediate release PO bid-tid, or 400 mg of sustained release PO q am or q evening with or after food. Reduce dose in renal insufficiency or dialysis. The 400 mg SR tablet should not be used if CrCl <60 ml/min or creat >1.5 mg/dL.

PEDS - Not approved in children.

FORMS - Trade: Immediate release tab: 200 mg. Sustained release tab: 400 mg.

NOTES - Cholestyramine decreases absorption; space doses by 2 hour interval if used concurrently. Increased risk of myopathy and rhabdomyolysis when used with a statin. May increase the effect of warfarin; reduce oral anticoagulant dose by ~50%; monitor INR. Do not use in primary biliary cirrhosis.

ezetimibe (*Zetia*, ✖*Ezetrol*) ▶L ♀C ▶? $$$

WARNING - May increase cyclosporine levels.

ADULT - Hyperlipidemia: 10 mg PO qd alone or in combination with statin

PEDS - Not approved in children.

FORMS - Trade: Tabs non-scored 10 mg

NOTES - Take either ≥2 hours before or ≥4 hours after bile acid sequestrants. May increase cyclosporine levels. When used with statin, monitor LFTs per statin instructions.

fenofibrate (*Tricor, Lofibra*, ✖*Lipidil Micro, Lipidil Supra*) ▶LK ♀C ▶- $$$

ADULT - Hypertriglyceridemia: Tablets: Start 54-160 mg PO qd with a meal (max 160 mg/day. Micronized, capsules: 134-200 mg PO qd. Hypercholesterolemia & mixed dyslipidemia: 160 mg PO qd. Renal impairment, elderly: Start 54 mg PO qd.

PEDS - Not approved in children.

FORMS - Trade (Tricor): Tabs, non-scored 54, 160 mg. Generic/Trade (Lofibra): Micronized caps, 67,134,200 mg.

NOTES - Conversion from micronized caps to tabs: 160 mg tab = 200 mg cap. Monitor LFTs, dose related hepatotoxicity. Increased risk of myopathy and rhabdomyolysis when used with a statin. May increase the effect of warfarin, monitor INR.

gemfibrozil (*Lopid*) ▶LK ♀C ▶? $$$

ADULT - Hypertriglyceridemia / primary prevention of artery heart disease: 600 mg PO bid 30 minutes before meals.

PEDS - Not approved in children.

FORMS - Generic/Trade: Tabs, scored 600 mg.

NOTES - Increased risk of myopathy and rhabdomyolysis when used with a statin or with moderate/severe renal dysfunction. May increase the effect of warfarin, monitor INR. Increased risk of hypoglycemia when used with repaglinide: Do not start in those taking gemfibrozil. Similarly do not start gemfibrozil in those taking repaglinide. Avoid itraconazole with combined gemfibrozil and repaglinide.

niacin (*nicotinic acid, vitamin B3, Niacor, Nicolar, Niaspan*) ▶K ♀C ▶? $

ADULT - Hyperlipidemia: Start 50-100 mg PO bid-tid with meals, increase slowly, usual maintenance range 1.5-3 g/day, max 6 g/day. Extended-release (Niaspan): Start 500 mg qhs with a low-fat snack for 4 weeks, increase as needed every 4 weeks to max 2000 mg.

PEDS - Not approved in children.

FORMS - Generic (OTC): Tabs, scored 25,50, 100,150,500 mg. Trade: Tabs, immediate-release, scored (Niacor), 500 mg; ext'd-release, non-scored (Niaspan), 500,750,1000 mg.

NOTES - Extended-release formulations not listed here may have greater hepatotoxicity. Do not break, chew, or crush extended-release niacin, swallow whole. Aspirin or ibuprofen, 30 minutes before niacin doses may decrease flushing reaction. Titrate niacin slowly to avoid flushing events. Niacin may worsen glucose control, peptic ulcer disease, gout, headaches, and menopausal flushing. Significantly lowers LDL-cholesterol and triglycerides, raises HDL-cholesterol. Increased risk of myopathy and rhabdomyolysis when used with a fibric acid agent or a statin.

omega-3 fatty acid (fish oil, Promega, Cardio-Omega 3, Sea-Omega, Marine Lipid Concentrate, MAX EPA, SuperEPA 1200) ▶L ♀? ▶? $$

PEDS - Not approved in children.

UNAPPROVED ADULT - Hypertriglyceridemia: 2-4 g EPA+DHA content daily under physician's care. Secondary prevention of CHD: 1000 mg EPA+DHA content daily.

FORMS - Trade/Generic: cap, shown as EPA+ DHA mg content, 240 (Promega Pearls), 300 (Cardi-Omega 3, Max EPA), 320 (Sea-Omega), 400 (Promega), 500 (Sea-Omega), 600 (Marine Lipid Concentrate, SuperEPA 1200), 875 mg (SuperEPA 2000).

NOTES - Dose dependent GI upset, may increase LDL-cholesterol, excessive bleeding, hyperglycemia. Marine Lipid Concentrate, Super EPA 1200 mg cap contains EPA 360 mg + DHA 240 mg, daily dose = 5-8 Caps. Treatment doses lowers triglycerides by 30-50%. Safe to use with other cholesterol lowering drugs. Caps may contain vitamin E. Vitamin E content varies with cap strength.

CARDIOVASCULAR: Antihypertensive Combinations

ACE Inhibitor/Diuretic: Accuretic, Capozide, Inhibace Plus, Lotensin HCT, Monopril HCT, Prinzide, Uniretic, Vaseretic, Zestoretic. *Calcium Channel Blocker / ACE Inhibitor:* Lexxel, Lotrel, Tarka. *ARB/Diuretic:* Atacand HCT, Avalide, Benicar HCT, Diovan HCT, Hyzaar, Micardis HCT, Teveten HCT. *Beta-blocker/Diuretic:* Corzide, Inderide, Lopressor HCT, Tenoretic, Timolide, Ziac. *Diuretic combinations:* Aldactazide, Dyazide, Maxzide, Maxzide-25, Moduretic. *Diuretic/miscellaneous antihypertensive:* Aldoril, Apresazide, Combipres, Diutensin-R, Enduronyl, Minizide, Rauzide, Renese-R, Ser-Ap-Es.

NOTE: Dosage should first be adjusted by using each drug separately. See component drugs for metabolism, pregnancy, and lactation.

Accuretic (quinapril + hydrochlorothiazide) $$

ADULT - HTN: Establish dose using component drugs first. Dosing interval: qd.

PEDS - Not approved in children.

FORMS - Generic/Trade: Tabs, 10/12.5, 20/12.5, 20/25.

Aldactazide (spironolactone + hydrochlorothiazide) $$

ADULT - HTN: Establish dose using component drugs first. Dosing interval: qd-bid.

PEDS - Not approved in children.

FORMS - Generic/Trade: Tabs, non-scored 25/25, scored 50/50 mg.

Aldoril (methyldopa + hydrochlorothiazide) $$

ADULT - HTN: Establish dose using component drugs first. Dosing interval: bid.

PEDS - Not approved in children.

FORMS - Generic/Trade: Tabs, non-scored, 250/15 (Aldoril-15), 250/25 mg (Aldoril-25). Trade: Tabs, non-scored, 500/30 (Aldoril D30), 500/50 mg (Aldoril D50).

Apresazide (hydralazine + hydrochlorothiazide) $$

ADULT - HTN: Establish dose using component drugs first. Dosing interval: bid.

PEDS - Not approved in children.

FORMS - Generic only: Caps 25/25, 50/50 mg.

Atacand HCT (candesartan + hydrochlorothiazide, ♥Atacand Plus) $$$

ADULT - HTN: Establish dose using component drugs first. Dosing interval: qd.

PEDS - Not approved in children.

FORMS - Trade: tab, non-scored 16/12.5, 32/12.5 mg.

Avalide (irbesartan + hydrochlorothiazide) $$$

ADULT - HTN: Establish dose using component drugs first. Dosing interval: qd.

PEDS - Not approved in children.

FORMS - Trade: Tabs, non-scored 150/12.5, 300/12.5 mg.

Benicar HCT (olmesartan + hydrochlorothiazide) $$$

ADULT - HTN: Establish dose using component drugs first. Dosing interval: qd.

PEDS - Not approved in children.

FORMS - Trade: Tabs, non-scored 20/12.5, 40/12.5, 40/25

Capozide (captopril + hydrochlorothiazide) $$

ADULT - HTN: Establish dose using component drugs first. Dosing interval: bid-tid.

PEDS - Not approved in children.

FORMS - Generic/Trade: Tabs, scored 25/15, 25/25, 50/15, 50/25 mg.

Combipres (clonidine + chlorthalidone) $$$
ADULT - HTN: Establish dose using component drugs first. Dosing interval: bid-tid.
PEDS - Not approved in children.
FORMS - Generic/Trade: Tabs, non-scored 0.1/15, 0.2/15, 0.3/15 mg.

Corzide (nadolol + bendroflumethiazide) $$$
ADULT - HTN: Establish dose using component drugs first. Dosing interval: qd.
PEDS - Not approved in children.
FORMS - Trade: Tabs, scored 40/5, 80/5 mg.

Diovan HCT (valsartan + hydrochlorothiazide) $$
ADULT - HTN: Establish dose using component drugs first. Dosing interval: qd.
PEDS - Not approved in children.
FORMS - Trade: Tabs, non-scored 80/12.5, 160/12.5, 160/25 mg.

Diutensen-R (reserpine + methyclothiazide) $$$$
ADULT - HTN: Establish dose using component drugs first. Dosing interval: qd.
PEDS - Not approved in children.
FORMS - Trade: Tabs, non-scored, 0.1/2.5 mg.

Dyazide (triamterene + hydrochlorothiazide) $
ADULT - HTN: Establish dose using component drugs first. Dosing interval: qd.
PEDS - Not approved in children.
FORMS - Generic/Trade: Caps, (Dyazide) 37.5/25, (generic only) 50/25 mg.
NOTES - Dyazide 37.5/25 cap same combination as Maxzide-25 tab.

Enduronyl (deserpidine + methyclothiazide) $$$
ADULT - HTN: Establish dose using component drugs first. Dosing interval: qd.
PEDS - Not approved in children.
FORMS - Trade: Tabs, non-scored, 0.25/5 (Enduronyl), 0.5/5 mg (Enduronyl Forte).

Hyzaar (losartan + hydrochlorothiazide) $$
ADULT - HTN: Establish dose using component drugs first. Dosing interval: qd. Severe HTN: Start 50/12.5 PO qd, may increase to 100/25 PO qd after 2-4 weeks.
PEDS - Not approved in children.
FORMS - Trade: Tabs, non-scored 50/12.5, 100/25 mg.

Inderide (propranolol + hydrochlorothiazide) $$

ADULT - HTN: Establish dose using component drugs first. Dosing interval: qd-bid.
PEDS - Not approved in children.
FORMS - Generic/Trade: Tabs, scored 40/25, 80/25.
NOTES - Do not crush or chew cap contents. Swallow whole.

Inhibace Plus (cilazapril + hydrochlorothiazide) $$
ADULT - Canada only, HTN: Establish dose using component drugs first. Dosing interval qd.
PEDS - Not approved in children.
FORMS - Trade: Scored tabs 5 mg cilazapril + 12.5 mg HCTZ.

Lexxel (enalapril + felodipine) $$
ADULT - HTN: Establish dose using component drugs first. Dosing interval: qd.
PEDS - Not approved in children.
FORMS - Trade: Tabs, non-scored 5/2.5, 5/5 mg.
NOTES - Do not crush or chew, swallow whole.

Lopressor HCT (metoprolol + hydrochlorothiazide) $$$
ADULT - HTN: Establish dose using component drugs first. Dosing interval: qd-bid.
PEDS - Not approved in children.
FORMS - Trade: Tabs, scored 50/25, 100/25, 100/50 mg.

Lotensin HCT (benazepril + hydrochlorothiazide) $$
ADULT - HTN: Establish dose using component drugs first. Dosing interval: qd.
PEDS - Not approved in children.
FORMS - Trade: Tabs, scored 5/6.25, 10/12.5, 20/12.5, 20/25 mg.

Lotrel (amlodipine + benazepril) $$$
ADULT - HTN: Establish dose using component drugs first. Dosing interval: qd.
PEDS - Not approved in children.
FORMS - Trade: cap, 2.5/10, 5/10, 5 /20 10/20 mg.

Maxzide (triamterene + hydrochlorothiazide) $
ADULT - HTN: Establish dose using component drugs first. Dosing interval: qd.
PEDS - Not approved in children.
FORMS - Generic/Trade: Tabs, scored (Maxzide-25) 37.5/25 (Maxzide) 75/50 mg.

Maxzide-25 (triamterene + hydrochlorothiazide) $
ADULT - HTN: Establish dose using component drugs first. Dosing interval: qd.
PEDS - Not approved in children.
FORMS - Generic/Trade: Tabs, scored (Maxzide-25) 37.5/25 (Maxzide) 75/50 mg.

Micardis HCT (telmisartan + hydrochlorothiazide, ✢*Micardis Plus*) $$
ADULT - HTN: Establish dose using component drugs first. Dosing interval: qd.
PEDS - Not approved in children.
FORMS - Trade: Tabs, non-scored 40/12.5, 80/12.5, 80/25 mg.
NOTES - Swallow tabs whole, do not break or crush. Caution in hepatic insufficiency.

Minizide (prazosin + polythiazide) $$$
ADULT - HTN: Establish dose using component drugs first. Dosing interval: bid-tid.
PEDS - Not approved in children.
FORMS - Trade: cap, 1/0.5, 2/0.5, 5/0.5 mg.

Moduretic (amiloride + hydrochlorothiazide, ✢*Moduret*) $
ADULT - HTN: Establish dose using component drugs first. Dosing interval: qd.
PEDS - Not approved in children.
FORMS - Generic/Trade: Tabs, scored 5/50 mg.

Monopril HCT (fosinopril + hydrochlorothiazide) $$
ADULT - HTN: Establish dose using component drugs first. Dosing interval: qd.
PEDS - Not approved in children.
FORMS - Trade: Tabs, non-scored 10/12.5, scored 20/12.5 mg.

Prinzide (lisinopril + hydrochlorothiazide) $$
ADULT - HTN: Establish dose using component drugs first. Dosing interval: qd.
PEDS - Not approved in children.
FORMS - Generic/Trade: Tabs, non-scored 10/12.5, 20/12.5, 20/25 mg.

Rauzide (rauwolfia + bendroflumethiazide) $$
ADULT - HTN: Establish dose using component drugs first. Dosing interval: qd.
PEDS - Not approved in children.
FORMS - Trade: Tabs, non-scored, 50/4 mg.

Renese-R (reserpine + polythiazide) $$
ADULT - HTN: Establish dose using component drugs first. Dosing interval: qd.
PEDS - Not approved in children.
FORMS - Trade: Tabs, scored, 0.25/2 mg.

Ser-Ap-Es (hydralazine + hydrochlorothiazide + reserpine) $
ADULT - HTN: Establish dose using component drugs first. Dosing interval: qd-bid.
PEDS - Not approved in children.
FORMS - Generic: Tabs, non-scored, 25/15/0.1 mg.

Tarka (trandolapril + verapamil) $$$
ADULT - HTN: Establish dose using component drugs first. Dosing interval: qd.
PEDS - Not approved in children.
FORMS - Trade: Tabs, non-scored 2/180, 1/240, 2/240, 4/240 mg.
NOTES - Contains extended release form of verapamil. 'Do not chew or crush, swallow whole.

Tenoretic (atenolol + chlorthalidone) $$
ADULT - HTN: Establish dose using component drugs first. Dosing interval: qd.
PEDS - Not approved in children.
FORMS - Generic/Trade: Tabs, scored 50/25, non-scored 100/25 mg.

Teveten HCT (eprosartan + hydrochlorothiazide) $$
ADULT - HTN: Establish dose using component drugs first. Dosing interval: qd.
PEDS - Not approved in children.
FORMS - Trade: Tabs, non-scored 600/12.5, 600/25 mg.

Timolide (timolol + hydrochlorothiazide) $$
ADULT - HTN: Establish dose using component drugs first. Dosing interval: qd-bid.
PEDS - Not approved in children.
FORMS - Trade: Tabs, non-scored 10/25 mg.

Uniretic (moexipril + hydrochlorothiazide) $$
ADULT - HTN: Establish dose using component drugs first. Dosing interval: qd-bid.
PEDS - Not approved in children.
FORMS - Trade: Tabs, scored 7.5/12.5, 15/12.5, 15/25 mg.

Vaseretic (enalapril + hydrochlorothiazide) $$
ADULT - HTN: Establish dose using component drugs first. Dosing interval: qd-bid.
PEDS - Not approved in children.
FORMS - Generic/Trade: Tabs, non-scored 5/12.5, 10/25 mg.

Zestoretic (lisinopril + hydrochlorothiazide) $$
ADULT - HTN: Establish dose using component drugs first. Dosing interval: qd.
PEDS - Not approved in children.
FORMS - Generic/Trade: Tabs, non-scored 10/12.5, 20/12.5, 20/25 mg.

Ziac (bisoprolol + hydrochlorothiazide) $$
ADULT - HTN: Establish dose using component drugs first. Dosing interval: qd.
PEDS - Not approved in children.
FORMS - Generic/Trade: Tabs, non-scored 2.5/6.25, 5/6.25, 10/6.25 mg.

CARDIOVASCULAR: Antihypertensives - Miscellaneous

bosentan (*Tracleer*) ▶L ♀X ▶-? $$$$$

WARNING - Hepatotoxicity; monitor LFTs prior to starting therapy & monthly thereafter. Contraindicated in pregnancy due to birth defects; women of child bearing age must use reliable contraception and have monthly pregnancy tests. Oral, injectable, and implanted contraception must be supplemented with another method.

ADULT - Pulmonary arterial hypertension: Start 62.5 mg PO bid for 4 weeks, increase to 125 mg bid maintenance dose.

PEDS - Not approved in children.

FORMS - Trade: Tabs, non-scored 62.5, 125 mg.

NOTES - Available only through access program by calling 866-228-3546. Concomitant use with glyburide contraindicated due to hepatotoxic risk. Ketoconazole and cyclosporine inhibit metabolism of bosentan via cytochrome P450 3A4; concomitant cyclosporine contraindicated. Induces metabolism of other drugs (eg, contraceptives, simvastatin, lovastatin, atorvastatin). May decrease warfarin plasma concentration; monitor INR.

diazoxide (*Hyperstat*) ▶L ♀C ▶- $$$$

ADULT - Severe HTN: 1-3 mg/kg (up to 150 mg) IV q5-15 min until BP is controlled.

PEDS - Severe HTN: same as adult.

UNAPPROVED ADULT - Preeclampsia/eclampsia: 30 mg IV every few minutes until control of BP is achieved.

NOTES - Severe hyperglycemia possible. Monitor for edema and CHF exacerbation during administration; diuretic therapy may be needed. See endocrine section for diazoxide use in managing hypoglycemia.

epoprostenol (*Flolan*) ▶Plasma ♀B ▶? $$$$$

ADULT - Pulmonary arterial hypertension: Acute dose ranging, 2 ng/kg/min increments via IV infusion until the patient develops symptomatic intolerance (mean maximal dose without symptoms 8.6 ng/kg/min), start continuous IV infusion at 4 ng/kg/min or less than the patient's maximum-tolerated infusion (MTI) rate for acute dose ranging. If the MTI rate is <5 ng/kg/min, start chronic IV infusion at one-half the MTI.

PEDS - Not approved in children.

NOTES - Administer by continuous IV infusion via a central venous catheter. Temporary peripheral IV infusions may be used until central access is established.

fenoldopam (*Corlopam*) ▶LK ♀B ▶? $$$$$

ADULT - Severe HTN: 10 mg in 250 ml D5W (40 mcg/mL), start at 0.1 mcg/kg/min (for 70 kg adult = 11 mL/h), titrate q15 min, usual effective dose 0.1-1.6 mcg/kg/min. Lower initial doses (0.03-0.1 mcg/kg/min) associated with less reflex tachycardia.

PEDS - Reduce BP: Start 0.2 mcg/kg/min, increase by up to 0.3-0.5 mcg/kg/min q 20-30 min. Max infusion 0.8 mcg/kg/min. Administer in hospital by continuous infusion pump; use max 4 hrs; monitor BP & HR continuously. Refer to package insert for dilution instructions & infusion rates.

UNAPPROVED ADULT - Prevention of contrast nephropathy in those at risk (conflicting evidence of efficacy): Start 0.03 mcg/kg/min infusion 60 min prior to dye. Titrate infusion q15min up to 0.1 mcg/kg/min if BP tolerates. Maintain infusion (with concurrent saline) up to 4-6 hours after procedure.

NOTES - Avoid combined use with beta blockers; if must be done, watch for unexpected hypotension. Patients at high-risk for contrast nephropathy include age >70, creat >1.5 mg/dL, HTN, DM, CHF. Use cautiously with glaucoma or increased intraocular HTN. Concurrent acetaminophen may increase fenoldopam levels.

hydralazine (*Apresoline*) ▶LK ♀C ▶+ $

ADULT - HTN: Start 10 mg PO bid-qid for 2-4 days, increase to 25 mg bid-qid, then 50 mg bid-qid if necessary, max 300 mg/day. Hypertensive emergency: 10-50 mg IM or 10-20 mg IV. Use lower doses initially & repeat prn to control BP. Preeclampsia/eclampsia: 5-10 mg IV initially, followed by 5-10 mg IV every 20-30 min as needed to control BP.

PEDS - Not approved in children.

UNAPPROVED ADULT - CHF: Start 10-25 mg PO tid, target dose 75 mg tid, max 100 mg tid. Use in combination with isosorbide dinitrate for patients intolerant to ACE inhibitors

UNAPPROVED PEDS - HTN: Start 0.75-1 mg/kg/day PO divided bid-qid, increase slowly over 3-4 weeks up to 7.5 mg/kg/day; initial IV dose 1.7-3.5 mg/kg/day divided in 4-6 doses. HTN urgency: 0.1-0.2 mg/kg IM/IV q4-6 h as needed. Max single dose, 25 mg PO and 20 mg IV.

FORMS - Generic/Trade: Tabs, non-scored 10,25,50,100 mg.

NOTES - Headache, nausea, dizziness, tachycardia, peripheral edema, lupus-like syndrome. Usually used in combination with diuretic and beta-blocker to counter side effects.

mecamylamine (*Inversine*) ▶K ♀C ▶- $$$$$
ADULT - Severe HTN: Start 2.5 mg PO bid, increase as needed by 2.5 mg increments no sooner than every 2 days, usual maintenance dose 25 mg/day divided tid.
PEDS - Not approved in children.
FORMS - Trade: Tabs, scored, 2.5 mg.
NOTES - Orthostatic hypotension, especially during dosage titration. Monitor BP standing and supine. Rebound, severe hypertension with sudden drug withdrawal. Discontinue slowly and use other antihypertensives.

metyrosine (*Demser*) ▶K ♀C ▶? $$$$$
ADULT - Pheochromocytoma: Start 250 mg PO qid, increase by 250-500 mg/day as needed, max dose 4 g/day.
PEDS - Pheochromocytoma >12 yo: Same as adult.
FORMS - Trade: Caps, 250 mg.

minoxidil (*Loniten*) ▶K ♀C ▶+ $$
ADULT - Refractory HTN: Start 2.5-5 mg PO qd, increase at no less than 3 day intervals, usual dose 10-40 mg qd, max 100 mg/day.
PEDS - Not approved in children <12 yo.
UNAPPROVED PEDS - HTN: Start 0.2 mg/kg PO qd, increase every 3 days as needed up to 0.25-1 mg/kg/day qd or divided bid; max 50 mg/day.
FORMS - Generic/Trade: Tabs, scored, 2.5,10 mg.
NOTES - Edema, weight gain, hypertrichosis, may exacerbate CHF. Usually used in combination with a diuretic and a beta-blocker to counteract side effects .

nitroprusside (*Nipride, Nitropress*) ▶RBC's ♀C ▶- $
WARNING - May cause significant hypotension. Reconstituted solution must be protected before use. Cyanide toxicity may occur, especially with high infusion rates (10 mcg/kg/min), hepatic/renal impairment, and prolonged infusions (>3-7 days). Protect from light.
ADULT - Hypertensive emergency: 50 mg in 250 ml D5W (200 mcg/mL), start at 0.3 mcg/kg/min (for 70 kg adult = 6 mL/h) via IV infusion, titrate slowly, usual range 0.3-10 mcg/kg/min, max 10 mcg/kg/min.
PEDS - Severe HTN: Same as adult.
NOTES - Discontinue if inadequate response to 10 mcg/kg/min after 10 minutes. Cyanide toxicity with high doses, hepatic/renal impairment, and prolonged infusions, check thiocyanate

levels. Protect IV infusion minibag from light.

phenoxybenzamine (*Dibenzyline*) ▶KL ♀C ▶? $$$$$
ADULT - Pheochromocytoma: Start 10 mg PO bid, increase slowly qod as needed, usual dose 20-40 mg bid-tid, max 120 mg/day.
PEDS - Not approved in children.
UNAPPROVED PEDS - Pheochromocytoma: 0.2 mg/kg/day PO qd, initial dose ≤10 mg, increase slowly qod as needed, usual dose 0.4-1.2 mg/kg/day.
FORMS - Trade: Caps, 10 mg.
NOTES - Patients should be observed after each dosage increase for symptomatic hypotension and other adverse effects. Do not use for essential HTN.

phentolamine (*Regitine, Rogitine*) ▶Plasma ♀C ▶? $$
ADULT - Diagnosis of pheochromocytoma: 5 mg IV/IM. Rapid IV administration is preferred. An immediate, marked decrease in BP should occur, typically, 60 mm Hg SBP and 25 mm Hg DBP decrease in 2 minutes. HTN during pheochromocytoma surgery: 5 mg IV/IM 1-2h pre-op, 5 mg IV during surgery prn.
PEDS - Diagnosis of pheochromocytoma: 0.05-0.1 mg/kg IV/IM, up to 5 mg per dose. Rapid IV administration is preferred. An immediate, marked decrease in BP should occur, typically, 60 mm Hg SBP and 25 mm Hg DBP decrease in 2 minutes. HTN during pheochromocytoma surgery: 0.05-0.1 mg/kg IV/IM 1-2h pre-op, repeat q2-4h prn.
UNAPPROVED ADULT - IV extravasation of catecholamines: 5-10 mg in 10 mL NS, inject 1-5 mL (in divided doses) around extravasation site. Hypertensive crisis: 5-15 mg IV.
UNAPPROVED PEDS - IV extravasation of catecholamines: neonates, 2.5-5 mg in 10 mL NS, inject 1 mL (in divided doses) around extravasation site; children, same as adult.
NOTES - Weakness, flushing, hypotension; priapism with intracavernous injection. Use within 12h of extravasation. Distributed to hospital pharmacies, at no charge, only for use in life-threatening situations. Call (888) 669-6682 for ordering.

treprostinil (*Remodulin*) ▶KL ♀B ▶? $$$$$
ADULT - Continuous subcutaneous infusion in pulmonary arterial HTN with NYHA Class II to IV symptoms: Start 1.25 ng/kg/minute based on ideal body weight. Reduce to 0.625 ng/kg/minute if initial dose not tolerated. Dose based on clinical response & tolerance. Increase by no more than 1.25 ng/kg/minute/week in first 4

weeks, then increase by no more than 2.5 ng/kg/minute/week. Max 40 ng/ kg/minute.
PEDS - Not approved in children.
NOTES - Use cautiously in the elderly and those with liver or renal dysfunction. Initiate in setting

with personnel & equipment for physiological monitoring & emergency care. Administer by continuous SQ infusion using infusion pump. Patient must have access to backup infusion pump and SQ infusion sets.

CARDIOVASCULAR: Antiplatelet Drugs

abciximab (*ReoPro*) ▶Plasma ♀C ▶? $$$$$
ADULT - Platelet aggregation inhibition, prevention of acute cardiac ischemic events associated with PTCA: 0.25 mg/kg IV bolus over 1 min via separate infusion line 10-60 min before procedure, then 0.125 mcg/kg/min up to 10 mcg/min infusion for 12h. Unstable angina not responding to standard therapy: 0.25 mg/kg IV bolus over 1 min via separate infusion line, followed by 10 mcg/min IV infusion for 18-24h, concluding 1h after PTCA.
PEDS - Not approved in children.
NOTES - Thrombocytopenia possible. Discontinue abciximab, heparin, and aspirin if uncontrollable bleeding occurs.

Aggrenox (dipyridamole + aspirin) ▶LK ♀D ▶? $$$$
ADULT - Platelet aggregation inhibition/prevention of TIAs and strokes: 1 cap bid.
PEDS - Not approved in children.
FORMS - Trade: Caps, 200/25 mg.
NOTES - The dipyridamole component is extended-release. Do not crush or chew Caps. May need supplemental aspirin for prevention of MI.

aspirin (*Ecotrin, Empirin, Halfprin, Bayer, ASA, ✤Entrophen, Asaphen, Novasen*) ▶K ♀D ▶? $
ADULT - Platelet aggregation inhibition: 81-325 mg PO qd.
PEDS - See analgesic section for pain/antipyretic doses.
UNAPPROVED ADULT - Post ST-elevation MI: 162-325 mg PO on day 1, continue indefinitely at 75-162 mg/day. Primary prevention of cardiovascular events (patients with 10-year CHD risk >6-10% based on Framingham risk scoring): 75-325 mg PO qd. Long-term antithrombotic therapy in atrial fib with risk factors for stroke & contraindication to warfarin or no risk factors for stroke: 325 mg PO qd. Prevention of thrombosis/restenosis after percutaneous coronary intervention: 81-325 mg PO qd.
FORMS - Generic/Trade (OTC): tabs, 325,500 mg; chewable 81 mg; enteric-coated 81,165 mg (Halfprin), 81,325,500 mg (Ecotrin), 650, 975 mg. Trade only: tabs, controlled-release 650,800 mg (ZORprin, Rx). Generic only

(OTC): suppository 120,200,300,600 mg.
NOTES - Crush or chew tabs (including enteric-coated products) in first dose with acute MI. Higher doses of aspirin (1.3 g/day) have not been shown to be superior to low doses in preventing TIAs and strokes. Do not withhold before coronary artery bypass (CAB) surgery; may prescribe 75-325 mg qd within 24 hours after CAB surgery.

clopidogrel (*Plavix*) ▶LK ♀B ▶? $$$$
WARNING - Rarely may cause life-threatening thrombotic thrombocytopenia purpura (TTP), usually during the first 2 weeks of therapy.
ADULT - Reduction of thrombotic events: after recent AMI, recent stroke, established peripheral arterial disease: 75 mg PO qd with or without food; acute coronary syndrome (unstable angina or non Q-wave MI): 300 mg loading dose, then 75 mg PO qd in combination with aspirin PO qd.
PEDS - Not approved in children.
UNAPPROVED ADULT - Post percutaneous coronary artery intervention: 75 mg qd in combination with aspirin for ≥1 month after bare metal stenting, for several months after drug-eluting stenting (3 months sirolimus, 6 months paclitaxel), & preferably up to 12 months in patients not at high risk for bleeding. Post percutaneous coronary brachytherapy: 75 mg qd for ≥9 months. Post ST-elevation MI with aspirin allergy: 75 mg PO qd. Reduction of thrombotic events in high-risk patient after TIA: 75 mg PO qd.
FORMS - Trade: Tab, non-scored 75 mg.
NOTES - Prolongs bleeding time. Discontinue use 7 days before surgery. Loading dose 300 mg PO >6 hours prior to procedure may be used for prevention of cardiac stent occlusion. Contraindicated with active pathologic bleeding (peptic ulcer or intracranial bleed). Concomitant ASA increases bleeding risk.

dipyridamole (*Persantine*) ▶L ♀B ▶? $
ADULT - Prevention of thromboembolic complications of cardiac valve replacement: 75-100 mg PO qid. Used as adjunctive agent to warfarin.
PEDS - Not approved in children <12 yo.

UNAPPROVED ADULT - Platelet aggregation inhibition: 150-400 mg/day PO divided tid-qid.
FORMS - Generic/Trade: Tabs, non-scored 25,50,75 mg.
NOTES - Not effective for angina.

eptifibatide (Integrilin) ▸K ♀B ▶? $$$$$
ADULT - Acute coronary syndrome (unstable angina/non-ST-segment elevation MI): Load 180 mcg/kg IV bolus, then IV infusion 2 mcg/kg/min for up to 72 hr. If percutaneous coronary intervention (PCI) occurs during the infusion, continue infusion for 18-24 hr after procedure. PCI in patients not presenting with acute coronary syndrome: Load 180 mcg/kg IV bolus just before procedure, followed by infusion 2 mcg/kg/min and a second 180 mcg/kg IV bolus 10 min after the first bolus. Continue infusion for up to 18-24 hr (minimum 12 hr) after the procedure. Renal impairment (CrCl <50 ml/min; if CrCl not available, serum creat >2mg/dl): No change in bolus dose; decrease infusion to 1 mcg/kg/min. Obese patient (>121 kg): Max bolus dose 22.6 mg; max infusion rate 15 mg/hr. Renal impairment and obese: Max bolus dose 22.6 mg; max infusion rate 7.5 mg/hr.
PEDS - Not approved in children.
NOTES - Discontinue infusion prior to CABG. Thrombocytopenia possible. Concomitant aspirin & heparin/enoxaparin use recommended, unless contraindicated. Contraindicated in dialysis patients.

ticlopidine (Ticlid) ▸L ♀B ▶? $$$$
WARNING - May cause life-threatening neutropenia, agranulocytosis, and thrombotic thrombocytopenia purpura (TTP). TTP usually occurs during the first two weeks of treatment. Monitor CBC routinely.
ADULT - Due to adverse effects, clopidogrel preferred. Platelet aggregation inhibition/reduction of thrombotic stroke: 250 mg PO bid with food. Prevention of cardiac stent occlusion: 250 mg PO bid in combo with aspirin 325 mg PO qd for up to 30 days post stent implantation.
PEDS - Not approved in children.
UNAPPROVED ADULT - Due to adverse effects, clopidogrel preferred. Prevention of graft occlusion with CABG: 250 mg PO bid.
FORMS - Generic/Trade: Tab, non-scored 250 mg.
NOTES - Check CBC every 2 weeks during the first 3 months of therapy. Neutrophil counts usually return to normal within 1-3 weeks following discontinuation. Loading dose 500 mg PO on day 1 may be used for prevention of cardiac stent occlusion.

tirofiban (Aggrastat) ▸K ♀B ▶? $$$$$
ADULT - Acute coronary syndromes (unstable angina and non-Q wave MI): Start 0.4 mcg/kg/min IV infusion for 30 mins, then decrease to 0.1 mcg/kg/min for 48-108 hr or until 12-24 hr after coronary intervention.
PEDS - Not approved in children.
NOTES - Thrombocytopenia possible. Concomitant aspirin & heparin/enoxaparin use recommended, unless contraindicated. Dose heparin to keep PTT twice normal. Decrease bolus dose and rate of infusion by 50% in patients with CrCl <30 mL/min. Dilute concentrate solution before using.

CARDIOVASCULAR: Beta Blockers

NOTE: See also antihypertensive combinations. Abrupt discontinuation may precipitate angina, myocardial infarction, arrhythmias, or rebound hypertension; discontinue by tapering over 2 weeks. Avoid using nonselective beta-blockers and use agents with beta1 selectivity cautiously in asthma/COPD. Beta 1 selectivity diminishes at high doses. Avoid in decompensated CHF.

acebutolol (Sectral, ♥Rhotral, Monitan) ▸LK ♀B ▶- $
ADULT - HTN: Start 400 mg PO qd or 200 mg PO bid, usual maintenance 400-800 mg/day, max 1200 mg/day. Twice daily dosing appears to be more effective than qd dosing.
PEDS - Not approved in children <12.
UNAPPROVED ADULT - Angina: Start 200 mg PO bid, increase as needed up to 800 mg/day.
FORMS - Generic/Trade: Caps, 200,400 mg.
NOTES - Has mild intrinsic sympathomimetic activity (partial beta agonist activity). Beta1 receptor selective.

atenolol (Tenormin) ▸K ♀D ▶- $
WARNING - Avoid abrupt cessation in coronary heart disease or HTN.
ADULT - Acute MI: 5 mg IV over 5 min, repeat in 10 min, follow with 50 mg PO 10 min after IV dosing in patients tolerating the total IV dose, increase as tolerated to 100 mg/day given qd or divided bid. HTN: Start 25-50 mg PO qd or divided bid, maximum 100 mg/day. Renal impairment, elderly: Start 25 mg PO qd, increase as needed. Angina: Start 50 mg PO qd or divided bid, increase as needed to max of 200

mg/day.

PEDS - Not approved in children.

UNAPPROVED ADULT - Reduce perioperative cardiac events (death) in high risk patients undergoing noncardiac surgery: Start 5-10 mg IV prior to anesthesia, then 50-100 mg PO qd during hospitalization (max 7 days). Maintain HR between 55-65 bpm. Hold dose for HR <55 bpm and SBP <100 mm Hg. Reentrant PSVT associated w/ ST-elevation MI (after carotid massage, IV adenosine): 2.5-5 mg over 2 min to 10 mg max over 10-15 min. Rate control of atrial fibrillation/flutter: Start 25 mg PO qd, titrate to desired heart rate.

UNAPPROVED PEDS - HTN: 1-1.2 mg/kg/dose PO qd, max 2 mg/kg/day.

FORMS - Generic/Trade: Tabs, non-scored 25, 100; scored, 50 mg.

NOTES - Doses >100 mg/day usually do not provide further BP lowering. Beta1 receptor selective. Risk of hypoglycemia to neonates born to mothers using atenolol at parturition or while breastfeeding.

betaxolol (*Kerlone*) ▶LK ♀C ▶? $$

ADULT - HTN: Start 5-10 mg PO qd, max 20 mg/day. Renal impairment, elderly: Start 5 mg PO qd, increase as needed.

PEDS - Not approved in children.

FORMS - Trade: Tabs, scored 10, non-scored 20 mg.

NOTES - Beta1 receptor selective.

bisoprolol (*Zebeta*, ✿*Monocor*) ▶LK ♀C ▶? $$

ADULT - HTN: Start 2.5-5 mg PO qd, max 20 mg/day. Renal impairment: Start 2.5 mg PO qd, increase as needed.

PEDS - Not approved in children.

UNAPPROVED ADULT - Compensated heart failure: Start 1.25 mg PO qd, double dose every 2 weeks as tolerated up to max 10 mg/day. Reduce perioperative cardiac events (death, MI) in high risk patients undergoing noncardiac surgery: Start 5 mg PO qd, at least 1 week prior to surgery, increase to 10 mg qd to maintain HR <60 bpm, continue for 30 days postop. Hold dose for HR <50 bpm or SBP <100 mm Hg.

FORMS - Generic/Trade: Tabs, scored 5, non-scored 10 mg.

NOTES - Monitor closely for CHF exacerbation and hypotension when titrating dose. Avoid use in patients with decompensated CHF (i.e. NYHA class IV heart failure). Stabilize dose of digoxin, diuretics, and ACEI before starting bisoprolol. Beta1 receptor selective.

carteolol (*Cartrol*) ▶K ♀C ▶? $$

ADULT - HTN: Start 2.5 mg PO qd, usual maintenance dose 2.5-5 mg qd, max 10 mg qd. Doses >10 mg daily generally do not produce additional BP lowering.

PEDS - Not approved in children.

FORMS - Trade: Tabs, non-scored, 2.5,5 mg.

NOTES - Decrease dosing frequency with renal impairment - CrCl 20-60 ml/min, q48 hours; CrCl <20 ml/min, q72 hours. Avoid in asthma and obstructive lung disease. Has mild intrinsic sympathomimetic activity (partial beta agonist activity).

carvedilol (*Coreg*) ▶L ♀C ▶? $$$$

ADULT - CHF: Start 3.125 mg PO bid with food, double dose q2 weeks as tolerated up to max of 25 mg bid (if <85 kg) or 50 mg bid (if >85 kg). Reduce cardiovascular risk in post-MI with LV dysfunction: Start 6.25 mg PO bid, double dose q 3-10 days as tolerated to max of 25 mg bid. HTN: Start 6.25 mg PO bid, maximum 50 mg/day. Not first line agent for HTN.

PEDS - Not approved in children.

FORMS - Trade: Tabs, non-scored 3.125, scored, 6.25,12.5,25 mg.

NOTES - Do not initiate in decompensated CHF. Monitor closely for CHF exacerbation and hypotension (particularly orthostatic) when titrating dose. Stabilize dose of digoxin, diuretics, and ACEI before starting carvedilol. Avoid use in severe hepatic impairment. Alpha1, beta1, and beta2 receptor blocker. Contraindicated in asthma and hepatic impairment. May reversibly elevate LFTs.

esmolol (*Brevibloc*) ▶K ♀C ▶? $$

ADULT - SVT/HTN emergency: Mix infusion 5 g in 500 mL (10 mg/mL), load with 500 mcg/kg IV over 1 minute (70 kg: 35 mg or 3.5 mL) then IV infusion 50 mcg/kg/min for 4 min (70 kg: 100 mcg/kg/min = 40 mL/h). If optimal response is not attained, repeat IV load and increase IV infusion to 100 mcg/kg/min for 4 min. If necessary, additional boluses (500 mcg/kg/min over 1 min) may be given followed by IV infusion with increased dose by 50 mcg/kg/min for 4 min. Max IV infusion rate 200 mcg/kg/min.

PEDS - Not approved in children.

UNAPPROVED PEDS - Same schedule as adult except loading dose 100-500 mcg/kg IV over 1 min and IV infusion 25-100 mcg/kg/min. IV infusions may be increased by 25-50 mcg/kg/min every 5-10 min. Titrate dose based on patient response.

NOTES - Hypotension. Beta1 receptor selective. Half-life = 9 minutes.

labetalol (*Trandate, Normodyne*) ▶LK ♀C ▶+ $$$

ADULT - HTN: Start 100 mg PO bid, usual maintenance dose 200-600 mg bid, max 2400 mg/day. HTN emergency: Start 20 mg slow IV injection, then 40-80 mg IV q10min as needed up to 300 mg total cumulative dose or start 0.5-2 mg/min IV infusion, adjust rate as needed up to total cumulative dose 300 mg.

PEDS - Not approved in children.

UNAPPROVED PEDS - HTN: 4 mg/kg/day PO divided bid, increase as needed up to 40 mg/kg/day. IV: Start 0.3-1 mg/kg/dose (max 20 mg) slow IV injection q10 min or 0.4-1 mg/kg/h IV infusion up to 3 mg/kg/hr.

FORMS - Generic/Trade: Tabs, scored 100,200 (Trandate, Normodyne), 300 (Trandate), non-scored 300 mg (Normodyne).

NOTES - Hypotension. Contraindicated in asthma/COPD. Alpha1, beta1, and beta2 receptor blocker.

metoprolol (*Lopressor, Toprol-XL*, ✿*Be-taloc*) ▶L ♀C ▶? $$

WARNING - Avoid abrupt cessation in ischemic heart disease or HTN.

ADULT - Acute MI: 5 mg IV q5-15 min up to 15 mg. If tolerated, start 50 mg PO q6h for 48h, then 100 mg PO bid. If usual IV dose is not tolerated, start 25-50 mg PO q6h. If early IV therapy is contraindicated, patient should be titrated to 100 mg PO bid as soon as possible. HTN (immediate release): Start 100 mg PO qd or 50 mg bid, increase as needed up to 450 mg/day. HTN (extended release): Start 50-100 mg PO qd, increase as needed up to 400 mg/day. CHF: Start 12.5-25 mg (extended-release) PO qd, double dose every 2 weeks as tolerated up to max 200 mg/day. Angina: Start 50 mg PO bid (immediate release) or 100 mg PO qd (extended-release), increase as needed up to 400 mg/day.

PEDS - Not approved in children.

UNAPPROVED ADULT - CHF: Start 6.25 (immediate release) PO bid, max 75 mg bid. Atrial tachyarrhythmia, except with Wolff-Parkinson-White syndrome: 2.5-5 mg IV q2-5 min as needed to control rapid ventricular response, max 15 mg over 10-15 min. Reentrant PSVT associated w/ ST-elevation MI (after carotid massage, IV adenosine): 2.5-5 mg q 2-5 min to 15 mg max over 10-15 min. Reduce perioperative cardiac events (death) in high-risk patients undergoing noncardiac surgery: Start 5-10 mg IV prior to anesthesia, then 50-100 mg (extended release) PO qd during hospitalization (max 7 days). Maintain HR between 55-65 bpm. Hold dose for HR <55 bpm and SBP <100 mm Hg. Rate control of atrial fibrillation/flutter: Start 25 mg PO bid, titrate to desired heart rate.

FORMS - Generic/Trade: tabs, scored 50,100 mg. Trade only: tabs, extended-release (Toprol-XL) 25,50,100,200 mg.

NOTES - Monitor closely for CHF exacerbation and hypotension when titrating dose. Avoid use in patients with decompensated CHF (i.e. NYHA class IV heart failure or pulmonary edema). Stabilize dose of digoxin, diuretics, and ACEI before starting metoprolol. Beta1 receptor selective. Extended-release tabs may be broken in half, but do not chew or crush. Avoid using extended release tabs with verapamil, diltiazem, or peripheral vascular disease. May need lower doses in elderly.

nadolol (*Corgard*) ▶K ♀C ▶- $$

ADULT - HTN: Start 20-40 mg PO qd, usual maintenance dose 40-80 mg/day, max 320 mg/day. Renal impairment: Start 20 mg PO qd, adjust dosage interval based on severity of renal impairment - CrCl 31-50 mL/min, q24-36h; CrCl 10-30 mL/min, q24-48h; CrCl <10 mL/min, q40-60h. Angina: Start 40 mg PO qd, usual maintenance dose 40-80 mg/day, max 240 mg/day.

PEDS - Not approved in children.

UNAPPROVED ADULT - Rebleeding esophageal varices: 40-160 mg/day PO. Titrate dose to reduce heart rate to 25% below baseline. Ventricular arrhythmia: 10-640 mg/day PO.

FORMS - Generic/Trade: Tabs, scored 20,40, 80,120,160 mg.

NOTES - Beta1 and beta2 receptor blocker.

oxprenolol (✿*Trasicor, Slow-Trasicor*) ▶L ♀D ▶- $$

ADULT - Canada only. Mild to moderate HTN, usually in combination with a thiazide-type diuretic: Regular release: Initially 20 mg PO tid, titrate upwards prn to usual maintenance 120-320 mg/day divided bid-tid. Alternatively, may substitute an equivalent qd dose of sustained release product; do not exceed 480 mg/day.

PEDS - Not approved in children.

FORMS - Trade: Regular release tabs: 40, 80 mg. Sustained release tabs: 80, 160 mg.

NOTES - Caution in bronchospasm, diabetes, or heart failure. Has mild intrinsic sympathomimetic activity (partial beta agonist activity). No dose adjustment in impaired renal function. Empty matrix of sustained release tablet may be excreted and found in the feces.

penbutolol (*Levatol*) ▶LK ♀C ▶? $$$
ADULT - HTN: Start 20 mg PO qd, usual maintenance dose 20-40 mg, max 80 mg/day.
PEDS - Not approved in children.
FORMS - Trade: Tabs, scored 20 mg.
NOTES - Has mild intrinsic sympathomimetic activity (partial beta agonist activity). Beta1 and beta2 receptor blocker.

pindolol ▶K ♀B ▶? $$$
ADULT - HTN: Start 5 mg PO bid, usual maintenance dose 10-30 mg/day, max 60 mg/day.
PEDS - Not approved in children.
UNAPPROVED ADULT - Angina: 15-40 mg/day PO in divided doses tid-qid.
FORMS - Generic: Tabs, scored 5,10 mg.
NOTES - Has intrinsic sympathomimetic activity (partial beta agonist activity). Beta1 and beta2 receptor blocker. Contraindicated with thioridazine.

propranolol (*Inderal, Inderal LA, InnoPran XL*) ▶L ♀C ▶+ $$
WARNING - Avoid abrupt cessation in coronary heart disease or HTN.
ADULT - HTN: Start 20-40 mg PO bid, usual maintenance dose 160-480 mg/day, max 640 mg/day; extended-release (Inderal LA): start 60-80 mg PO qd, usual maintenance dose 120-160 mg/day, max 640 mg/day; extended-release (InnoPran XL): start 80 mg qhs (10 PM), max 120 mg qhs. Angina: Start 10-20 mg PO tid/qid, usual maintenance 160-240 mg/day, max 320 mg/day; extended-release (Inderal LA): start 80 mg PO qd, same usual dosage range and max for HTN. Migraine prophylaxis: Start 40 mg PO bid or 80 mg PO qd (extended-release), max 240 mg/day. Supraventricular tachycardia or rapid atrial fibrillation/flutter: 10-30 mg PO tid/qid. MI: 180-240 mg/day PO in divided doses bid-qid. Pheochromocytoma surgery: 60 mg PO in divided doses bid-tid beginning 3 days before surgery, use in combination with an alpha blocking agent. IV: reserved for life-threatening arrhythmia, 1-3 mg IV, repeat dose in 2 min if

needed, additional doses should not be given in <4h. Not for use in hypertensive emergency.
PEDS - HTN: Start 1 mg/kg/day PO divided bid, usual maintenance dose 2-4 mg/kg/day PO divided bid, max 16 mg/kg/day.
UNAPPROVED ADULT - Rebleeding esophageal varices: 20-180 mg PO bid. Titrate dose to reduce heart rate to 25% below baseline.
UNAPPROVED PEDS - Arrhythmia: 0.01-0.1 mg/kg/dose (max 1 mg/dose) by slow IV push. Manufacturer does not recommend IV propranolol in children.
FORMS - Generic/Trade: Tabs, scored 10,20, 40,60,80. Generic only: Solution 20,40 mg/5 mL. Concentrate 80 mg/mL. Trade: Caps, extended-release (Inderal LA qd) 60,80,120,160 mg, (InnoPran XL qhs) 80,120 mg.
NOTES - Do not substitute extended-release product for immediate-release product on mg-for-mg basis. Dosage titration may be necessary with extended-release product when converting from immediate-release Tabs. Extended-release Caps (Inderal LA) may be opened, and the contents sprinkled on food for administration. Cap contents should be swallowed whole without crushing or chewing. Beta1 and beta2 receptor blocker. Contraindicated with thioridazine.

timolol (*Blocadren*) ▶LK ♀C ▶+ $$
ADULT - HTN: Start 10 mg PO bid, usual maintenance 20-40 mg/day, max 60 mg/day. MI: 10 mg PO bid, started 1-4 weeks post-MI. Migraine headaches: Start 10 mg PO bid, use 20 mg/day qd or divided bid for prophylaxis, increase as needed up to max 60 mg/day. Stop therapy if satisfactory response not obtained after 6-8 weeks of max dose.
PEDS - Not approved in children.
UNAPPROVED ADULT - Angina: 15-45 mg/day PO divided tid-qid.
FORMS - Generic/Trade: Tabs, non-scored 5, scored 10,20 mg.
NOTES - Beta1 and beta2 receptor blocker.

CARDIOVASCULAR: Calcium Channel Blockers (CCBs) - Dihydropyridines

NOTE: See also antihypertensive combinations. Peripheral edema, especially with higher doses. Extended / controlled / sustained-release tabs should be swallowed whole; do not chew or crush. Avoid concomitant grapefruit / grapefruit juice, which may enhance effect. Avoid in decompensated CHF.

amlodipine (*Norvasc*) ▶L ♀C ▶? $$

ADULT - HTN: Start 2.5 to 5 mg PO qd, max 10 qd. Angina: Start 5 mg PO qd, usual maintenance dose 10 mg PO qd.
PEDS - HTN (6-17 yo): 2.5-5 mg PO qd.
UNAPPROVED PEDS - HTN: Start 0.1-0.2 mg/kg/day PO qd, max 0.3 mg/kg/day.
FORMS - Trade: Tabs, non-scored 2.5,5,10 mg.
NOTES - HTN control improved with 5-10 mg

PO qd in patients with CHF (already on ACEI, digoxin, and diuretics) without worsening morbidity or mortality.

felodipine (Plendil, ✦Renedil) ▶L ♀C ▶? $$
ADULT - HTN: Start 2.5-5 mg PO qd, usual maintenance dose 5-10 mg/day, max 10 mg/day.
PEDS - Not approved in children.
FORMS - Trade: Tabs, extended-release, non-scored 2.5,5,10 mg.
NOTES - Extended-release tab. HTN control improved with 5-10 mg PO qd in patients with CHF (already on ACEI, digoxin, and diuretics) without worsening CHF. May increase tacrolimus concentration; monitor level.

isradipine (DynaCirc, DynaCirc CR) ▶L ♀C ▶? $$$
ADULT - HTN: Start 2.5 mg PO bid, usual maintenance 5-10 mg/day, max 20 mg/day divided bid (max 10 mg/day in elderly). Controlled-release (DynaCirc CR): Start 5 mg PO qd, usual maintenance dose 5-10 mg/day, max 20 mg/day.
PEDS - Not approved in children.
FORMS - Caps 2.5,5 mg; tab, controlled-release 5,10 mg.

nicardipine (Cardene, Cardene SR) ▶L ♀C ▶? $$
ADULT - HTN: sustained-release (Cardene SR), Start 30 mg PO bid, usual maintenance dose 30-60 mg PO bid, max 120 mg/day; immediate-release, Start 20 mg PO tid, usual maintenance dose 20-40 mg PO tid, max 120 mg/day. Hypertensive emergency/short-term management of acute HTN: Begin IV infusion at 5 mg/h, titrate infusion rate by 2.5 mg/h q15min as needed, max 15 mg/h. Angina: immediate-release, Start 20 mg PO tid, usual maintenance dose 20-40 mg tid.
PEDS - Not approved in children.

UNAPPROVED PEDS - HTN: 0.5-3 mcg/kg/min IV infusion.
FORMS - Generic/Trade: caps, immediate-release 20,30 mg. Trade only: caps, sustained-release 30,45,60 mg.
NOTES - Hypotension, especially with immediate-release Caps and IV. Decrease dose if hepatically impaired. Use sustained-release Caps for HTN only, not for angina.

nifedipine (Procardia, Adalat, Procardia XL, Adalat CC, ✦Adalat XL) ▶L ♀C ▶+ $$
ADULT - HTN: extended-release, Start 30-60 mg PO qd, max 120 mg/day. Angina: extended-release, Start 30-60 mg PO qd, max 120 mg/day; immediate-release, Start 10 mg PO tid, usual maintenance dose 10-20 mg tid, max 120 mg/day.
PEDS - Not approved in children.
UNAPPROVED PEDS - HTN: 0.25-0.5 mg/kg/dose PO q4-6 h as needed, max 10 mg/dose or 3 mg/kg/day. Doses <0.25 mg/kg may be effective.
FORMS - Generic/Trade: Caps, 10,20 mg. Tabs, extended-release 30,60,90 mg.
NOTES - Avoid sublingual administration of immediate-release cap, may cause excessive hypotension, stroke. Do not use immediate-release caps for treating HTN, hypertensive emergencies, or ST-elevation MI. Extended-release tabs can be substituted for immediate-release caps at the same dose in patients whose angina is controlled.

nisoldipine (Sular) ▶L ♀C ▶? $$
ADULT - HTN: Start 20 mg PO qd, usual maintenance 20-40 mg/day, max 60 mg/day. Impaired hepatic function, elderly: Start 10 mg PO qd, titrate as needed.
PEDS - Not approved in children.
FORMS - Trade: Tabs, extended-release 10,20, 30,40 mg.

CARDIOVASCULAR: Calcium Channel Blockers (CCBs) - Other

NOTE: See also antihypertensive combinations. Avoid in decompensated CHF.

diltiazem (Cardizem, Cardizem SR, Cardizem LA, Cardizem CD, Cartia XT, Dilacor XR, Diltiazem CD, Diltia XT, Tiazac, Taztia XT) ▶L ♀C ▶+ $$
ADULT - Rapid atrial fibrillation: 20 mg (0.25 mg/kg) IV bolus over 2 min. If needed and patient tolerated IV bolus with no hypotension, rebolus 15 min later with 25 mg (0.35 mg/kg). IV infusion: Start 10 mg/h, increase by 5 mg/h

(usual range 5-15 mg/h). Once daily, extended-release (Cardizem CD, Cartia XT, Dilacor XR, Diltia XT, Taztia XT, Tiazac), HTN: Start 120-240 mg PO qd, usual maintenance range 240-360 mg/day, max 540 mg/day. Once daily, graded extended release (Cardizem LA), HTN: Start 180-240 mg, max 540 mg/day. Twice daily, sustained-release (Cardizem SR), HTN: Start 60-120 mg PO bid, max 360 mg/day. Immediate-release, angina: Start 30 mg PO qid, max 360 mg/day divided tid-qid. Extended-release, angina: 120-180 mg PO qd, max 540 mg/day. Once daily, graded extended release (Cardizem LA), angina: Start 180 mg PO qd, doses >360 mg may provide no additional benefit.

PEDS - Not approved in children. Diltiazem injection should be avoided in neonates due to potential toxicity from benzyl alcohol in the injectable product .

UNAPPROVED ADULT - Control heart rate at rest or during exercise with chronic A-fib: titrate up to 360 mg/day PO alone or with digoxin. Reentrant PSVT associated w/ ST-elevation MI (after carotid massage, IV adenosine, beta blocker): 20 mg (0.25 mg/kg) IV over 2 min, then 10 mg/hr IV infusion.

UNAPPROVED PEDS - HTN: Start 1.5-2 mg/kg/ day PO divided tid-qid, max 3.5 mg/kg/day.

FORMS - Generic/Trade: Immediate-release tabs, non-scored (Cardizem) 30, scored 60, 90, 120 mg; extended-release caps (Cardizem CD, Taztia XT qd) 120, 180, 240, 300, 360 mg, (Cartia XT, Dilt-CD qd) 120, 180, 240, 300, (Tiazac qd) 120, 180, 240, 300, 360, 420 mg, (Dilacor XR, Diltia XT qd) 120, 180, 240 mg. Trade only: Sustained-release caps (Cardizem SR q12h) 60, 90, 120 mg; extended-release grade tabs (Cardizem LA qd) 120, 180, 240, 300, 360, 420 mg.

NOTES - Contraindicated in acute MI and pulmonary congestion, hypotension, sick sinus syndrome without pacemaker, second or third degree AV block without pacemaker, Wolff-Parkinson-White syndrome with rapid A-fib/flutter. Contents of extended-release caps may be sprinkled over food (eg, apple sauce). Do not chew or crush cap contents. May accumulate with hepatic impairment; dose based on clinical response.

verapamil (*Isoptin, Calan, Covera-HS, Verelan, Verelan PM, ♥Chronovera*) ▶L ♀C ▶+ $$
ADULT - SVT: 5-10 mg (0.075-0.15 mg/kg) IV over 2 min. A second dose of 10 mg IV may be given 15-30 min later if needed. PSVT/rate control with atrial fibrillation: 240-480 mg/day PO divided tid-qid. Angina: Start 40-80 mg PO tid-qid, max 480 mg/day; sustained-release (Isoptin SR, Calan SR, Verelan), start 120-240 mg PO qd, max 480 mg/day (use bid dosing for doses >240 mg/day with Isoptin SR and Calan SR); extended-release (Covera-HS), start 180 mg PO qhs, max 480 mg/day. HTN: Same as angina, except (Verelan PM) start 100-200 mg PO qhs, max 400 mg/day; (Covera-HS) start 180 mg PO qhs, max 480 mg/day; immediate-release tabs should be avoided in treating HTN.

PEDS - SVT: (1-15 yo) 2-5 mg (0.1-0.3 mg/kg) IV, max dose 5 mg. Repeat dose once in 30 min if needed, max second dose 10 mg. Immediate-release and sustained-release tabs not approved in children.

FORMS - Generic/Trade: tabs, immediate-release, scored 40,80,120 mg; sustained-release, non-scored (Calan SR, Isoptin SR) 120, scored 180,240 mg; caps, sustained-release (Verelan) 120,180,240,360 mg. Trade only: tabs, extended-release (Covera HS) 180,240 mg; caps, extended-release (Verelan PM) 100, 200,300 mg.

NOTES - Contraindicated in severe LV dysfunction, hypotension, sick sinus syndrome, second or third degree AV block without pacemaker, A-fib/flutter conducted via accessory pathway (ie, Wolff-Parkinson-White). Avoid concomitant grapefruit juice (enhances effect). Scored, sustained-release tabs (Calan SR, Isoptin SR) may be broken and each piece swallowed whole, do not chew or crush. Other extended-release tabs (Covera HS) should be swallowed whole. Contents of sustained-release caps may be sprinkled on food (eg, apple sauce). Do not chew or crush cap contents. Coadministration with aspirin may increase bleeding times. Use cautiously with impaired renal/hepatic function.

CARDIOVASCULAR: Diuretics – Carbonic Anhydrase Inhibitors

acetazolamide (*Diamox*) ▶LK ♀C ▶+ $
ADULT - Edema: Rarely used, start 250-375 mg IV/PO qam given intermittently (qod or 2 consecutive days followed by none for 1-2 days) to avoid loss of diuretic effect. Acute mountain sickness: 125-250 mg PO bid-tid, beginning 1-2 days prior to ascent and continuing ≥5 days at higher altitude.

PEDS - Diuretic: 5 mg/kg PO/IV qam.

FORMS - Generic only: Tabs, 125,250 mg; Trade only: cap, sustained-release 500 mg.

NOTES - A suspension (250 mg/5 mL) can be made by crushing and mixing tabs in flavored syrup. The susp is stable for 7 days at room temperature. One tab may be softened in 2 teaspoons of hot water, then add to 2 teaspoons of honey or syrup, and swallowed at once. Tabs and compounded susp may have a bitter taste. Use cautiously in sulfa allergy. Prompt descent is necessary if severe forms of high altitude sickness occur (eg, pulmonary or cerebral edema). Test the drug for tolerance/allergies 1-2 weeks before initial dosing prior to ascent.

CARDIOVASCULAR: Diuretics – Loop

NOTE: Give second dose of bid schedule in mid afternoon to avoid nocturia. Rare hypersensitivity in patients allergic to sulfa-containing drugs.

bumetanide (*Bumex*, ✱*Burinex*) ▶K♀C▷? $
ADULT - Edema: 0.5-2 mg PO qd, repeat doses at 4-5 hr intervals as needed until desired response is attained, max 10 mg/day; 0.5-1 mg IV/IM, repeat doses at 2-3 hr intervals as needed until desired response is attained, max 10 mg/day. Dosing for 3-4 consecutive days followed by no drug for 1-2 days is acceptable. BID dosing may enhance diuretic effect. IV injections should be over 1-2 min. An IV infusion may be used, change bag every 24 hours.
PEDS - Not approved in children.
UNAPPROVED PEDS - Edema: 0.015-0.1 mg/kg/dose PO/IV/IM qd or qod.
FORMS - Generic/Trade: Tabs, scored 0.5,1,2 mg.
NOTES - 1 mg bumetanide is roughly equivalent to 40 mg furosemide. IV administration is preferred when GI absorption is impaired.

ethacrynic acid (*Edecrin*) ▶K♀C▷? $$
ADULT - Edema: 0.5-1 mg/kg IV, max 50 mg IV; 25 mg PO qd on day one, followed by 50 mg PO bid on day two, followed by 100 mg PO in the morning and 50-100 mg PO in the evening depending on the response to the morning dose, max 400 mg/day.
PEDS - Not approved in children.
UNAPPROVED ADULT - HTN: 25 mg PO qd, max 100 mg/day divided bid-tid.
UNAPPROVED PEDS - Edema: 1 mg/kg IV; 25 mg PO qd, increase slowly by 25 mg increments as needed. Ethacrynic acid should not be administered to infants.
FORMS - Trade: Tabs, scored 25
NOTES - Rarely used. Ototoxicity possible.

Does not contain a sulfonamide group; may be useful in sulfonamide-allergic patients. Do not administer SC or IM due to local irritation. IV ethacrynic acid should be reconstituted to a concentration of 50 mg/mL and given slowly by IV infusion over 20-30 min.

furosemide (*Lasix*) ▶K ♀C ▷? $
ADULT - Edema: Start 20-80 mg IV/IM/PO, increase dose by 20-40 mg every 6-8h until desired response is achieved, max 600 mg/day. Give maintenance dose qd or divided bid. IV infusion: 0.05 mg/kg/h, titrate rate to desired response. HTN: Start 20-40 mg bid, adjust dose as needed based on BP response. Thiazide diuretics generally preferred for HTN.
PEDS - Edema: 0.5-2 mg/kg/dose IV/IM/PO q6-12h, max 6 mg/kg/dose. IV infusion: 0.05 mg/kg/h, titrate rate to achieve desired response.
FORMS - Generic/Trade: Tabs, non-scored 20, scored 40,80 mg. Generic only: Oral solution 10 mg/mL, 40 mg/5 mL.
NOTES - Loop diuretics are agent of choice for edema with decreased renal function (CrCl <30 mL/min or creat >2.5 mg/dl).

torsemide (*Demadex*) ▶LK ♀B ▷? $
ADULT - Edema: Start 5-20 mg IV/PO qd, double dose as needed to desired response, max 200 mg as a single dose. HTN: Start 5 mg PO qd, increase as needed every 4-6 weeks, max 100 mg PO qd or divided bid. Thiazide diuretics generally preferred for HTN.
PEDS - Not approved in children.
FORMS - Generic/Trade: Tabs, scored 5,10,20, 100 mg.
NOTES - Loop diuretics are agent of choice for edema with decreased renal function (CrCl <30 mL/min or creat >2.5 mg/dl).

CARDIOVASCULAR: Diuretics – Potassium Sparing

NOTE: See also antihypertensive combinations and aldosterone antagonists. Beware of hyperkalemia. Use cautiously with other agents that may cause hyperkalemia (ie. ACEIs, ARBs).

amiloride (*Midamor*) ▶LK ♀B ▷? $$
ADULT - Diuretic-induced hypokalemia: Start 5 mg PO qd, increase prn based on potassium,

max 20 mg/day. Edema/HTN: Start 5 mg PO qd in combination with another diuretic, usually a thiazide for HTN, increase prn based on potassium, max 20 mg/day. Other diuretics may need to be added when treating edema.
PEDS - Not approved in children.
UNAPPROVED ADULT - Hyperaldosteronism:

10-40 mg PO qd. Do not use combination product (Moduretic) for treatment of hyperaldosteronism.
UNAPPROVED PEDS - Edema: 0.625 mg/kg qd for children weighing 6-20 kg.
FORMS - Generic/Trade: Tabs, non-scored 5 mg.
NOTES - Spironolactone is generally preferred for treating primary hyperaldosteronism. Thiazide diuretics may worsen hypokalemia in patients with hyperaldosteronism.
triamterene (*Dyrenium*) ▶LK ♀B ▶- $$$

ADULT - Edema (cirrhosis, nephrotic syndrome, CHF): Start 100 mg PO bid, max 300 mg/day. Most patients can be maintained on 100 mg PO qd or qod after edema is controlled. Other diuretics may be needed.
PEDS - Not approved in children.
UNAPPROVED PEDS - Edema: 4 mg/kg/day divided bid after meals, increase to 6 mg/kg/day if needed, max 300 mg/day.
FORMS - Trade: Caps, 50,100 mg.
NOTES - Combo product with HCTZ (eg, Dyazide, Maxzide) available for HTN.

HYPERTENSION RISK STRATIFICATION AND TREATMENT (JNC 7)*

Normal <120/<80 mmHg	*Lifestyle modifications*: ↓Weight, diet modifi-
Prehypertension 120-139/80-89 mmHg	cation, ↓dietary sodium, physical activity, al-
Hypertension ≥140/≥90 mmHg	cohol moderation

Not at goal BP of <140/90 mmHg? (<130/80 if diabetes or chronic kidney disease)

Compelling Indication	*Compelling indication*	*Diuretic*	*BB*	*ACEI*	*ARB*	*CCB*	*AA*
	Heart failure	√	√	√	√		√
	Post-myocardial infarction		√	√			√
	High coronary disease risk	√	√	√		√	
	Diabetes	√	√	√	√	√	
	Chronic kidney disease			√	√		
	Recurrent stroke prevention	√		√			

No such indication	*Stage 1 Hypertension* 140-159/90-99 mmHg	Thiazide-type diuretics for most. Alternatives: ACEI, ARB, BB, CCB, or combination.
	Stage 2 Hypertension ≥160/≥100 mmHg	Two-drug combination for most: usually a thiazide plus either ACEI, ARB, BB, or CCB

Not at goal BP?	Optimize doses, add drugs, consider HTN specialist consult

*JNC 7 *JAMA* 2003; 289:2560. BB=beta blocker; ACEI = angiotensin converting enzyme inhibitor; ARB = angiotensin-receptor blocker; BB = beta-blocker; CCB = calcium-channel blocker; AA = aldosterone antagonist

CARDIOVASCULAR: Diuretics – Thiazide Type

NOTE: See also antihypertensive combinations. Possible hypersensitivity in sulfa allergy. Should be used for most patients with HTN, alone or combined with other anti-hypertensive agents. Thiazides are not recommended for pregnancy-induced HTN.
bendroflumethiazide (*Naturetin-5*) ▶L ♀C, D if used in pregnancy-induced HTN ▶? $$$
ADULT - HTN/Edema: Start 5 mg PO qam, usual maintenance dose 5-20 mg/day qd or divided bid.
PEDS - Not approved in children.
FORMS - Trade: Tabs, scored, 5 mg.

NOTES - May dose qod or 3-5 days/week as maintenance therapy to control edema.
chlorothiazide (*Diuril*) ▶L ♀C, D if used in pregnancy-induced HTN ▶+ $
ADULT - HTN: Start 125-250 mg PO qd or divided bid, max 1000 mg/day divided bid. Edema: 500-2000 mg PO/IV qd or divided bid. Dosing on alternate days or for 3-4 consecutive days followed by no drug for 1-2 days is acceptable.
PEDS - Edema: Infants: Start 10-20 mg/kg/day PO qd or divided bid, up to 30 mg/kg/day divided bid. Children 6 mo-2 yo: 10-20 mg/kg/day

PO qd or divided bid, max 375 mg/day. Children 2-12 yo: start 10-20 mg/kg/day PO qd or divided bid, up to 1g/day. IV formulation not recommended for infants or children.

FORMS - Generic/Trade: Tabs, scored 250,500 mg. Trade only: suspension, 250 mg/5 ml.

NOTES - Do not administer SC or IM.

chlorthalidone (*Thalitone*) ▶L ♀B, D if in pregnancy-induced HTN ▶+ $

ADULT - HTN: Start 12.5-25 mg PO qd, usual maintenance dose 12.5-50 mg/day, max 50 mg/day. (Thalitone) Start 15 mg PO qd, usual maintenance 30-45 mg/day, max 50 mg/day. Edema: Start 50-100 mg PO qd after breakfast or 100 mg qod or 100 mg 3 times/week, usual maintenance dose 150-200 mg/day, max 200 mg/day. (Thalitone) Start 30-60 mg PO qd or 60 mg qod, usual maintenance dose 90-120 mg PO qd or qod.

PEDS - Not approved in children.

UNAPPROVED ADULT - Nephrolithiasis: 25-50 mg PO qd.

UNAPPROVED PEDS - Edema: 2 mg/kg PO 3 times weekly.

FORMS - Trade only: Tabs, non-scored (Thalitone) 15 mg. Generic only: Tabs 25,50 mg.

NOTES - Thalitone has greater bioavailability than Hygroton product, do not interchange. Doses greater than 50 mg/day for HTN are usually associated with hypokalemia with little added BP control.

hydrochlorothiazide (*HCTZ, Oretic, Microzide*) ▶L ♀B, D if used in pregnancy-induced HTN ▶+ $

ADULT - HTN: Start 12.5-25 mg PO qd, usual maintenance dose 12.5-25 mg/day, max 50 mg/day. Edema: 25-100 mg PO qd or in divided doses or 50-100 mg PO qod or 3-5 days/week, max 200 mg/day.

PEDS - Edema: 1-2 mg/kg/day PO qd or divided bid, max 37.5 mg/day in infants up to 2 yo, max 100 mg/day in children 2-12 yo.

UNAPPROVED ADULT - Nephrolithiasis: 50-100 mg PO qd.

FORMS - Generic/Trade: Tabs, scored 50 mg; Cap 12.5 mg. Generic: Tabs, scored 25,100 mg. Solution 50 mg/5 mL.

NOTES - Doses as low as 6.25 mg qd may be effective in combination with other antihypertensives. Doses greater than 50 mg/day for HTN may cause hypokalemia with little added BP control.

indapamide (*Lozol*, ♣*Lozide*) ▶L ♀B, D if used in pregnancy-induced HTN ▶? $

ADULT - HTN: Start 1.25-2.5 mg PO qd, max 5 mg/day. Edema/CHF: 2.5-5 mg PO qam.

PEDS - Not approved in children.

FORMS - Generic/Trade: Tabs, non-scored 1.25, 2.5 mg.

methyclothiazide (*Enduron, Aquatensen*) ▶L ♀B, D if used in pregnancy-induced HTN ▶? $

ADULT - HTN: Start 2.5 mg PO qd, usual maintenance dose 2.5-5 mg/day. Edema: Start 2.5 mg PO qd, usual maintenance dose 2.5-10 mg/day.

PEDS - Not approved in children.

FORMS - Generic/Trade: Tabs, scored, 5 mg.

NOTES - May dose qod or 3-5 days/week as maintenance therapy to control edema.

metolazone (*Zaroxolyn*) ▶L ♀B, D if used in pregnancy-induced HTN ▶? $$$

ADULT - Edema (CHF, renal disease): 5-10 mg PO qd, max 10 mg/day in CHF, 20 mg/day in renal disease . If used with loop diuretic, start with 2.5 mg PO qd. Reduce to lowest effective dose as edema resolves. May be given qod as edema resolves.

PEDS - Not approved in children.

UNAPPROVED PEDS - Edema: 0.2-0.4 mg/kg/day qd or divided bid.

FORMS - Generic/Trade: tabs 2.5,5,10 mg.

NOTES - Generally used for CHF, not HTN. When used with furosemide or other loop diuretics, administer metolazone 30 min before loop diuretic. Cross-allergy may occur if allergic to sulfonamides or thiazides.

polythiazide (*Renese*) ▶L ♀C, D if used in pregnancy-induced HTN ▶? $

ADULT - HTN: Start 2 mg PO qd, usual maintenance dose 2-4 mg qd. Edema: 1-4 mg PO qd.

PEDS - Not approved in children.

FORMS - Trade: Tabs, scored, 1,2,4 mg.

NOTES - May dose qod or 3-5 days/week as maintenance therapy to control edema.

CARDIOVASCULAR: Nitrates

NOTE: Avoid if systolic BP <90 mmHg or ≥30 mmHg below baseline, severe bradycardia (<50 bpm), tachycardia (>100 bpm) or right ventricular infarction. Avoid in those who have received erectile dysfunction therapy in the last 24 (sildenafil, vardenafil) to 48 (tadalafil) hours.

amyl nitrite ▶Lung ♀X ▶- $

ADULT - Angina: 0.3 ml inhaled as needed.

PEDS - Not approved in children.

NOTES - May cause headache and flushing. Flammable. Avoid use in areas with open flames. To avoid syncope, use only when lying down.

isosorbide dinitrate (*Isordil, Dilatrate-SR*, ♣*Cedocard SR*) ▶L ♀C ▶? $

ADULT - Acute angina: 2.5-10 mg SL or chewed immediately, repeat as needed every 5-10 minutes up to 3 doses in 30 min. SL and chew Tabs may be used prior to events likely to provoke angina. Angina prophylaxis: Start 5-20 mg PO tid (7 am, noon, & 5 pm), max 40 mg tid. Sustained-release (Dilatrate SR): Start 40 mg PO bid, max 80 mg PO bid (8 am & 2 pm).

PEDS - Not approved in children.

UNAPPROVED ADULT - CHF: 10-40 mg PO tid (7 am, noon, & 5 pm), max 80 mg tid. Use in combination with hydralazine.

FORMS - Generic/Trade: Tabs, scored 5,10,20, 30,40, chewable, scored 5,10, sublingual tabs, non-scored 2.5,5,10 mg. Trade only: cap, sustained-release (Dilatrate-SR) 40 mg. Generic only: tab, sustained-release 40 mg.

NOTES - Headache possible. Use SL or chew Tabs for an acute angina attack. Extended-release tab may be broken, but do not chew or crush, swallow whole. Allow for a nitrate-free period of 10-14 h each day to avoid nitrate tolerance.

isosorbide mononitrate (*ISMO, Monoket, Imdur*) ▶L ♀C ▶? $$

ADULT - Angina: 20 mg PO bid (8 am and 3 pm). Extended-release (Imdur): Start 30-60 mg PO qd, max 240 mg/day.

PEDS - Not approved in children.

FORMS - Generic/Trade: Tabs, non-scored (ISMO, bid dosing) 20, scored (Monoket, bid dosing) 10,20, extended-release, scored (Imdur, qd dosing) 30,60, non-scored 120 mg.

NOTES - Headache. Extended-release tab may be broken, but do not chew or crush, swallow whole. Do not use for acute angina.

nitroglycerin intravenous infusion (*Tridil*) ▶L ♀C ▶? $

ADULT - Perioperative HTN, acute MI/CHF, acute angina: mix 50 mg in 250 mL D5W (200 mcg/mL), start at 10-20 mcg/min IV (3-6 mL/h), then titrate upward by 10-20 mcg/min every 3-5 min until desired effect is achieved.

PEDS - Not approved in children.

UNAPPROVED ADULT - Hypertensive emergency: Start 10-20 mcg/min IV infusion, titrate

up to 100 mcg/min. Antihypertensive effect is usually evident in 2-5 min. Effect may persist for only 3-5 min after infusion is stopped.

UNAPPROVED PEDS - IV infusion: start 0.25-0.5 mcg/kg/min, increase by 0.5-1 mcg/kg/min q3-5 min as needed, max 5 mcg/kg/min.

FORMS - Brand name "Tridil" no longer made, but retained herein for name recognition.

NOTES - Nitroglycerin migrates into polyvinyl chloride (PVC) tubing. Use lower initial doses (5 mcg/min) with non-PVC tubing. Use with caution in inferior/right ventricular myocardial infarction. Nitroglycerin-induced venodilation can cause severe hypotension.

nitroglycerin ointment (*Nitrol, Nitro-BID*) ▶L ♀C ▶? $

ADULT - Angina prophylaxis: Start 0.5 inch q8h applied to non-hairy skin area, maintenance 1-2 inches q8h, maximum 4 inches q4-6h.

PEDS - Not approved in children.

FORMS - Trade: Ointment, 2%, tubes 1,30,60g (Nitro-BID).

NOTES - 1 inch ointment is approximately 15 mg nitroglycerin. Allow for a nitrate-free period of 10-14 h each day to avoid nitrate tolerance. Generally change to oral tabs or transdermal patch for long-term therapy. Do not use topical therapy (ointment, transdermal system) for acute angina.

nitroglycerin spray (*Nitrolingual*) ▶L ♀C ▶? $$

ADULT - Acute angina: 1-2 sprays under the tongue at the onset of attack, repeat as needed, max 3 sprays in 15 min.

PEDS - Not approved in children.

FORMS - Trade: Solution, 0.4 mg/spray (200 sprays/canister).

NOTES - May be preferred over SL Tabs in patients with dry mouth. Patient can see how much medicine is left in bottle.

nitroglycerin sublingual (*Nitrostat, Nitro-Quick*) ▶L ♀C ▶? $

ADULT - Acute angina: 0.4 mg under tongue or between the cheek and gum, repeat dose every 5 min as needed up to 3 doses in 15 min. A dose may be given 5-10 min before activities that might provoke angina.

PEDS - Not approved in children.

FORMS - Generic/Trade: Sublingual tabs, non-scored 0.3,0.4,0.6 mg; in bottles of 100 or package of 4 bottles with 25 tabs each.

NOTES - Headache. May produce a burning/tingling sensation when administered, although this should not be used to assess potency. Store in original glass bottle to maintain potency/stability. Traditionally, unused Tabs should be discarded 6 months after the original bottle is opened; however the Nitrostat product is stable for 24 months after the bottle is opened or until the expiration date on the bottle, whichever is earlier. If used rarely, prescribe package with 4 bottles with 25 Tabs each.

nitroglycerin sustained release ▶L ♀C ▶? $
ADULT - Angina prophylaxis: Start 2.5 or 2.6 mg PO bid-tid, then titrate upward as needed.
PEDS - Not approved in children.
FORMS - Generic only: cap, extended-release 2.5, 6.5, 9 mg.
NOTES - Headache. Extended-release tab may be broken, but do not chew or crush, swallow whole. cap should be swallowed whole. Do not use extended-release Tabs or Caps for acute angina attack. Allow for a nitrate-free period of 10-14 h each day to avoid nitrate tolerance.

nitroglycerin transdermal (*Minitran, Nitro-Dur,* ✲*Trinipatch*) ▶L ♀C ▶? $$$
ADULT - Angina prophylaxis: Start with lowest dose and apply 1 patch for 12-14 h each day to

non-hairy skin.
PEDS - Not approved in children.
FORMS - Trade: Transdermal system, doses in mg/h: Nitro-Dur 0.1,0.2,0.3,0.4,0.6,0.8; Minitran 0.1,0.2,0.4,0.6. Generic only: Transdermal system, doses in mg/h: 0.1,0.2,0.4,0.6.
NOTES - Do not use topical therapy (ointment, transdermal system) for acute angina attack. Allow for a nitrate-free period of 10-14 h each day to avoid nitrate tolerance. Elderly are at more risk of hypotension and falling; start at lower doses.

nitroglycerin transmucosal (*Nitroguard*) ▶L ♀C ▶? $$$
ADULT - Acute angina and prophylaxis: 1-3 mg PO, between lip and gum or between cheek and gum, q 3-5 h while awake.
PEDS - Not approved in children.
FORMS - Trade: Tabs, controlled-release 2,3 mg.
NOTES - May cause headache and flushing. Allow for a nitrate-free period of 10-14 h each day to avoid nitrate tolerance.

CARDIAC PARAMETERS AND FORMULAS	*Normal*
Cardiac output (CO) = heart rate x stroke volume	4-8 l/min
Cardiac index (CI) = CO/BSA	2.8-4.2 l/min/m2
MAP (mean arterial press) = [(SBP - DBP)/3] + DBP	80-100 mmHg
SVR (systemic vasc resis) = (MAP - CVP)x(80)/CO	800-1200 dyne/sec/cm5
PVR (pulm vasc resis) = (PAM - PCWP)x(80)/CO	45-120 dyne/sec/cm5
QT_C = QT / square root of RR [calculate using both measures in sec]	≤0.44
Right atrial pressure (central venous pressure)	0-8 mmHg
Pulmonary artery systolic pressure (PAS)	20-30 mmHg
Pulmonary artery diastolic pressure (PAD)	10-15 mmHg
Pulmonary capillary wedge pressure (PCWP)	8-12 mmHg (post-MI ~16 mmHg)

CARDIOVASCULAR: Pressors / Inotropes

dobutamine (*Dobutrex*) ▶Plasma ♀D ▶- $
ADULT - Inotropic support in cardiac decompensation (CHF, surgical procedures): 250 mg in 250 ml D5W (1 mg/mL) at 2-20 mcg/kg/min. 70 kg: 5 mcg/kg/min = 21 mL/h.
PEDS - Not approved in children.
UNAPPROVED PEDS - Same as adult. Use lowest effective dose.
NOTES - For short-term use, up to 72 hours.

dopamine (*Intropin*) ▶Plasma ♀C ▶- $
ADULT - Pressor: 400 mg in 250 ml D5W (1600 mcg/ mL), start 5 mcg/kg/min, increase as needed by 5-10 mcg/kg/min increments at 10 min intervals, max 50 mcg/kg/min. 70 kg: 5 mcg/kg/min = 13 mL/h.
PEDS - Not approved in children.

UNAPPROVED ADULT - Symptomatic bradycardia unresponsive to atropine: 5-20 mcg/kg/min IV infusion.
UNAPPROVED PEDS - Pressor: same as adult.
NOTES - Doses in mcg/kg/min: 2-4 = (traditional renal dose; recent evidence suggests ineffective) dopaminergic receptors; 5-10 = (cardiac dose) dopaminergic and beta1 receptors; >10 = dopaminergic, beta1, and alpha1 receptors.

ephedrine ▶K ♀C ▶? $
ADULT - Pressor: 10-25 mg IV slow injection, with repeat doses every 5-10 min as needed, max 150 mg/day. Orthostatic hypotension: 25 mg PO qd-qid. Bronchospasm: 25-50 mg PO q3-4h prn.
PEDS - Not approved in children.

UNAPPROVED PEDS - Pressor: 3 mg/kg/day SC or IV in 4-6 divided doses.

FORMS - Generic: Caps, 25,50 mg.

epinephrine (adrenalin) ▶Plasma ♀C ▶- $

ADULT - Cardiac arrest: 0.5-1 mg (1:10,000 solution) IV, repeat every 3-5 minutes if needed; infusion 1 mg in 250 ml D5W (4 mcg/mL) at 1-4 mcg/min (15-60 mL/h). Anaphylaxis: 0.1-0.5 mg SC/IM (1:1,000 solution), may repeat SC dose every 10-15 minutes for anaphylactic shock.

PEDS - Cardiac arrest: 0.01 mg/kg IV/IO or 0.1 mg/kg ET, repeat 0.1-0.2 mg/kg IV/IO/ET every 3-5 minutes if needed. Neonates: 0.01-0.03 mg/kg IV/ET, repeat every 3-5 minutes if needed; IV infusion start 0.1 mcg/kg/min, increase in increments of 0.1 mcg/kg/min if needed, max 1 mcg/kg/min. Anaphylaxis: 0.01 mg/kg (0.01 ml/kg of 1:1000 injection) SC, may repeat SC dose at 20 minute to 4 hour intervals depending on severity of condition.

UNAPPROVED ADULT - Symptomatic bradycardia unresponsive to atropine: 2-10 mcg/min IV infusion. ET administration prior to IV access: 2-2.5 x the recommended IV dose in 10 ml of NS or distilled water.

NOTES - Use the 1:10,000 injectable solution for IV use in cardiac arrest (10 mL = 1 mg). Use the 1:1000 injectable solution for SC/IM use in anaphylaxis (0.1 mL = 0.1 mg).

inamrinone (*Amrinone*) ▶K ♀C ▶? $$$$$

ADULT - CHF (NYHA class III,IV): 0.75 mg/kg bolus IV over 2-3 min, then infusion 100 mg in 100 mL NS (1 mg/mL) at 5-10 mcg/kg/min. 70 kg: 5 mcg/kg/min = 21 mL/h. An additional IV bolus of 0.75 mg/kg may be given 30 min after initiating therapy if needed. Total daily dose should not exceed 10 mg/kg.

PEDS - Not approved in children.

UNAPPROVED ADULT - CPR: 0.75 mg/kg bolus IV over 2-3 min, followed by 5-15 mcg/kg/min.

UNAPPROVED PEDS - Inotropic support: 0.75 mg/kg IV bolus over 2-3 minutes, followed by 3-5 mcg/kg/min (neonates) or 5-10 mcg/kg/min (children) maintenance infusion.

NOTES - Thrombocytopenia possible. Children may require higher bolus doses, 3-4.5 mg/kg. Name changed from "amrinone" to avoid medication errors.

mephentermine (*Wyamine*) ▶Plasma ♀C ▶- $$$$

ADULT - Hypotension during anesthesia: 0.5 mg/kg/dose, usually 15-30 mg IM, max 80 mg/dose. Spinal anesthesia: 30-45 mg IV, repeat 30 mg dose prn to maintain BP. Spinal anesthesia in cesarean section: 15 mg IV, repeat dose prn to maintain BP.

PEDS - Not approved in children.

UNAPPROVED PEDS - Hypotension during anesthesia: 0.4 mg/kg/dose IM.

metaraminol (*Aramine*) ▶Plasma ♀C ▶- $

ADULT - Acute hypotension during spinal anesthesia: 500-1500 mcg IV bolus followed by 100 mg in 250 ml D5W (400 mcg/mL) IV infusion, start 5 mcg/kg/min (70 kg = 53 mL/h). Prevention of hypotension: 2-10 mg IM/SC.

PEDS - Not approved in children.

UNAPPROVED PEDS - Acute hypotension during spinal anesthesia: 0.1 mg/kg SC/IM, wait at least 10 min before repeat dose. Severe hypotension/shock: 0.01 mg/kg IV and, if needed, continue with IV infusion 0.4 mg/kg diluted and administered at a rate to maintain BP.

midodrine (*ProAmatine*, ♣*Amatine*) ▶LK ♀C ▶? $$$$$

WARNING - May cause significant HTN. Clinical benefits (ie, improved activities of daily living) have not been verified. Use in patients where nonpharmacological treatment fails.

ADULT - Orthostatic hypotension: Start 10 mg PO tid while awake, increase dose as needed to max 40 mg/day. Renal impairment: Start 2.5 mg tid while awake, increase dose as needed.

PEDS - Not approved in children.

FORMS - Generic/Trade: Tabs, scored 2.5,5,10 mg.

NOTES - The last daily dose should be no later than 6 pm to avoid supine HTN during sleep.

milrinone (*Primacor*) ▶K ♀C ▶? $$$$$

ADULT - CHF (NYHA class III,IV): Load 50 mcg/kg IV over 10 min, then begin IV infusion of 0.375-0.75 mcg/kg/min. Renal impairment: reduce IV infusion rate (mcg/kg/min) as follows, CrCl 50-41 mL/min, 0.43; CrCl 40-31 mL/min, 0.38; CrCl 30-21 mL/min, 0.33; CrCl 20-11 mL/min, 0.28; CrCl 10-6 mL/min, 0.23; CrCl ≤5 mL/min, 0.2.

PEDS - Not approved in children.

UNAPPROVED PEDS - Inotropic support: Limited data, 50 mcg/kg IV bolus over 10 minutes, followed by 0.5-1 mcg/kg/min IV infusion, titrate to effect within dosing range.

norepinephrine (*Levophed*) ▶Plasma ♀C ▶? $

ADULT - Acute hypotension: 4 mg in 500 mL D5W (8 mcg/mL), start IV infusion 8-12 mcg/min, ideally through central line, adjust rate to maintain BP, average maintenance dose 2-4 mcg/min. 3 mcg/min = 22.5 mL/h.

PEDS - Not approved in children.

UNAPPROVED PEDS - Acute hypotension: Start 0.05-0.1mcg/kg/min IV infusion, titrate to desired effect, max dose 2 mcg/kg/min.

NOTES - Avoid extravasation, do not administer IV push or IM.

phenylephrine (*Neo-Synephrine*) ▶Plasma ♀C ▶- $

ADULT - Mild to moderate hypotension: 0.1-0.2 mg slow IV injection, do not exceed 0.5 mg in initial dose, repeat dose as needed no less than every 10-15 min; 1-10 mg SC/IM, initial

dose should not exceed 5 mg. Infusion for severe hypotension: 20 mg in 250 ml D5W (80 mcg/mL), start 100-180 mcg/min (75-135 mL/h), usual dose once BP is stabilized 40-60 mcg/min.

PEDS - Not approved in children.

UNAPPROVED PEDS - Mild to moderate hypotension: 5-20 mcg/kg IV bolus every 10-15 minutes as needed; 0.1-0.5 mcg/kg/min IV infusion, titrate to desired effect.

NOTES - Avoid SC or IM administration during shock, use IV route to ensure drug absorption.

THROMBOLYTIC THERAPY FOR ACUTE MI (if high-volume cath lab unavailable)

- *Indications*: Clinical history & presentation strongly suggestive of MI within 12 hours plus ≥1 of the following: 1 mm ST↑ in ≥2 contiguous leads; new left BBB; or 2 mm ST↓ in V1-4 suggestive of true posterior MI.
- *Absolute contraindications*: Previous cerebral hemorrhage, known cerebral aneurysm or arteriovenous malformation, known intracranial neoplasm, recent (<3 months) ischemic stroke (except acute ischemic stroke <3 hours), aortic dissection, active bleeding or bleeding diathesis (excluding menstruation), significant closed head or facial trauma (<3 months).
- *Relative contraindications*: Severe uncontrolled HTN (>180/110 mmHg) on presentation or chronic severe HTN; prior ischemic stroke (>3 months), dementia, other intracranial pathology; traumatic/prolonged (>10 minutes) cardiopulmonary resuscitation; major surgery (<3 weeks); recent (within 2-4 weeks) internal bleeding; puncture of non-compressible vessel; pregnancy; active peptic ulcer disease; current use of anticoagulants. For streptokinase/anistreplase: prior exposure (>5 days ago) or prior allergic reaction. *Circulation* 2004;110:588-636

CARDIOVASCULAR: Thrombolytics

alteplase (tpa, t-PA, *Activase*, *Cathflo*, ♣*Activase rt-PA*) ▶L ♀C ▶? $$$$$

ADULT - Acute MI: (patients >67 kg) 15 mg IV bolus, then 50 mg IV over 30 min, then 35 mg IV over the next 60 min; (patients ≤67 kg) 15 mg IV bolus, then 0.75 mg/kg (not to exceed 50 mg) IV over 30 min, then 0.5 mg/kg (not to exceed 35 mg) IV over the next 60 min. Concurrent heparin infusion. Acute ischemic stroke: 0.9 mg/kg up to 90 mg infused over 60 min, with 10% of dose as initial IV bolus over 1 minute; start within 3 h of symptom onset. Acute pulmonary embolism: 100 mg IV over 2h, then restart heparin when PTT ≤twice normal. Occluded central venous access device: 2 mg/ml in catheter for 2 hr. May use second dose if needed.

PEDS - Occluded central venous access device: ≥10 kg and <30 kg: Dose equal to 110% of the internal lumen volume, not to exceed 2 mg/2 ml. Other uses not approved in children.

NOTES - Must be reconstituted. Solution must be used within 8h after reconstitution.

reteplase (*Retavase*) ▶L ♀C ▶? $$$$$

ADULT - Acute MI: 10 units IV over 2 minutes; repeat dose in 30 min.

PEDS - Not approved in children.

NOTES - Must be reconstituted with sterile water for injection to 1 mg/ml concentration. Soln must be used within 4 h after reconstitution.

streptokinase (*Streptase*, *Kabikinase*) ▶L ♀C ▶? $$$$$

ADULT - Acute MI: 1.5 million units IV over 60 min. Pulmonary embolism: 250,000 units IV loading dose over 30 min, followed by 100,000 units/h IV infusion for 24 h (maintain infusion for 72 h if concurrent DVT suspected). DVT: 250,000 units IV loading dose over 30 min, followed by 100,000 units/h IV infusion for 24 hours. Occluded arteriovenous catheter: 250,000 units instilled into the catheter, remove solution containing 250,000 units of drug from catheter after 2 h using a 5-mL syringe.

PEDS - Not approved in children.

NOTES - Must be reconstituted. Solution must be used within 8 h of reconstitution. Do not shake vial. Do not repeat use in less than one year. Do not use with history of severe allergic reaction to anistreplase/streptokinase.

tenecteplase (*TNKase*) ▶L ♀C ▶? $$$$$
ADULT - Acute MI: Single IV bolus dose over 5 seconds based on body weight; <60 kg, 30 mg; 60-69 kg, 35 mg; 70-79 kg, 40 mg; 80-89 kg, 45 mg; ≥90kg, 50 mg.
PEDS - Not approved in children.
NOTES - Must be reconstituted. Solution must be used within 8h after reconstitution.

urokinase (*Abbokinase, Abbokinase Open -Cath*) ▶L ♀B ▶? $$$$$
ADULT - Pulmonary embolism: 4400 units/kg IV loading dose over 10 min, followed by IV infusion 4400 units/kg/h for 12 hours. Occluded IV catheter: 5000 units instilled into the catheter with a tuberculin syringe, remove solution containing 5000 units of drug from catheter after 5

min using a 5-mL syringe. Aspiration attempts may be repeated q5min. If unsuccessful, cap catheter and allow 5000 unit solution to remain in catheter for 30-60 min before again attempting to aspirate solution and residual clot.
PEDS - Not approved in children.
UNAPPROVED ADULT - Acute MI: 2-3 million units IV infusion over 45-90 min. Give one-half the total dose as a rapid initial IV injection over 5 min.
UNAPPROVED PEDS - Arterial or venous thrombosis: 4400 units/kg IV loading dose over 10 minutes, followed by 4400 units/kg/hr for 12-72 hours. Occluded IV catheter: same as adult.
NOTES - Must be reconstituted. Do not shake vial.

CARDIOVASCULAR: Volume Expanders

albumin (*Albuminar, Buminate, Albumarc, ♣Plasbumin*) ▶L ♀C ▶? $$$$
ADULT - Shock, burns: 500 mL of 5% solution (50 mg/mL) infused as rapidly as tolerated. Repeat infusion in 30 min if response is inadequate. 25% solution may be used with or without dilution if necessary. Undiluted 25% solution should be infused at 1 ml/min to avoid too rapid plasma volume expansion.
PEDS - Shock, burns: 10-20 mL/kg IV infusion at 5-10 mL/min using 50 mL of 5% solution.
UNAPPROVED PEDS - Shock/hypovolemia: 1 g/kg/dose IV rapid infusion. Hypoproteinemia: 1 g/kg/dose IV infusion over 30-120 min.
NOTES - Fever, chills. Monitor for plasma volume overload (dyspnea, fluid in lungs, abnormal increase in BP or CVP). Less likely to cause hypotension than plasma protein fraction, more purified. In treating burns, large volumes of crystalloid solutions (0.9% sodium chloride) are used to maintain plasma volume with albumin. Use 5% solution in pediatric hypovolemic patients. Use 25% solution in pediatric patients with volume restrictions.

dextran (*Rheomacrodex, Gentran, Macrodex*) ▶K ♀C ▶? $$$$
ADULT - Shock/hypovolemia: Dextran 40, Dextran 70 and 75, up to 20 mL/kg during the first 24 hours, up to 10 mL/kg/day thereafter, do not continue for longer than 5 days. The first 500 mL may be infused rapidly with CVP monitoring. DVT/PE prophylaxis during surgery: Dextran 40, 50-100 g IV infusion the day of surgery, continue for 2-3 days post-op with 50 g/day. 50 g/day may be given every 2nd or 3rd

day thereafter up to 14 days.
PEDS - Total dose should not exceed 20 mL/kg.
UNAPPROVED ADULT - DVT/PE prophylaxis during surgery: Dextran 70 and 75 solutions have been used. Other uses: to improve circulation with sickle cell crisis, prevention of nephrotoxicity with radiographic contrast media, toxemia of late pregnancy.
NOTES - Monitor for plasma volume overload (dyspnea, fluid in lungs, abnormal increase in BP or CVP) and anaphylactoid reactions. May impair platelet function. Less effective that other agents for DVT/PE prevention.

hetastarch (*Hespan, Hextend*) ▶K ♀C ▶? $$$
ADULT - Shock/hypovolemia: 500-1000 mL IV infusion, total daily dose usually should not exceed 20 mL/kg (1500 mL). Renal impairment: CrCl <10 mL/min, usual initial dose followed by 20-25% of usual dose.
PEDS - Not approved in children.
UNAPPROVED PEDS - Shock/hypovolemia: 10 ml/kg/dose; do not exceed 20 mL/kg/day.
NOTES - Monitor for plasma volume overload (dyspnea, fluid in lungs, abnormal increase in BP or CVP). Little or no antigenic properties compared to dextran.

plasma protein fraction (*Plasmanate, Protenate, Plasmatein*) ▶L ♀C ▶? $$$$
ADULT - Shock/hypovolemia: Adjust initial rate according to clinical response and BP, but rate should not exceed 10 mL/min. As plasma volume normalizes, infusion rate should not exceed 5-8 mL/min. Usual dose 250-500 mL. Hypoproteinemia: 1000-1500 mL/day IV infusion.

PEDS - Shock/hypovolemia: Initial dose 6.6-33 mL/kg infused at a rate of 5-10 mL/min.
NOTES - Fever, chills, hypotension with rapid

infusion. Monitor for plasma volume overload (dyspnea, fluid in lungs, abnormal increase in BP or CVP). Less pure than albumin products.

CARDIOVASCULAR: Other

alprostadil (*Prostin VR Pediatric,* prostaglandin E1) ▶Lung ♀- ▶- $$$$$
PEDS - Temporary maintenance of patent ductus arteriosus in neonates: Start 0.1 mcg/kg/min IV infusion. Reduce dose to minimal amount that maintains therapeutic response. Max dose 0.4 mcg/kg/min.

cilostazol (*Pletal*) ▶L ♀C ▶? $$$$
WARNING - Contraindicated in CHF of any severity.
ADULT - Intermittent claudication: 100 mg PO bid on empty stomach. 50 mg PO bid with cytochrome P450 3A4 inhibitors (like ketoconazole, itraconazole, erythromycin, diltiazem) or cytochrome P450 2C19 inhibitors (like omeprazole). Beneficial effect may take up to 12 weeks.
PEDS - Not approved in children.
FORMS - Trade: Tabs 50, 100 mg.
NOTES - Avoid grapefruit juice.

indomethacin (*Indocin IV,* ✚*Indocid*) ▶KL ♀- ▶- $$
ADULT - See analgesics section
PEDS - Closure of patent ductus arteriosus in neonates: Initial dose 0.2 mg/kg IV, if additional doses necessary, dose and frequency (q12h or q24h) based on age and urine output.
NOTES - Administer prepared IV solution over 5-10 seconds.

isoxsuprine (*Vasodilan*) ▶KL ♀C ▶? $
ADULT - Adjunctive therapy for cerebral vascular insufficiency and PVD: 10-20 mg PO tid-qid.
PEDS - Not approved in children.
FORMS - Generic/Trade: Tabs, 10,20 mg.
NOTES - Drug has questionable therapeutic effect.

nesiritide (*Natrecor*) ▶K, plasma ♀C ▶? $$$$$
ADULT - Decompensated CHF: 2 mcg/kg IV bolus over 60 seconds, then 0.01 mcg/kg/min IV infusion for up to 48 hours. Do not initiate at

higher doses. Limited experience with increased doses: 0.005 mcg/kg/min increments, preceded by 1 mcg/kg bolus, no more frequently than q3h up to max infusion dose 0.03 mcg/kg/min. 1.5 mg vial in 250mL D5W (6 mcg/mL). 70 kg: 2 mcg/kg bolus = 23.3 ml, 0.01 mcg/kg/min infusion = 7 mL/h.
PEDS - Not approved in children.
NOTES - Contraindicated as primary therapy for cardiogenic shock and when SBP <90 mmHg. Discontinue if dose-related symptomatic hypotension occurs and support BP prn. May restart infusion with dose reduced by 30% (no bolus dose) once BP stabilized. Do not shake reconstituted vial, and dilute vial prior to administration. Incompatible with heparin and most other injectable drugs; administer agents using separate IV lines. Do not measure BNP levels while infusing; may measure BNP at least 2-6 hrs after infusion completion.

papaverine ▶LK ♀C ▶? $
ADULT - Cerebral and peripheral ischemia: Start 150 mg PO bid, increase to max 300 mg bid if needed. Start 30 mg IV/IM, dose range 30-120 mg q3h prn. Give IV doses over 1-2 min.
PEDS - Not approved in children.
FORMS - Generic: cap, extended-release, 150 mg.

pentoxifylline (*Trental*) ▶L ♀C ▶? $$$
ADULT - Intermittent claudication: 400 mg PO tid with meals. For CNS/GI adverse effects, decrease dose to 400 mg PO bid. Beneficial effect may take up to 8 weeks. May be less effective in relieving cramps, tiredness, tightness, and pain during exercise.
PEDS - Not approved in children.
FORMS - Generic/Trade: Tabs 400 mg.
NOTES - Contraindicated with recent cerebral/retinal bleed. Increases theophylline levels. Increases INR with warfarin.

CONTRAST MEDIA: MRI Contrast

gadodiamide (*Omniscan*) ▶K ♀C ▶? $$$$
ADULT - Non-iodinated, non-ionic IV contrast for MRI.
PEDS - Non-iodinated, non-ionic IV contrast for

MRI.
NOTES - Use caution if renal disease. May falsely lower serum calcium.

gadopentetate (*Magnevist*) ▶K ♀C ▶? $$$

ADULT - Non-iodinated IV contrast for MRI.
PEDS - >2 yo: Non-iodinated IV MRI contrast.

NOTES - Caution in sickle cell, renal disease.

CONTRAST MEDIA: Radiography Contrast

NOTE: Beware of allergic or anaphylactoid reactions. Avoid IV contrast in renal insufficiency or dehydration. Hold metformin (Glucophage) prior to or at the time of iodinated contrast dye use and for 48 h after procedure. Restart after procedure only if renal function is normal.

barium sulfate ▶Not absorbed ♀? ▶+ $
ADULT, PEDS - Non-iodinated GI (eg, oral, rectal) contrast.
NOTES - Contraindicated if suspected gastric or intestinal perforation. Use with caution in GI obstruction. May cause abdominal distention, cramping, and constipation with oral use.

diatrizoate (*Hypaque, Renografin, Gastrografin, MD-Gastroview, Cystografin***)** ▶K ♀C ▶? $
WARNING - Not for intrathecal or epidural use.
ADULT, PEDS - Iodinated, ionic, high osmolality IV or GI contrast.
NOTES - High osmolality contrast may cause tissue damage if infiltrated/extravasated. IV: Hypaque, Renografin. GI: Gastrografin, MD-Gastroview.

iodixanol (*Visipaque***)** ▶K ♀B ▶? $$$
ADULT, PEDS - Iodinated, non-ionic, low osmolality IV contrast.
NOTES - Not for intrathecal use.

iohexol (*Omnipaque***)** ▶K ♀B ▶? $$$
ADULT, PEDS - Iodinated, non-ionic, low osmolality IV and oral/body cavity contrast.

iopamidol (*Isovue***)** ▶K ♀? ▶? $$
ADULT, PEDS - Iodinated, non-ionic, low osmolality IV contrast.

iothalamate (*Conray***)** ▶K ♀B ▶- $
ADULT, PEDS - Iodinated, ionic, high osmolality IV contrast.
NOTES - High osmolality contrast may cause tissue damage if infiltrated/extravasated.

ioversol (*Optiray***)** ▶K ♀B ▶? $$
ADULT, PEDS - Iodinated, non-ionic, low osmolality IV contrast.

ioxaglate (*Hexabrix***)** ▶K ♀B ▶- $$$
ADULT, PEDS - Iodinated, ionic, low osmolality IV contrast.

CONTRAST MEDIA: Ultrasound Contrast

perflexane (*Imagent***)** ▶Respiratory ♀C ▶? ?
ADULT - Echocardiography contrast: 0.125 mg/kg (0.00625 ml/kg) IV over ≥10 seconds followed by saline flush. Effect 0.7 to 2.6 minutes following injection.

PEDS - Not approved in children.
NOTES - Avoid in those with possible cardiac shunts; caution with severe COPD, pulmonary vasculitis, history of PE. Use ≤30 minutes after reconstitution.

CONTRAST MEDIA: Other

acetylcysteine (*Mucomyst***, ♣ ***Parvolex***)** ▶L ♀B ▶? $
ADULT, PEDS - Acetaminophen toxicity: See toxicology section.
UNAPPROVED ADULT - Contrast nephropathy

prophylaxis: 600 mg PO bid on the day before and on the day of contrast.
FORMS - Generic/Trade: solution 10%, 20%.
NOTES - May be diluted with water or soft drink to a 5% solution; use diluted soln within 1 hour.

DERMATOLOGY: Acne Preparations

NOTE: For topical agents, wash area prior to application. Wash hands before & after application; avoid eye area.

adapalene (*Differin***)** ▶Bile ♀C ▶? $$
ADULT - Acne: apply qhs.
PEDS - Not approved in children.
UNAPPROVED PEDS - Acne: apply qhs.

FORMS - Trade only: gel 0.1% (15,45 g) cream 0.1% (15,45 g), soln 0.1% (30 mL).
NOTES - During early weeks of therapy, acne exacerbation may occur. May cause erythema, scaling, dryness, pruritus, and burning in up to 40% of patients. Therapeutic results take 8-12 weeks.

azelaic acid (*Azelex, Finacea, Finevin*) ▶K ♀B ▶? $$$

ADULT - Acne (Azelex, Finevin): apply bid. Rosacea (Finacea): apply bid.

PEDS - Not approved in children.

UNAPPROVED ADULT - Melasma: apply bid.

UNAPPROVED PEDS - Acne: apply qhs.

FORMS - Trade only: cream 20%, 30g, 50g (Azelex, Finevin), gel 15% 30g (Finacea).

NOTES - Improvement occurs within 4 weeks. Monitor for hypopigmentation esp in patients with dark complexions. Avoid use of occlusive dressings.

BenzaClin (clindamycin + benzoyl peroxide) ▶K ♀C ▶+ $$$

ADULT - Acne: apply bid.

PEDS - Not approved in children.

UNAPPROVED PEDS - Acne: apply qhs.

FORMS - Trade only: gel clindamycin 1% + benzoyl peroxide 5%; 19.7 g.

NOTES - Expires 10 weeks after mixing.

Benzamycin (erythromycin + benzoyl peroxide) ▶LK ♀C ▶? $$$

ADULT - Acne: apply bid.

PEDS - Not approved in children.

UNAPPROVED PEDS - Acne: apply qhs.

FORMS - Trade only: gel erythromycin 3% + benzoyl peroxide 5%; 23.3, 46.6 g.

NOTES - Must be refrigerated, expires 3 months after pharmacy dispensing.

benzoyl peroxide (*Benzac, Desquam, Clearasil, ✦Acetoxyl, Solugel, Benoxyl, Oxyderm*) ▶LK ♀C ▶? $

ADULT - Acne: Cleansers: wash qd-bid. Creams/gels/lotion: apply qd initially, gradually increase to bid-tid if needed.

PEDS - Not approved in children.

UNAPPROVED PEDS - Acne: Cleansers: wash qd-bid. Creams/gels/lotion: apply qd initially, gradually increase to bid-tid if needed.

FORMS - OTC and Rx generic: liquid 2.5,5, 10%, bar 5,10%, mask 5%, lotion 5,5.5,10%, cream 5,10%, cleanser 10%, gel 2.5,4,5, 6,10, 20%.

NOTES - If excessive drying or peeling occurs, reduce frequency of application. Use with PABA-containing sunscreens may cause transient skin discoloration. May bleach fabric.

Clenia (sodium sulfacetamide + sulfur) ▶K ♀C ▶? $$

ADULT - Acne, rosacea, seborrheic dermatitis: apply cream/gel qd-tid, foaming wash qd-bid.

PEDS - Not approved in children.

FORMS - Generic: lotion (sodium sulfacetamide 10% & sulfur 5%) 25 g. Trade only (sodium sulfacetamide 10% & sulfur 5%): cream 28 g, foaming wash 170,340 g.

NOTES - Avoid with sulfa allergy, renal failure.

clindamycin (*Cleocin T, ✦Dalacin T*) ▶L ♀B ▶- $

ADULT - Acne: apply bid.

PEDS - Not approved in children.

UNAPPROVED ADULT - Rosacea: apply lotion bid.

UNAPPROVED PEDS - Acne: apply bid.

FORMS - Generic/Trade: gel 10 mg/ml 7.5, 30g, lotion 10 mg/ml 60 ml, soln 10 mg/ml 30,60 ml.

NOTES - Concomitant use with erythromycin may decrease effectiveness. Most common adverse effects dryness, erythema, burning, peeling, oiliness and itching. Pseudomembranous colitis has been reported with topical use.

Diane-35 (cyproterone + ethinyl estradiol) ▶L ♀X ▶- $$

WARNING - Not recommended in women who smoke. Increased risk of thromboembolism, stroke, MI, hepatic neoplasia & gallbladder disease. Nausea, breast tenderness, & breakthrough bleeding are common, transient side effects. Nighttime dosing may minimize nausea. Effectiveness is reduced by hepatic enzyme-inducing drugs such as certain anticonvulsants and barbiturates, rifampin, rifabutin, griseofulvin & protease inhibitors. Antibiotics or products that contain St. John's wort may reduce efficacy.

ADULT - Canada only. In women, severe acne unresponsive to oral antibiotics and other treatments, with associated symptoms of androgenization, including seborrhea and mild hirsutism: 1 tab PO qd for 21 consecutive days, stop for 7 days, repeat cycle.

PEDS - Not approved in children.

FORMS - Rx: Trade: blister pack of 21 tabs 2 mg/0.035 mg cyproterone acetate/ethinyl estradiol.

NOTES - Higher thromboembolic risk than other oral contraceptives, therefore only indicated for acne, and not solely for contraception (although effective for the latter). Same warnings, precautions, and contraindications as other oral contraceptives.

doxycycline (*Vibramycin, Doryx, ✦Doxycin*) ▶LK ♀D ▶+ $$

ADULT - Acne vulgaris: 100 mg PO bid.

PEDS - Avoid in children <8 yo due to teeth staining.

UNAPPROVED PEDS - Acne vulgaris: children >8 y: 2.2 mg/kg PO given as a single daily dose or divided bid; maximum 100 mg PO bid.

FORMS - Generic/Trade: Tabs 75, 100 mg, caps 50,100 mg. Trade only: susp 25 mg/5 ml, syrup 50 mg/5 ml (contains sulfites).

NOTES - Photosensitivity, pseudotumor cerebri, increased BUN. Decreased efficacy of oral contraceptives. Increased INR with warfarin. Do not give antacids or calcium supplements within 2 h of doxycycline. Barbiturates, carbamazepine, and phenytoin may decrease doxycycline levels.

Duac (clindamycin + benzoyl peroxide) ▶K ♀C ▶+ $$$

ADULT - Acne: apply qhs.

PEDS - Not approved in children.

UNAPPROVED PEDS - Acne: apply qhs.

FORMS - Trade only: gel clindamycin 1% + benzoyl peroxide 5%; 45 g.

NOTES - Expires 2 months after pharmacy dispensing.

erythromycin (Eryderm, Erycette, Erygel, A/T/S, ✦Sans-Acne, Erysol) ▶L ♀B ▶? $$

ADULT - Acne: apply bid.

PEDS - Not approved in children.

UNAPPROVED PEDS - Acne: apply bid.

FORMS - Generic: solution 1.5% 60 ml, 2% 60,120 ml, pads 2%, gel 2% 30,60 g, ointment 2% 25 g.

NOTES - May be more irritating when used with other acne products. Concomitant use with clindamycin may decrease effectiveness.

isotretinoin (Accutane, ✦Isotrex) ▶LK ♀X ▶- $$$$$

WARNING - Contraindicated in pregnant women or in women who may become pregnant. If used in a woman of childbearing age, patient must have severe, disfiguring acne, be reliable, comply with mandatory contraceptive measures, receive written and oral instructions about hazards of taking during pregnancy, have 2 negative pregnancy tests prior to beginning therapy. Must use 2 forms of effective contraception, unless absolute abstinence is chosen or patient has undergone a hysterectomy, from 1 month prior until 1 month after discontinuation of therapy. Men should not father children. May cause depression, suicidal thought, and aggressive or violent behavior; monitor for symptoms. Obtain written informed consent. Write prescription for no more than a 1 month supply. Informed consent documents available from the manufacturer.

ADULT - Severe, recalcitrant cystic acne: 0.5-2 mg/kg/day PO divided bid for 15-20 weeks. Typical target dose is 1 mg/kg/day. May repeat second course of therapy after >2 months off therapy.

PEDS - Not approved in children.

UNAPPROVED ADULT - Prevention of second primary tumors in patients treated for squamous-cell carcinoma of the head and neck: 50-100 mg/m²/day PO. Also been used in keratinization disorders.

UNAPPROVED PEDS - Severe, recalcitrant cystic acne: 0.5-2 mg/kg/day PO divided bid for 15-20 weeks. Typical target dose is 1 mg/kg/day. Maintenance therapy for neuroblastoma: 100-250 mg/m²/day PO in 2 divided doses.

FORMS - Trade/generic: caps 10,20,40 mg.

NOTES - Can only be prescribed by healthcare professionals who have undergone specific training. Prescription must have a "qualification sticker" attached. Prescription can be for a maximum of a 1 month supply. May cause headache, cheilitis, drying of mucous membranes including eyes, nose, mouth, hair loss, abdominal pain, pyuria, joint and muscle pain/stiffness, conjunctivitis, elevated ESR, and changes in serum lipids and LFTs. Effect on bone loss unknown; use caution in patients predisposed to osteoporosis. In children in whom skeletal growth is not complete, do not exceed the recommended dose for the recommended duration of treatment. Pseudotumor cerebri has occurred during therapy. May cause corneal opacities, decreased night vision, and inflammatory bowel disease. Avoid concomitant vitamin A, tetracycline and minocycline. May decrease carbamazepine concentrations. Avoid exposure to sunlight.

Rosula (sodium sulfacetamide + sulfur) ▶K ♀C ▶? $$

ADULT - Acne, rosacea, seborrheic dermatitis: apply cream / gel / aqueous cleanser qd-tid, foaming wash qd-bid.

PEDS - Not approved in children.

FORMS - Generic: lotion (sodium sulfacetamide 10% & sulfur 5%) 25 g. Trade only: gel (sodium sulfacetamide 10% & sulfur 5%) 45 ml, aqueous cleanser (sodium sulfacetamide 10% & sulfur 5%) 355 ml.

NOTES - Avoid with sulfa allergy, renal failure.

sodium sulfacetamide (Klaron) ▶K ♀C ▶? $$

ADULT - Acne: apply bid.

PEDS - Not approved in children.

FORMS - Trade only: lotion 10% 59 ml.

NOTES - Cross-sensitivity with sulfa or sulfite allergy.

Sulfacet-R (sodium sulfacetamide + sulfur) ▶K ♀C ▶? $$

ADULT - Acne, rosacea, seborrheic dermatitis: apply cream/gel qd-tid, foaming wash qd-bid.
PEDS - Not approved in children.
FORMS - Trade (Sulfacet-R) and generic: lotion (sodium sulfacetamide 10% & sulfur 5%) 25 g.
NOTES - Avoid with sulfa allergy, renal failure.

tazarotene (*Tazorac, Avage*) ▶L ♀X ▶? $$$
ADULT - Acne (Tazorac): apply 0.1% cream qhs. Palliation of fine facial wrinkles, mottled hyper- and hypopigmentation, benign facial lentigines (Avage): apply qhs. Psoriasis: see Antipsoriatic section.
PEDS - Not approved in children.
UNAPPROVED PEDS - Acne: apply 0.1% cream qhs.
FORMS - Trade only (Tazorac): cream 0.05% 30,100g, 0.1% 30, 100g. Trade only (Avage): cream 0.1% 15,30g.
NOTES - Desquamation, burning, dry skin, erythema, pruritus may occur in up to 30% of patients. May cause photosensitivity.

tretinoin (*Retin-A, Retin-A Micro, Renova, Retisol-A, ♣Stieva-A*) ▶LK ♀C ▶? $$
ADULT - Acne (Retin A, Retin-A Micro): apply qhs. Wrinkles, hyperpigmentation, tactile roughness (Renova): apply qhs.
PEDS - Not approved in children.
UNAPPROVED ADULT - Used in skin cancer and lamellar ichthyosis, mollusca contagiosa, verrucae plantaris, verrucae planae juvenilis, hyperpigmented lesions in black individuals, ichthyosis vulgaris, and pityriasis rubra pilaris.
FORMS - Generic/Trade: cream 0.025% 20,45 g, 0.05% 20,45 g, 0.1% 20,45 g, gel 0.025% 15,45 g, 0.1% 15,45 g, liquid 0.05% 28 ml. Trade only: Renova cream 0.02%, 0.05% 40, 60 g, Retin-A Micro gel 0.04%, 0.1% 20,45 g.
NOTES - May induce erythema, peeling. Minimize sun exposure. Concomitant use with sulfur, resorcinol, benzoyl peroxide, or salicylic acid may result in skin irritation. Gel preps are flammable.

DERMATOLOGY: Actinic Keratosis Preparations

diclofenac (*Solaraze*) ▶L ♀B ▶? $$$$
ADULT - Actinic/solar keratoses: apply bid to lesions x 60-90 days.
PEDS - Not approved in children.
FORMS - Trade only: gel 3% 25, 50 g.
NOTES - Avoid exposure to sun and sunlamps. Use caution in aspirin-sensitive patients.

fluorouracil (*5-FU, Carac, Efudex, Fluoroplex*) ▶L ♀X ▶- $$$$$
ADULT - Actinic or solar keratoses: apply bid to lesions x 2-6 wks. Superficial basal cell carcinomas: apply 5% cream/solution bid.

PEDS - Not approved in children.
UNAPPROVED ADULT - Condylomata acuminata: a 1% solution in 70% ethanol and the 5% cream has been used.
FORMS - Trade only: cream 0.5% 30 g (Carac), 5% 25 g (Efudex), 1% 30 g (Fluoroplex), solution 1% 30 ml (Fluoroplex), 2% 10 ml (Efudex), 5% 10 ml (Efudex).
NOTES - May cause severe irritation & photosensitivity. Contraindicated in women who are or who may become pregnant during therapy. Avoid application to mucous membranes.

DERMATOLOGY: Antibacterials

bacitracin (♣*Baciguent*) ▶Not absorbed ♀C ▶? $
ADULT - Minor cuts, wounds, burns or skin abrasions: apply qd-tid.
PEDS - Not approved in children.
UNAPPROVED PEDS - Minor cuts, wounds, burns or skin abrasions: apply qd-tid.
FORMS - OTC Generic/Trade: ointment 500 units/g 1,15,30g.
NOTES - May cause contact dermatitis or anaphylaxis.

fusidic acid (*Fucidin*) ▶L ♀? ▶? $
ADULT - Canada only. Skin infections: Apply tid-qid.
PEDS - Canada only. Skin infections: Apply tid-

qid.
FORMS - Trade: cream 2% fusidic acid 15,30 g, ointment 2% sodium fusidate 15,30 g.
NOTES - Contains lanolin; possible hypersensitivity.

gentamicin (*Garamycin*) ▶K ♀D ▶? $
ADULT - Skin infections: apply tid-qid.
PEDS - Skin infections >1 yo: apply tid-qid.
FORMS - Generic/Trade: ointment 0.1% 15,30 g, cream 0.1% 15,30 g.

mafenide (*Sulfamylon*) ▶LK ♀C ▶? $$$
ADULT - Adjunctive treatment of burns: apply qd-bid.
PEDS - Adjunctive treatment of burns: apply qd-bid.

FORMS - Trade only: cream 37, 114, 411 g, 5% topical solution 50 g packets.

NOTES - Can cause metabolic acidosis. Contains sulfonamides.

metronidazole (*Noritate, MetroCream, MetroGel, MetroLotion, ♥Rosasol*) ▶KL ♀B(- in 1st trimester) ▶- $$$

ADULT - Rosacea: apply bid.

PEDS - Not approved in children.

UNAPPROVED ADULT - A 1% solution prepared from the oral Tabs has been used in the treatment of infected decubitus ulcers.

FORMS - Trade only: gel (MetroGel) 0.75% 29 g, cream (Noritate) 1% 30, 60 g, lotion (MetroLotion) 0.75% 59 ml. Trade/Generic: cream 0.75% 45 g.

NOTES - Results usually noted within 3 weeks, with continuing improvement through 9 weeks. Avoid using vaginal prep on face due to irritation because of formulation differences.

mupirocin (*Bactroban*) ▶Not absorbed ♀B ▶? $$

ADULT - Impetigo: apply tid x 3-5 days. Infected wounds: apply tid x 10 days. Nasal MRSA eradication: 0.5 g in each nostril bid x 5 days.

PEDS - Impetigo (mupirocin cream/ointment): apply tid. Infected wounds: apply tid x 10 days. Nasal form not approved in children <12 yo.

FORMS - Trade/Generic: cream/ointment 2% 15, 22, 30 g. Trade only: 2% nasal ointment 1 g single-use tubes (for MRSA eradication).

Neosporin cream (neomycin + polymyxin) ▶K ♀C ▶? $

ADULT - Minor cuts, wounds, burns or skin abrasions: apply qd-tid.

PEDS - Not approved in children.

UNAPPROVED PEDS - Minor cuts, wounds, burns or skin abrasions: apply qd-tid.

FORMS - OTC trade only: neomycin 3.5 mg/g + polymyxin 10,000 units/g 15 g and unit dose 0.94 g.

NOTES - Neomycin component can cause contact dermatitis.

Neosporin ointment (bacitracin + neomycin + polymyxin) ▶K ♀C ▶? $

ADULT - Minor cuts, wounds, burns or skin abrasions: apply qd-tid.

PEDS - Not approved in children.

UNAPPROVED PEDS - Minor cuts, wounds, burns or skin abrasions: apply qd-tid.

FORMS - OTC Generic/Trade: bacitracin 400 units/g + neomycin 3.5 mg/g + polymyxin 5,000 units/g 2.4,9.6,14.2,15,30 g & unit dose 0.94 g.

NOTES - Also known as triple antibiotic ointment. Neomycin component can cause contact dermatitis.

Polysporin (bacitracin + polymyxin, ♥Polytopic) ▶K ♀C ▶? $

ADULT - Minor cuts, wounds, burns or skin abrasions: apply qd-tid.

PEDS - Not approved in children.

UNAPPROVED PEDS - Minor cuts, wounds, burns or skin abrasions: apply qd-tid.

FORMS - OTC trade only: ointment 15,30 g and unit dose 0.9 g, powder 10 g, aerosol 90 g.

silver sulfadiazine (*Silvadene, ♥Dermazin, Flamazine*) ▶LK ♀B ▶- $

ADULT - Burns: apply qd-bid.

PEDS - Not approved in children.

UNAPPROVED ADULT - Has been used for pressure ulcers.

UNAPPROVED PEDS - Burns: apply qd-bid.

FORMS - Generic/Trade: cream 1% 20,50,85, 400,1000g.

NOTES - Avoid in sulfa allergy. Leukopenia, primarily decreased neutrophil count in up to 20% of patients. Significant absorption may occur and serum sulfa concentrations approach therapeutic levels. Avoid in G6PD deficiency. Use caution in pregnancy nearing term, premature infants, infants ≤2 months and in patients with renal or hepatic dysfunction.

DERMATOLOGY: Antifungal Preparations

butenafine (*Lotrimin Ultra, Mentax*) ▶L ♀B ▶? $$$

ADULT - Treatment of tinea pedis: apply qd for 4 weeks or bid x 7 days. Tinea corporis, tinea versicolor, or tinea cruris: apply qd for 2 weeks.

PEDS - Not approved in children.

FORMS - Trade only. Rx: cream 1% 15,30 g (Mentax). OTC: cream 1% (Lotrimin Ultra).

NOTES - Most common adverse effects include contact dermatitis, burning, and worsening of condition. If no improvement in 4 weeks, re-evaluate diagnosis.

ciclopirox (*Loprox, Penlac*) ▶K ♀B ▶? $$

ADULT - Tinea pedis, cruris, corporis, and versicolor, candidiasis (cream, lotion): apply bid. Onychomycosis of fingernails/toenails (nail solution): apply daily to affected nails; apply over previous coat; remove with alcohol every 7 days. Seborrheic dermatitis (Loprox shampoo): shampoo twice/week x 4 weeks.

PEDS - Onychomycosis of fingernails/toenails in children ≥12 yo (nail solution): apply daily to af-

fected nails; apply over previous coat; remove with alcohol every 7 days (Penlac). Not approved in children <12 yo.
FORMS - Trade only: cream (Loprox) 0.77% 15,30,90 g, gel (Loprox) 0.77% 30,45 g, shampoo (Loprox) 1% 120 ml, nail solution (Penlac) 8% 6.6 ml. Trade/generic: lotion (Loprox) 0.77% 30,60 ml.
NOTES - Clinical improvement of tinea usually occurs within first week. Patients with tinea versicolor usually exhibit clinical and mycological clearing after 2 weeks. If no improvement in 4 weeks, reevaluate diagnosis. Do not get shampoo in eyes. For nail solution, infected portion of each nail should be removed by health care professional as frequently as monthly. Oral antifungal therapy is more effective for onychomycosis than Penlac.

clotrimazole (*Lotrimin, Mycelex, ♣Canesten, Clotrimaderm*) ▶L ♀B ▶? $
ADULT - Treatment of tinea pedis, cruris, corporis, and versicolor, and cutaneous candidiasis: apply bid.
PEDS - Treatment of tinea pedis, cruris, corporis, versicolor, cutaneous candidiasis: apply bid.
FORMS - Note that *Lotrimin* brand cream, lotion, solution are clotrimazole, while *Lotrimin* powders and liquid spray are miconazole. OTC & Rx generic/Trade: cream 1% 15, 30, 45, 90 g, solution 1% 10,30 ml. Trade only: lotion 1% 30 ml.
NOTES - If no improvement in 4 weeks, reevaluate diagnosis.

econazole (*Spectazole, ♣Ecostatin*) ▶Not absorbed ♀C ▶? $$
ADULT - Treatment of tinea pedis, cruris, corporis, and versicolor: apply qd. Cutaneous candidiasis: apply bid.
PEDS - Not approved in children.
FORMS - Trade/Generic: cream 1% 15,30, 85g.
NOTES - Treat candidal infections, tinea cruris and tinea corporis for 2 weeks and tinea pedis for 1 month to reduce risk of recurrence.

ketoconazole (*Nizoral, ♣Ketoderm*) ▶L ♀C ▶? $
ADULT - Shampoo (2%): Tinea versicolor: apply to affected area, leave on for 5 min, rinse. Cream: cutaneous candidiasis, tinea corporis, cruris, and versicolor: apply qd. Seborrheic dermatitis: apply cream (2%) bid. Dandruff: apply shampoo (1%) twice a week.
PEDS - Not approved in children <12 years.
UNAPPROVED ADULT - Seborrheic dermatitis: apply cream (2%) qd.
UNAPPROVED PEDS - Shampoo (2%): Tinea versicolor: apply to affected area, leave on for 5 min, rinse. Cream: cutaneous candidiasis, tinea corporis, cruris, and versicolor: apply qd. Seborrheic dermatitis: apply cream (2%) bid. Dandruff: apply shampoo (1%) twice a week.
FORMS - Trade only: shampoo 1% (OTC), 2%, 120 ml. Trade/Generic: cream 2% 15,30,60 g.
NOTES - Treat candidal infections, tinea cruris, corporis and versicolor for 2 weeks. Treat seborrheic dermatitis for 4 weeks. Treat tinea pedis for 6 weeks.

miconazole (*Monistat-Derm, Micatin, Lotrimin, ♣Micozole*) ▶L ♀+ ▶? $
ADULT - Tinea pedis, cruris, corporis, and versicolor, cutaneous candidiasis: apply bid.
PEDS - Not approved in children.
UNAPPROVED PEDS - Tinea pedis, cruris, corporis, and versicolor, cutaneous candidiasis: apply bid.
FORMS - Note that Lotrimin brand cream, lotion, solution are clotrimazole, while Lotrimin powders and liquid spray are miconazole. OTC generic: ointment 2% 29 g, spray 2% 105 ml, solution 2% 7.39, 30 ml. Generic/Trade: cream 2% 15,30,90 g, powder 2% 90 g, spray powder 2% 90,100 g, spray liquid 2% 105,113 ml.
NOTES - Symptomatic relief generally occurs in 2-3 days. Treat candida, tinea cruris, tinea corporis for 2 weeks, tinea pedis for 1 month to reduce risk of recurrence.

naftifine (*Naftin*) ▶LK ♀B ▶? $$
ADULT - Tinea pedis, cruris, and corporis: apply qd (cream) or bid (gel).
PEDS - Not approved in children.
FORMS - Trade only: cream 1% 15,30,60 g, gel 1% 20,40, 60 g.
NOTES - If no improvement in 4 weeks, reevaluate diagnosis.

nystatin (*Mycostatin, ♣Nilstat, Nyaderm, Candistatin*) ▶Not absorbed ♀C ▶? $
ADULT - Cutaneous or mucocutaneous Candida infections: apply bid-tid.
PEDS - Cutaneous or mucocutaneous Candida infections: apply bid-tid.
FORMS - Generic/Trade: cream 100,000 units/g 15,30,240 g, ointment 100,000 units/g 15,30 g, powder 100,000 units/g 15 g.
NOTES - Ineffective for dermatophytes/tinea. For fungal infections of the feet, dust feet and footwear with powder.

oxiconazole (*Oxistat, Oxizole*) ▶? ♀B ▶? $$
ADULT - Tinea pedis, cruris, and corporis: apply qd-bid. Tinea versicolor (cream only): apply qd.
PEDS - Cream: Tinea pedis, cruris, and corporis: apply qd-bid. Tinea versicolor: apply qd.

FORMS - Trade only: cream 1% 15,30,60 g, lotion 1% 30 ml.

sertaconazole (*Ertaczo*) ▶Not absorbed ♀C ▶? $$

ADULT - Tinea pedis: apply bid.

PEDS - Not approved for children <12 yo.

FORMS - Trade only: cream 2% 15,30g.

terbinafine (*Lamisil, Lamisil AT*) ▶L ♀B ▶? $$$

ADULT - Tinea pedis: apply bid. Tinea cruris and corporis: apply qd-bid. Tinea versicolor (solution): apply bid.

PEDS - Not approved in children.

UNAPPROVED ADULT - Cutaneous candidiasis.

UNAPPROVED PEDS - Tinea pedis: apply bid. Tinea cruris and corporis: apply qd-bid. Tinea versicolor (solution): apply bid.

FORMS - Trade only: cream 1% 15,30 g, gel 1% 5,15,30 g OTC: Trade only (Lamisil AT): cream 1% 12,24 g, spray pump soln 1% 30 ml.

NOTES - In many patients, improvement noted within 3-4 days, but therapy should continue for a minimum of 1 week, maximum of 4 weeks. Topical therapy not effective for nail fungus.

tolnaftate (*Tinactin*) ▶? ♀? ▶? $

ADULT - Tinea pedis, cruris, corporis, and versicolor: apply bid. Prevention of tinea pedis (powder and aerosol): apply prn.

PEDS - >2 yo: Tinea pedis, cruris, corporis, and versicolor: apply bid. Prevention of tinea pedis (powder and aerosol): apply prn.

FORMS - OTC Generic/Trade: cream 1% 15,30 g, solution 1% 10,15 ml, powder 1% 45,90 g, spray powder 1% 100,105,150 g, spray liquid 1% 60,120 ml. Trade only: gel 1% 15 g.

DERMATOLOGY: Antiparasitics (topical)

NOTE: See also acne preparations

A-200 (pyrethrins + piperonyl butoxide, ❧*R&C*) ▶L ♀C ▶? $

ADULT - Lice: Apply shampoo, wash after 10 min. Reapply in 5-7 days.

PEDS - Lice: Apply shampoo, wash after 10 min. Reapply in 5-7 days.

FORMS - OTC Generic/Trade: shampoo (0.33% pyrethrins, 4% piperonyl butoxide) 60,120,240 ml.

NOTES - Use caution if allergic to ragweed. Avoid contact with mucous membranes.

crotamiton (*Eurax*) ▶? ♀C ▶? $$

ADULT - Scabies: massage cream/lotion into entire body from chin down, repeat 24 h later, bathe 48 h later. Pruritus: massage into affected areas prn.

PEDS - Not approved in children.

UNAPPROVED PEDS - Scabies: massage cream/lotion into entire body from chin down, repeat 24h later, bathe 48h later. Pruritus: massage into affected areas prn.

FORMS - Trade only: cream 10% 60 g, lotion 10% 60,480 ml.

NOTES - Patients with scabies should change bed linen and clothing in am after second application and bathe 48h after last application. Consider treating entire family.

lindane (❧*Kwellada*) ▶L ♀B ▶? $

WARNING - For use only in patients who have failed other agents. Seizures and deaths have been reported with repeat or prolonged use. Use caution with infants, children, elderly, those who weigh <50 kg. Contraindicated in premature infants and patients with uncontrolled seizures.

ADULT - Head/crab lice: Lotion: apply 30-60 ml to affected area, wash off after 12h. Shampoo: apply 30-60 ml, wash off after 4 min. Scabies (lotion): apply 30-60 ml to total body from neck down, wash off after 8-12h.

PEDS - Lindane penetrates human skin and has potential for CNS toxicity. Studies indicate potential toxic effects of topical lindane are greater in young. Maximum dose for children <6 yo is 30 ml.

FORMS - Generic/Trade: lotion 1% 30,60,480 ml, shampoo 1% 30,60,480 ml.

NOTES - For lice, reapply if living lice noted after 7 days. After shampooing, comb with fine tooth comb to remove nits. Consider treating entire family.

malathion (*Ovide*) ▶? ♀B ▶? $$

ADULT - Head lice: apply to dry hair, let dry naturally, wash off in 8-12 hrs.

PEDS - Head lice in children >6 yo: apply to dry hair, let dry naturally, wash off in 8-12 hrs.

FORMS - Trade only: lotion 0.5% 59 ml.

NOTES - Do not use hair dryer; flammable. Avoid contact with eyes. Use a fine tooth comb to remove nits and dead lice. Application may be repeated in 7-9 days.

permethrin (*Elimite, Acticin, Nix*, ❧*Kwellada-P*) ▶L ♀B ▶? $$

ADULT - Scabies (cream): massage cream into entire body (avoid mouth, eyes, nose), wash off after 8-14h. 30 g is typical adult dose. Head lice (liquid): apply to clean, towel-dried hair, saturate hair and scalp, wash off after 10 min.

PEDS - Scabies (cream) >2 mo: massage cream into entire body (avoid mouth, eyes, nose), wash off after 8-14h. Head lice (liquid) in children >2 yo: saturate hair and scalp, wash off after 10 min.

FORMS - Trade only: cream (Elimite, Acticin) 5% 60 g. OTC Trade/generic: liquid creme rinse (Nix) 1% 60 ml.

NOTES - If necessary, may repeat application in 7 days. Consider treating entire family.

RID (pyrethrins + piperonyl butoxide) ▶L

♀C ▶? $

ADULT - Lice: Apply shampoo/mousse, wash after 10 min. Reapply in 5-10 days.

PEDS - Lice: Apply shampoo/mousse, wash after 10 min. Reapply in 5-10 days.

FORMS - OTC Generic/Trade: shampoo 60,120,240 ml. Trade only: mousse 5.5 oz.

NOTES - Use caution if ragweed allergy. Avoid contact with mucus membranes. Available alone or as part of a RID 1-2-3 kit containing shampoo, egg and nit comb-out gel and home lice control spray for non-washable items.

DERMATOLOGY: Antipsoriatic Preparations

acitretin (Soriatane) ▶L ♀X ▶- $$$$$

WARNING - Contraindicated in pregnancy and avoid pregnancy for 3 years following medication discontinuation. Major human fetal abnormalities have been reported. Females of child bearing age must avoid alcohol while on medication and for 2 months following therapy since alcohol prolongs elimination of a teratogenic metabolite. Use in reliable females of reproductive potential only if they have severe, unresponsive psoriasis, have received written and oral warnings of the teratogenic potential, are using 2 reliable forms of contraception, and have 2 negative pregnancy tests within 1 week prior to starting therapy. It is unknown whether residual acitretin in seminal fluid poses a risk to the fetus while a male patient is taking the drug or after it is discontinued.

ADULT - Severe psoriasis: initiate at 25-50 mg PO qd.

PEDS - Not approved in children.

UNAPPROVED ADULT - Lichen planus: 30 mg/day PO for 4 weeks, then titrate to 10-50 mg/day for 12 weeks total. Sjogren-Larsson syndrome: 0.47 mg/kg/day PO. Also used in Darier's disease, palmoplantar pustulosis, nonbullous and bullous ichthyosiform erythroderma, lichen sclerosus et atrophicus of the vulva and palmoplantar lichen nitidus.

UNAPPROVED PEDS - Has been used in children with lamellar ichthyosis. Pediatric use is not recommended. Adverse effects on bone growth are suspected.

FORMS - Trade only: cap 10,25 mg.

NOTES - Transient worsening of psoriasis may occur, and full benefit may take 2-3 mo. Elevated LFTs may occur in 1/3 of patients; monitor LFTs at 1-2 week intervals until stable and then periodically thereafter. Monitor serum lipid concentrations every 1-2 weeks until response

to drug is established. May decrease tolerance to contact lenses due to dry eyes. Avoid prolonged exposure to sunlight. May cause hair loss. May cause depression. May cause bone changes, especially with use >6 months. Many adverse drug reactions.

alefacept (Amevive) ▶? ♀B ▶? $$$$$

ADULT - Moderate to severe psoriasis: 7.5 mg IV or 15 mg IM once weekly x 12 doses. May repeat with 1 additional 12-week course after 12 weeks have elapsed from last dose.

PEDS - Not approved in children.

NOTES - Monitor CD4+ T lymphocyte cells weekly; withhold therapy if count <250/mcL and stop altogether if <250/mcL for one month. Do not give with other immunosuppressives or phototherapy.

anthralin (Anthra-Derm, Drithocreme, ♣Anthrascalp, Anthranol, Anthraforte, Micanol) ▶? ♀C ▶- $$

ADULT - Chronic psoriasis: apply qd.

PEDS - Not approved in children.

UNAPPROVED PEDS - Chronic psoriasis: apply qd.

FORMS - Trade only: ointment 0.1% 42.5 g, 0.25% 42.5 g, 0.4% 60 g, 0.5% 42.5 g, 1% 42.5 g, cream 0.1% 50 g, 0.2% 50 g, 0.25% 50 g, 0.5% 50 g. Generic/Trade: cream 1% 50 g.

NOTES - Short contact periods (i.e. 15-20 minutes) followed by removal with an appropriate solvent (soap or petrolatum) may be preferred. May stain fabric, skin or hair.

calcipotriene (Dovonex) ▶L ♀C ▶? $$$

ADULT - Moderate plaque psoriasis: apply bid.

PEDS - Not approved in children.

UNAPPROVED PEDS - Moderate plaque psoriasis: apply bid.

FORMS - Trade only: ointment 0.005% 30,60, 100 g, cream 0.005% 30,60,100 g, scalp solution 0.005% 60 ml.

NOTES - Avoid contact with face. Do not exceed 100 g/week to minimize risk of hypercalcemia, hypercalcuria. Burning, itching, and skin irritation may occur in 10-15% of patients.

efalizumab (*Raptiva*) ▶L ♀C ▶? $$$$$
ADULT - Moderate to severe plaque psoriasis: 0.7 mg/kg SC x 1 then 1 mg/kg SC q week.
PEDS - Not approved in children.
FORMS - Trade only: single use vials, 125 mg.
NOTES - Monitor platelets upon initiation and monthly thereafter.

methoxsalen (*8-MOP, Oxsoralen-Ultra*) ▶Skin ♀C ▶? $$$$$
ADULT - Psoriasis: dose based on weight (0.4 mg/kg/dose), 1½ to 2 hours before ultraviolet light exposure.
PEDS - Not approved in children.
FORMS - Trade only: soft gelatin cap 10 mg (Oxsoralen-Ultra), hard gelatin cap 10 mg (8-MOP).

NOTES - Oxsoralen-Ultra (soft gelatin cap) cannot be interchanged with 8-MOP (hard gelatin cap) due to significant bioavailability differences and photosensitization onset times. Take with food or milk. Wear ultraviolet light blocking glasses after ingestion and for remainder of day.

tazarotene (*Tazorac*) ▶L ♀X ▶? $$$
ADULT - Psoriasis: apply 0.05% cream qhs, increase to 0.1% prn. Acne: see Acne Preparation section.
PEDS - Not approved in children.
UNAPPROVED PEDS - Psoriasis: apply qhs.
FORMS - Trade only: gel 0.05% 30,100 g, 0.1% 30, 100 g.
NOTES - May reduce irritation and improve efficacy by using topical steroid in morning and tazarotene at bedtime. Desquamation, burning, dry skin, erythema, pruritus may occur in up to 30% of patients. May cause photosensitivity.

DERMATOLOGY: Antiviral Preparations (topical)

acyclovir (*Zovirax*) ▶K ♀C ▶? $$$
ADULT - Initial episodes of herpes genitalis: apply oint q3h (6 times/d) x 7 days. Non-life threatening mucocutaneous herpes simplex in immunocompromised patients: apply oint q3h (6 times/d) x 7 days. Recurrent herpes labialis: apply cream 5 times/day for 4 days.
PEDS - <12 yo: Not approved. ≥12 yo: Recurrent herpes labialis: apply cream 5 times/day for 4 days.
UNAPPROVED PEDS - Initial episodes of herpes genitalis: apply oint q3h (6 times/d) x 7 days. Non-life threatening mucocutaneous herpes simplex in immunocompromised patients: apply oint q3h (6 times/d) x 7 days.
FORMS - Trade only: ointment 5% 3,15 g, cream 5% 2 g.
NOTES - Use finger cot or rubber glove to apply ointment to avoid dissemination. Burning/stinging may occur in up to 28% of patients. Oral form more effective than topical for herpes genitalis.

docosanol (*Abreva*) ▶Not absorbed ♀B ▶? $
ADULT - Oral-facial herpes simplex: apply 5x/day until healed.
PEDS - Not approved in children.
FORMS - OTC: Trade only: cream 10% 2 g.

imiquimod (*Aldara*) ▶Not absorbed ♀C ▶? $$$$
ADULT - External genital and perianal warts: apply 3 times weekly at bedtime for up to 16 weeks. Wash off after 8 hours. Nonhyperkera-

totic, nonhypertrophic actinic keratoses on face /scalp in immunocompetent adults: apply to face or scalp (but not both) 2 times weekly for up to 16 weeks. Wash off after 8 hours. Primary superficial basal cell carcinoma: apply 5 times weekly x 6 weeks. Wash off after 8 hrs.
PEDS - Children >11 yo: External genital and perianal warts: apply 3 times/week at bedtime. Wash off after 6-10 hours.
UNAPPROVED ADULT - Giant molluscum contagiosum: apply 3 times weekly for 6-10 hours.
FORMS - Trade only: cream 5% 250 mg single use packets.
NOTES - May weaken condoms and diaphragms. Avoid sexual contact while cream is on when used for genital/perianal warts. Most common adverse effects include erythema, itching, erosion, burning, excoriation, edema and pain. Discard partially used packets.

penciclovir (*Denavir*) ▶Not absorbed ♀B ▶? $$$
ADULT - Recurrent herpes labialis: apply q2h while awake x 4 days.
PEDS - Not approved in children.
UNAPPROVED PEDS - Recurrent herpes labialis: apply q2h while awake x 4 days.
FORMS - Trade only: cream 1% 2 g tubes.
NOTES - Start therapy as soon as possible during prodrome. For moderate to severe cases of herpes labialis, systemic treatment with famciclovir or acyclovir may be preferred.

podofilox (*Condylox*, ✠*Condyline*) ▶? ♀C

▶? $$$
ADULT - External genital warts (gel and solution) and perianal warts (gel only): apply bid for 3 consecutive days of a week and repeat for up to 4 weeks.
PEDS - Not approved in children.
FORMS - Trade only: gel 0.5% 3.5 g, solution 0.5% 3.5 ml.

podophyllin (*Podocon-25, Podofin, Podofilm*) ▶? ♀- ▶- $$
ADULT - Genital wart removal: Initial application: apply to wart and leave on for 30-40 min to determine patient's sensitivity. Thereafter, use minimum contact time necessary (1-4h depending on result). Remove dried podophyllin with alcohol or soap and water.
PEDS - Not approved in children.
FORMS - Not to be dispensed to patients. For hospital/clinic use; not intended for outpatient prescribing. Trade only: liquid 25% 15 ml.
NOTES - Not to be dispensed to patients. Do not treat large areas or numerous warts all at once. Contraindicated in diabetics, pregnancy, patients using steroids or with poor circulation, and on bleeding warts.

DERMATOLOGY: Atopic Dermatitis Preparations

pimecrolimus (*Elidel*) ▶L ♀C ▶? $$$
ADULT - Atopic dermatitis: apply bid.
PEDS - Atopic dermatitis: ≥2 yo: apply bid.
UNAPPROVED PEDS - Atopic dermatitis: <2 yo: apply bid.
FORMS - Trade: cream 1% 15, 30, 100 g.

tacrolimus (*Protopic*) ▶Minimal absorption ♀C ▶? $$$$
ADULT - Atopic dermatitis: apply bid.
PEDS - Children <2 yo: not approved. 2-15 yo: Atopic dermatitis: apply 0.03% oint bid.
FORMS - Trade only: ointment 0.03% 30,60 g, 0.1% 30,60 g.
NOTES - Do not use with an occlusive dressing. Continue treatment for 1 week after clearing of symptoms.

DERMATOLOGY: Corticosteroids (topical)

NOTE: After long-term use, do not discontinue abruptly; switch to a less potent agent or alternate use of corticosteroids and emollient products. Monitor for hyperglycemia / adrenal suppression if used for long period of time or over a large area of the body, especially in children. Chronic administration may interfere with pediatric growth & development.

alclometasone dipropionate (*Aclovate*) ▶L ♀C ▶? $$
ADULT - Inflammatory and pruritic manifestations of corticosteroid-responsive dermatoses: apply sparingly 2-3 times/day.
PEDS - Inflammatory and pruritic manifestations of corticosteroid-responsive dermatoses in children ≥1 yo: apply sparingly 2-3 times/day. Safety and efficacy for >3 weeks have not been established.
FORMS - Trade/generic: ointment 0.05% 15,45, 60 g. Trade only: cream 0.05% 15,45,60 g.

amcinonide (*Cyclocort*) ▶L ♀C ▶? $$
ADULT - Inflammatory and pruritic manifestations of corticosteroid-responsive dermatoses: apply sparingly 2-3 times/day.
PEDS - Inflammatory and pruritic manifestations of corticosteroid-responsive dermatoses: apply sparingly 2-3 times/day.
FORMS - Trade only: ointment 0.1% 15,30,60 g, cream 0.1% 15,30,60 g, lotion 0.1% 20,60 ml.

augmented betamethasone dipropionate (*Diprolene, Diprolene AF, ♣Topilene Glycol*) ▶L ♀C ▶? $$
ADULT - Inflammatory and pruritic manifestations of corticosteroid-responsive dermatoses: apply sparingly 1-2 times/day.
PEDS - Not approved in children.
FORMS - Trade/generic only: Diprolene: ointment 0.05% 15,50 g. Trade/generic: Diprolene AF: cream 0.05% 15, 50, 90 g. Trade only: gel 0.05% 15,50g, lotion 0.05% 30,60 ml.
NOTES - Do not use occlusive dressings. Do not use for longer than 2 consecutive weeks and do not exceed a total dose of 45-50 g/week or 50 ml/week of the lotion.

betamethasone dipropionate (*Diprosone, Maxivate, Topisone, ♣Propiderm, TARO-sone*) ▶L ♀C ▶? $
ADULT - Inflammatory and pruritic manifestations of corticosteroid-responsive dermatoses: apply sparingly 1-2 times/day.
PEDS - Inflammatory and pruritic manifestations of corticosteroid-responsive dermatoses: apply sparingly 1-2 times/day.
FORMS - Generic/Trade: ointment 0.05% 15,45

g, cream 0.05% 15,45 g, lotion 0.05% 20,60 ml. Trade only: aerosol 0.1% 85 g.

NOTES - Do not use occlusive dressings.

betamethasone valerate (*Luxiq foam*, ✤*Betaderm, Betnovate, Celestoderm, Ectosone, Prevex-B, Valisone*) ▶L ♀C▶? $

ADULT - Inflammatory and pruritic manifestations of corticosteroid-responsive dermatoses: apply sparingly 1-2 times/day. Dermatoses of scalp: apply small amount of foam to scalp bid.

PEDS - Inflammatory and pruritic manifestations of corticosteroid-responsive dermatoses: apply sparingly 1-2 times/day.

FORMS - Generic: ointment 0.1% 15,45 g, cream 0.1% 15,45,110 g, lotion 0.1% 20,60 ml, foam (Luxiq) 0.12%100 g.

clobetasol (*Temovate, Dermovate, Olux, Clobex, Cormax,* ✤*Dermasone*) ▶L ♀C ▶? $$

ADULT - Inflammatory and pruritic manifestations of corticosteroid-responsive dermatoses: apply sparingly 2 times/day. For scalp apply foam 2 times/day.

PEDS - Not approved in children.

FORMS - Generic/Trade: ointment 0.05% 15,30,45,60 g, cream 0.05% 15,30,45,60 g, scalp application 0.05% 25,50 ml, gel 0.05% 15,30,60 g. Trade only: foam 0.05% (Olux) 50,100g, lotion 0.05% (Clobex) 30,59,118 ml.

NOTES - Adrenal suppression at doses as low as 2 g/day. Do not use occlusive dressings. Do not use for longer than 2 consecutive weeks and do not exceed a total dose of 50 g/week.

clocortolone pivalate (*Cloderm*) ▶L ♀C ▶? $$

ADULT - Inflammatory and pruritic manifestations of corticosteroid-responsive dermatoses: apply sparingly 3 times/day.

PEDS - Inflammatory and pruritic manifestations of corticosteroid-responsive dermatoses: apply sparingly 3 times/day.

FORMS - Trade/generic: cream 0.1% 15,45 g.

desonide (*DesOwen, Desocort, Tridesilon*) ▶L ♀C ▶? $

ADULT - Inflammatory and pruritic manifestations of corticosteroid-responsive dermatoses: apply sparingly 2-3 times/day.

PEDS - Inflammatory and pruritic manifestations of corticosteroid-responsive dermatoses: apply sparingly 2-3 times/day.

FORMS - Generic/Trade: cream 0.05% 15,60 g, ointment 0.05% 15,60 g. Trade only: lotion 0.05% 60,120 ml.

NOTES - Do not use with occlusive dressings.

desoximetasone (*Topicort, Topicort LP*) ▶L ♀C ▶? $$

ADULT - Inflammatory and pruritic manifestations of corticosteroid-responsive dermatoses: apply sparingly 2 times/day.

PEDS - Safety and efficacy have not been established for Topicort 0.25% ointment. For inflammatory and pruritic manifestations of corticosteroid-responsive dermatoses (cream and gel): apply sparingly 2 times/day.

FORMS - Generic/Trade: cream 0.05% 15,60 g, cream 0.25%15,60,120 g, gel 0.05% 15,60 g. Trade only: ointment 0.25% 15,60 g.

diflorasone (*Florone, Psorcon, Psorcon E, Maxiflor*) ▶L ♀C ▶? $$

ADULT - Inflammatory and pruritic manifestations of corticosteroid-responsive dermatoses: apply sparingly 1-3 times/day.

PEDS - Not approved in children.

FORMS - Generic/Trade: ointment 0.05% 15,30, 60 g, cream 0.05% 15,30,60 g.

NOTES - Doses of 30 g/day of diflorasone 0.05% cream for 1 week resulted in adrenal suppression in some psoriasis patients.

fluocinolone (*Synalar, Fluoderm, Derma-Smooth-FS,* ✤*Synamol*) ▶L ♀C ▶? $

ADULT - Inflammatory and pruritic manifestations of corticosteroid-responsive dermatoses: apply sparingly 2-4 times/day. Psoriasis of the scalp (Derma-Smoothe/FS): Massage into scalp, cover with shower cap and leave on ≥4 h or overnight and then wash off.

PEDS - Inflammatory and pruritic manifestations of corticosteroid-responsive dermatoses: apply sparingly 2-4 times/day.

FORMS - Generic/Trade: ointment 0.025% 15,30,60 g, cream 0.01% 15,30,60 g, cream 0.025% 15,30,60 g, shampoo 0.01% 180 ml, solution 0.01% 20,60 ml, shampoo 0.01% 180 ml, oil 0.01% 120 ml. Trade only (Derma-Smoothe/FS): topical oil 0.01% 120 ml.

fluocinonide (*Lidex, Lidex-E, Lyderm,* ✤*Topactin, Lidemol, Topsyn, Tiamol*) ▶L ♀C ▶? $

ADULT - Inflammatory and pruritic manifestations of corticosteroid-responsive dermatoses: apply sparingly 2-4 times/day.

PEDS - Inflammatory and pruritic manifestations of corticosteroid-responsive dermatoses: apply sparingly 2-4 times/day.

FORMS - Generic/Trade: cream 0.05% 15,30, 60,120 g, ointment 0.05% 15,30,60 g, solution 0.05% 20,60 ml, gel 0.05% 15,30,60,120 g.

flurandrenolide (*Cordran, Cordran SP*) ▶L ♀C ▶? $

ADULT - Inflammatory and pruritic manifestations of corticosteroid-responsive dermatoses: apply sparingly 2-3 times/day.

PEDS - Inflammatory and pruritic manifestations of corticosteroid-responsive dermatoses: apply sparingly 2-3 times/day.

FORMS - Trade only: ointment 0.025% 30,60 g, ointment 0.05% 15,30,60 g, cream 0.025% 30, 60 g, cream 0.05% 15,30,60 g, tape 4mcg/cm^2. Generic/Trade: lotion 0.05% 15,60 ml.

fluticasone propionate (*Cutivate*) ▶L ♀C ▶? $$

ADULT - Eczema: apply sparingly 1-2 times/day. Other inflammatory and pruritic manifestations of corticosteroid-responsive dermatoses: apply sparingly 2 times/day.

PEDS - Children >3 mo old: Eczema: apply sparingly 1-2 times/day. Other inflammatory and pruritic manifestations of corticosteroid-responsive dermatoses: apply sparingly 2 times/day.

FORMS - Trade/generic: cream 0.05% 15,30,60 g, ointment 0.005% 15,60 g.

NOTES - Do not use with an occlusive dressing.

halcinonide (*Halog*) ▶L ♀C ▶? $$

ADULT - Inflammatory and pruritic manifestations of corticosteroid-responsive dermatoses: apply sparingly 2-3 times/day.

PEDS - Inflammatory and pruritic manifestations of corticosteroid-responsive dermatoses: apply sparingly 2-3 times/day.

FORMS - Trade only: ointment 0.1% 15,30,60 g cream 0.1% 15,30,60 g, soln 0.1% 20,60 ml.

halobetasol propionate (*Ultravate*) ▶L ♀C ▶? $$

ADULT - Inflammatory and pruritic manifestations of corticosteroid-responsive dermatoses: apply sparingly 1-2 times/day.

PEDS - Not approved in children.

FORMS - Trade only: ointment 0.05% 15,45 g, cream 0.05% 15,45 g.

NOTES - Do not use occlusive dressings. Do not use for >2 consecutive weeks and do not exceed a total dose of 50 g/week.

hydrocortisone (*Cortizone, Hycort, Tegrin -HC, Dermolate, Synacort, ✚Cortoderm, Prevex-HC, Cortate, Emo-Cort, Sarna-HC*) ▶L ♀C ▶? $

ADULT - Inflammatory and pruritic manifestations of corticosteroid-responsive dermatoses: apply sparingly 2-4 times/day.

PEDS - Inflammatory and pruritic manifestations of corticosteroid-responsive dermatoses: apply sparingly 2-4 times/day.

FORMS - Products available OTC & Rx depending on labeling. 2.5% preparation available Rx

only. Generic: ointment 0.5% 30 g, ointment 1% 15, 20,30,60,120 g, ointment 2.5% 20,30 g, cream 0.5% 15,30,60 g, cream 1% 20,30,60, 90,120 g, cream 2.5% 15,20,30,60,120 g, lotion 0.25% 120 ml, lotion 0.5% 30,60,120 ml, lotion 1% 60,120 ml, lotion 2% 30 ml, lotion 2.5% 60 ml.

hydrocortisone acetate (*Cortaid, Corticaine, Micort-HC Lipocream, ✚Hyderm, Cortamed, Cortifoam*) ▶L ♀C ▶? $

ADULT - Inflammatory and pruritic manifestations of corticosteroid-responsive dermatoses: apply sparingly 2-4 times/day.

PEDS - Inflammatory and pruritic manifestations of corticosteroid-responsive dermatoses: apply sparingly 2-4 times/day.

FORMS - OTC Generic/Trade: ointment 0.5% 15,30 g, ointment 1% 30g, cream 0.5% 15,30 g. Rx only generic/trade: cream 1% 15,20, 30,120 g, 2.5% 30 g (Micort-HC Lipocream).

hydrocortisone butyrate (*Locoid*) ▶L ♀C ▶? $$

ADULT - Inflammatory and pruritic manifestations of corticosteroid-responsive dermatoses: apply sparingly 2-3 times/day. Seborrheic dermatitis (solution only): apply 2-3 times/day.

PEDS - Inflammatory and pruritic manifestations of corticosteroid-responsive dermatoses: apply sparingly 2-3 times/day. Seborrheic dermatitis (solution only): apply 2-3 times/day.

FORMS - Trade only: ointment 0.1% 15,45 g, cream 0.1% 15,45 g. Trade/generic: solution 0.1% 15,30,60 ml.

hydrocortisone probutate (*Pandel*) ▶L ♀C ▶? $

ADULT - Inflammatory and pruritic manifestations of corticosteroid-responsive dermatoses: apply sparingly 1-2 times/day.

PEDS - Not approved in children.

FORMS - Trade only: cream 0.1% 15,45 g, 1% 15,45 g.

hydrocortisone valerate (*Westcort, ✚Hydroval*) ▶L ♀C ▶? $$

ADULT - Inflammatory and pruritic manifestations of corticosteroid-responsive dermatoses: apply sparingly 2-3 times/day.

PEDS - Safety and efficacy of Westcort ointment have not been established in children. Inflammatory and pruritic manifestations of corticosteroid-responsive dermatoses (cream only): apply sparingly 2-3 times/day.

FORMS - Generic/Trade: ointment 0.2% 15,45, 60 g, cream 0.2% 15,45,60 g.

mometasone furoate (*Elocon, ✚Elocom*) ▶L ♀C ▶? $

ADULT - Inflammatory and pruritic manifestations of corticosteroid-responsive dermatoses: apply sparingly once daily.

PEDS - Inflammatory and pruritic manifestations of corticosteroid-responsive dermatoses ≥2 yo: apply sparingly once daily. Safety and efficacy for >3 weeks have not been established.

FORMS - Trade only: cream 0.1% 15,45 g, lotion 0.1% 30,60 ml. Trade/Generic: ointment 0.1% 15,45 g.

NOTES - Do not use an occlusive dressing.

prednicarbate (*Dermatop*) ►L ♀C ▶? $$

ADULT - Inflammatory and pruritic manifestations of corticosteroid-responsive dermatoses: apply sparingly 2 times/day.

PEDS - Inflammatory and pruritic manifestations of corticosteroid-responsive dermatoses in children ≥1 yo: apply sparingly 2 times/day. Safety and efficacy for >3 weeks have not

been established.

FORMS - Trade only: cream 0.1% 15,60 g, ointment 0.1% 15, 60 g.

triamcinolone (*Kenalog, Aristocort, ♥Triaderm*) ►L ♀C ▶? $

ADULT - Inflammatory and pruritic manifestations of corticosteroid-responsive dermatoses: apply sparingly 3-4 times/day.

PEDS - Inflammatory and pruritic manifestations of corticosteroid-responsive dermatoses: apply sparingly 3-4 times/day.

FORMS - Generic/Trade: ointment 0.025% 15, 28,57,80,113 g, ointment 0.1% 15,28,57,60,80, 113 g, ointment 0.5% 15,20,28,57,113 g, cream 0.025% 15,20, 30,60,80,90,120 g, cream 0.5% 15,20,30,60,120 g, cream 0.1% 15,60,80 g, lotion 0.025% 60 ml, lotion 0.1% 15,60 ml. Trade only: aerosol 23,63 g.

CORTICOSTEROIDS – TOPICAL*

	Agent	Strength/Formulation*	Freq
Low Potency	alclometasone dipropionate (*Aclovate*)	0.05% C O	bid-tid
	clocortolone pivalate (*Cloderm*)	0.1% C	tid
	desonide (*DesOwen, Tridesilon*)	0.05% C L O	bid-tid
	hydrocortisone (*Hytone*, others)	0.25% CL; 0.5% CLO; 1% CLOS; 2% L; 2.5% CLO	bid-qid
	hydrocortisone acetate (*Cortaid, Corticaine*)	0.5% C O, 1% C O	bid-qid
Medium Potency	betamethasone valerate	0.1% CLO; 0.12% F (*Luxiq*)	qd-bid
	desoximetasone‡ (*Topicort*)	0.05% C	bid
	fluocinolone acetonide (*Synalar*)	0.01% C S; 0.025% C O	bid-qid
	flurandrenolide (*Cordran*)	0.025% C; 0.05% CLO; T	bid-qid
	fluticasone propionate (*Cutivate*)	0.005% O; 0.05% C	qd-bid
	hydrocortisone butyrate (*Locoid*)	0.1% C O	bid-tid
	hydrocortisone valerate (*Westcort*)	0.2% C O	bid-tid
	mometasone furoate (*Elocon*)	0.1% C L O	qd
	triamcinolone‡ (*Aristocort, Kenalog*)	0.025% C L O; 0.1% C L O	bid-tid
High Potency	amcinonide (*Cyclocort*)	0.1% C L O	bid-tid
	betamethasone dipropionate‡ (*Maxivate*)	0.05% CLO (non-*Diprolene*)	qd-bid
	desoximetasone‡ (*Topicort*)	0.05% G; 0.25% C O	bid
	diflorasone diacetate‡ (*Maxiflor*)	0.05% C 0.05% O (*Maxiflor*)	bid
	fluocinonide (*Lidex*)	0.05% C G O S	bid-qid
	halcinonide (*Halog*)	0.1% C O S	bid-tid
	triamcinolone‡ (*Aristocort, Kenalog*)	0.5% C O	bid-tid
Very high	betamethasone dipropionate‡ (*Diprolene, Diprolene AF*)	0.05% C G L O	qd-bid
	clobetasol (*Temovate, Cormax*)	0.05% C O S	bid
	diflorasone diacetate‡ (*Psorcon*)	0.05% C O (*Psorcon*)	qd-tid
	halobetasol propionate (*Ultravate*)	0.05% C O	qd-bid

*C-cream, G-gel, L-lotion, O-ointment, S-solution, T-tape, F-foam. Potency based on vasoconstrictive assays, which may not correlate with efficacy. Not all available products are listed, including those lacking potency ratings. ‡These drugs have formulations in more than once potency category.

DERMATOLOGY: Corticosteroid / Antimicrobial Combinations

***Cortisporin* (neomycin + polymyxin + hydrocortisone)** ▶LK ♀C ▶? $

ADULT - Corticosteroid-responsive dermatoses with secondary infection: apply bid-qid.

PEDS - Not approved in children.

UNAPPROVED PEDS - Corticosteroid-responsive dermatoses with secondary infection: apply bid-qid.

FORMS - Generic/Trade: cream 7.5 g, ointment 15 g.

NOTES - Due to concerns about nephrotoxicity and ototoxicity associated with neomycin, do not use over wide areas or for prolonged periods of time.

***Fucidin H* (fusidic acid + hydrocortisone)** ▶L ♀? ▶? $

ADULT - Canada only. Atopic dermatitis: apply tid.

PEDS - Canada only. Children >3 yo, atopic dermatitis: apply tid.

FORMS - Trade: cream 2% fusidic acid, 1% hydrocortisone acetate 30 g.

***Lotrisone* (clotrimazole + betamethasone, ♣*Lotriderm*)** ▶L ♀C ▶? $$$

ADULT - Tinea pedis, cruris, and corporis: apply bid.

PEDS - Not approved in children.

FORMS - Trade/generic: cream (clotrimazole 1% + betamethasone 0.05%) 15,45 g, lotion (clotrimazole 1% + betamethasone 0.05%) 30 ml.

NOTES - Treat tinea cruris and corporis for 2 weeks and tinea pedis for 4 weeks. Do not use for diaper dermatitis.

***Mycolog II* (nystatin + triamcinolone)** ▶L ♀C ▶? $

ADULT - Cutaneous candidiasis: apply bid.

PEDS - Not approved in children.

UNAPPROVED PEDS - Sometimes used for diaper dermatitis, but this is not recommended due to risk of adrenal suppression.

FORMS - Generic/Trade: cream 15,30,60,120 g, ointment 15,30,60,120 g.

NOTES - Avoid occlusive dressings.

DERMATOLOGY: Hemorrhoid Care

dibucaine (*Nupercainal*) ▶L ♀? ▶? $

ADULT - Hemorrhoids or other anorectal disorders: apply tid-qid prn.

PEDS - Not approved in children.

UNAPPROVED PEDS - Hemorrhoids or other anorectal disorders; children >2yo or >35 pounds: apply tid-qid prn.

FORMS - OTC Generic/Trade: ointment 1% 30 g.

NOTES - Do not use if <2 yo or <35 pounds.

hydrocortisone (*Anusol-HC, Cortifoam*, ♣*Hemcort HC, Egozinc-HC*) ▶L ♀? ▶? $

ADULT - External anal itching: apply cream tid-qid prn or supp bid or rectal foam qd-bid.

PEDS - Not approved in children.

FORMS - Generic/Trade: cream 1% (Anusol HC -1), 2.5% 30 g (Anusol HC), suppository 25 mg (Anusol HC), 10% rectal foam (Cortifoam) 15g.

pramoxine (*Anusol Hemorrhoidal Ointment, Fleet Pain Relief, Proctofoam NS*) ▶Not absorbed ♀+ ▶+ $

ADULT - Hemorrhoids: apply ointment, pads, or foam up to 5 times/day prn.

PEDS - Not approved in children.

FORMS - OTC Trade only: ointment (Anusol Hemorrhoidal Ointment), pads (Fleet Pain Relief), aerosol foam (ProctoFoam NS).

starch (*Anusol Suppositories*) ▶Not absorbed ♀+ ▶+ $

ADULT - Hemorrhoids: 1 suppository PR up to 6 times/day prn or after each bowel movement.

PEDS - Not approved in children.

FORMS - OTC Trade only: suppositories (51% topical starch; soy bean oil, tocopheryl acetate).

witch hazel (*Tucks*) ▶? ♀+ ▶+ $

ADULT - Hemorrhoids: Apply to anus/perineum up to 6 times/day prn.

PEDS - Not approved in children.

FORMS - OTC Generic/Trade: pads, gel.

DERMATOLOGY: Other Dermatologic Preparations

alitretinoin (*Panretin*) ▶Not absorbed ♀D ▶- $$$$$

WARNING - May cause fetal harm if significant absorption were to occur. Women of childbearing age should be advised to avoid becoming pregnant during treatment.

ADULT - Cutaneous lesions of AIDS-related Kaposi's sarcoma: apply bid-qid.

PEDS - Not approved in children.

FORMS - Trade only: gel 60 g.

aluminum chloride (*Drysol, Certain Dri*) ▶K ♀? ▶? $

ADULT - Hyperhidrosis: apply qhs. For maximum effect, cover area with plastic wrap held in place with tight shirt and wash area following morning. Once excessive sweating stopped, use once or twice weekly.

PEDS - Not approved in children.

FORMS - Rx: Trade/Generic: solution 20%: 37.5 ml bottle, 35, 60 ml bottle with applicator. OTC: Trade (Certain Dri): solution 12.5%: 36 ml bottle.

NOTES - To prevent irritation, apply to dry area.

aminolevulinic acid (*Levulan Kerastick*) ▶Not absorbed ♀C ▶? $$$

ADULT - Non-hyperkeratotic actinic keratoses: apply solution to lesions on scalp or face; expose to special light source 14-18 h later.

PEDS - Not approved in children.

FORMS - Trade only: 20% solution single use ampules.

NOTES - Solution should be applied by healthcare personnel. Advise patients to avoid sunlight during 14-18 h period before blue light illumination.

azelaic acid (*Finacea*) ▶K ♀B ▶? $$$

ADULT - Rosacea: apply bid.

PEDS - Not approved in children.

FORMS - Trade only: gel 15%, 30g.

NOTES - Monitor for hypopigmentation esp in patients with dark complexions. Avoid use of occlusive dressings.

becaplermin (*Regranex*) ▶Minimal absorption ♀C ▶? $$$$$

ADULT - Diabetic neuropathic ulcers: apply qd and cover with saline-moistened gauze for 12 hours. Rinse after 12 h and cover with saline gauze without medication.

PEDS - Not approved in children.

FORMS - Trade only: gel 0.01% 2,7.5,15 g.

NOTES - Length of gel to be applied calculated by size of wound (length x width x 0.6 = amount of gel in inches). If ulcer does not decrease by 30% in size by 10 weeks, or complete healing has not occurred by 20 weeks, continued therapy should be reassessed.

botulinum toxin (*Botox, Botox Cosmetic*) ▶Not absorbed ♀C ▶? $$$$$

ADULT - Blepharospasm: 1.25-2.5 units injected into orbicularis oculi of upper and lower lids. Strabismus: 1.25-5.0 units depending on diagnosis, injected into extraocular muscles. Cervical dystonia: Individualize dose. Primary axillary hyperhidrosis: Inject 50 units/axilla. Moderate to severe glabellar lines in patients ≤65 yo: inject 0.1 mL into 5 sites.

PEDS - Not approved in children.

FORMS - Trade only: 100 unit single-use vials.

calamine ▶? ♀? ▶? $

ADULT - Itching due to poison ivy/oak/sumac, insect bites, or minor irritation: apply up to tid-qid prn.

PEDS - Itching due to poison ivy/oak/sumac, insect bites, or minor irritation (>2 yo): apply up to tid-qid prn.

FORMS - OTC Generic: lotion 120, 240, 480 ml.

capsaicin (*Zostrix, Zostrix-HP*) ▶? ♀? ▶? $

ADULT - Pain due to rheumatoid arthritis, osteoarthritis, and neuralgias such as zoster or diabetic neuropathies: apply to affected area up to tid-qid.

PEDS - Children >2yo: Pain due to rheumatoid arthritis, osteoarthritis, and neuralgias such as zoster or diabetic neuropathies: apply to affected area up to tid-qid.

UNAPPROVED ADULT - Psoriasis and intractable pruritus, postmastectomy/ postamputation neuromas (phantom limb pain), vulvar vestibulitis, apocrine chromhidrosis and reflex sympathetic dystrophy.

FORMS - OTC Generic/Trade: cream 0.025% 45,60 g, 0.075% 30,60 g, lotion 0.025% 59 ml, 0.075% 59 ml, gel 0.025% 15,30 g, 0.05% 43 g, roll-on 0.075% 60 ml.

NOTES - Burning occurs in ≥30% patients but diminishes with continued use. Pain more commenly occurs when applied <3-4 times/day. Wash hands immediately after application.

coal tar (*Polytar, Tegrin, Cutar, Tarsum*) ▶? ♀? ▶? $

ADULT - Dandruff, seborrheic dermatitis: apply shampoo at least twice a week. Psoriasis: apply to affected areas qd to qid or use shampoo on affected areas.

PEDS - Children >2 yo: Dandruff, seborrheic dermatitis: apply shampoo at least twice a week. Psoriasis: apply to affected areas qd to qid or use shampoo on affected areas.

FORMS - OTC Generic/Trade: shampoo, conditioner, cream, ointment, gel, lotion, soap, oil.

NOTES - May cause photosensitivity for up to 24 h after application.

doxepin (*Zonalon*) ▶L ♀B ▶- $

ADULT - Pruritus associated with atopic dermatitis, lichen simplex chronicus, eczematous dermatitis: apply qid for up to 8 days.

PEDS - Not approved in children.

FORMS - Trade only: cream 5% 30,45 g.

NOTES - Risk of systemic toxicity increased if applied to >10% of body. Can cause contact dermatitis.

eflornithine (Vaniqa) ▶K ♀C ▶? $$

ADULT - Reduction of facial hair: apply to face bid at least 8 h apart.

PEDS - Not approved in children.

FORMS - Trade only: cream 13.9% 30 g.

NOTES - Takes ≥4-8 weeks to see an effect.

EMLA (lidocaine + prilocaine) ▶LK ♀B ▶? $$

ADULT - Topical anesthesia for minor dermal procedures (eg, IV cannulation, venipuncture) apply 2.5 g over 20-25 cm² area or 1 disc at least 1 hour prior to procedure, for major dermal procedures (ie, skin grafting harvesting) apply 2 g per 10 cm² area ≥2h prior to procedure.

PEDS - Prior to circumcision in infants >37 weeks gestation: apply a max dose 1g over max of 10 cm². Topical anesthesia: Children age 1-3 mo or <5 kg: apply a max 1 g over max of 10 cm²; age 4-12 mo and >5kg: apply max 2 g over a max of 20 cm²; age 1-6 yo and >10kg: apply max 10g over max of 100 cm²; age 7-12 yo and >20kg: apply max 20g over max of 200 cm².

FORMS - Trade only: cream (2.5% lidocaine + 2.5% prilocaine) 5, g, disc 1 g. Trade/generic: cream (2.5% lidocaine + 2.5% prilocaine) 30 g.

NOTES - Cover cream with an occlusive dressing. Do not use in children <12 mo if child is receiving treatment with methemoglobin-inducing agents. Patients with glucose-6-phosphate deficiencies are more susceptible to methemoglobinemia. Dermal analgesia increases for up to 3 h under occlusive dressings, and persists for 1-2 h after removal.

finasteride (Propecia) ▶L ♀X ▶- $$

ADULT - Androgenetic alopecia in men: 1 mg PO qd.

PEDS - Not approved in children.

UNAPPROVED ADULT - Androgenetic alopecia in postmenopausal women (no evidence of efficacy): 1 mg PO qd.

FORMS - Trade only: tab 1 mg.

NOTES - May require ≥3 months before benefit seen. Monitor PSA before therapy; finasteride will decrease PSA by 50% in patients with BPH, even with prostate cancer. Contraindicated in pregnancy or possible pregnancy. Women should not handle crushed or broken tabs if they are or could be pregnant.

hyaluronic acid (Restylane) ▶? ♀? ▶? $$$$$

ADULT - Moderate to severe facial wrinkles: inject into wrinkle/fold.

PEDS - Not approved in children.

FORMS - Rx: 0.4 mL and 0.7 mL syringe.

NOTES - Do not use more than 1.5 mL per treatment area. Contains trace amounts of gram positive bacterial proteins; contraindicated if history of anaphylaxis or severe allergy.

hydroquinone (Eldopaque, Eldoquin, Eldoquin Forte, EpiQuin Micro, Esoterica, Lustra, Melanex, Solaquin) ▶? ♀C ▶? $$$

ADULT - Temporary bleaching of hyperpigmented skin conditions (ie, chloasma, melasma, freckles, senile lentigines, ultraviolet-induced discoloration from oral contraceptives, pregnancy, or hormone replacement therapy): apply bid to affected area.

PEDS - Not approved in children.

FORMS - OTC Generic/Trade: cream 1.5%, lotion 2%. Rx Generic/Trade: solution 3%, gel 4%, cream 4%.

NOTES - Responses may take 3 weeks - 6 months. Use a sunscreen on treated, exposed areas.

lactic acid (Lac-Hydrin) ▶? ♀? ▶? $$

ADULT - Ichthyosis vulgaris and xerosis (dry, scaly skin): apply bid to affected area.

PEDS - Ichthyosis vulgaris and xerosis (dry, scaly skin) in children >2 yo: apply bid to affected area.

FORMS - Trade only: lotion 12% 150,360 ml. Trade/Generic: cream 12% 140,385 g.

NOTES - Frequently causes irritation in non-intact skin.

lidocaine (Xylocaine, Lidoderm, Numby Stuff, ELA-Max) ▶LK ♀B ▶? $$

ADULT - Topical anesthesia: apply to affected area prn. Dose varies with anesthetic procedure, degree of anesthesia required and individual patient response. Post-herpetic neuralgia (patch): apply up to 3 patches for up to 12h within a 24h period.

PEDS - Topical anesthesia: apply to affected area prn. Dose varies with anesthetic procedure, degree of anesthesia required and individual patient response. Max 3 mg/kg/dose, do not repeat dose within 2 hours.

UNAPPROVED PEDS - Topical anesthesia prior to venipuncture: apply 30 min prior to procedure (ELA-Max 4%).

FORMS - For membranes of mouth and pharynx: spray 10%, ointment 5%, liquid 5%, solution 2,4%, dental patch. For urethral use: jelly 2%. Patch (Lidoderm) 5%. OTC: Trade: liposomal lidocaine 4%, 5% (ELA-Max).

methylaminolevulinate ▶Not absorbed ♀C ▶?

ADULT - Non-hyperkeratotic actinic keratoses of face/scalp: Apply cream 1 mm thick (max 1 g) to lesion & 5 mm surrounding area; cover with dressing x 3h; remove dressing and cream and perform illumination therapy. Repeat in 7 days.

PEDS - Not approved in children.

FORMS - Trade only: cream: 16.8%, 2 g.

NOTES - Use in immunocompetent individuals. Lesion debridement should be performed prior to application. Made with peanut & almond oil; has not been tested in peanut allergy.

minoxidil (*Rogaine, Rogaine Forte, Rogaine Extra Strength, Minoxidil for Men*, ♣*Minox, Apo-Gain*) ▶K ♀C ▶- $$

ADULT - Androgenetic alopecia in men or women: 1 ml to dry scalp bid.

PEDS - Not approved in children.

UNAPPROVED ADULT - Alopecia areata.

UNAPPROVED PEDS - Alopecia: Apply to dry scalp bid.

FORMS - OTC Trade only: solution 2%, 60 ml, 5%, 60 ml, 5% (Rogaine Extra Strength - for men only) 60 ml.

NOTES - 5% strength for men only. Alcohol content may cause burning and stinging. Evidence of hair growth usually takes ≥4 months. If treatment is stopped, new hair will be shed in a few months.

oatmeal (*Aveeno*) ▶Not absorbed ♀? ▶? $

ADULT - Pruritus from poison ivy/oak, varicella: apply lotion qid prn. Also available in packets to be added to bath.

PEDS - Pruritus from poison ivy/oak, varicella: apply lotion qid prn. Also available in bath packets for tub.

FORMS - OTC Generic/Trade: lotion, packets.

poly-L-lactic acid (*Sculptra*) ▶Not absorbed ♀? ▶? ?

ADULT - Restoration of facial fat loss due to HIV lipoatrophy: dose based on degree of correction needed.

PEDS - Not approved in children <18 yo.

***Pramosone* (pramoxine + hydrocortisone)** ▶Not absorbed ♀X ▶? $$$

ADULT - Inflammatory and pruritic manifestations of corticosteroid-responsive dermatoses: Apply tid-qid.

PEDS - Apply bid-tid.

FORMS - Trade only: 1% pramoxine/1% hydrocortisone acetate: cream 30, 60 g, oint 30 g, lotion 60, 120, 240 mL. 1% pramoxine/2.5% hydrocortisone acetate: cream 30, 60 g, oint 30 g, lotion 60, 120 mL.

NOTES - Monitor for hyperglycemia / adrenal suppression if used for long period of time or over a large area of the body, especially in children. Chronic administration may interfere with pediatric growth & development.

selenium sulfide (*Selsun, Exsel, Versel*) ▶? ♀C ▶? $

ADULT - Dandruff, seborrheic dermatitis: Massage 5-10 ml of shampoo into wet scalp, allow to remain 2-3 minutes, rinse. Apply twice a week for 2 weeks. For maintenance, less frequent administration needed. Tinea versicolor: Apply 2.5% shampoo/lotion to affected area, allow to remain on skin 10 min, rinse. Repeat qd x 7days.

PEDS - Dandruff, seborrheic dermatitis: Massage 5-10 ml of shampoo into wet scalp, allow to remain 2-3 minutes, rinse. Apply twice a week for 2 weeks. For maintenance, less frequent administration needed. Tinea versicolor: Apply 2.5% lotion/shampoo to affected area, allow to remain on skin 10 min, rinse. Repeat qd x 7days.

FORMS - OTC Generic/Trade: lotion/shampoo 1% 120,210,240, 330 ml, 2.5% 120 ml. Rx generic/trade: lotion/shampoo 2.5% 120 ml.

***Solag* (mequinol + tretinoin, ♣*Solagé*)** ▶Not absorbed ♀X ▶? $$$$

ADULT - Solar lentigines: apply bid separated by at least 8 hrs.

PEDS - Not approved in children.

FORMS - Trade only: soln 30 ml (mequinol 2% + tretinoin 0.01%).

NOTES - Use in non-Caucasians has not been evaluated. Avoid in patients taking photosensitizers. Minimize exposure to sunlight.

thalidomide (*Thalomid*) ▶Plasma ♀X ▶? $$$$$

WARNING - Pregnancy category X. Has caused severe, life-threatening human birth defects. Available only through special restricted distribution program. Prescribers and pharmacists must be registered in this program in order to prescribe or dispense.

ADULT - Erythema nodosum leprosum: 100-400 mg PO qhs. Initial episodes, patients <50 kg should be started on low end of dosing range.

PEDS - Not approved in children.

FORMS - Trade only: cap 50, 100, 200 mg.

***Tri-Luma* (fluocinolone + hydroquinone + tretinoin)** ▶Minimal absorption ♀C ▶? $$$

ADULT – Facial melasma: apply qhs x 4-8 wks.

PEDS - Not approved in children.

FORMS - Trade only: soln 30 g (fluocinolone 0.01% + hydroquinone 4% + tretinoin 0.05%).

NOTES - Minimize exposure to sunlight. Not intended for melasma maintenance therapy.

ENDOCRINE & METABOLIC: Androgens / Anabolic Steroids

NOTE: Monitor LFTs & lipids. See OB/GYN section for other hormones.

fluoxymesterone (*Halotestin*) ▶L ♀X ▶? ©III $$$

ADULT - Palliative treatment of androgen-responsive recurrent breast cancer in women who are 1-5 years postmenopausal: 5-10 mg PO bid-qid x 1-3 months. Hypogonadism: 5-20 mg PO qd.

PEDS - Delayed puberty in males: 2.5-10 mg PO qd x 4-6 months.

FORMS - Trade: Tabs (scored) 2, 5 mg . Generic/Trade: Tabs (scored) 10 mg.

NOTES - Transdermal or injectable therapy preferred for hypogonadism. Pediatric use by specialists who monitor bone maturation q6 months. Prolonged high-dose use may cause hepatic adenomas, hepatocellular carcinoma, and peliosis hepatitis. Monitor bone maturation q6 months during treatment of prepubertal male.

methyltestosterone (*Android, Methitest, Testred, Virilon*) ▶L ♀X ▶? ©III $$$

ADULT - Advancing inoperable breast cancer in women who are 1-5 years postmenopausal: 50-200 mg/day PO in divided doses. Hypogonadism: 10-50 mg PO qd.

PEDS - Delayed puberty in males: 10 mg PO qd x 4-6 months.

FORMS - Trade: Caps 10 mg. Generic/Trade: Tabs 10, 25 mg.

NOTES - Transdermal or injectable therapy preferred to oral for hypogonadism. Pediatric use by specialists who monitor bone maturation q6 months. Prolonged high-dose use may cause hepatic adenomas, hepatocellular carcinoma, peliosis hepatitis. Monitor bone maturation q6 months during treatment of prepubertal male.

nandrolone (*Deca-Durabolin*) ▶L ♀X ▶- ©III $$$

WARNING - Peliosis hepatitis, liver cell tumors, and lipid changes have occurred secondary to anabolic steroid use.

ADULT - Anemia of renal insufficiency: women 50-100 mg IM q wk, men 100-200 mg IM q wk.

PEDS - Anemia of renal disease age 2- 13 yo: 25- 50 mg IM q3-4 weeks.

FORMS - Generic/Trade: injection 100 mg/ml, 200 mg/ml. Trade only: injection 50 mg/ml.

NOTES - Pediatric use by specialists who monitor bone maturation q6 months. Long-term use may cause hepatic adenomas, hepatocellular carcinoma, and peliosis hepatitis.

oxandrolone (*Oxandrin*) ▶L ♀X ▶? ©III $$$$$

WARNING - Peliosis hepatitis, liver cell tumors, and lipid changes have occurred secondary to anabolic steroid use.

ADULT - To promote weight gain following extensive surgery, chronic infection, or severe trauma; in some patients who fail to gain or maintain weight without a physiologic cause; to offset protein catabolism associated with long-term corticosteroid therapy: 2.5 mg PO bid-qid for 2-4 wks. Max 20 mg/day. May repeat therapy intermittently as indicated.

PEDS - Weight gain: ≤0.1 mg/kg or ≤0.045 mg/pound PO divided bid-qid for 2-4 wks. May repeat therapy intermittently as indicated.

FORMS - Trade: Tabs 2.5, 10 mg.

NOTES - Contraindicated in known or suspected prostate/breast cancer. Not shown to enhance athletic ability. Associated with dyslipidemia. Pediatric use by specialists who monitor bone maturation q6 months. Long-term use may cause hepatic adenomas, hepatocellular carcinoma, and peliosis hepatitis. May increase anticoagulant effects of warfarin.

stanozolol (*Winstrol*) ▶L ♀X ▶- ©III $

WARNING - Peliosis hepatitis, liver cell tumors, and lipid changes have occurred secondary to anabolic steroid use.

ADULT - Hereditary Angioedema: Start 2 mg PO tid. After favorable response, decrease dose at interval of 1-3 months to a maintenance dose of 2 mg qd or 2 mg every other day.

PEDS - Not approved in children.

FORMS - Trade: tabs 2 mg

NOTES - Long-term use may cause hepatic adenomas. Hepatocellular neoplasm & peliosis hepatitis may occur. Monitor LFTS & hemoglobin periodically. May increase effects of anticoagulants.

testosterone (*Androderm, Androgel, Delatestryl, Depo-Testosterone, Depotest, Everone, Striant, Testim, Testopel, Testro AQ, Testro-L.A., Virilon IM, ♥Androil*) ▶L ♀X ▶? ©III $$$$

ADULT - Hypogonadism: injectable enanthate or cypionate- 50-400 mg IM q2-4 weeks. Androderm- 5 mg patch qhs to clean, dry area of skin on back, abdomen, upper arms, or thighs. Non-virilized patients start with 2.5 mg patch qhs. AndroGel 1% (5 g): apply 1 foil packet of gel qd to clean, dry, intact skin of the shoulders, upper arms, or abdomen. May increase dose to 7.5-10 g after 2 weeks. Testim: One tube (5 g) qd to the clean, dry intact skin of the shoulders or upper arms. May increase dose to 2 tubes (10 g) after 2 weeks. For topical administration, obtain serum testosterone level 2 weeks after initiation, then increase dose if necessary. Testopel: 2-6 pellets (150-450 mg testosterone) pellets SC q 3-6 months. 2 pellets for each 25 mg testosterone propionate required weekly. Buccal- Striant: 30 mg q12 hours on upper gum above the incisor tooth; alternate sides for each application.

PEDS - Not approved in children.

FORMS - Trade only: Patch 2.5, 5 mg (Androderm). Gel 1% 2.5, 5 g (AndroGel). Gel 1%, 5 g (Testim). Pellet 75mg (Testopel). Buccal: blister packs - 30 mg (Striant). Injection 200 mg/ml (enanthate). Generic/Trade: injection 100, 200 mg/ml (cypionate).

NOTES - Do not apply Androderm, or AndroGel to scrotum. Do not apply Testim to the scrotum or abdomen. Pellet implantation is less flexible for dosage adjustment, therefore, take great care when estimating the amount of testosterone. Prolonged high-dose use may cause hepatic adenomas, hepatocellular carcinoma, and peliosis hepatitis. May promote the development of prostatic hyperplasia or prostate cancer. Monitor hemoglobin and PSA. Advise patient to regularly inspect the gum region where Striant is applied; report any abnormality.

ENDOCRINE & METABOLIC: Bisphosphonates

NOTE: Supplemental Vit D and calcium are recommended for osteoporosis prevention & treatment.

alendronate (*Fosamax*) ▶K ♀C ▶- $$$
ADULT - Postmenopausal osteoporosis prevention (5 mg PO qd or 35 mg PO weekly) & treatment (10 mg qd or 70 mg PO weekly). Glucocorticoid-induced osteoporosis: 5 mg PO qd or 10 mg PO qd (postmenopausal women not taking estrogen). Treatment of osteoporosis in men: 10 mg PO qd or consider 70 mg PO weekly. Paget's disease: 40 mg PO qd x 6 months.

PEDS - Not approved in children.

UNAPPROVED ADULT - Glucocorticoid-induced osteoporosis prevention: 5 mg PO qd or 35 mg PO weekly; 10 mg PO qd or 70 mg PO weekly (postmenopausal women not taking estrogen).

FORMS - Trade: Tabs 5,10,35,40,70 mg. Oral soln 70 mg/75 mL (single dose bottle).

NOTES - May cause esophagitis, esophageal ulcers and esophageal erosions, occasionally with bleeding and rarely followed by esophageal stricture or perforation. Monitor frequently for dysphagia, odynophagia, and retrosternal pain. Take 30 minutes before first food, beverage, or medication of the day with a full glass of water only. Remain in upright position for ≥30 minutes following dose. Caution if CrCl <35 ml/min.

clodronate (♣*Ostac, Bonefos*) ▶K ♀D ▶- $$$
ADULT - Canada only. Hypercalcemia of malignancy; management of osteolysis resulting from bone metastases of malignant tumors: IV single dose - 1500 mg slow infusion over ≥4 hours. IV multiple dose - 300 mg slow infusion qd over 2-6 hours up to 10 days. Oral - following IV therapy, maintenance 1600-2400 mg/day in single or divided doses. Max PO dose 3200 mg/day; duration of therapy is usually 6 months.

PEDS - Not approved in children.

FORMS - Trade: Capsules 400 mg.

NOTES - Contraindicated if creat >5 mg/dl or if severe GI tract inflammation. Avoid rapid bolus which may cause severe local reactions, thrombophlebitis, or renal failure. Do not mix with calcium-containing infusions. Ensure adequate hydration prior to infusion. Normocalcemia usually occurs within 2-5 days after initiation of therapy with multiple dose infusion. Monitor serum calcium, renal function in those with renal insufficiency, LFTs & hematological parameters.

etidronate (*Didronel*) ▶K ♀C ▶? $$$$
ADULT - Hypercalcemia: 7.5 mg/kg in 250 ml NS IV over ≥2h qd for 3 days. May start oral therapy the day following the last IV dose at 20 mg/kg/day x 30 days. Paget's disease: 5-10 mg/kg PO qd x 6 months or 11-20 mg/kg qd x 3 months. Heterotopic ossification with hip replacement: 20 mg/kg/day PO x 1 month before and 3 months after surgery. Heterotopic ossification with spinal cord injury: 20 mg/kg/day PO x 2 weeks, then 10 mg/kg/day PO x 10 weeks.

PEDS - Not approved in children.

UNAPPROVED ADULT - Postmenopausal osteoporosis: 400 mg PO qd x 14 days every 3 months (intermittent cyclical therapy).

FORMS - Generic/Trade: Tabs 200, 400 mg.

NOTES - Divide oral dose if GI discomfort occurs. Avoid food, vitamins with minerals, or antacids within 2 h of dose.

ibandronate (Boniva) ▶K ♀C ▶? ?
ADULT - Approved, but not yet marketed. Treatment/Prevention of postmenopausal osteoporosis: 2.5 mg PO qd.
PEDS - Not approved in children.
FORMS - Trade: 2.5 mg tabs.
NOTES - May cause esophagitis. Take 1 hr before first food/drink; remain in upright position 1 hr after taking. Avoid if CrCl <30 mL/min.

pamidronate (Aredia) ▶K ♀D ▶? $$$$$
WARNING - Single dose should not exceed 90 mg due to risk of renal impairment/failure.
ADULT - Hypercalcemia of malignancy, moderate (corrected Ca= 12-13.5 mg/dl): 60-90 mg IV single dose infused over 2-24 h. Hypercalcemia of malignancy, severe (Ca >13.5 mg/dl): 90 mg IV single dose infused over 2-24 h. Wait ≥7 days before considering retreatment. Paget's disease: 30 mg IV over 4h qd x 3 days. Osteolytic bone lesions: 90 mg IV over 4 h once monthly. Osteolytic bone metastases: 90 mg IV over 2 h q3-4 weeks.
PEDS - Not approved in children.
UNAPPROVED ADULT - Mild hypercalcemia: 30 mg IV single dose over 4 h. Osteoporosis treatment: 30 mg IV q 3 months.
UNAPPROVED PEDS - Osteogenesis imperfecta: 3.0 mg/kg IV over 4 hr q4-6 month.
NOTES - Fever occurs in 20% of patients. Monitor creatinine prior to each dose. Withhold dose in patients with bone metastases if renal function deteriorates. Longer infusions (>2 h) may reduce renal toxicity.

risedronate (Actonel) ▶K ♀C ▶? $$$
ADULT - Paget's disease: 30 mg PO qd x 2 months. Postmenopausal and glucocorticoid-induced osteoporosis prevention and treatment: 5 mg PO qd or 35 mg PO weekly.
PEDS - Not approved in children.
UNAPPROVED ADULT - Glucocorticoid-induced osteoporosis treatment and preven-
tion: 35 mg PO weekly.
FORMS - Trade: Tabs 5, 30 mg.
NOTES - May cause esophagitis, monitor frequently for dysphagia, odynophagia, and retrosternal pain; take 30 minutes before first food, beverage, or medication of the day with a full glass of water only. Remain in upright position for ≥30 minutes following dose.

tiludronate (Skelid) ▶K ♀C ▶? $$$$$
ADULT - Paget's disease: 400 mg PO qd x 3 months.
PEDS - Not approved in children.
FORMS - Trade: Tabs 200 mg.
NOTES - May cause esophagitis; take 30 minutes before first food, beverage, or medication of the day with a full glass of water only. Remain in upright position for ≥30 minutes following dose.

zoledronic acid (Zometa) ▶K ♀D ▶? $$$$$
WARNING - Avoid single doses >4 mg, infusions <15 min, and use in those with bone metastases with severe renal impairment.
ADULT - Hypercalcemia of malignancy (corrected Ca ≥12 mg/dL): 4 mg single dose IV infusion over ≥15 min. Wait ≥7 days before considering retreatment. Multiple myeloma and metastatic bone lesions from solid tumors: 4 mg IV infusion over ≥15 min q3-4 weeks. Metastatic hormone-resistant prostate cancer: 4 mg IV q3-4 weeks.
PEDS - Not approved in children.
UNAPPROVED ADULT - Osteoporosis: 4 mg IV dose once yearly. Metastatic hormone-sensitive prostate cancer: 4 mg IV q3-4 weeks.
NOTES - Monitor serum creatinine (before each dose), lytes, calcium, phosphate, magnesium and Hb/HCT (regularly). Avoid use in severe renal impairment and hold dosing with worsening renal function. Maintain adequate hydration for those with hypercalcemia of malignancy, and give 500 mg calcium supplement and vitamin D 400 IU PO qd to those with multiple myeloma or metastatic bone lesions.

ENDOCRINE & METABOLIC: Corticosteroids

NOTE: See also dermatology, ophthalmology.
betamethasone (Celestone, Celestone Soluspan, ✚Betnesol) ▶L ♀C ▶- $$$$$
ADULT - Anti-inflammatory/Immunosuppressive: 0.6-7.2 mg/day PO divided bid-qid or up to 9 mg/day IM. 0.25-2.0 ml intraarticular depending on location and size of joint.
PEDS - Dosing guidelines have not been established.
UNAPPROVED PEDS - Anti-inflammatory/ Immunosuppressive: 0.0175-0.25 mg/kg/day PO divided tid-qid. Fetal lung maturation, maternal antepartum: 12 mg IM q24h x 2 doses.
FORMS - Trade: Syrup 0.6 mg/5 ml.
NOTES - Avoid prolonged use in children due to

possible bone growth retardation. Monitor growth & development if prolonged therapy is necessary.

cortisone (*Cortone*) ▶L ♀D ▶- $

ADULT - Adrenocortical insufficiency: 25-300 mg PO qd.

PEDS - Dosing guidelines have not been established.

UNAPPROVED PEDS - Adrenocortical insufficiency: 0.5-0.75 mg/kg/day PO divided q8h.

FORMS - Generic/Trade: Tabs 5, 10, 25 mg.

dexamethasone (*Decadron*, *Dexone*, *♣Dexasone, Hexadrol*) ▶L ♀C ▶- $

ADULT - Anti-inflammatory/Immunosuppressive: 0.5-9 mg/day PO/IV/IM divided bid- qid. Cerebral edema: 10-20 mg IV load, then 4 mg IM q6h (off-label IV use common) or 1-3 mg PO tid.

PEDS - Dosage in children <12 yo of age has not been established.

UNAPPROVED ADULT - Initial treatment of immune thrombocytopenic purpura: 40 mg PO qd x 4 days.

UNAPPROVED PEDS - Anti-inflammatory/ immunosuppressive: 0.08-0.3 mg/kg/day PO/IV/ IM divided q6-12h. Croup: 0.15-0.6 mg/kg PO/IV/IM x 1. Bacterial meningitis: 0.15 mg/kg/dose IV q6h x 16 doses.

FORMS - Generic/Trade: Tabs 0.25, 0.5, 0.75, 1.0, 1.5, 2, 4, 6 mg. elixir/ solution 0.5 mg/5 ml. Trade only: oral solution 0.5 mg/ 0.5 ml. Decadron unipak (0.75 mg-12 tabs).

NOTES - Avoid prolonged use in children due to possible bone growth retardation. Monitor growth & development if prolonged therapy is necessary.

fludrocortisone (*Florinef*) ▶L ♀C ▶? $

ADULT - Adrenocortical insufficiency/ Addison's disease: 0.1 mg PO 3 times weekly to 0.2 mg PO qd. Salt-losing adrenogenital syndrome: 0.1-0.2 mg PO qd.

PEDS - Not approved in children.

UNAPPROVED ADULT - Postural hypotension: 0.05-0.4 mg PO qd.

UNAPPROVED PEDS - Adrenocortical insufficiency: 0.05-0.2 mg PO qd.

FORMS - Generic/Trade: Tabs 0.1 mg.

NOTES - Usually given in conjunction with cortisone or hydrocortisone for adrenocortical insufficiency.

hydrocortisone (*Cortef, Hydrocortone, Solu-Cortef*) ▶L ♀C ▶- $

ADULT - Adrenocortical insufficiency: 20-240 mg/day PO divided tid-qid or 100-500 mg IV/IM q2-10h prn (sodium succinate).

PEDS - Dosing guidelines not established.

UNAPPROVED PEDS - Chronic adrenocortical insufficiency: 0.5-0.75 mg/kg/day PO divided q8h or 0.25-0.35 mg/kg/day IM qd. Acute adrenocortical insufficiency: infants & young children 1-2 mg/kg IV bolus, then 25-150 mg/day divided q6-8 hours. Older children 1-2 mg/kg IV bolus, then 150-250 mg/day IV q6-8 hours.

FORMS - Trade: Tabs 5 mg. Generic/Trade: Tabs 10, 20 mg.

NOTES - Agent of choice for adrenocortical insufficiency because of mixed glucocorticoid and mineralocorticoid properties at doses >100 mg/day.

methylprednisolone (*Solu-Medrol, Medrol, Depo-Medrol*) ▶L ♀C ▶- $$$

ADULT - Anti-inflammatory/Immunosuppressive: Parenteral (Solu-Medrol) 10- 250 mg IV/IM q4h prn. Oral (Medrol) 4- 48 mg PO qd. Medrol Dosepak tapers 24 to 0 mg PO over 7d. IM/ joints (Depo-Medrol) 4- 120 mg IM q1-2 weeks.

PEDS - Dosing guidelines not established.

UNAPPROVED PEDS - Anti-inflammatory/ Immunosuppressive: 0.5-1.7 mg/kg/day PO/IV/IM divided q6-12h.

FORMS - Trade only: Tabs 2, 8, 16, 24, 32 mg. Generic/Trade: Tabs 4 mg. Medrol Dosepak (4 mg-21 tabs).

prednisolone (*Delta-Cortef, Prelone, Pediapred, Orapred*) ▶L ♀C ▶+ $$

ADULT - Anti-inflammatory/ Immunosuppressive: 5- 60 mg/day PO/IV/IM.

PEDS - Dosing guidelines not established.

UNAPPROVED PEDS - Anti-inflammatory/ Immunosuppressive: 0.1-2 mg/kg/day PO divided qd-qid or 0.04-0.25 mg/kg/day IV/IM divided qd-bid. Early active rheumatoid arthritis: 10 mg/day PO.

FORMS - Generic/Trade: Tabs 5 mg; syrup 5 mg/5 ml, 15 mg/5 ml (Prelone; wild cherry flavor). Generic/Trade: solution 5 mg/5 ml (Pediapred; raspberry flavor); solution 15 mg/5 ml (Orapred; grape flavor).

prednisone (*Deltasone, Meticorten, Pred-Pak, Sterapred, ♣Winpred*) ▶L ♀C ▶+ $

ADULT - Anti-inflammatory/ Immunosuppressive: 5-60 mg/day PO qd or divided bid-qid.

PEDS - Dosing guidelines have not been established.

UNAPPROVED PEDS - Anti-inflammatory/ Immunosuppressive: 0.05-2 mg/kg/day divided qd-qid.

FORMS - Generic/Trade: Tabs 1, 5, 10, 20, 50 mg. Trade only: Tabs 2.5 mg. Sterapred (5 mg tabs: tapers 30 to 5 mg PO over 6d or 30 to 10

mg over 12d), Sterapred DS (10 mg tabs: tapers 60 to 10 mg over 6d, or 60 to 20 mg PO over 12d) & Pred-Pak (5 mg 45 & 79 tabs) taper packs. Solution 5 mg/5 ml & 5 mg/ml (Prednisone Intensol).
NOTES - Conversion to prednisolone may be impaired in liver disease.

triamcinolone (Aristocort, Kenalog, ♣Aristospan) ▶L ♀C ▶- $$$$
ADULT - Anti-inflammatory/ Immunosuppressive: 4-48 mg/day PO divided qd-qid. 2.5-60 mg IM qd (Kenalog). 40 mg IM q week (Aristocort).
PEDS - Dosing guidelines not established.
UNAPPROVED PEDS - Anti-inflammatory/ Immunosuppressive: 0.117-1.66 mg/kg/day PO divided qid.
FORMS - Generic/Trade: Tabs 4 mg. Trade only: injection 10 mg/ml, 25 mg/ml, 40 mg/ml.
NOTES - Parenteral form not for IV use.

CORTICOSTEROIDS	Approximate equivalent dose (mg)	Relative anti-inflammatory potency	Relative mineralocorti-coid potency	Biologic Half-life (hours)
betamethasone	0.6-0.75	20-30	0	36-54
cortisone	25	0.8	2	8-12
dexamethasone	0.75	20-30	0	36-54
fludrocortisone	--	10	125	18-36
hydrocortisone	20	1	2	8-12
methylprednisolone	4	5	0	18-36
prednisolone	5	4	1	18-36
prednisone	5	4	1	18-36
triamcinolone	4	5	0	12-36

ENDOCRINE & METABOLIC: Diabetes-Related – Alphaglucosidase Inhibitors

acarbose (Precose, ♣Prandase) ▶Gut/K ♀B ▶- $$
ADULT - Diabetes: initiate therapy with 25 mg PO tid with the first bite of each meal. Start with 25 mg PO qd to minimize GI adverse effects. May increase to 50 mg PO tid after 4-8 weeks. Usual range is 50-100 mg PO tid. Maximum dose for patients ≤60 kg is 50 mg tid, >60 kg is 100 mg tid.
PEDS - Not approved in children.
FORMS - Trade: Tabs 25, 50, 100 mg.
NOTES - Acarbose alone should not cause hypoglycemia. If hypoglycemia occurs, treat with oral glucose rather than sucrose (table sugar). Adverse GI effects (eg, flatulence, diarrhea,

abdominal pain) may occur with initial therapy.
miglitol (Glyset) ▶K ♀B ▶- $$$
ADULT - Diabetes: Initiate therapy with 25 mg PO tid with the first bite of each meal. Use 25 mg PO qd to start if GI adverse effects. May increase dose to 50 mg PO tid after 4-8 weeks, max 300 mg/day.
PEDS - Not approved in children.
FORMS - Trade: Tabs 25, 50, 100 mg.
NOTES - Miglitol administered alone should not cause hypoglycemia. If hypoglycemia occurs, treat with oral glucose rather than sucrose (table sugar). Adverse GI effects (i.e. flatulence, diarrhea, abdominal pain) may occur with initial therapy.

ENDOCRINE & METABOLIC: Diabetes-Related – Biguanides & Combinations

NOTE: Metformin-containing products may cause life-threatening lactic acidosis, usually in setting of decreased tissue perfusion, hypoxia, hepatic dysfunction, or impaired renal clearance. Hold prior to IV contrast agents and for 48 h after. Avoid if ethanol abuse, heart failure (requiring treatment), hepatic or renal insufficiency (creat ≥1.4 mg/dl in women, ≥1.5 mg/dl in men), or hypoxic states (cardiogenic shock, septicemia, acute MI).

Avandamet (rosiglitazone + metformin) ▶KL ♀C ▶? $$$$
ADULT - 1 tablet PO bid. If inadequate control with metformin monotherapy, select tab strength based on adding 4 mg/day rosiglitazone to existing metformin dose. If inadequate control with rosiglitazone monotherapy, select tab strength based on adding 1000 mg/day metformin to existing rosiglitazone dose. Max 8/2000 mg/day.

PEDS - Not approved in children.

FORMS - Trade: Tabs 1/500, 2/500, 4/500, 2/1000, 4/1000 mg.

NOTES - May be given concomitantly with sulfonylureas or insulin. Caution with ethanol abuse & hypoxic states. Full effect may not be apparent for up to 12 weeks. May cause edema, weight gain, new CHF, or exacerbate existing CHF (avoid in NYHA Class III or IV). May cause resumption of ovulation in premenopausal anovulatory patients; recommend contraception use. Avoid if liver disease or ALT >2.5 x upper normal limit. Monitor LFTs before therapy, and periodically thereafter. Discontinue if ALT >3x upper normal limit. Initial GI upset may be minimized by starting with lower dose of metformin component.

Glucovance (glyburide + metformin) ▶KL ♀B ▶? $$

ADULT - Diabetes, initial therapy: Start 1.25/250 mg PO qd or bid with meals; maximum 10/2000 mg daily. Diabetes, second-line therapy: Start 2.5/500 or 5/500 mg PO bid with meals; maximum 20/2000 mg daily.

PEDS - Not approved in children.

FORMS - Trade/Generic: Tabs 1.25/250, 2.5/500, 5/500 mg

NOTES - May add thiazolidinedione if glycemic control is not obtained.

Metaglip (glipizide + metformin) ▶KL ♀C ▶? $$$

ADULT - Diabetes, as initial therapy: Start 2.5/250 mg PO qd to 2.5/500 mg PO bid with meals; max 10/2000 mg daily. Diabetes, as second-line therapy: Start 2.5/500 or 5/500 mg PO bid with meals; max 20/2000 mg daily.

PEDS - Not approved in children.

FORMS - Trade: tabs 2.5/250,2.5/500,5/500mg.

NOTES - May add thiazolidinedione if glycemic control is not obtained.

metformin (*Glucophage, Glucophage XR, Fortamet, Riomet*) ▶K ♀B ▶? $$$

ADULT - Diabetes: Glucophage: Start 500 mg PO qd-bid or 850 mg PO qd with meals. Increase by 500 mg q week or 850 mg q other week to a maximum of 2550 mg/day. Higher doses may be divided tid with meals. Glucophage XR: 500 mg PO qd with evening meal; increase by 500 mg q week to max 2000 mg/day (may divide 1000 mg PO bid). Fortamet: 500-1000 mg qd with evening meal; increase by 500 mg q week to max 2500 mg/day.

PEDS - Diabetes ≥10 yo: Start 500 mg PO qd-bid (Glucophage) with meals, increase by 500 mg q week to max 2000 mg/day in divided doses (10-16 yo). Glucophage XR & Fortamet are indicated in ≥17 yo.

UNAPPROVED ADULT - Polycystic ovary syndrome: 500 mg PO tid.

FORMS - Generic/Trade: Tabs 500, 625, 750, 850,1000 mg, extended release 500 mg. Trade only: 750 mg (Glucophage XR); 500, 1000 mg (Fortamet). Trade only: oral soln 500 mg/5 mL (Riomet).

NOTES - May be given concomitantly with sulfonylureas, thiazolidinedione or insulin.

ENDOCRINE & METABOLIC: Diabetes-Related – "Glitazones" (Thiazolidinediones)

pioglitazone (*Actos*) ▶L ♀C ▶- $$$$

ADULT - Diabetes monotherapy or in combination with a sulfonylurea, metformin, or insulin: Start 15-30 mg PO qd, may adjust dose after 3 months to max 45 mg/day.

PEDS - Not approved in children.

FORMS - Trade: Tabs 15, 30, 45 mg.

NOTES - May cause edema, weight gain, new CHF, or exacerbate existing CHF (avoid in NYHA Class III or IV). Full effect may not be apparent for up to 12 weeks. May cause resumption of ovulation in premenopausal anovulatory women; recommend contraception use. Avoid if liver disease or ALT >2.5 x normal. Monitor LFTs before therapy & periodically thereafter. Discontinue if ALT >3 x upper normal limit.

rosiglitazone (*Avandia*) ▶L ♀C ▶- $$$

ADULT - Diabetes monotherapy or in combo with metformin, sulfonylurea or insulin: Start 4 mg PO qd or divided bid, may increase after 12 weeks to max 8 mg/day as monotherapy or in combination with metformin. Max 4 mg/day when used with insulin or a sulfonylurea.

PEDS - Not approved in children <18 yo.

FORMS - Trade: Tabs 2, 4, 8 mg.

NOTES – May cause edema, weight gain, new CHF, or exacerbate existing CHF (avoid in NYHA Class III or IV). Full effect may not be apparent for up to 12 weeks. May cause resumption of ovulation in premenopausal anovulatory women; recommend contraception use. Avoid if liver disease or ALT >2.5 x normal. Monitor LFTs before therapy & periodically thereafter. Discontinue if ALT >3x upper normal limit.

ENDOCRINE & METABOLIC: Diabetes-Related - Meglitinides

nateglinide (*Starlix*) ▶L ♀C ▶? $$$
ADULT - Diabetes, monotherapy or in combination with metformin or thiazolidinedione: 120 mg PO tid ≤30 min before meals; use 60 mg PO tid in patients who are near goal A1C.
PEDS - Not approved in children.
FORMS - Trade: Tabs 60, 120 mg.
NOTES - Not to be used as monotherapy in patients inadequately controlled with glyburide or other anti-diabetic agents previously. Patients with severe renal impairment are at risk for hypoglycemic episodes.

repaglinide (*Prandin*, ♥*Gluconorm*) ▶L ♀C ▶? $$$
ADULT - Diabetes: 0.5- 2 mg PO tid within 30 minutes before a meal. Allow 1 week between dosage adjustments. Usual range is 0.5-4 mg PO tid-qid, max 16 mg/day.
PEDS - Not approved in children.
FORMS - Trade: Tabs 0.5, 1, 2 mg.
NOTES - May take dose immediately preceding meal to as long as 30 minutes before the meal. Gemfibrozil and itraconazole increase blood repaglinide levels and may result in an increased risk of hypoglycemia.

ENDOCRINE & METABOLIC: Diabetes-Related – Sulfonylureas – 1st Generation

chlorpropamide (*Diabinese*) ▶LK ♀C ▶- $
ADULT - Initiate therapy with 100-250 mg PO qd. Titrate after 5-7 days by increments of 50-125 mg at intervals of 3-5 days to obtain optimal control. Max 750 mg/day.
PEDS - Not approved in children.
FORMS - Generic/Trade: Tabs 100, 250 mg.
NOTES - Clinical use in the elderly has not been properly evaluated. Elderly are more prone to hypoglycemia and/or hyponatremia possibly from renal impairment or drug interactions. May cause disulfiram-like reaction with alcohol.

tolazamide (*Tolinase*) ▶LK ♀C ▶? $
ADULT - Initiate therapy with 100 mg PO qd in patients with FBS <200 mg/dl, and in patients who are malnourished, underweight, or elderly.
Initiate therapy with 250 mg PO qd in patients with FBS >200 mg/dl. Give with breakfast or the first main meal of the day. If daily doses exceed 500 mg, divide the dose bid. Max 1,000 mg/day.
PEDS - Not approved in children.
FORMS - Generic/Trade: Tabs 100, 250, 500 mg.

tolbutamide (*Orinase, Tol-Tab*) ▶LK ♀C ▶+ $
ADULT - Start 1g PO qd. Maintenance dose is usually 250 mg to 2 g PO qd. Total daily dose may be taken in the morning, divide doses if GI intolerance occurs. Max 3 g/day.
PEDS - Not approved in children.
FORMS - Generic/Trade: Tabs 500 mg.

DIABETES NUMBERS*		Criteria for diagnosis of diabetes	
Self-monitoring glucose goals		*(repeat to confirm on subsequent day)*	
Preprandial	90-130 mg/dL	Fasting glucose	≥126 mg/dL
Postprandial	< 180 mg/dL	Random glucose with symptoms	≥200 mg/dL

Management schedule: Aspirin" (75–162 mg/day) in Type 1 & Type 2 adults for primary prevention (those with an increased cardiovascular risk, including >40 yo or with additional risk factors) & secondary prevention (those with any vascular disease) unless contraindicated; statin therapy to achieve 30% LDL reduction for >40 yo & total cholesterol ≥135mg/dL.† *At every visit*: Measure weight & BP (goal <130/80 mmHg); visual foot exam; review self-monitoring glucose record; review/adjust meds; review self-management skills, dietary needs, and physical activity; counsel on smoking cessation. *Twice a year*: A1c in those meeting treatment goals with stable glycemia (quarterly if not); dental exam. *Annually*: Fasting lipid profile (goal LDL <100 mg/dL, LDL <70mg/dL with cardiovascular disease, HDL >40 mg/dL, TG <150 mg/dL†) every 2 years with low-risk lipid values; creatinine; albumin to creatinine ratio spot collection; dilated eye exam; flu vaccine; comprehensive foot exam.

	A1c
Control	
Normal	<6%
Goal	<7%
Action	>8%

*See recommendations at the Diabetes Care website (http://care.diabetesjournals.org)
†ADA. *Diabetes Care* 2004;27 (Suppl 1):S15-S35, *Circulation*. 2004; 110:235
"Avoid aspirin below the age of 21 due to Reye's Syndrome risk. Use in those <30 yo has not been studied.

ENDOCRINE & METABOLIC: Diabetes-Related – Sulfonylureas – 2nd Generation

gliclazide (*Diamicron, Diamicron MR*) ▶KL ♀C ▶? $

ADULT - Canada only, diabetes type 2: Immediate release: Start 80-160 mg PO qd, max 320 mg PO qd (≥160 mg in divided doses). Modified release: Start 30 mg PO qd, max 120 mg PO qd.

PEDS - Not approved in children.

FORMS - Generic/Trade: Tab 80 mg (Diamicron). Trade only: Tab 30 mg (Diamicron MR).

NOTES - Immediate and modified release not equipotent; 80 mg of immediate release can be changed to 30 mg of modified release.

glimepiride (*Amaryl*) ▶LK ♀C ▶- $

ADULT - Diabetes: initiate therapy with 1-2 mg PO qd. Start with 1 mg PO qd in elderly, malnourished patients or those with renal or hepatic insufficiency. Give with breakfast or the first main meal of the day. Titrate in increments of 1-2 mg at 1-2 week intervals based on response. Usual maintenance dose is 1-4 mg PO qd, max 8 mg/day.

PEDS - Not approved in children.

FORMS - Trade: Tabs 1, 2, 4 mg.

glipizide (*Glucotrol, Glucotrol XL*) ▶LK ♀C ▶? $

ADULT - Diabetes: initiate therapy with 5 mg PO qd. Give 2.5 mg PO qd to geriatric patients or those with liver disease. Adjust dose in increments of 2.5-5 mg to a usual maintenance dose of 10-20 mg/day, max 40 mg/day. Doses >15 mg should be divided bid. Extended release (Glucotrol XL): initiate therapy with 5 mg PO qd. Usual dose is 5-10 mg PO qd, max 20 mg/day.

PEDS - Not approved in children.

FORMS - Generic/Trade: Tabs 5, 10 mg; extended release tabs (Glucotrol XL) 2.5, 5, 10 mg. Trade only: Glucotrol XL 2.5 mg.

NOTES - Maximum effective dose is generally 20 mg/day.

glyburide (*Micronase, DiaBeta, Glynase PresTab, ♣Euglucon*) ▶LK ♀B ▶? $

ADULT - Diabetes: initiate therapy with 2.5-5 mg PO qd. Start with 1.25 mg PO qd in elderly or malnourished patients or those with renal or hepatic insufficiency. Give with breakfast or the first main meal of the day. Titrate in increments of ≤2.5 mg at weekly intervals based on response. Usual maintenance dose is 1.25-20 mg PO qd or divided bid, max 20 mg/day. Micronized tabs: initiate therapy with 1.5-3 mg PO qd. Start with 0.75 mg PO qd in elderly, malnourished patients or those with renal or hepatic insufficiency. Give with breakfast or the first main meal of the day. Titrate in increments of ≤1.5 mg at weekly intervals based on response. Usual maintenance dose is 0.75-12 mg PO qd, max 12 mg/day. May divide dose bid if >6 mg/day.

PEDS - Not approved in children.

FORMS - Generic/Trade: Tabs (scored) 1.25, 2.5, 5 mg. micronized Tabs (scored) 1.5, 3, 4.5 6 mg.

NOTES - Maximum effective dose is generally 10 mg/day.

INSULIN*	Preparation	Onset (h)	Peak (h)	Duration (h)
Rapid-acting:	Insulin aspart (*Novolog*)	<0.2	1-3	3-5
	Insulin glulisine (*Apidra*)	0.30-0.4	1	4-5
	Insulin lispro (*Humalog*)	0.25-0.5	0.5-2.5	≤ 5
Short-acting:	Regular	0.5-1	2-3	3-6
Intermediate-acting:	NPH	2-4	4-10	10-16
	Lente	3-4	4-12	12-18
Long-acting:	Ultralente	6-10	10-16	18-20
	Insulin glargine (*Lantus*)	2-4	peakless	24
Mixtures:	Insulin aspart protamine suspension/insulin aspart (70/30)	0.25	2.4	up to 24
	Insulin lispro protamine suspension/insulin lispro (75/25)	<0.25	1-3 (biphasic)	10-20
	NPH/Reg (50/50 or 70/30)	0.5-1	2-10 (biphasic)	10-20

*These are general guidelines, as onset, peak, and duration of activity are affected by the site of injection, physical activity, body temperature, and blood supply.

ENDOCRINE & METABOLIC: Diabetes-Related – Other

A1C home testing (*Metrika A1CNow*)
▶None ♀+ ▶+ $

ADULT - Use for home A1C testing

PEDS - Use for home A1C testing

FORMS - Fingerstick blood

NOTES - Result displays in 8 minutes.

dextrose (*Glutose, B-D Glucose, Insta-Glucose*) ▶L ♀C ▶? $

ADULT - Hypoglycemia: 0.5-1 g/kg (1-2 ml/kg) up to 25 g (50 ml) of 50% solution by slow IV injection. Hypoglycemia in conscious diabetics: 10-20 g PO q10-20 min prn.

PEDS - Hypoglycemia in neonates: 0.25-0.5 g/kg/dose (5-10 ml of 25% dextrose in a 5 kg infant). Severe hypoglycemia or older infants may require larger doses up to 3 g (12 ml of 25% dextrose) followed by a continuous IV infusion of 10% dextrose. Non-neonates may require 0.5-1.0 g/kg.

FORMS - OTC/Trade only: chew Tabs 5 g. gel 40%.

NOTES - Do not exceed 0.5 g/kg/hr infusion.

diazoxide (*Proglycem*) ▶L ♀C ▶- $$$$$

ADULT - Hypoglycemia: initially 3 mg/kg/day PO divided equally q8h, usual maintenance dose 3-8 mg/kg/day divided equally q8-12 hours, max 10-15 mg/kg/day.

PEDS - Hypoglycemia: neonates and infants, initially 10 mg/kg/day divided equally q8h, usual maintenance dose 8-15 mg/kg/day divided equally q8-12h; children, same as adult.

FORMS - Trade: susp 50 mg/ ml.

glucagon (*Glucagon, GlucaGen*) ▶LK ♀B ▶? $$$

ADULT - Hypoglycemia in adults: 1 mg IV/IM/SC. If no response within 15 in 5-20 minutes, may repeat dose 1-2 times. Diagnostic aid for radiography of the GI tract: 1 mg IV/IM/SC.

PEDS - Hypoglycemia in children >20 kg: same as adults. Hypoglycemia in children <20 kg: 0.5 mg IV/IM/SC or 20-30 mcg/kg. If no response in 5-20 minutes, may repeat dose 1-2 times.

UNAPPROVED ADULT - The following indications are based upon limited data. Esophageal obstruction caused by food: 1 mg IV over 1-3 minutes. Symptomatic bradycardia/hypotension, especially with beta blocker therapy: 3-10 mg IV bolus (0.05 mg/kg general recommendation) may repeat in 10 minutes; may be followed by continuous infusion of 1-5 mg/hour or 0.07 mg/kg/hour. Infusion rate should be titrated to the desired response.

FORMS - Trade: injection 1 mg.

NOTES - Should be reserved for refractory/severe cases or when IV/IM dextrose cannot be administered. Advise patients to educate family members and co-workers how to administer a dose. Give supplemental carbohydrates when patient responds.

glucose home testing (*Chemstrip bG, Dextrostix, Diascan, Glucometer, Glucostix, Clinistix, Clinitest, Diastix, Tes-Tape, GlucoWatch*) ▶None ♀+ ▶+ $$

ADULT - Use for home glucose monitoring

PEDS - Use for home glucose monitoring

FORMS - Blood: Chemstrip bG, Dextrostix, Diascan, Glucometer, Glucostix; Urine: Clinistix, Clinitest, Diastix, Tes-Tape, GlucoWatch

NOTES - GlucoWatch measures glucose levels q10 min and reports an average of 2 readings q20 min for 12 h by sending small electric currents through the skin (a thin plastic sensor is attached to the back of the watch each time it is strapped on to extract glucose from fluid in skin cells). GlucoWatch may cause skin irritation. A1C monitors also available for home use.

insulin (*Apidra, Novolin, NovoLog, Humulin, Humalog, Lantus, ✿NovoRapid*) ▶LK ♀B/C ▶+ $$

ADULT - Diabetes: Humalog/NovoLog: maintenance dose 0.5-1 unit/kg/day SC in divided doses, but doses vary. Apidra: 1 unit = 1 unit regular insulin, doses vary, administer 15 min before meals or within 20 mins after starting a meal. Lantus: Start 10 units SC qd (same time everyday) in insulin naïve patients, adjust to usual dose of 2-100 units/day. When transferring from twice daily NPH human insulin, the initial Lantus dose should be reduced by ~20% from the previous total daily NPH dose, then adjust dose based on patient response. Other insulins are OTC products and have no FDA approved indications. Critical care protocol for intensive insulin: titrate to achieve serum glucose 80-110 mg/dL.

PEDS - Diabetes age >3 yo (Humalog): maintenance dose 0.5-1 unit/kg/day SC in divided doses, but doses vary. Age 6-15 yo (Lantus): Start 10 units SC qd (same time everyday) in insulin naïve patients, adjust to usual dose of 2-100 units/day. When transferring from twice daily NPH human insulin, the initial Lantus dose should be reduced by ~20% from the previous total daily NPH dose, then adjust dose based on patient response. Other insulins are not approved in children.

UNAPPROVED ADULT - Diabetes: 0.3-0.5 unit/kg/day SC in divided doses (Type 1), and 1-1.5 unit/kg/day SC in divided doses (Type 2), but doses vary. Severe hyperkalemia: 5-10 units regular insulin plus concurrent dextrose IV. Profound hyperglycemia (eg, DKA): 0.1 unit/kg regular insulin IV bolus, then IV infusion 100 units in 100 ml NS (1 unit/ml) at 0.1 units/kg/hr. 70 kg: 7 units/h (7 ml/h). Titrate to clinical effect.

UNAPPROVED PEDS - Diabetes: maintenance: 0.5-1 unit/kg/day SC, but doses vary. Humalog may be given after meals. Profound hyperglycemia (eg, DKA): 0.1 unit/kg regular insulin IV bolus, then IV infusion 100 units in 100 ml NS

(1 unit/ml) at 0.1 units/kg/hr. Titrate to clinical effect. Severe hyperkalemia: 0.1 units/kg regular insulin IV with glucose over 30 min. May repeat in 30-60 min or start 0.1 units/kg/hr.

FORMS - Trade: injection NPH, regular, lente, ultralente, insulin lispro (Humalog), insulin lispro protamine suspension/ insulin lispro (Humalog Mix 75/25), insulin glargine (Lantus), insulin aspart (NovoLog), insulin aspart protamine suspension/insulin aspart (NovoLog Mix 70/30), NPH and regular mixtures (70/30 or 50/50).

NOTES - Do not mix Lantus with other insulins in a syringe. Do not mix Apidra with other insulin when used in a pump.

ENDOCRINE & METABOLIC: Gout-Related

allopurinol (*Zyloprim*) ▶K ♀C ▶+ $

ADULT - Mild gout or recurrent calcium oxalate stones: 200-300 mg PO qd (start with 100 mg PO qd). Moderately severe gout: 400-600 mg PO qd. Secondary hyperuricemia: 600-800 mg PO qd. Doses in excess of 300 mg should be divided. Max 800 mg/day. Reduce dose in renal insufficiency (CrCl 10-20 ml/ min= 200 mg/day, CrCl <10 ml/min = 100 mg/day).

PEDS - Secondary hyperuricemia: age <6 yo = 150 mg PO qd; age 6-10 yo = 300 mg PO qd or 1 mg/kg/day divided q6h to a maximum of 600 mg/day.

FORMS - Generic/Trade: Tabs 100, 300 mg.

NOTES - Since may precipitate an acute gout flare use NSAIDs or colchicine initially. Start with 100 mg PO qd and increase weekly to target serum uric acid of <6 mg/d. Incidence of rash and allopurinol hypersensitivity syndrome is increased in renal impairment. Discontinue if rash or allergic symptoms. Drug interaction with warfarin and azathioprine. Normal serum uric acid levels are usually achieved after 1-3 weeks of therapy.

Colbenemid (colchicine + probenecid) ▶KL ♀C ▶? $$

ADULT - Chronic gouty arthritis: start 1 tab PO qd x 1 week, then 1 tab PO bid.

PEDS - Not approved in children.

FORMS - Generic/Trade: Tabs 0.5 mg colchicine + 500 mg probenecid.

NOTES - Maintain alkaline urine.

colchicine ▶L ♀C ▶? $

ADULT - Older FDA-approved dosing no longer recommended; see "unapproved adult" section.

PEDS - Not approved in children.

UNAPPROVED ADULT - Rapid treatment of

acute gouty arthritis: 0.6 mg PO q1h for up to 3h (max 3 tablets). Gout prophylaxis: 0.6 mg PO bid if CrCl ≥50 ml/min, 0.6 mg PO qd if CrCl 35-49 ml/min, 0.6 mg PO q2-3 days if CrCl 10-34 ml/min. Familial Mediterranean fever: 1 mg in divided doses daily, may increase to 2-3 mg/day if needed.

FORMS - Generic/Trade: Tabs 0.6 mg.

NOTES - Colchicine is most effective when initiated on the first day of gouty arthritis. IV route no longer recommended due to serious adverse effects including death.

probenecid (✤*Benuryl*) ▶KL ♀B ▶? $

ADULT - Gout: 250 mg PO bid x 7 days, then 500 mg PO bid. May increase by 500 mg/day q4 weeks not to exceed 2 g/day. Adjunct to penicillin: 2 g/day PO in divided doses. Reduce dose to 1 g/day in renal impairment.

PEDS - Adjunct to penicillin in children 2-14 yo: 25 mg/kg PO initially, then 40 mg/kg/day divided qid. For children >50 kg, use adult dose. Contraindicated in children <2 yo.

FORMS - Generic: Tabs 500 mg.

NOTES - Decrease dose if GI intolerance occurs. Maintain alkaline urine. Begin therapy 2-3 weeks after acute gouty attack subsides.

rasburicase (*Elitek*) ▶L ♀C ▶- $$$$$

WARNING - May cause hypersensitivity reactions including anaphylaxis, hemolysis (G6PD-deficient patients), methemoglobinemia, interference with uric acid measurements

ADULT - Not approved in adults.

PEDS - Uric acid elevation prevention in children (1 mo-17 yr) with leukemia, lymphoma, and solid tumor malignancies receiving anticancer therapy: 0.15 or 0.20 mg/kg IV over 30 min qd x 5 days. Initiate chemotherapy 4 to 24 hrs after the first dose.

NOTES - Safety and efficacy have been established only for one 5 day treatment course. Hydrate IV if at risk for tumor lysis syndrome. Screen for G6PD deficiency if high risk.

sulfinpyrazone (*Anturane*) ▶K ♀? ▶? $$

ADULT - Gout: start 100-200 mg PO bid with meals, titrate over 1 week to 400-800 mg/day.

PEDS - Not approved in children.

FORMS - Generic: Tabs 100 mg. Caps 200 mg.

NOTES - May precipitate an acute gouty flare; continue treatment throughout exacerbation. Maintain adequate fluid intake and alkaline urine.

INTRAVENOUS SOLUTIONS		(ions in mEq/l)						
Solution	*Dextrose*	*Cal/l*	*Na*	*K*	*Ca*	*Cl*	*Lactate*	*Osm*
0.9 NS	0 g/l	0	154	0	0	154	0	310
LR	0 g/l	9	130	4	3	109	28	273
D5 W	50 g/l	170	0	0	0	0	0	253
D5 0.2 NS	50 g/l	170	34	0	0	34	0	320
D5 0.45 NS	50 g/l	170	77	0	0	77	0	405
D5 0.9 NS	50 g/l	170	154	0	0	154	0	560
D5 LR	50 g/l	179	130	4	3	109	28	527

ENDOCRINE & METABOLIC: Minerals

calcium acetate (*PhosLo*) ▶K ♀+ ▶? $

ADULT - Hyperphosphatemia in end-stage renal failure: initially 2 tabs/caps PO tid with each meal. Titrate dose based on serum phosphorus.

PEDS - Not approved in children.

UNAPPROVED PEDS - Titrate to response.

FORMS - Trade only: Tab/Cap 667 mg (169 mg elem Ca).

NOTES - Higher doses more effective, but beware of hypercalcemia, especially if given with vitamin D. Most patients require 3-4 tabs/meal.

calcium carbonate (*Tums, Os-Cal, Caltrate, Viactiv*, ✿*Calsan*) ▶K ♀+ ▶+ $

ADULT - 1-2 g elem Ca/day or more PO with meals divided bid-qid. Prevention of osteoporosis: 1000-1500 mg elem Ca/day PO divided bid-tid with meals. The adequate intake in most adults is 1000-1200 mg elem Ca/day.

PEDS - Hypocalcemia: Neonates: 50-150 mg elem Ca/kg/day PO in 4-6 divided doses; Children: 45-65 mg elem Ca/kg/day PO divided qid. Adequate intake for children (in elem calcium): <6 mo: 210 mg/day when fed human milk and 315 mg/day when fed cow's milk; 6-12 mo: 270 mg/day when fed human milk+solid food and 335 mg/day when fed cow's milk+solid food; 1-3 yo: 500 mg/day; 4-8 yo: 800 mg/day; 9-18 yo 1300 mg/day.

UNAPPROVED ADULT - May lower BP in patients with HTN. May reduce PMS symptoms such as fluid retention, pain, and negative affect.

FORMS - OTC Generic/Trade: tab 650,667,

1250,1500 mg, chew tab 750,1250 mg, cap 1250 mg, susp 1250 mg/5 ml. Calcium carbonate is 40% elem Ca and contains 20 mEq of elem Ca/g calcium carbonate. Not more than 500-600 mg elem Ca/dose. Os-Cal 250 + D contains 125 units vitamin D/tab, Os-Cal 500 + D contains 200 units vitamin D/tab, Caltrate 600 + D contains 200 units vitamin D/tab. Viactiv (chew candy) 500 +100 units vitamin D + 40 mcg vitamin K/tab.

NOTES - Decreases absorption of levothyroxine, tetracycline, and fluoroquinolones.

calcium chloride ▶K ♀+ ▶+ $

ADULT - Hypocalcemia: 500-1000 mg slow IV q1-3 days. Magnesium intoxication: 500 mg IV. Hyperkalemic ECG changes: dose based on ECG.

PEDS - Hypocalcemia: 0.2 ml/kg IV up to 10 ml/day. Cardiac resuscitation: 0.2 ml/kg IV.

UNAPPROVED ADULT - Has been used in calcium channel blocker toxicity and to treat or prevent calcium channel blocker-induced hypotension.

UNAPPROVED PEDS - Has been used in calcium channel blocker toxicity.

FORMS - Generic: injectable 10% (1000 mg/10 ml) 10 ml ampules, vials, syringes.

NOTES - Calcium chloride contains 14.4 mEq Ca/g versus calcium gluconate 4.7 mEq Ca/g. For IV use only; do not administer IM or SC. Avoid extravasation. Administer no faster than 0.5-1 ml/min. Use cautiously in patients receiving digoxin; inotropic and toxic effects are synergistic and may cause arrhythmias. Usually not recommended for hypocalcemia associated with renal insufficiency because calcium chloride is an acidifying salt.

calcium citrate (*Citracal*) ▶K ♀+ ▶+ $

ADULT - 1-2 g elem Ca/day or more PO with meals divided bid-qid. Prevention of osteoporosis: 1000-1500 mg elem Ca/day PO divided bid-tid with meals. The adequate intake in most adults is 1000-1200 mg elem Ca/day.

PEDS - Not approved in children.

FORMS - OTC: Trade (mg elem Ca): tab 200 mg, 250 mg with 125 units vitamin D, 315 mg with 200 units vitamin D, 250 mg with 62.5 units magnesium stearate vitamin D, effervescent tab 500 mg.

NOTES - Calcium citrate is 21% elem Ca. Not more than 500-600 mg elem Ca/dose. Decreases absorption of levothyroxine, tetracycline and fluoroquinolones.

calcium gluconate ▶K ♀+ ▶+ $

ADULT - Emergency correction of hypocalcemia: 7-14 mEq slow IV prn. Hypocalcemic tetany: 4.5-16 mEq IM prn. Hyperkalemia with cardiac toxicity: 2.25-14 mEq IV while monitoring ECG. May repeat after 1-2 minutes. Magnesium intoxication: 4.5-9 mEq IV, adjust dose based on patient response. If IV not possible, give 2-5 mEq IM. Exchange transfusions: 1.35 mEq calcium gluconate IV concurrent with each 100 ml of citrated blood. Oral calcium gluconate: 1-2 g elem Ca/day or more PO with meals divided bid-qid. Prevention of osteoporosis: 1000-1500 mg elem Ca/day PO with meals in divided doses.

PEDS - Emergency correction of hypocalcemia: Children: 1-7 mEq IV prn. Infants: 1 mEq IV prn. Hypocalcemic tetany: Children: 0.5-0.7 mEq/kg IV tid-qid. Neonates: 2.4 mEq/kg/day IV in divided doses. Exchange transfusions: Neonates: 0.45 mEq IV/100 ml of exchange transfusions. Oral calcium gluconate: Hypocalcemia: Neonates: 50-150 mg elem Ca/kg/day PO in 4-6 divided doses; children: 45-65 mg elem Ca/kg/day PO divided qid.

UNAPPROVED ADULT - Has been used in calcium channel blocker toxicity and to treat or prevent calcium channel blocker-induced hypotension.

UNAPPROVED PEDS - Has been used in calcium channel blocker toxicity.

FORMS - Generic: injectable 10% (1000 mg/10 ml, 4.65mEq/10 ml) 10,50,100,200 ml. OTC generic: tab 500,650,975,1000 mg.

NOTES - Calcium gluconate is 9.3% elem Ca and contains 4.6 mEq elem Ca/g calcium glu-

conate. Administer IV calcium gluconate not faster than 0.5-2 ml/min. Use cautiously in patients receiving digoxin; inotropic and toxic effects are synergistic and may cause arrhythmias.

ferrous gluconate (*Fergon*) ▶K ♀+ ▶+ $

ADULT - Iron deficiency: 800-1600 mg ferrous gluconate (100-200 mg elem iron) PO divided tid. Iron supplementation: RDA (elem iron) is: adult males (≥19 yo): 8 mg; adult premenopausal females (11-50 yo) 18 mg; adult females (≥51yo): 8 mg; pregnancy: 27 mg; lactation: 14-18 yo: 10 mg; 19-50 yo: 9 mg. Upper limit: 45 mg/day.

PEDS - Mild-moderate iron deficiency: 3 mg/kg/day of elem iron PO in 1-2 divided doses; severe iron deficiency: 4-6 mg/kg/day PO in 3 divided doses. Iron supplementation: RDA (elem iron) is: <6 mo: 0.27 mg; 7-12 mo: 11 mg; 1-3 yo: 7 mg; 4-8 yo: 10 mg; 9-13 yo: 8 mg; males 14-18 yo: 11 mg; females 14-18 yo: 15 mg.

UNAPPROVED ADULT - Adjunct to epoetin to maximize hematologic response: 200 mg elem iron/day PO.

UNAPPROVED PEDS - Adjunct to epoetin to maximize hematologic response: 2-3 mg/kg elem iron/day PO.

FORMS - OTC Generic/Trade: tab (ferrous gluconate) 240,300,324,325 mg.

NOTES - Ferrous gluconate is 12% elem iron. For iron deficiency, 4-6 months of therapy generally necessary to replete stores even after hemoglobin has returned to normal. Do not take within 2 h of antacids, tetracyclines, levothyroxine or fluoroquinolones. May cause black stools, constipation or diarrhea.

ferrous sulfate (*Fer-in-Sol, FeoSol Tabs, ♣Ferodan, Slow-Fe, Fero-Grad*) ▶K ♀+ ▶+ $

ADULT - Iron deficiency: 500-1000 mg ferrous sulfate (100-200 mg elem iron) PO divided tid. Liquid: 5-10 ml tid. Iron supplementation: RDA (elem iron) is: adult males (≥19 yo): 8 mg; adult premenopausal females (11-50 yo): 18 mg; adult females (≥51 yo): 8 mg; pregnancy: 27 mg; lactation: 14-18 yo: 10 mg; 19-50 yo: 9 mg. Upper limit: 45 mg/day.

PEDS - Mild-moderate iron deficiency: 3 mg/kg/day of elem iron PO in 1-2 divided doses; severe iron deficiency: 4-6 mg/kg/day PO in 3 divided doses. For iron supplementation RDA see ferrous gluconate.

UNAPPROVED ADULT - Adjunct to epoetin to maximize hematologic response: 200 mg elem iron/day PO.

UNAPPROVED PEDS - Adjunct to epoetin to maximize hematologic response: 2-3 mg/kg elem iron/day PO.

FORMS - OTC Generic/Trade (mg ferrous sulfate): tab 324,325 mg, liquid 220 mg/5 ml, drops 75 mg/0.6 ml.

NOTES - Iron sulfate is 20% elem iron. For iron deficiency, 4-6 months of therapy generally necessary. Do not take within 2 h of antacids, tetracyclines, levothyroxine or fluoroquinolones. May cause black stools, constipation or diarrhea.

fluoride (*Luride*, ❦*Fluor-A-Day*, *Fluotic*) ▶K ♀? ▶? $

ADULT - Prevention of dental cavities: 10 ml of topical rinse swish and spit qd.

PEDS - Prevention of dental caries: Dose based on age and fluoride concentrations in water. See table below.

FORMS - Generic: chew tab 0.5,1 mg, tab 1 mg, drops 0.125 mg, 0.25 mg, and 0.5 mg/dropperful, lozenges 1 mg, solution 0.2 mg/ml, gel 0.1%, 0.5%, 1.23%, rinse (sodium fluoride) 0.05%,0.1%,0.2%).

NOTES - In communities without fluoridated water, fluoride supplementation should be used until 13-16 years of age. Chronic overdosage of fluorides may result in dental fluorosis (mottling of tooth enamel) and osseous changes. Use rinses and gels after brushing and flossing and before bedtime.

FLUORIDE: Peds qd dose is based on drinking water fluoride (shown in ppm)			
Age	<0.3	0.3-0.6	>0.6
(years)	ppm	ppm	ppm
0-0.5	none	none	none
0.5-3	0.25mg	none	none
3-6	0.5mg	0.25mg	none
6-16	1 mg	0.5 mg	none

iron dextran (*InFed, DexFerrum*, ❦*Dexiron, Infufer*) ▶KL ♀- ▶? $$$$

WARNING - Parenteral iron therapy has resulted in anaphylactic reactions. Potentially fatal hypersensitivity reactions have been reported with iron dextran injection. Facilities for CPR must be available during dosing. Use only when clearly warranted.

ADULT - Iron deficiency: Dose based on patient weight and hemoglobin. Total dose (ml) = 0.0442 x (desired hgb - observed hgb) x weight (kg) + [0.26 x weight (kg)]. For weight, use lesser of lean body weight or actual body weight. Iron replacement for blood loss: re-

placement iron (mg) = blood loss (ml) x hematocrit. Maximum daily IM dose 100 mg.

PEDS - Not recommended for infants <4 months of age. Iron deficiency in children >5 kg: Dose based on patient weight and hemoglobin. Dose (ml) = 0.0442 x (desired hgb - observed hgb) x weight (kg) + [0.26 x weight (kg)]. For weight, use lesser of lean body weight or actual body weight. Iron replacement for blood loss: replacement iron (mg) = blood loss (ml) x hematocrit. Maximum daily IM dose: infants <5 kg: 25 mg; children 5-10 kg: 50 mg; children >10 kg 100 mg.

UNAPPROVED ADULT - Adjunct to epoetin to maximize hematologic response. Has been given by slow IV infusion. Total dose (325-1500 mg) as a single, slow (6 mg/min) IV infusion has been used.

UNAPPROVED PEDS - Adjunct to epoetin to maximize hematologic response.

NOTES - A 0.5 ml IV test dose (0.25 ml in infants) over ≥30 seconds should be given at least 1 h before therapy. Infuse ≤50 mg/min. For IM administration, use Z-track technique.

iron polysaccharide (*Niferex, Niferex-150, Nu-Iron, Nu-Iron 150*) ▶K ♀+ ▶+ $

ADULT - Iron deficiency: 50-200 mg PO divided qd-tid. Iron supplementation: RDA (elem iron) is: adult males (≥19 yo) 10 mg; adult females (11-50 yo) 15 mg; adult females (≥51 yo) 10 mg; pregnancy 30 mg; lactation 15 mg.

PEDS - Mild-moderate iron deficiency: 3 mg/kg/day of elem iron PO in 1-2 divided doses. Severe iron deficiency: 4-6 mg/kg/day PO in 3 divided doses. For iron supplementation RDA see ferrous gluconate.

UNAPPROVED ADULT - Adjunct to epoetin to maximize hematologic response: 200 mg elem iron/day PO.

UNAPPROVED PEDS - Adjunct to epoetin to maximize hematologic response: 2-3 mg/kg elem iron/day PO.

FORMS - OTC Trade only: tab 50 mg (Niferex). Trade/Generic: cap 150 mg (Niferex-150, Nu-Iron 150), liquid 100 mg/5 ml (Niferex, Nu-Iron). 1 mg iron polysaccharide=1 mg elemental iron.

NOTES - For iron deficiency, 4-6 months of therapy generally necessary. Do not take within 2 h of antacids, tetracyclines, levothyroxine, or fluoroquinolones. May cause black stools, constipation or diarrhea.

iron sucrose (*Venofer*) ▶KL ♀B ▶? $$$$

WARNING - Potentially fatal hypersensitivity reactions have been rarely reported with iron sucrose injection. Facilities for CPR must be available during dosing.

ADULT - Iron deficiency in chronic hemodialysis patients: 5 ml (100 mg elem iron) IV over 5 min or diluted in 100 ml NS IV over ≥15 minutes.

PEDS - Not approved in children.

UNAPPROVED ADULT - Iron deficiency: 5 ml (100 mg elem iron) IV over 5 min or diluted in 100 ml NS IV over ≥15 min.

NOTES - Most hemodialysis patients require 1 g of elem iron over 10 consecutive hemodialysis sessions.

magnesium chloride (*Slow-Mag*) ▶K♀A▶+ $

ADULT - Dietary supplement: 2 tabs PO qd. RDA (elem Mg): Adult males: 400 mg if 19-30 yo, 420 mg if >30 yo. Adult females: 310 mg if 19-30 yo, 320 mg if >30 yo.

PEDS - Not approved in children.

UNAPPROVED ADULT - Hypomagnesemia: 300 mg elem magnesium PO divided qid.

UNAPPROVED PEDS - Hypomagnesemia: 10-20 mg elem magnesium/kg/dose PO qid. For RDA (elem Mg) see magnesium gluconate.

FORMS - OTC Trade: enteric coated tab 64 mg. 64 mg tab Slow-Mag = 64 mg elem Mg.

NOTES - May cause diarrhea. May accumulate in renal insufficiency.

magnesium gluconate (*Almora, Magtrate, Maganate, ♥Maglucate*) ▶K♀A▶+ $

ADULT - Dietary supplement: 500-1000 mg/day PO divided tid. RDA (elem Mg): Adult males: 19-30 yo: 400 mg; >30 yo: 420 mg. Adult females: 19-30 yo: 310 mg; >30 yo: 320 mg.

PEDS - Not approved in children.

UNAPPROVED ADULT - Hypomagnesemia: 300 mg elem magnesium PO divided qid. Unproven efficacy for oral tocolysis following IV magnesium sulfate.

UNAPPROVED PEDS - Hypomagnesemia: 10-20 mg elem magnesium/kg/dose PO qid. RDA (elem Mg): Age 0-6 mos: 30 mg/day; 7-12 mos: 75 mg/day; 1-3 yo: 80 mg; 4-8 yo: 130 mg; 9-13 yo: 240 mg; 14-18 yo (males): 410 mg; 14-18 yo (females): 360 mg.

FORMS - OTC Generic: tab 500 mg, liquid 54 mg elem Mg/5 ml.

NOTES - 500 mg tabs of magnesium gluconate contain 27-29 mg elem magnesium. May cause diarrhea. Use caution in renal failure; may accumulate.

magnesium oxide (*Mag-200, Mag-Ox 400*) ▶K♀A▶+ $

ADULT - Dietary supplement: 400-800 mg PO qd. RDA (elem Mg): Adult males: 19-30 yo: 400 mg;>30 yo 420 mg. Adult females: 19-30 yo: 310 mg; >30yo: 320 mg.

PEDS - Not approved in children.

UNAPPROVED ADULT - Hypomagnesemia: 300 mg elem magnesium PO qid. Has also been used as oral tocolysis following IV magnesium sulfate (unproven efficacy) and in the prevention of calcium-oxalate kidney stones.

UNAPPROVED PEDS - Hypomagnesemia: 10-20 mg elem magnesium/kg/dose PO qid. For RDA (elem Mg) see magnesium gluconate.

FORMS - OTC Generic/Trade: cap 140,250, 400,420,500 mg.

NOTES - Magnesium oxide is approximately 60% elem magnesium. May accumulate in renal insufficiency.

magnesium sulfate ▶K♀A▶+ $

ADULT - Hypomagnesemia: mild deficiency: 1 IM q6h x 4 doses; severe deficiency: 2 g IV over 1 h (monitor for hypotension). Hyperalimentation: maintenance requirements not precisely known; adults generally require 8-24 mEq/day.

PEDS - Not approved in children.

UNAPPROVED ADULT - Has been used for inhibition of premature labor (tocolysis), as an adjunctive bronchodilator in very severe acute asthma (2 g IV over 10-20 min), to reduce early mortality when given ASAP after acute MI (controversial), & in chronic fatigue syndrome.

UNAPPROVED PEDS - Hypomagnesemia: 25-50 mg/kg IV/IM q4-6h for 3-4 doses, maximum single dose 2 g. Hyperalimentation: maintenance requirements not precisely known; infants require 2-10 mEq/day. Acute nephritis: 20-40 mg/kg (in 20% solution) IM prn. Adjunctive bronchodilator in very severe acute asthma: 25-100 mg/kg IV over 10-20 min.

NOTES - 1000 mg magnesium sulfate contains 8 mEq elem magnesium. Do not give faster than 1.5 ml/min (of 10% solution) except in eclampsia or seizures. Use caution in renal insufficiency; may accumulate. Monitor urine output, patellar reflex, respiratory rate and serum magnesium level. IM administration must be diluted to a 20% soln.

phosphorus (*Neutra-Phos, K-Phos*) ▶K♀C ▶? $

ADULT - Dietary supplement: 1 cap/packet (Neutra-Phos) PO qid or 1-2 tab (K-Phos) PO qid after meals and at bedtime. Severe hypophosphatemia (<1 mg/dl): 0.08-0.16 mmol/kg IV over 6 h. In TPN, 310-465 mg/day (10-15 mM) IV is usually adequate, although higher amounts may be necessary in hypermetabolic states. RDA for adults is 800 mg.

PEDS - RDA (elem phosphorus): 0-6 mo: 100

mg; 6-12 mo: 275 mg; 1-3 yo: 460 mg; 4-8 yo: 500 mg; 9-18: 1,250 mg. Severe hypophosphatemia (<1 mg/dl): 0.25-0.5 mmol/kg IV over 4-6 h. Infant TPN: 1.5-2 mmol/kg/day in TPN.

FORMS - OTC: Trade: (Neutra-Phos, Neutra-Phos K) tab/cap/packet 250 mg (8 mmol) phosphorus. Rx: Trade: (K-Phos) tab 250 mg (8 mmol) phosphorus.

NOTES - Dissolve caps/tabs/powder in 75 ml water prior to ingestion.

potassium (*Cena-K, Effer-K, K+8, K+10, Kaochlor, Kaon, Kaon Cl, Kay Ciel, Kaylixir, K+Care, K+Care ET, K-Dur, K-G Elixir, K-Lease, K-Lor, Klor-con, Klorvess, Klorvess Effervescent, Klotrix, K-Lyte, K-Lyte Cl, K-Norm, Kolyum, K-Tab, K-vescent, Micro-K, Micro-K LS, Slow-K, Ten-K, Tri-K,*) ▶K ♀C ▶? $

ADULT - Hypokalemia: 20-40 mEq/day or more PO/IV. Intermittent infusion: 10-20 mEq/dose IV over 1-2 h prn. Prevention of hypokalemia: 20-40 mEq/day PO qd-bid.

PEDS - Not approved in children.

UNAPPROVED ADULT - Diuretic-induced hypokalemia: 20-60 mEq/day PO.

UNAPPROVED PEDS - Hypokalemia: 2.5 mEq/kg/day given IV/PO qd-bid. Intermittent infusion: 0.5-1 mEq/kg/dose IV at 0.3-0.5 mEq/kg/h prn. Infusions faster than 0.5 mEq/kg/h require continuous monitoring.

FORMS - Injectable, many different products in a variety of salt forms (i.e. chloride, bicarbonate, citrate, acetate, gluconate), available in tabs, caps, liquids, effervescent tabs, packets. Potassium gluconate is available OTC.

NOTES - Use potassium chloride for hypokalemia associated with alkalosis; use potassium bicarbonate, citrate, acetate, or gluconate when associated with acidosis.

sodium ferric gluconate complex (*Ferrlecit*) ▶KL ♀B ▶? $$$$$

WARNING - Potentially fatal hypersensitivity reactions rarely reported with sodium ferric gluconate complex. Facilities for CPR must be available during dosing.

ADULT - Iron deficiency in chronic hemodialysis patients: 125 mg elem iron IV over 10 min or diluted in 100 ml NS IV over 1 h. Most hemodialysis patients require 1 g of elem iron over 8 consecutive hemodialysis session.

PEDS - Not approved in children.

UNAPPROVED ADULT - Iron deficiency: 125 mg elem iron IV over 10 min or diluted in 100 ml NS IV over 1 hr.

NOTES - Serious hypotensive events occur in 1.3% of patients.

POTASSIUM, oral forms

Effervescent Tablets	
20 mEq:	K+Care ET, Klorvess
25 mEq:	Effer-K, K+Care ET, K-Lyte, K-Lyte/Cl, Klor-Con/EF
50 mEq:	K-Lyte DS, K-Lyte/Cl 50
Effervescent Granules	
20 mEq:	Klorvess Effervescent, K-vescent
Liquids	
20 mEq/15 ml:	Cena-K, Kaochlor S-F, K-G Elixir, Kaochlor 10%, Kay Ciel, Kaon, Kaylixir, Klorvess,Kolyum, Potasalan, Twin-K
30 mEq/15 ml:	Rum-K
40 mEq/15 ml:	Cena-K, Kaon-Cl 20%
45 mEq/15 ml:	Tri-K
Powders	
15 mEq/pack:	K+Care
20 mEq/pack:	Gen-K,K+Care, Kay Ciel, K-Lor, Klor-Con, Klorvess, Micro-K LS
25 mEq/pack:	K+Care, Klor-Con 25
Tablets/Capsules	
6.7 mEq:	Kaon-CL
8 mEq:	K+8, Klor-Con 8,, Slow-K, Micro-K
10 mEq:	K+10, K-Lease, K-Norm, Kaon-Cl 10, Klor-Con 10, Klotrix, K-Tab, K-Dur 10, Micro-K 10,Ten-K
20 mEq:	K-Dur 20

ENDOCRINE & METABOLIC: Nutritionals

banana bag ▶KL ♀+ ▶+ $

UNAPPROVED ADULT - Alcoholic malnutrition (one formula): Add thiamine 100 mg + folic acid 1 mg + IV multivitamins to 1 liter NS and infuse over 4h. Magnesium sulfate 2g may be added. "Banana bag" is jargon and not a valid drug order; also known as "rally pack"; specify individual components.

fat emulsion (*Intralipid, Liposyn*) ▶L ♀C ▶? $$$$$

WARNING - Deaths have occurred in preterm infants after infusion of IV fat emulsions. Autopsy results showed intravascular fat accumulation in the lungs. Strict adherence to total daily dose and administration rate is mandatory. Premature and small for gestational age infants have poor clearance of IV fat emulsion. Monitor infant's ability to eliminate fat (i.e. triglycerides or plasma free fatty acid levels).

ADULT - Calorie and essential fatty acids

source: As part of TPN, fat emulsion should be no more than 60% of total calories. Initial infusion rate 1 ml/min IV (10% fat emulsion) or 0.5 ml/min (20% fat emulsion) IV for first 15-30 min. If tolerated increase rate. If using 10% fat emulsion infuse 500 ml first day and increase the next day. Maximum daily dose 2.5 g/kg. If using 20% fat emulsion, infuse 250 ml (Liposyn II) or 500 ml (Intralipid) first day and increase the next day. Maximum daily dose 3 g/day.

PEDS - Calorie and essential fatty acids source: As part of TPN, fat emulsion should be no more than 60% of total calories. Initial infusion rate 0.1 ml/min IV (10% fat emulsion) or 0.05 ml/min (20% fat emulsion) for first 10-15 min. If tolerated increase rate to 1 g/kg in 4 h. Max daily dose 3g/kg. For premature infants, start at 0.5 g/kg/day and increase based on infant's ability to eliminate fat.

NOTES - Do not use in patients with severe egg allergy; contains egg yolk phospholipids. Use caution in severe liver disease, pulmonary disease, anemia, blood coagulation disorders, when there is the danger of fat embolism or in jaundiced or premature infants. Monitor CBC, blood coagulation, LFTs, plasma lipid profile and platelet count.

formulas - infant (*Enfamil, Similac, Isomil, Nursoy, Prosobee, Soyalac, Alsoy*) ▶L ♀+ ▶+ $

ADULT - Not used in adults.
PEDS - Infant meals.
FORMS - OTC: Milk-based (Enfamil, Similac, SMA) or soy-based (Isomil, Nursoy, ProSobee, Soyalac, Alsoy).

levocarnitine (*Carnitor*) ▶KL ♀B ▶? $$$$$

ADULT - Prevention of levocarnitine deficiency in dialysis patients: 10-20 mg/kg IV at each dialysis session. Titrate dose based on serum concentration.

PEDS - Prevention of deficiency in dialysis patients: 10-20 mg/kg IV at each dialysis session. Titrate dose based on serum concentration.

NOTES - Adverse neurophysiologic effects may occur with long term, high doses of oral levocarnitine in patients with renal dysfunction. Only the IV formulation is indicated in patients receiving hemodialysis.

omega-3 fatty acid (*Promega, Max EPA*) ▶L ♀- ▶? $

ADULT - Dietary supplement in patients at risk for early coronary artery disease: 1-2 caps PO tid with meals.

PEDS - Not approved in children.

UNAPPROVED ADULT - Adjunctive treatment in rheumatoid arthritis: 20 g/day PO. Psoriasis: 10-15 g/day PO. Prevention of early restenosis after coronary angioplasty in combination with dipyridamole and aspirin: 18 g/day PO. Secondary prevention of coronary heart disease in those who do not consume fish: 2 g/day (1g EPA+DHA).

FORMS - OTC Generic/Trade: Cap 600,1000,1200 mg (with varying ratios of EPA:DHA).

NOTES - May increase bleeding time and inhibit platelet aggregation; use caution in patients receiving anticoagulants or aspirin. Monitor blood sugar in NIDDM patients.

rally pack ▶KL ♀C ▶- $

UNAPPROVED ADULT – See "banana bag" on prior page.

PEDIATRIC REHYDRATION SOLUTIONS (ions in mEq/l)

Brand	Glucose	Cal/l	Na	K	Cl	Citrate	Phos	Ca	Mg
Infalyte	30 g/l	140	50	25	45	34	0	0	0
Kao Lectrolyte*	20 g/l	90	50	20	40	30	0	0	0
Lytren†	20 g/l	80	50	25	45	30	0	0	0
Naturalyte	25 g/l	0	45	20	35	48	0	0	0
Pedialyte‡	25 g/l	100	45	20	35	30	0	0	0
Rehydralyte	25 g/l	100	75	20	65	30	0	0	0
Resol	20 g/l	80	50	20	50	34	5	4	4

*Available in premeasured powder packet. †Canada. ‡and Pedialyte Freezer Pops

ENDOCRINE & METABOLIC: Thyroid Agents

levothyroxine (*T4, Synthroid, Levoxyl, Thyro-Tabs, Unithroid, Levothroid, Levo -T, L-thyroxine, Novothyrox, ♥Eltroxin*) ▶L ♀A ▶+ $

WARNING - Do not use for obesity/weight loss.
ADULT - Hypothyroidism : Start 100-200 mcg PO qd (healthy adults) or 12.5-50 mcg PO qd (elderly or CV disease), increase by 12.5-25

mcg/day at 3-8 week intervals. Usual maintenance 100-200 mcg PO qd, max 300 mcg/day.

PEDS - Hypothyroidism 0-6 months: 8-10 mcg/kg/day PO; 6-12 months: 6-8 mcg/kg/day PO; 1-5 yo: 5-6 mcg/kg/day PO; 6-12 yo: 4-5 mcg/kg/day PO; >12 yo: 2-3 mcg/kg/day PO, max 300 mcg/day.

UNAPPROVED ADULT - Hypothyroidism: 1.6 mcg/kg/day PO; start with lower doses (25 mcg PO qd) in elderly and patients with cardiac disease.

FORMS - Generic/Trade: Tabs 25, 50, 75, 100, 125, 150, 200, 300 mcg. Trade only: Tabs 88, 112, 137, 175 mcg.

NOTES - May crush tabs for infants and children. May give IV or IM at ½ oral dose in adults and ½ - ¾ oral dose in children; then adjust based on tolerance and therapeutic response.

liothyronine (T3, Cytomel) ▶L ♀A ▶? $

WARNING - Do not use for obesity/weight loss.

ADULT - Mild hypothyroidism: 25 mcg PO qd, increase by 12.5-25 mcg/day at 1-2 week intervals to desired response. Usual maintenance dose 25-75 mcg PO qd. Goiter: 5 mcg PO qd, increase by 5-10 mcg/day at 1-2 week intervals. Usual maintenance dose 75 mcg qd. Myxedema: 5 mcg PO qd, increase by 5-10 mcg/day at 1-2 week intervals. Usual maintenance dose 50-100 mcg/day.

PEDS - Congenital hypothyroidism: 5 mcg PO qd, increase by 5 mcg/day at 3-4 day intervals to desired response.

FORMS - Trade only: Tabs 5 mcg. Generic/Trade: Tabs 25, 50 mcg.

NOTES - Start therapy at 5 mcg/d in children & elderly and increase by 5 mcg increments only. Rapidly absorbed from the GI tract. Monitor T3 and TSH. Elderly may need lower doses due to potential decreased renal function

methimazole (Tapazole) ▶L ♀D ▶+ $$$

ADULT - Mild hyperthyroidism: 5 mg PO tid. Moderate hyperthyroidism: 10 mg PO tid. Severe hyperthyroidism: 20 mg PO tid (q8h intervals). Maintenance dose = 5-30 mg/day.

PEDS - Hyperthyroidism: 0.4 mg/kg/day PO divided q8h. Maintenance dose = ½ initial dose, max 30 mg/day.

UNAPPROVED ADULT - Start 10-30 mg PO qd, then adjust.

FORMS - Generic/Trade: Tabs 5, 10 mg.

NOTES - Monitor CBC for evidence of marrow suppression if fever, sore throat, or other signs of infection. Propylthiouracil preferred over methimazole in pregnancy.

potassium iodide (Thyro-Block, Lugol's Solution, Pima Syrup, SSKI, iodine) ▶L ♀D ▶- $

WARNING - Do not use for obesity.

ADULT - Thyroidectomy preparation: 50-250 mg PO tid x 10-14 days prior to surgery. Thyroid storm: 1 ml (Lugol's) PO tid at least 1h after initial propylthiouracil or methimazole dose. Thyroid blocking in radiation emergency: 130 mg PO qd x 10 days or as directed by state health officials.

PEDS - Thyroid blocking in radiation emergency age 3-18 years: 65 mg (one-half of a 130 mg tab) PO qd, or 130 mg PO qd in adolescents >70 kg. 1 mo to 3 years: 32 mg (one-quarter of a 130 mg tab) PO qd. Birth to 1 mo: 16 mg (one-eighth of a 130 mg tab) PO qd. Duration is until risk of exposure to radioiodines no longer exists.

FORMS - Trade: Tabs (Thyro-Block) 130 mg. Soln: 325 mg/5 ml (Pima Syrup), 1 g/ml (SSKI). Strong iodine soln 50 mg iodine/ml and 100 mg potassium iodide/ml (Lugol's Solution).

NOTES - Tabs available to state and federal authorities only. Recommendations for radiation emergencies at FDA website (www.fda.gov).

propylthiouracil (PTU, ♣Propyl Thyracil) ▶L ♀D (but preferred over methimazole) ▶+ $

ADULT - Hyperthyroidism: 100-150 mg PO tid. Severe hyperthyroidism and/or large goiters: 200-400 mg PO tid. Continue initial dose for approximately 2 months. Adjust dose to desired response. Usual maintenance dose 100-150 mg/day. Thyroid storm: 200 mg PO q4-6h x 1 day, decrease dose gradually to usual maintenance dose.

PEDS - Hyperthyroidism in children age 6-10 yo: 50 mg PO qd-tid. Children ≥10 yo: 50-100 mg PO tid. Continue initial dose for 2 months, then maintenance dose is 1/3 to 2/3 initial dose.

UNAPPROVED PEDS - Hyperthyroidism in neonates: 5-10 mg/kg/day PO divided q8h. Children: 5-7 mg/kg/day PO divided q8h.

FORMS - Generic: Tabs 50 mg.

NOTES - Monitor CBC for marrow suppression if fever, sore throat, or other signs of infection. Vasculitic syndrome with positive anti-neutrophilic cytoplasmic antibodies (ANCA) reported requiring discontinuation. Propylthiouracil preferred over methimazole in pregnancy.

sodium iodide I-131 (Iodotope, Sodium Iodide I-131 Therapeutic) ▶K ♀X ▶- $$$$$

WARNING - Not usually used if age <30 yo.

ADULT - Specialized dosing for hyperthyroidism and thyroid carcinoma.

PEDS - Not approved in children.

FORMS - Generic/Trade: Capsules & oral solution: radioactivity range varies at the time of calibration.

NOTES - Avoid if preexisting vomiting or diarrhea. Discontinue antithyroid therapy ≥3 days before starting. Low serum chloride or nephrosis may increase uptake; renal insufficiency may decrease excretion and thus increase radiation exposure. Ensure adequate hydration before and after administration. Follow low iodine diet for 1-2 weeks before treatment. Women should have negative pregnancy test prior to treatment and advise not to conceive for ≥6 months.

thyroid - dessicated (*Thyroid USP, Armour Thyroid*) ▶L ♀A ▶? $

WARNING - Do not use for obesity.

ADULT - Obsolete; use thyroxine instead. Hypothyroidism: Start 30 mg PO qd, increase by 15 mg/day at 2-3 week intervals to a maximum dose of 180 mg/day.

PEDS - Congenital hypothyroidism: 15 mg PO qd. Increase at 2 week intervals.

FORMS - Generic/Trade: Tabs 15,30,60,65,90, 120, 180, 300 mg. Trade only: Tabs 240 mg.

NOTES - 60 mg thyroid desiccated is roughly equivalent to 50-60 mcg thyroxine. Combination of levothyroxine (T4) and liothyronine (T3); content varies.

Thyrolar (levothyroxine + liothyronine) ▶L ♀A ▶? $

WARNING - Do not use for obesity.

ADULT - Hypothyroidism: 1 PO qd, starting with small doses initially (¼ - ½ strength), then increase at 2 week intervals.

PEDS - Not approved in children.

FORMS - Trade: Tabs T4/T3 12.5/3.1 (¼ strength), 25/6.25 (½ strength), 50/12.5 (#1), 100/25 (#2), 150/37.5 (#3) mcg.

NOTES - Combination of levothyroxine (T4) and liothyronine (T3).

ENDOCRINE & METABOLIC: Vitamins

ascorbic acid (vitamin C, *♥Redoxon*) ▶K ♀C ▶? $

ADULT - Prevention of scurvy: 70-150 mg/day PO. Treatment of scurvy: 300-1000 mg/day. RDA females 75 mg/day; males 90 mg/day. Smokers: add 35 mg/day more.

PEDS - Prevention of scurvy: Infants: 30 mg/day PO. Treatment of scurvy: Infants: 100-300 mg/day PO. Adequate daily intake for infants 0-6 mo: 40 mg; 7-12 mo: 50 mg. RDA for children: 1-3 yo: 15 mg; 4-8 yo: 25 mg; 9-13 yo: 45 mg; 14-18 yo: 75 mg (males), 65 mg (females).

UNAPPROVED ADULT - Urinary acidification with methenamine: >2 g/day PO. Idiopathic methemoglobinemia: 150 mg/day or more PO. Wound healing: 300-500 mg/day or more PO for 7-10 days. Severe burns: 1-2 g/day PO.

FORMS - OTC: Generic: tab 25,50,100,250, 500,1000 mg, chew tab 100,250,500 mg, time-released tab 500 mg, 1000,1500 mg, time-released cap 500 mg, lozenge 60 mg, liquid 35 mg/0.6 ml, oral solution 100 mg/ml, syrup 500 mg/5 ml.

NOTES - Use IV/IM/SC ascorbic acid for acute deficiency or when oral absorption is uncertain. Avoid excessive doses in diabetics, patients prone to renal calculi, those undergoing stool occult blood tests (may cause false-negative), those on sodium restricted diets and those taking anticoagulants (may decrease INR). Doses in adults >2 g/day may cause osmotic diarrhea.

calcitriol (*Rocaltrol, Calcijex*) ▶L ♀C ▶? $$

ADULT - Hypocalcemia in chronic renal dialysis: Oral - 0.25 mcg PO qd, increase by 0.25 mcg q 4-8 weeks until normocalcemia achieved. Most hemodialysis patients require 0.5-1 mcg/day PO. IV: 1-2 mcg, 3 times a week; increase dose by 0.5-1 mcg every 2-4 weeks. If PTH decreased <30% then increase dose; if PTH decreased 30-60% then maintain current dose; if PTH decreased >60% then decrease dose; if PTH 1.5-3 times the upper normal limit then maintain current dose. Hypoparathyroidism: 0.25 mcg PO qam; increase dose q 2-4 weeks if inadequate response. Most adults respond to 0.5-2 mcg/day PO. Secondary hyperparathyroidism in pre-dialysis patients: 0.25 mcg PO qam; may increase dose to 0.5 mcg qam.

PEDS - Hypoparathyroidism 1-5 yo: 0.25-0.75 mcg PO qam. If ≥6 yo then 0.25 mcg PO qam; increase dose in 2-4 weeks; usually respond to 0.5-2 mcg/day PO. Secondary hyperparathyroidism in pre-dialysis patients ≥3 yo: 0.25 mcg qam; may increase dose to 0.5 mcg qam. If <3 yo: 0.01-0.15 mcg/kg/day PO.

UNAPPROVED ADULT - Psoriatic vulgaris: 0.5 mcg/day PO or 0.5 mcg/g petrolatum topically qd.

FORMS - Generic/Trade: Cap 0.25, 0.5 mcg. Oral soln 1 mcg/ml. Injection 1,2 mcg/ml.

NOTES - Calcitriol is the activated form of vitamin D. During titration period, monitor serum calcium at least twice weekly. Successful therapy requires an adequate daily calcium intake. Topical preparation must be compounded (not commercially available).

cyanocobalamin (vitamin B12, *Nascobal*) ▶K ♀C ▶+ $

ADULT - See also "unapproved adult" dosing. Nutritional deficiency: 500 mcg intranasal weekly. Pernicious anemia: 100 mcg IM/SC qd, for 6-7 days, then qod for 7 doses, then q3-4 days for 2-3 weeks, then q month. Other patients with vitamin B12 deficiency: 30 mcg IM qd for 5-10 days, then 100-200 mcg IM q month. RDA for adults is 2.4 mcg.

PEDS - Nutritional deficiency: 100 mcg/24 hr deep IM/SC x 10-15 days then at least 60 mcg/month IM/deep SC. Pernicious anemia: 30-50 mcg/24 hr for ≥14 days to total dose of 1000-5000 mcg deep IM/SC then 100 mcg/month deep IM/SC. Adequate daily intake for infants: 0-6 mo: 0.4 mcg; 7-11 mo: 0.5 mcg. RDA for children: 1-3 yo: 0.9 mcg; 4-8 yo: 1.2 mcg; 9-13 yo: 1.8 mcg; 14-18 yo: 2.4 mcg.

UNAPPROVED ADULT - Pernicious anemia & nutritional deficiency states: 1000-2000 mcg PO qd for 1-2 weeks, then 1000 mcg PO qd. Prevention and treatment of cyanide toxicity associated with nitroprusside.

UNAPPROVED PEDS – Prevention/treatment of nitroprusside-associated cyanide toxicity.

FORMS - OTC Generic: tab 100,500,1000,5000 mcg; lozenges 100,250,500 mcg. Rx Trade only: nasal gel 500 mcg/0.1 ml.

NOTES - Pricing for nasal form (Nascobal) is $$$. Although official dose for deficiency states is 100-200 mcg IM q month, some give 1000 mcg IM periodically. Oral supplementation is safe & effective for B12 deficiency even when intrinsic factor is not present.

***Diatx* (folic acid + niacinamide + cobalamin + pantothenic acid + pyridoxine + d-biotin + thiamine + vitamin C + riboflavin)** ▶LK ♀? ▶? $$

ADULT - Nutritional supplement for end-stage renal failure, dialysis, hyperhomocysteinemia or inadequate dietary vitamin intake: 1 PO qd.

PEDS - Not approved in children.

FORMS - Trade: Each tab contains folic acid 5 mg + niacinamide 20 mg + cobalamin 1 mg + pantothenic acid 10 mg + pyridoxine 50 mg + d-biotin 300 mcg + thiamine 1.5 mg + vitamin C 60 mg + riboflavin 1.5 mg. Diatx Fe: adds 100 mg ferrous fumarate per tab.

NOTES - Cobalamin appears to prevent masking of pernicious anemia by folic acid.

dihydrotachysterol (vitamin D, DHT, ♥*Hytakerol*) ▶L ♀C ▶? $$

ADULT - Treatment of acute, chronic, and latent forms of postoperative tetany, idiopathic tetany and hypoparathyroidism: Initial dose 0.75-2.5 mg PO qd for several days, then 0.2-1.75 mg PO qd to maintain normocalcemia.

PEDS - Safe dosing exceeding the RDA and in children undergoing dialysis has not been established.

UNAPPROVED PEDS - Hypoparathyroidism: Neonates: 0.05-0.1 mg PO qd; Infants and young children: 1-5 mg PO qd × 4 days, then 0.5-1.5 mg PO qd; Older children: 0.75-2.5 mg PO qd × 4 days, then 0.2-1.5 mg PO qd. Nutritional rickets: 0.5 mg PO for 1 dose or 13-50 mcg/day PO until healing occurs. Renal osteodystrophy: 0.125-0.5 mg PO qd.

FORMS - Generic: tab 0.125,0.2, 0.4 mg, cap 0.125 mg, oral solution 0.2 mg/ml.

NOTES - Monitor serum calcium. Dose may be supplemented with calcium therapy.

doxercalciferol (*Hectorol*) ▶L ♀B ▶? $$$$

ADULT - Secondary hyperparathyroidism on dialysis: Oral: If PTH >400 pg/ml then start 10 mcg PO 3x/ week; if PTH >300 pg/ml then increase by 2.5 mcg/dose q8 weeks as necessary; if PTH 150-300 pg/ml then maintain current dose; if PTH <100 pg/ml then stop x 1 week, then resume at a dose at least 2.5 mcg lower. Max 60 mcg/week. IV: If PTH >400 pg/ml then 4 mcg IV 3x/ week; if PTH decreased by <50% & >300 pg/ml then increase by 1-2 mcg q8 weeks as necessary; if PTH 150-300 pg/ml then maintain current dose; if PTH <100 pg/ml then stop x1 week, then resume at a dose that is at least 1 mcg lower. Max 18 mcg/week. Secondary hyperparathyroidism not on dialysis: If PTH >70 pg/ml (Stage 3) or >110 pg/ml (Stage 4) then start 1 mcg PO qd; if PTH >70 pg/ml (Stage 3) or >110 pg/ml (Stage 4) then increase by 0.5 mcg/dose q2 weeks; if PTH 35-70 pg/ml (Stage 3) or 70-110 pg/ml (Stage 4) then maintain current dose; if <35 pg/ml (Stage 3) or <70 pg/ml (Stage 4) then stop x1 week, then resume at a dose that is at least 0.5mcg lower. Max 3.5 mcg/day.

PEDS - Not approved in children.

FORMS - Trade only: Caps 0.5, 2.5 mcg.

NOTES - Monitor PTH, serum calcium and phosphorus weekly during dose titration; may need to monitor patients with hepatic insufficiency more closely.

folic acid (folate, *Folvite*) ▶K ♀A ▶+ $

ADULT - Megaloblastic anemia: 1 mg PO/IM/IV/

SC qd. When symptoms subside and CBC normalizes, give maintenance dose of 0.4 mg PO qd and 0.8 mg PO qd in pregnant and lactating females. RDA for adults 0.4 mg, 0.6 mg for pregnant females, and 0.5 mg for lactating women. Max recommended daily dose 1 mg.

PEDS - Megaloblastic anemia: Infants: 0.05 mg PO qd, maintenance of 0.04 mg PO qd; Children: 0.5-1 mg PO qd, maintenance of 0.4 mg PO qd. Adequate daily intake for infants: 0-6 mo: 65 mcg; 7-12 mo: 80 mcg. RDA for children: 1-3 yo: 150 mcg; 4-8 yo: 200 mcg; 9-13 yo: 300 mcg, 14-18 yo: 400 mcg.

UNAPPROVED ADULT - Hyperhomocysteinemia: 0.5-1 mg PO qd.

FORMS - OTC Generic: Tab 0.4,0.8 mg. Rx Generic 1 mg.

NOTES - Folic acid doses >0.1 mg may obscure pernicious anemia. Prior to conception all women should receive 0.4 mg/day to reduce the risk of neural tube defects in infants. Consider high dose (up to 4 mg) in women with prior history of infant with neural tube defect. Use oral route except in cases of severe intestinal absorption.

***Foltx* (folic acid + cyanocobalamin + pyridoxine)** ▶K ♀A ▶+ $

ADULT - Nutritional supplement for end stage renal failure, dialysis, hyperhomocysteinemia, homocystinuria, nutrient malabsorption or inadequate dietary intake: 1 tab PO qd.

PEDS - Not approved in children.

FORMS - Trade: folic acid 2.5 mg/ cyanocobalamin 2 mg/ pyridoxine 25 mg tab.

NOTES - Folic acid doses >0.1 mg may obscure pernicious anemia, preventable with the concurrent cyanocobalamin.

multivitamins (*MVI*) ▶LK ♀+ ▶+ $

ADULT, PEDS - Dietary supplement: Dose varies by product.

FORMS - OTC & Rx: Many different brands and forms available with and without iron (tab, cap, chew tab, drops, liquid).

NOTES - Do not take within 2 h of antacids, tetracyclines, levothyroxine or fluoroquinolones.

***Nephrocap* (vitamin C + folic acid + niacin + thiamine + riboflavin + pyridoxine + pantothenic acid + biotin+ cyanocobalamin)** ▶K ♀? ▶? $

ADULT - Nutritional supplement for chronic renal failure, uremia, impaired metabolic functions of the kidney & to maintain levels when the dietary intake of vitamins is inadequate or excretion & loss are excessive: 1 cap PO qd. If on dialysis, take after treatment.

PEDS - Not approved in children.

FORMS - Trade/Generic: vitamin C 100 mg / folic acid 1 mg / niacin 20 mg / thiamine 1.5 mg / riboflavin 1.7 mg / pyridoxine 10 mg / pantothenic acid 5 mg / biotin 150 mcg / cyanocobalamin 6 mcg

NOTES - Folic acid doses >0.1 mg may obscure pernicious anemia, preventable with the concurrent cyanocobalamin.

***Nephrovite* (vitamin C + folic acid + niacin +thiamine + riboflavin + pyridoxine + pantothenic acid + biotin+ cyanocobalamin)** ▶K ♀? ▶? ?

ADULT - Nutritional supplement for chronic renal failure, dialysis, hyperhomocysteinemia or inadequate dietary vitamin intake: 1 tab PO qd. If on dialysis, take after treatment.

PEDS - Not approved in children.

FORMS - Trade/Generic: vitamin C 60 mg/folic acid 1 mg/ niacin 20 mg/ thiamine 1.5 mg/ riboflavin 1.7 mg/ pyridoxine 10 mg/ pantothenic acid 10 mg/ biotin 300 mcg/ cyanocobalamin 6 mcg

NOTES - Folic acid doses >0.1 mg may obscure pernicious anemia, preventable with the concurrent cyanocobalamin.

niacin (vitamin B3, *Niacor, Slo-Niacin, Niaspan*) ▶K ♀C ▶? $

ADULT - Niacin deficiency: 100 mg PO qd. Pellagra: up to 500 mg PO qd. RDA is 16 mg for males and 14 mg for females. See cardiovascular section for lipid-lowering dose.

PEDS - Safety and efficacy not established for doses that exceed nutritional requirements. Adequate daily intake for infants: 0-6 mo: 2 mg; 7-12 mo: 3 mg. RDA for children: 1-3 yo: 6 mg; 48 yo: 8 mg; 9-13 yo: 12 mg; 14-18 yo: 16 mg (males) and 14 mg (females).

FORMS - OTC: Generic: tab 50,100,250,500 mg, timed-release cap 125,250,400 mg, timed-release tab 250,500 mg, liquid 50 mg/5 ml. Trade: 250,500,750 mg (Slo-Niacin). Rx: Trade only: tab 500 mg (Niacor), timed-release cap 500 mg, timed-release tab 500,750,1000 mg (Niaspan, $$).

NOTES - Start with low doses and increase slowly to minimize flushing (usually <2h); 325 mg aspirin 30-60 min prior to niacin ingestion will minimize flushing. Use caution in diabetics, patients with gout, peptic ulcer, liver, or gallbladder disease.

paricalcitol (*Zemplar*) ▶L ♀C ▶? $$$$$

ADULT - Prevention/treatment of secondary hyperparathyroidism with renal failure: Initially 0.04-0.1 mcg/kg (2.8-7 mcg) IV 3 times/week during dialysis. Can increase dose 2-4 mcg based on PTH in 2-4 week intervals. If PTH level decreased <30% then increase dose; if PTH level decreased 30-60% then maintain current dose; if PTH level decreased >60% then decrease dose; if PTH level 1.5-3 times upper limit of normal then maintain current dose. Max dose 0.24 mcg/kg (16.8 mcg).

PEDS - Not approved in children.

NOTES - Monitor serum PTH, calcium and phosphorous.

phytonadione (vitamin K, *Mephyton, AquaMephyton*) ▶L ♀C ▶+ $

WARNING - Severe reactions, including fatalities, have occurred during and immediately after IV injection, even with diluted injection and slow administration. Restrict IV use to situations where other routes of administration are not feasible.

ADULT - Excessive oral anticoagulation: Dose varies based on INR. INR 5-9: 1-2.5 mg PO (2-4 mg PO may be given if rapid reversal necessary); INR >9 with no bleeding: 3-5 mg PO; INR >20: 10 mg slow IV. Hypoprothrombinemia due to other causes: 2.5-25 mg PO/IM/SC. Adequate daily intake 120 mcg (males) and 90 mcg (females).

PEDS - Hemorrhagic disease of the newborn: Prophylaxis: 0.5-1 mg IM 1 hr after birth; Treatment: 1 mg SC/IM.

UNAPPROVED PEDS - Nutritional deficiency: Children: 2.5-5m g PO qd or 1-2 mg IM/SC/IV. Excessive oral anticoagulation: Infants: 1-2 mg IM/SC/IV q4-8 hr; Children: 2.5-10 mg PO/IM/SC/IV, may be repeated 12-48 hr after PO dose or 6-8 hr after IM/SC/IV dose.

FORMS - Trade only: Tab 5 mg.

NOTES - Excessive doses of vitamin K in a patient receiving warfarin may cause warfarin resistance for up to a week. Avoid IM administration in patients with a high INR.

pyridoxine (vitamin B6) ▶K ♀A ▶+ $

ADULT - Dietary deficiency: 10-20 mg PO qd for 3 weeks. Prevention of deficiency due to isoniazid in high-risk patients: 10-25 mg PO qd. Treatment of neuropathies due to INH: 50-200 mg PO qd. INH overdose (>10 g): Give an equal amount of pyridoxine: 4 g IV followed by 1 g IM q 30 min. RDA for adults: 19-50 yo: 1.3 mg; >50 yo: 1.7 mg (males), 1.5 mg (females). Max recommended: 100 mg/day.

PEDS - Not approved in children. Adequate daily intake for infants: 0-6 mo: 0.1 mg; 7-12 mo: 0.3 mg. RDA for children: 1-3 yo: 0.5 mg; 4-8 yo: 0.6 mg; 9-13 yo: 1 mg; 14-18 yo: 1.3

(boys) and 1.2 mg (girls).

UNAPPROVED ADULT - PMS: 50-500 mg/day PO. Hyperoxaluria type I and oxalate kidney stones: 25-300 mg/day PO. Prevention of oral contraceptive-induced deficiency; 25-40 mg PO qd. Hyperemesis of pregnancy: 10-50 mg q8h. Has been used in hydrazine poisoning.

UNAPPROVED PEDS - Dietary deficiency: 5-10 mg PO qd for 3 weeks. Prevention of deficiency due to isoniazid: 1-2 mg/kg/day PO qd. Treatment of neuropathies due to INH: 10-50 mg PO qd. Pyridoxine-dependent epilepsy: neonatal: 25-50 mg/dose IV; older infants and children: 100 mg/dose IV for 1 dose then 100 mg PO qd.

FORMS - OTC Generic: Tab 25,50,100 mg, timed-release tab 100 mg.

riboflavin (vitamin B2) ▶K ♀A ▶+ $

ADULT - Deficiency: 5-25 mg/day PO. RDA for adults is 1.3 mg (males) and 1.1 mg (females), 1.4 mg for pregnant women and 1.6 mg for lactating women.

PEDS - Deficiency: 5-10 mg/day PO. Adequate daily intake for infants: 0-6 mo: 0.3 mg; 7-12 mo: 0.4 mg. RDA for children: 1-3 yo: 0.5 mg; 4-8 yo: 0.6 mg; 9-13 yo: 0.9 mg; 14-18 yo: 1.3 mg (males) and 1 mg (females).

UNAPPROVED ADULT - Prevention of migraine headaches: 400 mg PO qd.

FORMS - OTC Generic: tab 25,50,100 mg.

NOTES - May cause yellow/orange discoloration of urine.

thiamine (vitamin B1) ▶K ♀A ▶+ $

ADULT - Beriberi: 10-20 mg IM 3 times/week for 2 weeks. Wet beriberi with myocardial infarction: 10-30 mg IV tid. Wernicke encephalopathy: 50-100 mg IV and 50-100 mg IM for 1 dose then 50-100 mg IM qd until patient resumes normal diet. Give before starting glucose. RDA for adults is 1.2 mg (males) and 1.1 mg (females).

PEDS - Beriberi: 10-25 mg IM qd or 10-50 mg PO qd for 2 weeks then 5-10 mg PO qd for 1 month. Adequate daily intake infants: 0-6 mo: 0.2 mg; 7-12 mo: 0.3 mg. RDA for children: 1-3 yo: 0.5 mg; 4-8 yo: 0.6 mg; 9-13 yo: 0.9 mg; 14-18 yo: 1.2 mg (males), 1.0 mg (females).

FORMS - OTC Generic: tab 50,100,250,500 mg, enteric coated tab 20 mg.

tocopherol (vitamin E) ▶L ♀A ▶? $

ADULT - RDA is 22 units (natural, d-alpha-tocopherol) or 33 units (synthetic, d,l-alpha-tocopherol) or 15 mg (alpha-tocopherol). Max recommended 1000 mg (alpha-tocopherol).

PEDS - Adequate daily intake (alpha-tocopher-

ol): infants 0-6 mo: 4 mg; 7-12 mo: 6 mg. RDA for children (alpha-tocopherol): 1-3 yo: 6 mg; 4-8 yo: 7 mg; 9-13 yo: 11 mg; 14-18 yo: 15 mg.
UNAPPROVED ADULT - Alzheimer's disease: 1000 units PO bid (controversial based on limited data & efficacy).
UNAPPROVED PEDS - Nutritional deficiency: Neonates: 25-50 units PO qd; Children: 1 units/kg PO qd. Cystic fibrosis: 5-10 units/kg PO qd (use water soluble form), max 400 units/day.
FORMS - OTC Generic: tab 200,400 units, cap 73.5, 100, 147, 165, 200, 330, 400, 500, 600, 1000 units, drops 50 mg/ml.
NOTES - Natural vitamin E (d-alpha-tocopherol) recommended over synthetic (d,l-alpha-tocopherol). Do not exceed 1500 units natural vit E/day. Higher doses may increase risk of bleeding. Large randomized trials have failed to demonstrate cardioprotective effects.

vitamin A (✽*Aquasol A*) ▶L ♀A (C if exceed RDA, X in high doses) ▶+ $
ADULT - Treatment of deficiency states: 100,000 units IM qd x 3 days, then 50,000 units IM qd x 2 weeks. RDA: 1000 mcg RE (males), 800 mcg RE (females). Max recommended daily dose in non-deficiency 3000 mcg (see notes).
PEDS - Treatment of deficiency states: Infants: 7,500 - 15,000 units IM qd x 10 days; children 1-8 yo: 17,500 - 35,000 units IM qd x 10 days. Kwashiorkor: 30 mg IM of water-soluble palmitate followed by 5,000-10,000 units PO qd x 2 months. Xerophthalmia: >1 yo: 110 mg retinyl palmitate PO or 55 mg IM plus 110 mg PO next day. Administer another 110 mg PO prior to discharge. Vitamin E (40 units) should be co-administered to increase efficacy of retinol. RDA for children: 0-6 mos: 400 mcg (adequate intake); 7-12 mos: 500 mcg; 1-3 yrs: 300 mcg; 4-8 yrs: 400 mcg; 9-13 yrs: 600 mcg; 14-18 yrs: 900 mcg (males), 700 mcg (females).
UNAPPROVED ADULT - Test for fat absorption: 7000 units/kg (2100 RE/kg) PO x 1. Measure serum vitamin A concentrations at baseline and 4 hr after ingestion. Dermatologic disorders such as follicularis keratosis: 50,000 -

500,000 units PO qd x several weeks.
UNAPPROVED PEDS - Has been tried in reduction of malaria episodes in children >12 mo and to reduce the mortality in HIV-infected children.
FORMS - OTC: Generic: cap 10,000, 15,000 units. Trade: tab 5,000 units. Rx: Generic: 25,000 units. Trade: soln 50,000 units/ml.
NOTES - 1 RE (retinol equivalent) = 1 mcg retinol or 6 mcg beta-carotene. Continued Vitamin A/retinol intake of ≥2000 mcg/d may increase risk of hip fracture in postmenopausal women.

vitamin D (vitamin D2, ergocalciferol, *Calciferol, Drisdol*, ✽*Osteoforte*) ▶L ♀A (C if exceed RDA) ▶+ $
ADULT - Familial hypophosphatemia (Vitamin D Resistant Rickets): 12,000-500,000 units PO qd. Hypoparathyroidism: 50,000-200,000 units PO qd. Adequate daily intake adults: 19-50 yo: 5 mcg (200 units); 51-70 yo: 10 mcg (400 units); >70 yo: 15 mcg (600 units). Max recommended daily dose in non-deficiency 50 mcg (2000 units).
PEDS - Adequate daily intake infants and children: 5 mcg (200 units) . Hypoparathyroidism: 1.25-5 mg PO qd.
UNAPPROVED ADULT - Osteoporosis prevention: 400-800 units PO qd with calcium supplements. Fanconi syndrome: 50,000-200,000 units PO qd. Osteomalacia: 1000-5000 units PO qd. Anticonvulsant-induced osteomalacia: 2000-50,000 units PO qd. Vitamin D deficiency: 50,000 units PO q week to q month.
UNAPPROVED PEDS - Familial hypophosphatemia: 400,000-800,000 units PO qd, increased by 10,000-20,000 units/day q3-4 mo prn. Hypoparathyroidism: 50,000-200,000 units PO qd. Fanconi syndrome: 250-50,000 units PO qd.
FORMS - OTC: Trade: soln 8000 units/ml. Rx: Trade: cap 50,000 units, inj 500,000 units/ml.
NOTES - 1 mcg ergocalciferol = 40 units vitamin D. IM therapy may be necessary if malabsorption exists. Familial hypophosphatemia also requires phosphate supplementation; Hypoparathyroidism also requires calcium supplementation.

ENDOCRINE & METABOLIC: Other

agalsidase beta (*Fabrazyme*) ▶? ♀B ▶? $$$$$
WARNING - Infusion reactions occurred in many patients & some reactions were severe.
ADULT - Fabry disease: 1 mg/kg infused q 2 weeks. Initial infusion rate <0.25 mg/min. If tol-

erated, increase rate in increments of 0.05-0.08 mg/min each subsequent infusion. Pretreat with antipyretic and antihistamine.
PEDS - Not approved in children.
FORMS - Trade only: 35 mg single-use vial.
NOTES - When infusion reaction occurs, de-

crease infusion rate, temporarily stop the infusion, and/or give additional antipyretic, antihistamine and/or steroids; medical support should be readily available. Immunogenicity may develop ≤3 months; consider testing for IgE; determine risk & benefits of continued treatment with anti-Fabrazyme IgE. Orphan drug; available through specialty distributor; encourage enrollment in the Fabry disease registry.

aminoglutethimide (Cytadren) ▶K ♀D ▶? $$$$
WARNING - Used only as an interim measure until more definitive therapy such as surgery can be undertaken; only small numbers have been treated >3 months. Benefits are limited in ACTH-dependent Cushing's syndrome as high levels of ACTH overcome the drug's effect. Avoid alcohol. May cause adrenocortical hypofunction; may give hydrocortisone & mineralocorticoid supplements if indicated; dexamethasone should not be used. May cause orthostatic hypotension; monitor BP.
ADULT - Cushing's syndrome: 250 mg PO q6h (should be initiated in hospital). Increase dose in increments of 250 mg at intervals of 1-2 weeks if cortisol suppression is inadequate. Max dose 2 g/day.
PEDS - Not approved in children.
UNAPPROVED ADULT - Advanced breast cancer in postmenopausal women: Start 250 mg PO qd, then increase every couple of days to bid, tid, then to qid. Metastatic prostate carcinoma: Start 250 mg PO bid, then increase to 250 mg qid as tolerated. Response may take 4-6 weeks.
FORMS - Trade only: Tab 250 mg
NOTES - Monitor plasma cortisol levels (or to avoid daily variation instead monitor urinary free cortisol or other steroid metabolites) to determine if suppression is adequate. May need glucocorticoid & mineralocorticoid replacement if oversuppression. Dose reduction or temporary discontinuation may be required if adverse effects occurs. Discontinue if skin rash persists >5-8 days or becomes severe; may start at lower dose if rash is mild or moderate. Obtain baseline and monitor periodically hematologic studies, thyroid function tests, LFTs and electrolytes. Decreases effects of warfarin, dexamethasone, digoxin, medroxyprogesterone & theophylline.

bromocriptine (Parlodel) ▶L ♀B ▶- $$$$
ADULT - Start 1.25-2.5 mg PO qhs with food, increase q3-7 days, usual effective dose 2.5-15 mg/day, max 40 mg/day (hyperprolactinemia)

or 20-30 mg/day, max 100 mg/day (acromegaly). Doses >20 mg/day have been divided bid. Take with food to minimize dizziness, nausea.
PEDS - Not approved in children.
UNAPPROVED ADULT - Hyperprolactinemia: 2.5-7.5 mg vaginally qd if GI intolerance to PO.
FORMS - Generic/Trade: Tabs 2.5 mg. Caps 5 mg.
NOTES - Seizures, stroke, HTN, and MI have been reported. Should not be used for postpartum lactation suppression. Oral tablets can be used for vaginal insertion if retained until absorbed. Monitor serum prolactin levels.

cabergoline (Dostinex) ▶L ♀B ▶- $$$$$
ADULT - Hyperprolactinemia: initiate therapy with 0.25 mg PO twice weekly. Increase by 0.25 mg twice weekly at 4 week intervals up to a maximum of 1 mg twice weekly.
PEDS - Not approved in children.
FORMS - Trade: Tabs 0.5 mg.
NOTES - Monitor serum prolactin levels. Use with caution in hepatic insufficiency.

calcitonin (Calcimar, Miacalcin, ✦Caltine) ▶Plasma ♀C ▶? $$$
ADULT - Osteoporosis: 100 units SC/IM qd or 200 units intranasal qd (alternate nostrils). Paget's disease: 50-100 units SC/IM qd or 3 times weekly. Hypercalcemia: 4 units/kg SC/IM q12h. May increase after 2 days to maximum of 8 units/kg q6h.
PEDS - Not approved in children.
UNAPPROVED ADULT - Acute osteoporotic vertebral fracture pain: 100 units SC/IM qd or 200 units intranasal qd (alternate nostrils).
UNAPPROVED PEDS - Osteogenesis imperfecta age 6 mos-15 yo: 2 units/kg SC/IM three times weekly with oral calcium supplements.
FORMS - Trade: nasal spray 200 units/activation, 2 ml bottle (minimum of 14 doses/bottle).

NOTES - Skin test before using injection: 1 unit intradermally and observe for local reaction.

cinacalcet (Sensipar) ▶LK ♀C ▶? $$$$$
ADULT - Treatment of secondary hyperparathyroidism in dialysis patients: 30 mg PO qd. May titrate q 2-4 weeks through sequential doses of 60, 90, 120 & 180 mg qd to target intact parathyroid hormone level of 150-300 pg/mL. Treatment of hypercalcemia in parathyroid carcinoma: 30 mg PO bid. May titrate q 2-4 weeks through sequential does of 30 mg bid, 60 mg bid, 90 mg bid & 90 mg tid-qid as necessary to normalize serum calcium levels.
PEDS - Not approved in children.
FORMS - Trade: tab 30, 60, 90 mg

NOTES - Monitor calcium & phosphorus 1 week after initiation or dose adjustment, then monthly after maintenance dose established. Intact parathyroid hormone should be checked 1-4 weeks after initiation or dose adjustment, and then 1-3 months after a maintenance dose has been established. For parathyroid carcinoma, monitor serum calcium within 1 week after initiation or dose adjustment, then q 2 months after a maintenance dose has been established. Withhold if serum calcium falls below <7.5 mg/dL or if signs & symptoms of hypocalcemia. May restart when calcium level reaches 8.0 mg/dL or when signs & symptoms of hypocalcemia resolve. Re-initiate using the next lowest dose. Use calcium-containing phosphate binder and/or vitamin D to raise calcium if it falls between 7.5-8.4 mg/dL. Reduce dose or discontinue if intact parathyroid hormone level is <150-300 pg/mL to prevent adynamic bone disease. Dose adjustment may be needed when used with ketoconazole, erythromycin & itraconazole. Closely monitor parathyroid hormone & serum calcium if moderate to severe hepatic impairment.

cosyntropin (*Cortrosyn*, ♥*Synacthen*) ▶L ♀C ▶? $

ADULT - Rapid screen for adrenocortical insufficiency: 0.25 mg IM/ IV over 2 min; measure serum cortisol before & 30-60 min after.

PEDS - Rapid screen for adrenocortical insufficiency: 0.25 mg (0.125 mg if <2 yo) IM/IV over 2 min; measure serum cortisol before & 30-60 min after.

demeclocycline (*Declomycin*) ▶K, feces ♀D ▶- $$$$$

WARNING - Avoid in children <8 yo due to teeth staining. Long-term therapy may cause diabetes insipidus syndrome.

ADULT - FDA approved for anthrax, urinary tract infection & gonorrhea.

PEDS - >8 yo: FDA approved for anthrax, urinary tract infection & gonorrhea.

UNAPPROVED ADULT - SIADH: 600-1200 mg/day PO given in 3-4 divided doses.

FORMS - Trade only: Tabs 150, 300 mg

NOTES – Action onset within 5-14 days; do not increase dose more frequently than q3-4 days. May exacerbate renal insufficiency; use with caution. Hepatotoxicity. Do not give antacids or calcium supplements <2h of demeclocycline. Increased INR with warfarin. May decrease oral contraceptive effectiveness. Take with fluids (not milk) to decrease esophageal irritation.

desmopressin (*DDAVP*, *Stimate*, ♥*Minirin*) ▶LK ♀B ▶? $$$$

WARNING - Adjust fluid intake downward in elderly to decrease potential water intoxication and hyponatremia.

ADULT - Diabetes insipidus: 10-40 mcg (0.1-0.4 ml) intranasally qd -tid. or 0.05-1.2 mg PO daily or divided bid-tid. or 0.5-1 ml (2-4 mcg) SC/IV daily in 2 divided doses.

PEDS - Diabetes insipidus 3 mo-12 yo: 5-30 mcg (0.05-0.3 ml) intranasally qd-bid or 0.05 mg PO tid. Enuresis: See urology section.

UNAPPROVED PEDS - Hemophilia A and type 1 von Willebrand's disease: 2-4 mcg/kg intranasally or 0.2-0.4 mcg/kg IV over 15-30 min.

FORMS - Trade only: Tabs 0.1, 0.2 mg. Nasal soln 1.5 mg/ml (150 mcg/spray). Generic/ Trade: nasal soln 0.1 mg/ml (10 mcg/ spray). Note difference in concentration of nasal solns.

NOTES - Start at lowest dose with diabetes insipidus. Monitor sodium. Prime the nasal spray pump, stable for ≤3 wks at room temperature, otherwise refrigerate. IV/SC doses are approximately 1/10th the intranasal dose.

growth hormone human (*Protropin, Genotropin, Norditropin, Nutropin, Nutropin AQ, Humatrope, Serostim, Saizen, Somatropin, Zorbtive*) ▶LK ♀B/C ▶? $$$$$

WARNING - Avoid in Prader-Willi syndrome patients who are severely obese, have severe respiratory impairment or sleep apnea, or unidentified respiratory infection; fatalities have been reported.

ADULT - Somatotropin deficiency syndrome (Humatrope): 0.006 mg/kg/day SC. Max dose = 0.0125 mg/kg/day. AIDS wasting or cachexia (Serostim): >55 kg = 6 mg SC qhs, 45-55 kg = 5 mg SC qhs, 35-45 kg = 4 mg SC qhs, <35 kg = 0.1 mg/kg SC qhs. Short bowel syndrome (Zorbtive): 0.1mg/kg SC qd, max 8 mg qd. Use >4 weeks has not been studied. Replacement of endogenous growth hormone with either adult-onset or childhood-onset growth hormone deficiency (Saizen): Initiate no more than 0.005 mg/kg/day. Increase dose no more than 0.01 mg/kg/day after 4 weeks depending upon tolerance of treatment.

PEDS - Growth failure: doses vary according to product used. Turner syndrome (Nutropin, Humatrope): 0.375 mg/kg/week SC divided into 3-7 equal doses. Long-term treatment of idiopathic short stature: Up to 0.37 mg/kg/week SC divided into 6-7 equal doses.

FORMS - Single dose vials (powder for injection with diluent). Genotropin: 1.5, 5.8, 13.8 mg cartridges. Humatrope: 6, 12, 24 mg pen cartridges. Nutropin AQ: 10 mg multiple dose vial & 10 mg/pen cartridges. Norditropin: 5,10,15 mg pen cartridges. Saizen & Serostim: 8 mg pre-assembled reconstitution device with autoinjector pen.

NOTES - Use with caution in diabetics or family history of diabetes due to insulin resistance. Transient and dose-dependent fluid retention may occur in adults. May cause hypothyroidism. Evaluate patients with Prader-Willi syndrome for upper airway obstruction and sleep apnea prior to treatment; control weight and monitor for signs & symptoms of respiratory infection. Avoid initiating for short bowel syndrome in patients with acute critical illness.

laronidase (Aldurazyme) ▶? ♀B ▶? $$$$$
WARNING - Infusion-related hypersensitivity may occur.

ADULT - Hurler and Hurler-Scheie forms of mucopolysaccharidosis I and for patients with the Scheie form who have moderate to severe symptoms: 0.58 mg/kg infused q week with specialized weight-based infusion rate. Pretreat 60 minutes prior to infusion with antipyretics and/or antihistamines.

PEDS - Hurler and Hurler-Scheie forms of mucopolysaccharidosis I and for patients with the Scheie form who have moderate to severe symptoms >5 yo: 0.58 mg/kg infused q week with specialized weight-based infusion rate. Pretreat 60 minutes prior to infusion with antipyretics and/or antihistamines.

FORMS - Trade only: 2.9 mg single-use vial.

NOTES - Decrease infusion rate or give additional antipyretic and/or antihistamine when an infusion reaction occurs; stop infusion when severe hypersensitivity or anaphylactic reactions occur. Orphan drug; available through specialty distributor; encourage patient to enroll in the mucopolysaccharidosis I registry.

metyrapone (Metopirone) ▶KL ♀C ▶? $$
WARNING - May cause acute adrenal insufficiency.

ADULT - Diagnostic aid for testing hypothalamic-pituitary adrenocorticotropic hormone (ACTH) function: Specialized single- and multiple-test dose available.

PEDS - Diagnostic aid for testing hypothalamic-pituitary adrenocorticotropic hormone (ACTH) function: Specialized single- and multiple-test dose available.

FORMS - Trade only: Caps 250 mg.

NOTES - Ability of adrenals to respond to exogenous ACTH should be demonstrated before testing with metyrapone. In the presence of hypo- or hyperthyroidism, response to the test may be subnormal. May suppress aldosterone synthesis. May cause dizziness & sedation.

miglustat (Zavesca) ▶K ♀X ▶- $$$$$
ADULT - Treatment of mild to moderate type 1 Gaucher's disease when enzyme replacement therapy is not an option: 100 mg PO tid; may reduce dose to 100 mg PO qd-bid if adverse effects occur. Reduce dose in renal insufficiency (CrCl 50-70 ml/min = 100 mg PO bid; 30-50 ml/min = 100 mg PO qd; avoid use if <30ml/min).

PEDS - Not approved in children.

FORMS - Trade only: gelatin capsules 100 mg

NOTES - Requires effective birth control in men or women; including 3 months after stopping therapy for men. Tremors may occur but usually resolve within 1-3 months of treatment; may need to reduce dose and/or discontinue. Avoid high-carbohydrate foods if diarrhea occurs. Diarrhea frequently decreases over time.

nitisinone (Orfadin) ▶? ♀C ▶? $$$$$
WARNING - Elevation of plasma tyrosine level, transient thrombocytopenia and leukopenia.

ADULT - Hereditary tyrosinemia type I: 1-2 mg/kg/day PO divided bid.

PEDS - Hereditary tyrosinemia type I: 1-2 mg/kg/day PO divided bid.

FORMS - Trade: capsules 2, 5, 10 mg

NOTES - Orphan drug; keep tyrosine levels <500 micromoles/L; regular liver monitoring by imaging and LFTs, alpha-fetoprotein, serum tyrosine, phenylalanine, and urine succinylacetone (may use to guide dosing).

pegvisomant (Somavert) ▶? ♀B ▶? $$$$$
ADULT - Acromegaly unresponsive to other therapies: Load 40 mg SC on day 1, then maintenance 10 mg SC qd. Max 30 mg/day.

PEDS - Not approved in children.

FORMS - Trade only: 10,15,20 mg single-dose vials. Available only from manufacturer.

NOTES - Orphan drug. May cause elevations of growth hormone levels and pituitary tumor growth; periodically image sella turcica. May increase glucose tolerance. May cause IGF-1 deficiency, monitor IGF-1 4-6 weeks after initiation or dose change and q6 months after IGF-1 normalizes. May elevate LFTs; obtain baseline LFTs then check monthly x 6 months, quarterly for the next 6 months and biannually for the next year. Refer to manufacturer's guideline when initiating with abnormal LFTs. Dose adjustment should be every 4-6 weeks in 5-mg increment and based on IGF-1.

raloxifene (Evista) ▶L ♀X ▶- $$$

ADULT - Postmenopausal osteoporosis prevention and treatment: 60 mg PO qd.

PEDS - Not approved in children.

UNAPPROVED ADULT - Breast cancer prevention: 60 mg PO qd.

FORMS - Trade: Tabs 60 mg.

NOTES - Hot flashes and leg cramps may occur. Contraindicated if prior DVT. Discontinue use 72 h prior to and during prolonged immobilization because of DVT risk. Interactions with warfarin and cholestyramine. Triglyceride levels may increase in women with prior estrogen-associated hypertriglyceridemia (>500 mg/dL).

sevelamer (*Renagel*) ▶Not absorbed ♀C ▶? $$$$

ADULT - Hyperphosphatemia: 800-1600 mg PO tid with meals, adjust according to serum phosphorus concentration.

PEDS - Not approved in children.

FORMS - Trade: Caps 403 mg. Tabs 400, 800 mg.

NOTES - Titrate by one tab/cap per meal at 2 week intervals to keep phosphorus ≤6 mg/dl. Anti-arrhythmic & anti-seizure medications may have decreased absorption if not taken 1h before or 3h after sevelamer.

sodium polystyrene sulfonate (*Kayexalate*) ▶Fecal excretion ♀C ▶? $$$$

ADULT - Hyperkalemia: 15 g PO qd-qid or 30-50 g retention enema (in sorbitol) q6h prn. Retain for 30 minutes to several h. Irrigate with tap water after enema to prevent necrosis.

PEDS - Hyperkalemia: 1 g/kg PO q6h.

UNAPPROVED PEDS - Hyperkalemia: 1 g/kg PR q2-6h.

FORMS - Generic: Suspension 15 g/ 60 ml. Powdered resin.

NOTES - 1 g binds approximately 1 mEq of K+. Avoid in bowel obstruction or constipation.

spironolactone (*Aldactone*) ▶LK ♀D ▶? $

ADULT - Primary hyperaldosteronism, maintenance therapy: 100-400 mg/day PO until surgery or indefinitely if surgery not an option.

PEDS - Not approved in children.

UNAPPROVED ADULT - Hirsutism: 50-200 mg PO daily, maximal regression in 6 months.

FORMS - Generic/Trade: Tabs 25,50,100 mg.

NOTES - May cause menstrual irregularities.

tamoxifen (*Nolvadex*) ▶L ♀D ▶- $$$

WARNING - Uterine malignancies, stroke, and PE have been reported. Do not use during pregnancy.

ADULT - Breast cancer: 10-20 mg PO bid x 5 years. Breast cancer prevention: 20 mg PO qd x 5 years.

PEDS - Not approved in children.

UNAPPROVED ADULT - Mastalgia: 10 mg PO qd x 4 months. Anovulation: 5-40 mg PO bid x 4 days.

FORMS - Generic/Trade: Tabs 10,20 mg.

NOTES - Increased risk of uterine malignancies, CVA, & PE in those with ductal carcinoma in situ or at high risk for breast cancer. Use with caution in history of DVT. Safe for use in male breast cancer. Interacts with warfarin. May cause hot flashes.

teriparatide (*Forteo*) ▶LK ♀C ▶- $$$$$

WARNING - Possibility of osteosarcoma; avoid in those at risk (eg, Paget's disease, prior skeletal radiation).

ADULT - Treatment of postmenopausal women or men with primary or hypogonadal osteoporosis and high risk for fracture: 20 mcg SC qd in thigh or abdomen for ≤2 years.

PEDS - Not approved in children.

FORMS - Trade: 28-dose pen injector (20 mcg/dose).

NOTES - Take with calcium and vitamin D. Pen-like delivery device requires education, and should be discarded 28 days after first injection even if not empty.

vasopressin (*Pitressin*, ✚*Pressyn AR*) ▶LK ♀C ▶? $$$$$

ADULT - Diabetes insipidus: 5-10 units IM/SC bid-qid prn

PEDS - Diabetes insipidus: 2.5-10 units IM/SC bid-qid prn.

UNAPPROVED PEDS - Growth hormone and corticotropin provocative test: 0.3 units/kg IM, max 10 units. GI hemorrhage: start 0.002-0.005 units/kg/min IV, increase prn to 0.01 units/kg/min.

NOTES - Monitor serum sodium. Injectable form may be given intranasally.

ENT: Antihistamines – Nonsedating

NOTE: Antihistamines ineffective when treating the common cold.

desloratadine (*Clarinex*, ✚*Aerius*) ▶LK ♀C ▶+ $$$

ADULT - Allergic rhinitis/urticaria: 5 mg PO qd.

PEDS - Allergic rhinitis/urticaria: ≥12 yo: Use adult dose. 6-11 yo: 1 teaspoonful (2.5 mg) PO qd. 12 mo – 5 yo: ½ teaspoonful (1.25 mg) PO qd. 6-11 mo: 2 ml (1 mg) PO qd.

FORMS - Trade: Tabs 5 mg. Fast-dissolve Reditabs 5 mg. Syrup 0.5 mg/ml

NOTES - Increase dosing interval in liver or renal insufficiency to qod. Use a measured dropper for syrup.

fexofenadine (*Allegra*) ▸LK ♀C ▸+ $$$

ADULT - Allergic rhinitis: 60 mg PO bid or 180 mg PO qd. Urticaria: 60 mg PO bid; 60 mg PO qd if decreased renal function.

PEDS - Allergic rhinitis, urticaria: 6-12 yo: 30 mg PO bid; 30 mg qd if decreased renal function.

FORMS - Trade: Tabs 30, 60, & 180 mg. Caps 60 mg.

NOTES - Avoid taking with fruit juice due to a large decrease in bioavailability.

loratadine (*Claritin, Claritin Hives Relief, Claritin RediTabs, Alavert, Tavist ND*) ▸LK ♀B ▸+ $

ADULT - Allergic rhinitis/urticaria: 10 mg PO qd.

PEDS - Allergic rhinitis/urticaria ≥6 yo: Use adult dose. 2-5 yo: 5 mg PO qd (syrup).

FORMS - OTC: Generic/Trade: Tabs 10 mg. Fast-dissolve tabs (Alavert, Claritin RediTabs) 10 mg. Syrup 1 mg/ml.

NOTES - Decrease dose in liver failure or renal insufficiency. Fast-dissolve tabs dissolve on tongue without water. ND=non-drowsy (Tavist).

ENT: Antihistamines – Other

NOTE: Antihistamines ineffective when treating the common cold. Contraindicated in narrow angle glaucoma, BPH, stenosing peptic ulcer disease, & bladder obstruction. Use half the normal dose in the elderly. May cause drowsiness and/or sedation, which may be enhanced with alcohol, sedatives, and other CNS depressants.

azatadine (*Optimine*) ▸LK ♀B ▸- $$$

ADULT - Allergic rhinitis/urticaria: 1-2 mg PO bid.

PEDS - Allergic rhinitis/urticaria age ≥12 yo: 1-2 mg PO bid.

FORMS - Trade: Tabs 1 mg, scored.

cetirizine (*Zyrtec*, ♦*Reactine, Aller-Relief*) ▸LK ♀B ▸- $$$

ADULT - Allergic rhinitis/urticaria: 5-10 mg PO qd.

PEDS - Allergic rhinitis/urticaria: 6-11 yo: Use adult dose. 2-5 yo: 2.5 mg PO qd-bid or 5 mg PO qd. 6-23 mo: 2.5 mg PO qd. If >12 mo, may increase to 2.5 mg PO bid.

FORMS - Trade: Tabs 5, 10 mg. Syrup 5 mg/5 ml. Chewable tabs, grape-flavored 5, 10 mg.

NOTES - Decrease dose in renal or hepatic impairment.

chlorpheniramine (*Chlor-Trimeton, Chlo-Amine, Aller-Chlor*) ▸LK ♀B ▸- $

ADULT - Allergic rhinitis: 4 mg PO q4-6h. 8 mg PO q8-12h (timed release) or 12 mg PO q12h (timed release). Max 24 mg/day.

PEDS - Allergic rhinitis ≥12 yo: Use adult dose. 6-11 yo: 2 mg PO q4-6h. Max 12 mg/day.

UNAPPROVED PEDS - Allergic rhinitis 2-5 yo: 1 mg PO q4-6h. Max 6 mg/day. Timed release 6-11 yo: 8 mg PO q12h prn.

FORMS - OTC: Trade: Tabs chew 2 mg. Generic/Trade: Tabs 4 mg. Syrup 2 mg/5 ml. Generic/Trade: Tabs, Timed-release 8 mg. Trade only:

Tabs, Timed-release 12 mg.

clemastine (*Tavist*) ▸LK ♀B ▸- $

ADULT - Allergic rhinitis: 1.34 mg PO bid. Max 8.04 mg/day. Urticaria/angioedema: 2.68 mg PO qd-tid. Max 8.04 mg/day.

PEDS - Allergic rhinitis ≥12 yo: Use adult dose. 6-12 yo: 0.67 mg PO bid. Max 4.02 mg/day. Urticaria/angioedema ≥12 yo: Use adult dose. 6-12 yo: 1.34 mg PO bid. Max 4.02 mg/day.

UNAPPROVED PEDS - Allergic rhinitis <6 yo: 0.05 mg/kg/day (as clemastine base) PO divided bid-tid. Max dose 1 mg/day.

FORMS - OTC: Generic/Trade: Tabs 1.34 mg. Rx: Generic/Trade: Tabs 2.68 mg. Trade only: Syrup 0.67 mg/5 ml.

NOTES - 1.34 mg = 1 mg clemastine base

cyproheptadine (*Periactin*) ▸LK ♀B ▸- $

ADULT - Allergic rhinitis/urticaria: Start 4 mg PO tid, usual effective dose is 12-16 mg/day. Max 32 mg/day.

PEDS - Allergic rhinitis/urticaria: 2-6 yo: Start 2 mg PO bid-tid. Max 12 mg/day. 7-14 yo: Start 4 mg PO bid-tid. Max 16 mg/day.

UNAPPROVED ADULT - Appetite stimulant: 2-4 mg PO tid 1h ac. Prevention of cluster headache: 4 mg PO qid.

FORMS - Generic/Trade: Tabs 4 mg (trade scored). Syrup 2 mg/5 ml.

dexchlorpheniramine (*Polaramine*) ▸LK ♀? ▸- $$$

ADULT - Allergic rhinitis/urticaria: 2 mg PO q4-6h. Timed release tabs: 4 or 6 mg PO at qhs or q8-10h.

PEDS - Immediate Release tabs & syrup: ≥12 years: Use adult dose. 6-11 yo: 1 mg PO q4-6h. 2-5 yo: 0.5 mg PO q4-6h. Timed Release Tabs: 6-12 yo: 4 mg PO qd, preferably at qhs.

FORMS - Trade: Tabs, Immediate Release 2 mg. Syrup 2 mg/5 ml. Generic/Trade: Tabs,

Timed Release: 4, 6 mg.

diphenhydramine (Benadryl, ♥Allerdryl, Allernix) ▶LK ♀B ▶- $

ADULT - Allergic rhinitis, urticaria, hypersensitivity reactions: 25-50 mg PO/IM/IV q4-6h. Max 300-400 mg/day. Motion sickness: 25-50 mg PO pre-exposure & q4-6h prn. Drug-induced Parkinsonism: 10-50 mg IV/IM. Antitussive: 25 mg PO q4h. Max 100 mg/day.

PEDS - Hypersensitivity reactions: ≥12 yo: Use adult dose. 6-11 yo: 12.5-25 mg PO q4-6h or 5 mg/kg/day PO/IV/IM divided qid. Max 150 mg/day. Antitussive (syrup): 6-12 yo: 12.5 mg PO q4h. Max 50 mg/day. 2-5 yo: 6.25 mg PO q4h. Max 25 mg/day.

FORMS - OTC: Trade: Tabs 25, 50 mg, chew tabs 12.5 mg. OTC & Rx: Generic/Trade: Caps 25,50, softgel cap 25 mg. OTC: Generic/Trade: Liquid 6.25 mg/5 ml & 12.5 mg/5 ml.

NOTES - Anticholinergic side effects enhanced in the elderly.

hydroxyzine (Atarax, Vistaril) ▶L ♀C ▶- $

ADULT - Pruritus: 25-100 mg IM/PO qd-qid or prn.

PEDS - Pruritus: <6 yo: 50 mg/day PO divided qid. ≥6 yo: 50-100 mg/day PO divided qid.

FORMS - Generic/Trade: Tabs 10, 25, 50 mg. Trade only: 100 mg. Generic/Trade: Caps 25, 50, 100 mg. Syrup 10 mg/5 ml (Atarax). Trade: Suspension 25 mg/5 ml (Vistaril).

NOTES - Atarax (hydrochloride salt), Vistaril (pamoate salt).

promethazine (Phenergan) ▶LK ♀C ▶- $

ADULT - Hypersensitivity reactions: 25 mg IM/IV, may repeat in 2 hours. Allergic conditions: 12.5 mg PO/PR/IM/IV qid or 25 mg PO/PR qhs.

PEDS - Hypersensitivity reactions: >2 yo: 6.25-12.5 mg PO/PR/IM/IV q6h prn.

FORMS - Trade: Tabs 12.5 mg, scored. Generic/Trade: Tabs 25, 50 mg. Syrup 6.25 mg/5 ml. Trade only: Phenergan Fortis Syrup 25 mg/5 ml. Trade: Suppositories 12.5 & 25 mg. Generic/Trade: Suppositories 50 mg.

NOTES - Inject IV at ≤25 mg/min.

ENT: Antitussives / Expectorants

benzonatate (Tessalon, Tessalon Perles) ▶L ♀C ▶? $

ADULT - Cough: 100-200 mg PO tid. Max 600 mg/day.

PEDS - >10 yo: Use adult dose.

FORMS - Generic/Trade: Softgel caps:100, 200 mg.

NOTES - Swallow whole. Do not chew. Numbs mouth, possible choking hazard.

dextromethorphan (Benylin, Vick's, Delsym,) ▶L ♀+ ▶+ $

ADULT - Cough: 10- 20 mg PO q4h or 30 mg PO q6-8h. 60 mg PO q12h (Delsym).

PEDS - Cough >12 yo: Use adult dose. 6-12 yo: 5-10 mg PO q4h or 15 mg PO q6-8h. 30 mg PO q12h (sustained action liquid). 2-5 yo: 2.5-5 mg PO q4h or 7.5 mg PO q6-8h. 15 mg PO q12h (sustained action liquid).

FORMS - OTC: Trade: Caps 30 mg. Lozenges 2.5, 5, 7.5, 15 mg. Liquid 3.5, 5, 7.5, 10, 12.5, 15 mg/5 ml; 10 & 15 mg/15 ml (Generic/Trade). Trade (Delsym): Sustained-action liquid 30 mg/5 ml.

NOTES - Contraindicated with MAOIs due to potential for serotonin syndrome.

guaifenesin (Robitussin, Hytuss, Guiatuss, Mucinex) ▶L ♀C ▶+ $

ADULT - Expectorant: 100-400 mg PO q4h or 600-1200 mg PO q12h (extended release). Max 2.4g/day.

PEDS - Expectorant >12 yo: Use adult dose. 6-11 yo: 100-200 mg PO q4h. Max 1.2g/day. 2-5 yo: 50-100 mg PO q4h. Max 600 mg/day.

UNAPPROVED PEDS - Expectorant: 12-23 mo: 50 mg PO q4h. Max 300 mg/day. 6-11 mo: 25 mg PO q4h. Max 150 mg/day.

FORMS - OTC: Trade: Tabs 100, 200 mg. Caps 200 mg. Extended release tabs 600 & 1200 mg. Syrup 100 & 200 mg/5 ml. Generic: Syrup 100 mg/5 ml. Rx: Trade: Tabs 200, 1200 mg. Syrup 100 mg/5 ml.

NOTES - Lack of convincing studies to document efficacy.

ENT: Decongestants

NOTE: See ENT - Nasal Preparations for nasal spray decongestants (oxymetazoline, phenylephrine). Systemic decongestants are sympathomimetic and may aggravate HTN, anxiety and insomnia. Use cautiously in such patients.

pseudoephedrine (*Sudafed, Sudafed 12 Hour, Efidac/24, Dimetapp Decongestant Infant Drops, PediaCare Infants' Decongestant Drops, Triaminic Oral Infant Drops*) ▸L ♀C ▸+ $

ADULT - Nasal Congestion: 60 mg PO q4-6h. 120 mg PO q12h (extended release). 240 mg PO qd (extended release). Max 240 mg/day.

PEDS - Nasal Congestion: Use adult dose. 6-11 yo: 30 mg PO q4-6h. Max 120 mg/day. 2-5 yo: 15 mg PO q4-6h. Max 60 mg/day. Dimetapp, PediaCare, & Triaminic Infant Drops: Give PO q4-6h prn. Max 4 doses/day. 2-3 yo: 1.6 ml. 12-23 mo: 1.2 ml. 4-11 mo: 0.8 ml. ≤3 mo: 0.4 ml.

FORMS - OTC: Generic/Trade: Tabs 30, 60 mg. Chewable tabs 15 mg. Trade only: Tabs, extended release 120, 240 mg. Trade only: Liquid 15 mg/5 ml. Generic/Trade: Liquid 30 mg/5 ml. Infant drops 7.5 mg/0.8 ml.

NOTES - 12 to 24-hour extended release dosage forms may cause insomnia; use a shorter-acting form if this occurs.

ENT: Ear Preparations

Auralgan (benzocaine + antipyrine) ▸Not absorbed ♀C ▸? $

ADULT - Otitis media, adjunct: Instill 2-4 drops (or enough to fill the ear canal) tid-qid or q1-2h prn. Cerumen removal: Instill 2-4 drops or enough to fill the ear canal) tid x 2-3 days to detach cerumen, then prn for discomfort. Insert cotton plug moistened with soln after instillation.

PEDS - Otitis media, adjunct: Use adult dose. Cerumen removal: Use adult dose.

FORMS - Generic/Trade: Otic soln 10 & 15 ml.

carbamide peroxide (*Debrox, Murine Ear*) ▸Not absorbed ♀? ▸? $

ADULT - Cerumen removal: Instill 5-10 drops into ear bid x 4 days.

PEDS - Not approved in children.

FORMS - OTC: Trade: Otic soln 6.5%, 15 or 30 ml bottle.

NOTES - Drops should remain in ear >15 minutes. Do not use for >4 days. Remove excess wax by flushing with warm water using a rubber bulb ear syringe.

Cipro HC Otic (ciprofloxacin + hydrocortisone) ▸Not absorbed ♀C ▸- $$$

ADULT - Otitis externa: Instill 3 drops into affected ear(s) bid x 7 days.

PEDS - Otitis externa ≥1 yo: Use adult dose.

FORMS - Trade: Otic suspension 10 ml.

NOTES - Shake well. Contains benzyl alcohol.

Ciprodex Otic (ciprofloxacin + dexamethasone) ▸Not absorbed ♀C ▸- $$$

ADULT - Otitis externa: Instill 4 drops into affected ear(s) bid x 7 days.

PEDS - Otitis externa & otitis media w/ tympanostomy tubes, ≥6 mo: Instill 4 drops into affected ear(s) bid x 7 days.

FORMS - Trade: Otic suspension 5 & 7.5 ml.

NOTES - Shake well. Warm suspension by holding bottle in hands for 1-2 minutes before instilling.

Cortisporin Otic (hydrocortisone + polymyxin + neomycin) ▸Not absorbed ♀? ▸? $$

ADULT - Otitis externa: Instill 4 drops in affected ear(s) tid-qid up to 10 days.

PEDS - Otitis externa: Instill 3 drops in affected ear(s) tid-qid up to 10 days.

FORMS - Generic/Trade: Otic soln or suspension 7.5 & 10 ml.

NOTES - Caveats with perforated TMs or tympanostomy tubes: (1) Risk of neomycin ototoxicity, especially if use prolonged or repeated; (2) Use suspension rather than acidic soln.

Cortisporin TC Otic (hydrocortisone + neomycin + thonzonium + colistin) ▸Not absorbed ♀? ▸? $$$

ADULT - Otitis externa: Instill 5 drops in affected ear(s) tid-qid up to 10 days.

PEDS - Otitis externa: Instill 4 drops in affected ear(s) tid-qid up to 10 days.

FORMS - Trade: Otic suspension, 10 ml.

docusate sodium (*Colace*) ▸Not absorbed ♀+ ▸+ $

ADULT - See gastroenterology section

PEDS - Not approved in children.

UNAPPROVED ADULT - Cerumen removal: Instill 1 ml in affected ear.

UNAPPROVED PEDS - Cerumen removal: Instill 1 ml in affected ear.

FORMS - Generic/Trade: Liquid 150 mg/15 ml.

NOTES - Allow to remain in ear(s) for 10-15 min. Irrigate with 50 ml lukewarm NS if necessary. Use liquid, not syrup.

Domeboro Otic (acetic acid + aluminum acetate) ▸Not absorbed ♀? ▸? $

ADULT - Otitis externa: Instill 4-6 drops in affected ear(s) q2-3h.

PEDS - Otitis externa: Instill 2-3 drops in affected ear(s) q3-4h.

FORMS - Generic/Trade: Otic soln 60 ml.

NOTES - Insert a saturated wick. Keep moist x 24 hours.

ofloxacin (*Floxin Otic*) ▶Not absorbed ♀C ▶- $$

ADULT - Otitis externa: Instill 10 drops in affected ear(s) qd x 7 days. Chronic suppurative otitis media: Instill 10 drops in affected ear(s) bid x 14 days.

PEDS - Otitis externa >12 yo: Use adult dose. 1-12 yo: Instill 5 drops in affected ear(s) qd x 7 days. Chronic suppurative otitis media >12 yo: Use adult dose. Acute otitis media with tympanostomy tubes 1-12 yo: Instill 5 drops in affected ear(s) bid x 10 days.

FORMS - Trade: Otic soln 0.3% 5,10 ml. "Singles": single-dispensing containers 0.25 ml (5 drops), 2 per foil pouch.

Pediotic (hydrocortisone + polymyxin + neomycin) ▶Not absorbed ♀? ▶? $$

ADULT - Otitis externa: Instill 4 drops in affected ear(s) tid-qid up to 10 days.

PEDS - Otitis externa: Instill 3 drops in affected ear(s) tid-qid up to 10 days.

FORMS - Trade: Otic suspension 7.5 ml.

NOTES - Insert cotton plug prior to medication if TM perforation.

Swim-Ear (isopropyl alcohol + anhydrous glycerins) ▶Not absorbed ♀? ▶? $

ADULT - Otitis externa, prophylaxis: Instill 4-5 drops in ears after swimming, showering, or bathing.

PEDS - Otitis externa, prophylaxis: Use adult dose.

FORMS - OTC: Trade: Otic soln 30 ml.

triethanolamine (*Cerumenex*) ▶Not absorbed ♀C ▶- $$

ADULT - Cerumen removal: Fill ear canal with soln, insert cotton plug for 15-30 minutes, then flush with warm water.

PEDS - Not approved in children.

UNAPPROVED PEDS - Cerumen removal: Use adult dose.

FORMS - Trade: Otic soln 6 & 12 ml with dropper.

NOTES - Do not use for >4 days. Remove excess wax by flushing with warm water using a rubber bulb ear syringe.

VoSol otic (acetic acid + propylene glycol) ▶Not absorbed ♀? ▶? $

ADULT - Otitis externa: Instill 5 drops in affected ear(s) tid-qid. Insert cotton plug moistened with 3-5 drops q4-6h for the first 24 hours.

PEDS - Otitis externa >3 yo: Instill 3-4 drops in affected ear(s) tid-qid. Insert cotton plug moistened with 3-4 drops q4-6h for the first 24 hours.

FORMS - Generic/Trade: Otic soln 2%, 15 & 30 ml.

NOTES - VoSoL HC adds hydrocortisone 1%.

ENT: ENT Combination Products – Over the Counter

NOTE: Decongestants in some ENT combination products can increase BP, aggravate anxiety or cause insomnia (use caution). Some contain sedating antihistamines. Sedation can be enhanced by alcohol and other CNS depressants.

Actifed Cold & Allergy (pseudoephedrine + triprolidine) ▶L ♀C ▶+ $

ADULT - Allergic rhinitis/nasal congestion: 1 tab PO q4-6h. Max 4 tabs/day.

PEDS - Allergic rhinitis/nasal congestion: >12 yo: Use adult dose. 6-12 yo: 1/2 tab PO q4-6h. Max 2 tabs/day.

FORMS - OTC: Trade: Tabs 60 mg pseudoephedrine/2.5 mg triprolidine

NOTES - Cold & Sinus: 30 mg pseudoephedrine /1.25 mg triprolidine/500 mg acetaminophen.

Actifed Cold & Sinus (pseudoephedrine + chlorpheniramine + acetaminophen) ▶L ♀C ▶+ $

ADULT - Allergic rhinitis/nasal congestion/headache: 2 caplets PO q6h. Max 8 caplets/day.

PEDS - Allergic rhinitis/nasal congestion/headache: >12 yo: Use adult dose.

FORMS - OTC: Trade: tabs 30 mg pseudoephedrine/2 mg chlorpheniramine/500 mg acetamin.

Alavert D-12 (pseudoephedrine + loratadine) ▶LK ♀B ▶- $$

ADULT - Allergic rhinitis/nasal congestion: 1 tab PO bid.

PEDS - Not approved in children.

FORMS - OTC: Generic/Trade: Tabs, 12-hour extended release tabs: 120 mg pseudoephedrine/5 mg loratadine.

NOTES - Decrease dose to 1 tab PO qd with CrCl <30 ml/min. Avoid in hepatic insufficiency.

Aleve Cold & Sinus (naproxen + pseudoephedrine) ▶L ♀C (D in 3rd trimester) ▶+ $

ADULT - Nasal/sinus congestion, fever & pain: 1 cap PO q12h.

PEDS - Nasal/sinus congestion, fever & pain: >12 yo: Use adult dose.

FORMS - OTC: Generic/trade: Extended release caplets: 220 mg naproxen sodium/120 mg pseudoephedrine.

Allerfrim (pseudoephedrine + triprolidine) ▶L ♀C ▶+ $

ADULT - Allergic rhinitis/nasal congestion: 1 tab or 10 ml PO q4-6h. Max 4 tabs/day or 40 ml/day.

PEDS - Allergic rhinitis/nasal congestion: >12 yo: Use adult dose. 6-12 yo: 1/2 tab or 5 ml PO q4-6h. Max 2 tabs/day or 20 ml/day.

FORMS - OTC: Trade: Tabs 60 mg pseudoephedrine/2.5 mg triprolidine. Syrup 30 mg pseudoephedrine/1.25 mg triprolidine/5 ml.

Aprodine (pseudoephedrine + triprolidine) ▶L ♀C ▶+ $

ADULT - Allergic rhinitis/nasal congestion: 1 tab or 10 ml PO q4-6h. Max 4 tabs/day or 40 ml/day.

PEDS - Allergic rhinitis/nasal congestion: >12 yo: Use adult dose. 6-12 yo: 1/2 tab or 5 ml PO q4-6h. Max 2 tabs/day or 20 ml/day.

FORMS - OTC: Trade: Tabs 60 mg pseudoephedrine/2.5 mg triprolidine. Syrup 30 mg pseudoephedrine/1.25 mg triprolidine/5 ml.

Benadryl Allergy & Cold (pseudoephedrine + diphenhydramine + acetaminophen) ▶L ♀C ▶- $

ADULT - Allergic rhinitis/nasal congestion/headache: 2 tabs PO q6h. Max 8 tabs/day.

PEDS - Allergic rhinitis/nasal congestion/headache: >12 yo: Use adult dose.

FORMS - OTC: Trade: Tabs 30 mg pseudoephedrine/12.5 mg diphenhydramine/500 mg acetaminophen.

Benadryl-D Allergy & Sinus (pseudoephedrine + diphenhydramine) ▶L ♀C ▶- $

ADULT - Allergic rhinitis/nasal congestion: 1 tab PO q4-6h. Max 4 tabs/day.

PEDS - Allergic rhinitis/nasal congestion: >12 yo: Use adult dose.

FORMS - OTC: Trade: Tabs 60 mg pseudoephedrine/25 mg diphenhydramine.

Cheracol D Cough, ✱BenylinDME) (guaifenesin + dextromethorphan) ▶L ♀C ▶? $

ADULT - Cough: 10 ml PO q4h

PEDS - Cough ≥12 yo: Use adult dose. 6-11 yo: 5 ml PO q4h. 2- 5 yo: 2.5 ml PO q4h. Max 15 ml/day.

FORMS - OTC: Generic/Trade: Syrup 100 mg guaifenesin/10 mg dextromethorphan/5 ml.

Children's Advil Cold (ibuprofen + pseudoephedrine) ▶L ♀C (D in 3rd trimester) ▶+ $

ADULT - Not approved for use in adults

PEDS - Nasal congestion/sore throat/fever: 6-11 yo: 10 ml PO q6h. 2-5 yo: 5 ml PO q6h.

FORMS - OTC: Trade: Suspension: 100 mg ibuprofen/15 mg pseudoephedrine/ 5 ml. Grape flavor, alcohol-free.

NOTES - Shake well before using. Do not use for >7 days for cold, sinus, & flu symptoms.

Claritin-D 12 hr (pseudoephedrine + loratadine) ▶LK ♀B ▶+ $$

ADULT - Allergic rhinitis/nasal congestion: 1 tab PO bid.

PEDS - Not approved in children.

FORMS - OTC: Generic/Trade: Tabs, 12-hour extended-release tabs: 120 mg pseudoephedrine/5 mg loratadine.

NOTES - Decrease dose to 1 tab PO qd with CrCl <30 ml/min. Avoid in hepatic insufficiency.

Claritin-D 24 hr (pseudoephedrine + loratadine) ▶LK ♀B ▶+ $$

ADULT - Allergic rhinitis/nasal congestion: 1 tab PO qd.

PEDS - Not approved in children.

FORMS - OTC: Generic/Trade: Tabs, 24-hour extended release tabs: 240 mg pseudoephedrine/10 mg loratadine.

NOTES - Decrease dose to 1 tab PO qod with CrCl <30 ml/min. Avoid in patients with hepatic insufficiency.

Dimetapp Cold & Allergy (pseudoephedrine + brompheniramine) ▶LK ♀C ▶- $

ADULT - Allergic rhinitis/nasal congestion: 20 ml PO q4h. Max 4 doses/day.

PEDS - Allergic rhinitis/nasal congestion: ≥12 yo: Use adult dose. 6-11 yo: 10ml PO q4h. 2-5 yo: 5 ml PO q4h. Max 4 doses/day.

UNAPPROVED PEDS - Allergic rhinitis/nasal congestion: 12-23 mo: ¾ tsp PO q6-8h. 6-11mo: ½ tsp PO q6-8h. Max: 4 doses/day.

FORMS - OTC: Trade: Liquid 15 mg pseudoephedrine/1 mg brompheniramine/5 ml.

NOTES - Grape flavor, alcohol-free.

Dimetapp Decongestant Plus Cough Infant Drops (pseudoephedrine + dextromethorphan) ▶LK ♀C ▶- $

ADULT - Not recommended.

PEDS - Nasal congestion/cough: 2-3 yo: 1.6 ml PO q4-6h. Max: 4 doses/day.

UNAPPROVED PEDS - Nasal congestion/cough: 12-23 mo: 1.2 ml PO q6h. 6-11mo: 0.8 ml PO q6h. Max: 4 doses/day.

FORMS - OTC: Trade: Infant drops 7.5 mg pseudoephedrine/2.5 mg dextromethorphan/0.8 ml.

NOTES - Alcohol-free.

Dimetapp DM Cold & Cough (pseudoephedrine + brompheniramine + dextromethorphan) ▶LK ♀C ▶- $

ADULT - Nasal congestion/cough: 20 ml PO

q4h. Max 4 doses/day.

PEDS - Nasal congestion/cough: ≥12 yo: Use adult dose. 6-11 yo: 10 ml PO q4h. 2-5 yo: 5 ml PO q4h. Max: 4 doses/day.

UNAPPROVED PEDS - Nasal congestion/cough: 12-23 mo: ¾ tsp PO q6-8h. 6-11mo: ½ tsp PO q6-8h. Max: 4 doses/day.

FORMS - OTC: Trade: Elixir 15 mg pseudoephedrine/1 mg brompheniramine/5 mg dextromethorphan/5 ml.

NOTES - Red grape flavor, alcohol-free.

Dimetapp Multisymptom Cold & Allergy (pseudoephedrine + chlorpheniramine + acetaminophen) ▶LK ♀C ▶- $

ADULT - Allergic rhinitis/nasal congestion/headache: 2 tabs PO q4h. Max 12 tabs/day.

PEDS - Allergic rhinitis/nasal congestion/headache: ≥12 yo: Use adult dose.

FORMS - OTC: Trade: Tabs 5 mg phenylephrine/2 mg chlorpheniramine/325 mg acetaminophen.

Dimetapp Nighttime Flu (pseudoephedrine + dextromethorphan + acetaminophen + brompheniramine) ▶LK ♀C ▶- $

ADULT - Nasal congestion/runny nose/fever/cough/sore throat: 20 ml PO q4h. Max 4 doses/day.

PEDS - Nasal congestion/runny nose/fever/cough/sore throat ≥12 yo: Use adult dose. 6-11 yo: 10 ml PO q4h. 2-5 yo: 5 ml PO q4h. Max: 4 doses/day.

UNAPPROVED PEDS - Nasal congestion/runny nose/fever/cough/sore throat: 12-23 mo: ¾ tsp PO q6-8h. 6-11mo: ½ tsp PO q6-8h. Max: 4 doses/day.

FORMS - OTC: Trade: Syrup 15 mg pseudoephedrine/5 mg dextromethorphan/160 mg acetaminophen/1 mg brompheniramine/5 ml.

NOTES - Bubble gum flavor, alcohol-free.

Dimetapp Non-Drowsy Flu (pseudoephedrine + dextromethorphan + acetaminophen) ▶LK ♀C ▶- $

ADULT - Nasal congestion/fever/cough/sore throat: 20 ml PO q4h. Max 4 doses/day.

PEDS - Nasal congestion/fever/cough/sore throat ≥12 yo: Use adult dose. 6-11 yo: 10 ml PO q4h. 2-5 yo: 5 ml PO q4h. Max 4 doses/day.

UNAPPROVED PEDS - Nasal congestion/fever/cough/sore throat: 12-23 mo: ¾ tsp PO q6-8h. 6-11mo: ½ tsp PO q6-8h. Max: 4 doses/day.

FORMS - OTC: Trade: Syrup 15 mg pseudoephedrine/5 mg dextromethorphan/160 mg acetaminophen/5 ml.

NOTES - Fruit flavor, alcohol-free.

Drixoral Cold & Allergy (pseudoephedrine + dexbrompheniramine) ▶LK ♀C ▶- $

ADULT - Allergic rhinitis/nasal congestion: 1 tab PO q12h.

PEDS - Allergic rhinitis/nasal congestion ≥12 yo: Use adult dose.

FORMS - OTC: Trade: Tabs, sustained-action 120 mg pseudoephedrine/6 mg dexbrompheniramine.

Drixoral Cold & Flu (pseudoephedrine + dexbrompheniramine + acetaminophen) ▶LK ♀C ▶- $

ADULT - Allergic rhinitis/nasal congestion: 2 tabs PO q12h. Max dose 4 tabs/day.

PEDS - Allergic rhinitis/nasal congestion ≥12 yo: Use adult dose.

FORMS - OTC: Trade: Tabs, sustained-action 60 mg pseudoephedrine/3 mg dexbrompheniramine/500 mg acetaminophen.

Guiatuss PE (pseudoephedrine + guaifenesin) ▶L ♀C ▶- $

ADULT - Nasal congestion/cough: 10 ml PO q4h. Max 40 ml/day.

PEDS - Nasal congestion/cough: ≥12 yo: Use adult dose. 6-11 yo: 5 ml PO q4h. 2-5 yo: 2.5 ml PO q4h. Max 4 doses/day.

FORMS - OTC: Trade: Syrup 30 mg pseudoephedrine/100 mg guaifenesin/5 ml.

NOTES - PE = pseudoephedrine

Mytussin DM (guaifenesin + dextromethorphan) ▶L ♀C ▶? $

ADULT - Cough: 10 ml PO q4h. Max 60 ml/day.

PEDS - Cough: ≥12 yo: Use adult dose. 6-11 yo: 5 ml PO q4h. Max 30 ml/day. 2-5 yo: 2.5 ml PO q4h. Max 15 ml/day.

FORMS - OTC: Generic/Trade: Syrup 100 mg guaifenesin/10 mg dextromethorphan/5 ml.

NOTES - DM = dextromethorphan

Robitussin CF (pseudoephedrine + guaifenesin + dextromethorphan) ▶L ♀C ▶- $

ADULT - Nasal congestion/cough: 10 ml PO q4h.

PEDS - Nasal congestion/cough: ≥12 yo: Use adult dose. 6-11 yo: 5 ml PO q4h. 2-5 yo: 2.5 ml PO q4h.

UNAPPROVED PEDS - Nasal congestion/cough: 12-23 mo: 1.25 ml PO q6h. 6-11 mo: 1.25 ml PO q8h.

FORMS - OTC: Trade: Syrup 30 mg pseudoephedrine/100 mg guaifenesin/10 mg dextromethorphan/5 ml.

NOTES - CF= cough formula.

Robitussin DM (guaifenesin + dextromethorphan) ▶L ♀C ▶+ $

ADULT - Cough: 10 ml PO q4h. Max 60 ml/day.

PEDS - Cough: ≥12 yo: Use adult dose. 6-11 yo: 5 ml PO q4h. Max 30 ml/day. 2-5 yo: 2.5 ml PO q4h. Max 15 ml/day.

UNAPPROVED PEDS - Cough: 12-23 mo: 2.5 ml PO q8h. Max 7.5 ml/day. 6-11 mo: 1.25 ml PO q8h. Max 3.75 ml/day.

FORMS - OTC: Generic/Trade: Syrup 100 mg guaifenesin/10 mg dextromethorphan/5 ml.

NOTES - Alcohol-free. DM = dextromethorphan.

Robitussin PE (pseudoephedrine + guaifenesin) ▶L ♀C ▶- $

ADULT - Nasal congestion/cough: 10 ml PO q4h. Max 40 ml/day.

PEDS - Nasal congestion/cough: ≥12 yo: Use adult dose. 6-11 yo: 5 ml PO q4h. Max 20 ml/day. 2-5 yo: 2.5 ml PO q4h. Max 10 ml/day.

UNAPPROVED PEDS - Nasal congestion/cough: 12-23 mo: 1.25 ml PO q6h. Max 5 ml/day. 6-11 mo: 1.25 ml PO q8h. Max 3.75 ml/day.

FORMS - OTC: Trade: Syrup 30 mg pseudoephedrine/100 mg guaifenesin/5 ml.

NOTES - PE = pseudoephedrine.

Triaminic Chest Congestion (pseudoephedrine + guaifenesin) ▶LK ♀C ▶- $

ADULT - Chest/nasal congestion: 20 ml PO q4-6h.

PEDS - Chest/nasal congestion ≥12 yo: Use adult dose. 6-11 yo: 10 ml PO q4-6h. 2-5 yo: 5 ml PO q4-6h.

UNAPPROVED PEDS - Chest/nasal congestion: 13-23 mo: 2.5 ml PO q4-6h. 4-12 mo: 1.25 ml PO q4-6h.

FORMS - OTC: Trade: Syrup, 15 mg pseudoephedrine/50 mg guaifenesin/5 ml, citrus flavor.

Triaminic Cold & Allergy (pseudoephedrine + chlorpheniramine) ▶LK ♀C ▶- $

ADULT - Allergic rhinitis/nasal congestion: 20 ml PO q4-6h.

PEDS - Allergic rhinitis/nasal congestion ≥12 yo: Use adult dose. 6-11 yo: 10 ml PO q4-6h. Softchew tab: 6-11 yo: 2 tabs q4-6h.

UNAPPROVED PEDS - Allergic rhinitis/nasal congestion: Give PO q4-6h: 2-5 yo: 5 ml. 13-23 mo: 2.5 ml. 4-12 mo: 1.25 ml.

FORMS - OTC: Trade: Syrup, softchew tabs 15 mg pseudoephedrine/1 mg chlorpheniramine/5 ml, orange flavor.

Triaminic Cold & Cough (pseudoephedrine + chlorpheniramine + dextromethorphan) ▶LK ♀C ▶- $

ADULT - Nasal congestion/runny nose/cough: 20 ml PO q4h or 4 tabs q4-6h.

PEDS - Nasal congestion/runny nose/cough ≥12 yo: Use adult dose. 6-11 yo: 10 ml PO q4h. Softchew tab: 6-11 yo: 2 tabs q4-6h.

UNAPPROVED PEDS - Nasal congestion/runny nose/cough: 13-23 mo: 2.5 ml PO q4h. 4-12 mo: 1.25 ml PO q4h.

FORMS - OTC: Trade: Syrup, softchew tabs 15 mg pseudoephedrine/1 mg chlorpheniramine/5 mg dextromethorphan/5 ml, cherry flavor.

Triaminic Cough (pseudoephedrine + dextromethorphan) ▶LK ♀C ▶- $

ADULT - Nasal congestion/cough: 20 ml PO q4h.

PEDS - Nasal congestion/cough ≥12 yo: Use adult dose. 6-11 yo: 10 ml PO q4h. 2-5 yo: 5 ml PO q4h. Softchew tab: 6-11 yo: 2 tabs q4-6h.

UNAPPROVED PEDS - Nasal congestion/cough: 13-23 mo: 2.5 ml PO q4h. 4-12 mo: 1.25 ml PO q4h.

FORMS - OTC: Trade: Syrup, softchew tabs 15 mg pseudoephedrine/ 5 mg dextromethorphan/5 ml, berry flavor

Triaminic Cough & Sore Throat (pseudoephedrine + dextromethorphan + acetaminophen) ▶LK ♀C ▶- $

ADULT - Nasal congestion/cough/sore throat: 20 ml PO q4h.

PEDS - Nasal congestion/cough/sore throat ≥12 yo: Use adult dose. 6-11 yo: 10 ml PO q4h. 2-5 yo: 5 ml PO q4h. Softchew tab: 6-11 yo: 2 tabs q4-6h.

UNAPPROVED PEDS - Nasal congestion/cough/sore throat: 13-23 mo: 2.5 ml PO q4h. 4-12 mo: 1.25 ml PO q4h.

FORMS - OTC: Trade: Syrup, 15 mg pseudoephedrine/ 5 mg dextromethorphan / 160 mg acetaminophen /5 ml, berry flavor. Softchew tab, 15 mg pseudoephedrine/ 7.5 mg dextromethorphan/160 mg acetaminophen.

ENT: ENT Combination Products – Rx Only

NOTE: Decongestants in some ENT combination products can increase BP, aggravate anxiety or cause insomnia (use caution). Some contain sedating antihistamines. Sedation can be enhanced by alcohol and other CNS depressants.

Allegra-D (pseudoephedrine + fexofenadine) ▶LK ♀C ▶+ $$$

ADULT - Allergic rhinitis/nasal congestion: 1 tab PO q12h.

PEDS - Not approved in children.

FORMS - Trade: Tabs, extended release 120 mg pseudoephedrine/60 mg fexofenadine.

NOTES - Decrease dose to 1 tablet PO qd with decreased renal function. Take on an empty stomach. Avoid taking with fruit juice due to a large decrease in bioavailability.

Bromfenex (pseudoephedrine + brompheniramine) ▶LK ♀C ▶- $

ADULT - Allergic rhinitis/nasal congestion: 1 cap PO q12h. Max 2 caps/day.

PEDS - Allergic rhinitis/nasal congestion: >12 yo: Use adult dose. 6-11 yo: 1 cap PO qd.

FORMS - Generic/Trade: Caps, sustained release 120 mg pseudoephedrine/12 mg brompheniramine.

Bromfenex PD (pseudoephedrine + brompheniramine) ▶LK ♀C ▶- $

ADULT - Allergic rhinitis/nasal congestion: 1-2 caps PO q12h. Max 4 caps/day.

PEDS - Allergic rhinitis/nasal congestion: >12 yo: 1 cap PO q12h. Max 2 caps/day.

FORMS - Generic/Trade: Caps, sustained release 60 mg pseudoephedrine/6 mg brompheniramine.

NOTES - PD = pediatric.

Carbodec DM (pseudoephedrine + carbinoxamine + dextromethorphan) ▶L♀C▶- $

ADULT - Allergic rhinitis/nasal congestion/cough: 5 ml PO qid.

PEDS - Allergic rhinitis/nasal congestion/cough >6 yo: 5 ml PO qid. 18 mo-5 yo: 2.5 ml PO q6h. Infant Drops: Give PO qid: 1-3 mo: 0.25 ml. 4-6 mo: 0.5 ml. 7-9 mo: 0.75 ml. 10 mo-17 mo: 1 ml.

FORMS - Generic/Trade: Syrup 60 mg pseudoephedrine/4 mg carbinoxamine/15 mg dextromethorphan/5 ml (Carbodec DM Syrup). Generic/Trade: Drops 25 mg pseudoephedrine/2 mg carbinoxamine/4 mg dextromethorphan/ ml, grape flavor 30 ml w/dropper. Sugar-free (Carbodec DM Oral Infant Drops).

NOTES - Carbinoxamine has potential for sedation similar to diphenhydramine. DM = dextromethorphan.

Chlordrine SR (pseudoephedrine + chlorpheniramine) ▶LK ♀C ▶- $

ADULT - Allergic rhinitis/nasal congestion: 1 cap PO q12h. Max 2 caps/day.

PEDS - Allergic rhinitis/nasal congestion >12 yo: Use adult dose. 6-11 yo: 1 cap PO qd.

FORMS - Generic/Trade: Caps, sustained release 120 mg pseudoephedrine/8 mg chlorpheniramine.

Codeprex (chlorpheniramine + codeine) ▶LK ♀C ▶- ©III $

ADULT - Cough/rhinitis: 2 teaspoonfuls PO q12h. Max 4 tsp/day.

PEDS - Cough/rhinitis >12 yo: Use adult dose. 6-11 yo: 1 tsp PO q12h. Max 2 tsp/ day.

FORMS - Trade: Suspension, extended release 20 mg codeine + 4 mg chlorpheniramine per 5 mL. Cherry cream flavor.

NOTES - May increase phenytoin levels. Avoid MAO inhibitors. Shake well.

Cydec Drops (pseudoephedrine + carbinoxamine) ▶L ♀C ▶- $

PEDS - Allergic rhinitis/nasal congestion: Give PO qid: 1-3 mo: 0.25 ml. 3-6 mo: 0.5 ml. 6-9 mo: 0.75 ml. 9 mo-5 yo: 1.0 ml.

FORMS - Generic/Trade: Drops 25 mg pseudoephedrine/2 mg carbinoxamine/ml, raspberry flavor, 30 ml. Alcohol- & sugar-free.

NOTES - Carbinoxamine has potential for sedation similar to diphenhydramine.

Deconamine (pseudoephedrine + chlorpheniramine) ▶LK ♀C ▶- $

WARNING - Multiple strengths; write specific product on Rx.

ADULT - Allergic rhinitis/nasal congestion: 1 tab or 10 ml PO tid-qid. Max 6 tabs or 60 ml/day. Sustained release: 1 cap PO q12h. Max 2 caps /day.

PEDS - Allergic rhinitis/nasal congestion: >12 yo: Use adult dose. 6-11 yo: ½ tab or 5 ml PO tid-qid. Max 3 tabs or 30 ml/day.

FORMS - Trade: Tabs 60 mg pseudoephedrine/4 mg chlorpheniramine, scored (Deconamine). Syrup 30 mg pseudoephedrine/2 mg chlorpheniramine/5 ml (Deconamine). Generic/Trade: Caps, sustained release 120 mg pseudoephedrine/8 mg chlorpheniramine (Deconamine SR).

Deconsal II (pseudoephedrine + guaifenesin) ▶L ♀C ▶- $

ADULT - Nasal congestion/cough: 1-2 tabs PO q12h. Max 4 tabs/day.

PEDS - Nasal congestion/cough: >12 yo: Use adult dose. 6-12 yo: 1 tab PO q12h, max 2 tabs/day. 2-5 yo: ½ tab PO q12h. Max 1 tab/day.

FORMS - Generic/Trade: Tabs, sustained release 60 mg pseudoephedrine/600 mg guaifenesin, scored.

Defen-LA (pseudoephedrine + guaifenesin) ▶L ♀C ▶- $

ADULT - Nasal congestion/cough: 1-2 tabs PO q12h.

PEDS - Nasal congestion/cough: >12 yo: Use adult dose.

FORMS - Trade: Tabs, long-acting 60 mg pseudoephedrine/600 mg guaifenesin, scored.

Detussin (pseudoephedrine + hydro-codone, ♥Novahistex) ▶L ♀C ▶- ©III $
ADULT - Nasal congestion/cough: 5 ml PO qid prn.
PEDS - Nasal congestion/cough 22-40 kg: 2.5 ml PO qid prn. 12-22 kg: 1.25 ml PO qid prn.
FORMS - Generic/Trade: Liquid 60 mg pseudoephedrine/5 mg hydrocodone/5 ml.

Dimetane-DX Cough Syrup (pseudoephedrine + brompheniramine + dextromethorphan) ▶L ♀C ▶- $$
ADULT - Nasal congestion/rhinitis/cough: 10 ml PO q4h prn.
PEDS - Nasal congestion/rhinitis/cough: >12 yo: Use adult dose. 6-11 yo: 5 ml PO q4h. 2-5 yo: 2.5 ml PO q4h. 22-40 kg: 2.5 ml PO qid prn. 12-22 kg: 1.25 ml PO qid prn.
FORMS - Trade: Liquid 30 mg pseudoephedrine /2 mg brompheniramine/10 mg dextromethorphan/5 ml, butterscotch flavor. Sugar-free.

Duratuss (pseudoephedrine + guaifenesin) ▶L ♀C ▶- $
ADULT - Nasal congestion/cough: 1 tab PO q12h.
PEDS - Nasal congestion/cough: >12 yo: Use adult dose. 6-12 yo: ½ tab PO q12h.
FORMS - Trade: Tabs, long-acting 120 mg pseudoephedrine/600 mg guaifenesin, scored.

Duratuss GP (pseudoephedrine + guaifenesin) ▶L ♀C ▶- $
ADULT - Nasal congestion/cough: 1 PO q12h.
PEDS - Not approved in children.
FORMS - Trade: Tabs, long-acting 120 mg pseudoephedrine/1200 mg guaifenesin.

Duratuss HD (hydrocodone + pseudoephedrine + guaifenesin) ▶L ♀C ▶- ©III $$$
ADULT - Cough/nasal congestion: 10 ml PO q4-6h.
PEDS - Cough/nasal congestion: >12 yo: Use adult dose. 6-12 yo: 5 ml PO q4-6h.
FORMS - Trade: Elixir 2.5 mg hydrocodone/30 mg pseudoephedrine/ 100 mg guaifenensin/5 ml. 5% alcohol, fruit punch flavored.

Entex LA (phenylephrine + guaifenesin) ▶L ♀C ▶- $
ADULT - Nasal congestion/cough: 1 tab PO q12h.
PEDS - Nasal congestion/cough: ≥12 yo: Use adult dose. 6-11 yo: ½ tab PO q12h.
FORMS - Trade: Tabs, long-acting 30 mg phenylephrine/600 mg guaifenesin, scored.
NOTES - Do not crush or chew.

Entex Liquid (phenylephrine + guaifenesin) ▶L ♀C ▶- $$$

ADULT - Nasal congestion/cough: 5-10 ml PO q4-6h. Max 40 ml/day.
PEDS - Nasal congestion/cough: ≥12 yo: Use adult dose. 6-11 yo: 5 ml PO q4-6h. Max 20 ml/day. 2-5 yo: 2.5 ml PO q4-6h. Max 10 ml/day.
FORMS - Rx: Trade: Liquid 7.5 mg phenylephrine/100 mg guaifenesin/5 ml. Punch flavor, alcohol-free.

Entex PSE (pseudoephedrine + guaifenesin) ▶L ♀C ▶- $
ADULT - Nasal congestion/cough: 1 tab PO q12h.
PEDS - Nasal congestion/cough: >12 yo: Use adult dose. 6-12 yo: ½ tab PO q12h.
FORMS - Trade: Tabs, long-acting 120 mg pseudoephedrine/600 mg guaifenesin, scored.
NOTES - PSE = pseudoephedrine.

Fenesin DM (guaifenesin + dextromethorphan) ▶L ♀C ▶? $
ADULT - Cough: 1-2 tabs PO q12h. Max 4 tabs/day.
PEDS - Cough ≥12 yo: Use adult dose. 6-12 yo: 1 tab PO q12h. Max 2 tabs/day. 2-5 yo: ½ tab PO q12h. Max 1 tab/day.
FORMS - Trade: Tabs, sustained release 600 mg guaifenesin/30 mg dextromethorphan.
NOTES - DM = dextromethorphan.

Gani-Tuss NR (guaifenesin + codeine) ▶L ♀C ▶? ©V $
ADULT - Cough: 10 ml PO q4h. Max 60 ml/day.
PEDS - Cough ≥12 yo: Use adult dose. 6-11 yo: 5 ml PO q4h. Max 30 ml/day. 2-5 yo: 2.5-5 ml PO q4h. Max 30 ml/day. 6-23 mo: 1.25-2.5 ml PO q4h. Max 15 ml/day.
FORMS - Trade: Syrup 100 mg guaifenesin/10 mg codeine/5 ml, raspberry flavor. Sugar-free.

Guaifenex DM (guaifenesin + dextromethorphan) ▶L ♀C ▶? $
ADULT - Cough: 1-2 tabs PO q12h. Max 4 tabs/day.
PEDS - Cough ≥12 yo: Use adult dose. 6-12 yo: 1 tab PO q12h. Max 2 tabs/day. 2-6 yo: ½ tab PO q12h. Max 1 tab/day.
FORMS - Trade: Tabs, sustained release 600 mg guaifenesin/30 mg dextromethorphan, scored.
NOTES - DM = dextromethorphan.

Guaifenex PSE (pseudoephedrine + guaifenesin) ▶L ♀C ▶- $
WARNING - Multiple strengths; write specific product on Rx.
ADULT - Nasal congestion/cough: PSE 60: 1-2 tabs PO q12h. Max 4 tabs/day. PSE 120: 1 tab PO q12h.
PEDS - Nasal congestion/cough: PSE 60: >12

yo: Use adult dose. 6-12 yo: 1 tab PO q12h. Max 2 tabs/day. 2-6 yo: ½ tab PO q12h. Max 1 tab/day. PSE 120: >12 yo: Use adult dose. 6-12 yo: ½ tab PO q12h.

FORMS - Generic/Trade: Tabs, extended release 60 mg pseudoephedrine/600 mg guaifenesin, scored (Guaifenex PSE 60). Trade: Tabs, extended release 120 mg pseudoephedrine/600 mg guaifenesin (Guaifenex PSE 120).

NOTES - PSE = pseudoephedrine.

Guaitex II SR/PSE **(pseudoephedrine + guaifenesin)** ▶L ♀C ▶- $

WARNING - Multiple strengths; write specific product on Rx.

ADULT - Nasal congestion/cough: 1-2 tabs PO q12h. Max 4 tabs/day (Guaitex II SR). 1 tab PO q12h. Max 2 tabs/day (Guaitex PSE).

PEDS - Nasal congestion/cough: >12 yo: Use adult dose. 6-12 yo: 1 tab PO q12h. Max 2 tabs/day. 2-5 yo: ½ tab PO q12h. Max 1 tab/day (Guaitex II SR). >12 yo: Use adult dose. 6-12 yo: ½ tab PO q12h (Guaitex PSE).

FORMS - Generic/Trade: Tabs, sustained release 60 mg pseudoephedrine/600 mg guaifenesin (Guaitex II SR). Trade: Tabs, long-acting 120 mg pseudoephedrine/600 mg guaifenesin (Guaitex PSE).

NOTES - PSE=pseudoephedrine.

Guiatuss AC **(guaifenesin + codeine)** ▶L ♀C ▶? ©V $

ADULT - Cough: 10 ml PO q4h. Max 60 ml/day.

PEDS - Cough ≥12 yo: Use adult dose. 6-11 yo: 5 ml PO q4h. Max 30 ml/day.

FORMS - Generic/Trade: Syrup 100 mg guaifenesin/10 mg codeine/5 ml. Sugar-free.

NOTES - AC = and codeine

Guiatussin DAC **(pseudoephedrine + guaifenesin + codeine)** ▶L ♀C ▶- ©V $

ADULT - Nasal congestion/cough: 10 ml PO q4h. Max 40 ml/day.

PEDS - Nasal congestion/cough ≥12 yo: Use adult dose. 6-11 yo: 5 ml PO q4h. Max 20 ml/day.

FORMS - Trade: Syrup 30 mg pseudoephedrine/100 mg guaifenesin/10 mg codeine/5 ml. Sugar-free.

NOTES - DAC = decongestant and codeine.

Halotussin AC **(guaifenesin + codeine)** ▶L ♀C ▶? ©V $

ADULT - Cough: 10 ml PO q4h. Max 60 ml/day.

PEDS - Cough ≥12 yo: Use adult dose. 6-11 yo: 5 ml PO q4h. Max 30 ml/day.

FORMS - Trade: Syrup 100 mg guaifenesin/10 mg codeine/5 ml.

NOTES - AC = and codeine

Halotussin DAC **(pseudoephedrine + guaifenesin + codeine)** ▶L ♀C ▶- ©V $

ADULT - Nasal congestion/cough: 10 ml PO q4h. Max 40 ml/day.

PEDS - Nasal congestion/cough: ≥12 yo: Use adult dose. 6-11 yo: 5 ml PO q4h. Max 20 ml/day.

FORMS - Trade: Syrup 30 mg pseudoephedrine/100 mg guaifenesin/10 mg codeine/5 ml, cherry-raspberry flavor. Sugar-free.

NOTES - DAC = decongestant and codeine.

Histinex HC **(phenylephrine + chlorpheniramine + hydrocodone)** ▶L ♀C ▶- ©III $

ADULT - Allergic rhinitis/congestion/cough: 10 ml PO q4h. Max 40 ml/day.

PEDS - Allergic rhinitis/congestion/cough: >12 yo: Use adult dose. 6-12 yo: 5 ml PO q4h. Max 20 ml/day.

FORMS - Trade: Syrup 5 mg phenylephrine/2 mg chlorpheniramine/2.5 mg hydrocodone/5 ml. Alcohol- and sugar-free.

Histussin D **(pseudoephedrine + hydrocodone)** ▶L ♀C ▶- ©III $

ADULT - Nasal congestion/cough: 5 ml PO qid prn.

PEDS - Nasal congestion/cough: 22-40 kg: 2.5 ml PO qid prn. 12-22 kg: 1.25 ml PO qid prn.

FORMS - Generic/Trade: Liquid 60 mg pseudoephedrine/5 mg hydrocodone/5 ml, cherry/black raspberry flavor.

Histussin HC **(phenylephrine + chlorpheniramine + hydrocodone)** ▶L ♀C ▶- ©III $$

ADULT - Allergic rhinitis/congestion/cough: 10 ml PO q4h. Max 40 ml/day.

PEDS - Allergic rhinitis/congestion/cough: >12 yo: Use adult dose. 6-12 yo: 5 ml PO q4h. Max 20 ml/day.

FORMS - Trade: Syrup 5 mg phenylephrine/2 mg chlorpheniramine/2.5 mg hydrocodone/5 ml.

Humibid DM **(guaifenesin + guaiacolsulfonate + dextromethorphan)** ▶L ♀C ▶? $

ADULT - Cough: 1 cap PO q12h. Max 2 caps/day.

PEDS - Cough: ≥12 yo: Use adult dose. 6-12 yo: 1 cap PO qd.

FORMS - Trade: Caps, sustained release 400 mg guaifenesin + 200 mg guaiacolsulfonate + 50 mg dextromethorphan.

NOTES - DM = dextromethorphan.

Humibid LA **(guaifenesin + guaiacolsulfonate)** ▶L ♀C ▶+ $

ADULT - Expectorant: 1 tab PO q12h (extended release). Max 2/day.

PEDS - Expectorant >12 yo: Use adult dose.

FORMS - Trade: Tabs, extended release 600 mg guaifenesin + 300 mg guaiacolsulfonate.

Hycodan (hydrocodone + homatropine) ▶L ♀C ▶- ©III $

ADULT - Antitussive: 1 tab or 5 mL PO q4-6h. Max 6 doses/day.

PEDS - Antitussive >12: Use adult dose. 6-12 yo: 2.5 mg (based on hydrocodone) PO q4-6h prn. Max 15 mg/day.

FORMS - Trade: Tabs 5 mg hydrocodone/1.5 mg homatropine methylbromide. Generic/Trade; Syrup 5 mg hydrocodone/1.5 mg homatropine methylbromide/5 ml.

NOTES - May cause drowsiness/sedation. Dosing based on hydrocodone content.

Hycotuss (hydrocodone + guaifenesin) ▶L ♀C ▶- ©III $$

ADULT - Cough: 5 ml PO pc & qhs. Max 6 doses/day.

PEDS - Cough: >12 yo: Use adult dose. 6-12 yo: 2.5 ml PO pc & qhs. Max 6 doses/day.

FORMS - Trade: Syrup 5 mg hydrocodone/100 mg guaifenesin/5 ml. Butterscotch flavor.

Mucinex DM (guaifenesin + dextromethorphan) ▶L ♀C ▶? $

ADULT - Cough: 1-2 tabs (600/30) PO q12h; max 4 tabs/24 h. 1 tab (1200/60) PO q12h; max 2 tabs/24 h.

PEDS - Cough: ≥12 yo: Use adult dose.

FORMS - OTC: Trade: Tabs, extended release: 600 mg guaifenesin/30 mg dextromethorphan & 1200 mg guaifenesin/60 dextromethorphan.

NOTES - DM = dextromethorphan. Do not crush, chew or break the tablet. Take with a full glass of water.

Novafed A (pseudoephedrine + chlorpheniramine) ▶LK ♀C ▶- $

ADULT - Allergic rhinitis/nasal congestion: 1 cap PO q12h. Max 2 caps/day.

PEDS - Allergic rhinitis/nasal congestion: >12 yo: Use adult dose. 6-12 yo: 1 cap PO qd.

FORMS - Generic/Trade: Caps, sustained release 120 mg pseudoephedrine/8 mg chlorpheniramine.

Phenergan VC (phenylephrine + promethazine) ▶LK ♀C ▶? $

ADULT - Allergic rhinitis/congestion: 5 ml PO q4-6h. Max 30 ml/day.

PEDS - Allergic rhinitis/congestion: ≥12 yo: Use adult dose. 6-11 yo: 2.5-5 ml PO q4-6h. Max 20 ml/day. 2-5 yo: 1.25-2.5 ml PO q4-6h. Max 15 ml/day.

FORMS - Generic/Trade: Syrup 6.25 mg promethazine/5 mg phenylephrine/5 ml.

NOTES - VC = vasoconstrictor

Phenergan VC w/codeine (phenylephrine + promethazine + codeine) ▶LK♀C▶? ©V $

ADULT - Allergic rhinitis/congestion/cough: 5 ml PO q4-6h. Max 30 ml/day.

PEDS - Allergic rhinitis/congestion/cough: ≥12 yo: Use adult dose. 6-11 yo: 2.5-5 ml PO q4-6h. Max 20 ml/day. 2-5 yo: 1.25-2.5 ml PO q4-6h. Max 10 ml/day.

FORMS - Generic/Trade: Syrup 5 mg phenylephrine/6.25 mg promethazine/10 mg codeine/5 ml.

Phenergan/Dextromethorphan (promethazine + dextromethorphan) ▶LK ♀C ▶? $

ADULT - Allergic rhinitis/cough: 5 ml PO q4-6h. Max 30 ml/day.

PEDS - Allergic rhinitis/cough: ≥12 yo: Use adult dose. 6-11 yo: 2.5-5 ml PO q4-6h. Max 20 ml/day. 2-5 yo: 1.25-2.5 ml PO q4-6h. Max 10 ml/day.

FORMS - Generic/Trade: Syrup 6.25 mg promethazine/15 mg dextromethorphan/5 ml.

Polyhistine (phenyltoloxamine + pyrilamine + pheniramine) ▶L ♀? ▶? $

ADULT - Allergic/vasomotor rhinitis, allergic conjunctivitis, urticaria: 10 ml PO q4h.

PEDS - Allergic/vasomotor rhinitis, allergic conjunctivitis, urticaria: 6-12 yo: 5 ml PO q4h. 2-5 yo: 2.5 ml PO q4h.

FORMS - Trade: Elixir phenyltoloxamine 4 mg/pyrilamine 4 mg/pheniramine 4 mg/5 ml.

Pseudo-Chlor (pseudoephedrine + chlorpheniramine) ▶LK ♀C ▶- $

ADULT - Allergic rhinitis/nasal congestion: 1 cap PO q12h. Max 2 caps/day.

PEDS - Allergic rhinitis/nasal congestion: >12 yo: Use adult dose.

FORMS - Generic/Trade: Caps, sustained release 120 mg pseudoephedrine/8 mg chlorpheniramine.

Robitussin AC (guaifenesin + codeine) ▶L ♀C ▶? ©V $

ADULT - Cough: 10 ml PO q4h. Max 60 ml/day.

PEDS - Not approved in children.

UNAPPROVED PEDS - Cough: ≥12 yo: Use adult dose. 6-11 yo: 5-10 ml PO q4h. 2-5 yo: 2.5-5 ml PO q4h. 6-23 mo: 1.25-2.5 ml q4h.

FORMS - Generic/Trade: Syrup 100 mg guaifenesin/10 mg codeine/5 ml. Alcohol-free.

NOTES - AC = and codeine

Robitussin DAC (pseudoephedrine + guaifenesin + codeine) ▶L ♀C ▶- ©V $

ADULT - Nasal congestion/cough: 10 ml PO q4h. Max 40 ml/day.

PEDS - Nasal congestion/cough: ≥12 yo: Use adult dose. 6-11 yo: 5 ml PO q4h. Max 20 ml/

day.

FORMS - Trade: Syrup 30 mg pseudoephedrine/100 mg guaifenesin/10 mg codeine/5 ml. Sugar-free.

NOTES - DAC = decongestant and codeine.

***Rondec* (pseudoephedrine + brompheniramine)** ▶L ♀C ▶- $$

ADULT - Allergic rhinitis/nasal congestion: 5 ml syrup PO qid.

PEDS - Allergic rhinitis/nasal congestion >6 yo: 5 ml syrup PO qid. 18 mo-5 yo: 2.5 ml PO qid.

FORMS - Generic/Trade: Syrup 45 mg pseudoephedrine/4 mg brompheniramine/5 ml, berry flavor. Alcohol- & sugar-free.

***Rondec DM* (pseudoephedrine + brompheniramine + dextromethorphan)** ▶L ♀C ▶- $$

ADULT - Allergic rhinitis/nasal congestion/cough: 5 ml syrup PO qid.

PEDS - Allergic rhinitis/nasal congestion/cough >6 yo: 5 ml syrup PO qid. 18 mo-5 yo: 2.5 ml syrup PO qid.

FORMS - Generic/Trade: Syrup 45 mg pseudoephedrine/4 mg carbinoxamine/15 mg dextromethorphan/5 ml. Alcohol- & sugar-free.

NOTES - Carbinoxamine is a sedating antihistamine similar to diphenhydramine. DM = dextromethorphan.

***Rondec DM Infant Drops* (pseudoephedrine + carbinoxamine + dextromethorphan)** ▶L ♀C ▶- $$

PEDS - Allergic rhinitis/nasal congestion/cough: Give PO qid: 1-3 mo: 0.25 ml. 4-6 mo: 0.5 ml. 7-9 mo: 0.75 ml. 10 mo-17 mo: 1 ml.

FORMS - Generic/Trade: Drops 15 mg pseudoephedrine/1 mg carbinoxamine/4 mg dextromethorphan/ml, grape flavor, 30 ml w/dropper. Alcohol- & sugar-free.

NOTES - Carbinoxamine is a sedating antihistamine similar to diphenhydramine.

***Rondec Infant Drops* (pseudoephedrine + carbinoxamine)** ▶L ♀C ▶- $$

PEDS - Allergic rhinitis/nasal congestion: Give PO qid: 1-3 mo: 0.25 ml. 4-6 mo: 0.5 ml. 7-9 mo: 0.75 ml. 10 mo-17 mo: 1 ml.

FORMS - Trade: Drops 15 mg pseudoephedrine/1 mg carbinoxamine/ ml, berry flavor, 30 ml. Alcohol- & sugar-free.

NOTES - Carbinoxamine is a sedating antihistamine similar to diphenhydramine.

***Ryna-12 S* (phenylephrine + pyrilamine)** ▶L ♀C ▶- $$

PEDS - Nasal congestion, allergic rhinitis, sinusitis: >6 yo: 5-10 ml PO q12h. 2-6 yo 2.5-5 ml PO q12h. <2 yo titrate dose individually.

FORMS - Trade: Suspension 5 mg phenylephrine/30 mg pyrilamine/5 ml strawberry-currant flavor w/graduated oral syringe.

***Rynatan* (azatadine + pseudoephedrine)** ▶LK ♀C ▶- $$

ADULT - Allergic rhinitis/nasal congestion: 1-2 tabs PO q12h.

PEDS - Allergic rhinitis/nasal congestion: ≥12 yo: 1 tab PO q12h.

FORMS - Trade: Tabs, extended release: 25 mg phenylephrine tannate/9 mg chlorpheniramine tannate.

***Rynatan Pediatric Suspension* (phenylephrine + chlorpheniramine)** ▶L ♀C ▶- $$

PEDS - Nasal congestion, allergic rhinitis, sinusitis >6 yo: 5-10 ml PO q12h. 2-6 yo 2.5-5 ml PO q12h. <2 yo titrate dose individually.

FORMS - Trade: Suspension 5 mg phenylephrine/4.5 mg chlorpheniramine/5 ml strawberry-currant flavor.

***Semprex-D* (pseudoephedrine + acrivastine)** ▶LK ♀C ▶- $$$

ADULT - Allergic rhinitis/nasal congestion: 1 cap PO q4-6h. Max 4 caps/day.

PEDS - Not approved in children.

FORMS - Trade: Caps 60 mg pseudoephedrine/8 mg acrivastine.

***Tanafed* (pseudoephedrine + chlorpheniramine)** ▶L ♀C ▶- $$

ADULT - Allergic rhinitis/nasal congestion: 10-20 ml PO q12h. Max 40 ml/day.

PEDS - Allergic rhinitis/nasal congestion: ≥12 yo: Use adult dose. 6-11 yo: 5-10 ml PO q12h. Max 20 ml/day. 2-5 yo: 2.5-5 ml PO q12h. Max 10 ml/day.

FORMS - Trade: Suspension 75 mg pseudoephedrine/4.5 mg chlorpheniramine/5 ml, strawberry-banana flavor.

***Triacin-C* (pseudoephedrine + triprolidine + codeine)** ▶L ♀C ▶+ ©V $

ADULT - Allergic rhinitis/nasal congestion/cough: 10 ml PO q4-6h. Max 40 ml/day.

PEDS - Allergic rhinitis/nasal congestion/cough: ≥12 yo: Use adult dose. 6-11 yo: 2.5-5 ml PO q4-6h. Max 20 ml/day.

FORMS - Trade: Syrup 30 mg pseudoephedrine/1.25 mg triprolidine/10 mg codeine /5 ml.

***Tuss-HC* (phenylephrine + chlorpheniramine + hydrocodone)** ▶L ♀C ▶- ©III $

ADULT - Allergic rhinitis/congestion/cough: 10 ml PO q4h. Max 40 ml/day.

PEDS - Allergic rhinitis/congestion/cough: >12 yo: Use adult dose. 6-12 yo: 5 ml PO q4h. Max 20 ml/day.

FORMS - Trade: Syrup 5 mg phenylephrine/2

mg chlorpheniramine/2.5 mg hydrocodone/5 ml.

Tussionex (chlorpheniramine + hydrocodone) ▶L ♀C ▶- ©III $$

ADULT - Allergic rhinitis/cough: 5 ml PO q12h. Max 10 ml/day.

PEDS - Allergic rhinitis/cough: 6-12 yo: 2.5 ml PO q12h. Max 5 ml/day.

FORMS - Trade: Extended release susp 8 mg chlorpheniramine/10 mg hydrocodone/5 ml.

Zephrex-LA (pseudoephedrine + guaifenesin) ▶L ♀C ▶- $

ADULT - Nasal congestion/cough: 1 tab PO q12h.

PEDS - Nasal congestion/cough: >12 yo: Use adult dose. 6-12 yo: ½ tab PO q12h.

FORMS - Trade: Tabs, extended release 120 mg pseudoephedrine/600 mg guaifenesin.

Zyrtec-D (pseudoephedrine + cetirizine) ▶LK ♀C ▶- $$$

ADULT - Allergic rhinitis/nasal congestion: 1 tab PO q12h.

PEDS - Not approved in children.

FORMS - Trade: Tabs, extended release 120 mg pseudoephedrine/5 mg cetirizine.

NOTES - Decrease dose to 1 tablet PO qd with decreased renal or hepatic function. Take on an empty stomach.

ENT: Mouth & Lip Preparations

amlexanox (Aphthasol) ▶LK ♀B ▶? $

ADULT - Aphthous ulcers: Apply ¼ inch paste to ulcer in mouth qid after oral hygiene for up to 10 days.

PEDS - Not approved in children.

FORMS - Trade: Oral paste 5%, 5 g tube.

cevimeline (Evoxac) ▶L ♀C ▶- $$$

ADULT - Dry mouth due to Sjogren's syndrome: 30 mg PO tid.

PEDS - Not approved in children.

FORMS - Trade: Caps 30 mg.

NOTES - Contraindicated in narrow-angle glaucoma, acute iritis & severe asthma. May potentiate beta-blockers.

chlorhexidine gluconate (Peridex, Periogard) ▶Fecal excretion ♀B ▶? $

ADULT - Gingivitis: Bid as an oral rinse, morning & evening after brushing teeth. Rinse with 15 ml of undiluted soln for 30 seconds. Do not swallow. Spit after rinsing.

PEDS - Not approved in children.

FORMS - Trade: Oral rinse 0.12% 473-480 ml bottles.

clotrimazole (Mycelex) ▶L ♀C ▶? $$$

ADULT - Oral candidiasis: 1 troche dissolved slowly in mouth 5x/day x 14 days. Prevention of oropharyngeal candidiasis in immunocompromised patients: 1 troche dissolved slowly in mouth tid until end of chemotherapy/high-dose corticosteroids.

PEDS - Treatment of oropharyngeal candidiasis: ≥3 yo: Use adult dose.

FORMS - Trade: Oral troches 10 mg.

NOTES - Monitor LFTs.

Debacterol (sulfuric acid + sulfonated phenolics) ▶Not absorbed ♀C ▶+ $$

ADULT - Aphthous stomatitis, mucositis: Apply to dry ulcer. Rinse with water.

PEDS - Not approved in children <12 yo.

FORMS - Trade: 1 ml prefilled, single-use applicator.

NOTES - One application per ulcer treatment. Dry ulcer area with cotton swab. Apply to ulcer and ring of normal mucosa around it for 5 to 10 seconds. Rinse and spit. Return of ulcer pain right after rinsing indicates incomplete application; can be reapplied immediately one time. Avoid eye contact. If excess irritation, rinse with dilute bicarbonate soln.

docosanol (Abreva) ▶? ♀B ▶? $

ADULT - Herpes labialis (cold sores): At 1st sign of infection apply 5x/day until healed.

PEDS - Herpes labialis (cold sores): ≥12 yo: Use adult dose.

FORMS - OTC: Trade: 10% cream in 2 g tube.

NOTES - Dries clear. Cosmetics may be applied over docosanol using a separate applicator to avoid spreading the infection. Contains benzyl alcohol.

doxycycline (Periostat) ▶L ♀D ▶- $$$

ADULT - Adjunct to scaling & root planing in periodontitis: 20 mg PO bid.

PEDS - Not approved in children.

FORMS - Trade: Caps 20 mg.

NOTES - Used in studies for up to 9 months.

Gelclair (maltodextrin + propylene glycol) ▶Not absorbed ♀+ ▶+ $$$

ADULT - Aphthous ulcers, mucositis, stomatitis: Rinse mouth with 1 packet tid or prn.

PEDS - Not approved in children.

FORMS - Trade: 21 packets/box.

NOTES - Mix packet with 3 tablespoons of water. Swish for 1 minute, then spit. Do not eat or drink for 1 hour after treatment.

lidocaine viscous (Xylocaine) ▶LK ♀B ▶+ $

WARNING - Instruct patients not to swallow if

intended for oral or labial use. It may cause lidocaine toxicity from GI absorption. Tell patients to measure the dose exactly. Patients may apply to small areas in the mouth with a cotton-tipped applicator.
ADULT - Mouth or lip pain: 15-20 ml topically or swish & spit q3h. Max 8 doses/day.
PEDS - Use with extreme caution, as therapeutic doses approach potentially toxic levels. Use the lowest effective dose. Mouth or lip pain >3 yo: 3.75-5 ml topically or swish and spit up to q3h.
FORMS - Generic/Trade: soln 2%, 20 ml unit dose, 50, 100, 450 ml bottles.
NOTES - High risk of adverse effects and overdose in children. Consider benzocaine as a safer alternative. Clearly communicate the amount, frequency, max daily dose, & mode of administration (eg, cotton pledget to individual lesions, 1/2 dropper to each cheek q4h, or 20 minutes before meals). Do not prescribe on a "PRN" basis without specified dosing intervals.

"magic mouthwash" (*Benadryl* + *Mylanta* + *Carafate*) ▶LK ♀B(- in 1st trimester) ▶- $$$
ADULT - See components
PEDS - Not approved in children.
UNAPPROVED ADULT - Stomatitis: 5 ml PO swish & spit or swish & swallow tid before meals and prn.
UNAPPROVED PEDS - Stomatitis: Apply small amounts to lesions prn.
FORMS - Compounded suspension. A standard mixture is 30 ml diphenhydramine liquid (12.5 mg/5 ml) + 60 ml Mylanta or Maalox + 4 g Carafate.
NOTES - Variations of this formulation are available. The dose and decision to swish and spit or swallow may vary with the indication and/or ingredient. Some preparations may contain: Kaopectate, nystatin, tetracycline, hydrocortisone, 2% lidocaine, cherry syrup (for children). Check local pharmacies for customized formulations. Avoid diphenhydramine formulations that contain alcohol - may cause stinging of mouth sores.

nystatin (*Mycostatin*, ❧*Nilstat*) ▶Not ab-

sorbed ♀C ▶? $$
ADULT - Thrush: 5 ml PO swish & swallow qid with ½ of dose in each cheek or 1-2 oral lozenges 4-5 times/day for up to 14 days.
PEDS - Thrush in infants: 1 ml PO in each cheek qid. Premature and low birth weight infants: 0.5 ml PO in each cheek qid.
FORMS - Generic/Trade: Suspension 100,000 units/ml 60 & 480 ml bottle. Trade: Oral lozenges (Pastilles) 200,000 units.
NOTES - Allow oral lozenge to dissolve on tongue. May apply oral suspension in infants using a cotton swab.

penciclovir (*Denavir*) ▶Not absorbed ♀B ▶- $
ADULT - Herpes labialis (cold sores): apply cream q2h while awake x 4 days. Start at first sign of symptoms.
PEDS - Not approved in children.
FORMS - Trade: Cream 1%, 1.5 g tube.
NOTES - For moderate to severe cases of herpes labialis, systemic treatment with acyclovir, famciclovir, or valacyclovir may be preferred.

pilocarpine (*Salagen*) ▶L ♀C ▶- $$$
ADULT - Dry mouth due to radiation of head & neck: 5 mg PO tid. May increase to 10 mg PO tid. Dry mouth due to Sjogren's syndrome: 5 mg PO qid. Hepatic dysfunction: 5 mg PO bid.
PEDS - Not approved in children.
UNAPPROVED ADULT - Dry mouth due to Sjogren's syndrome: 2% pilocarpine eye drops: Swish & swallow 4 drops diluted in water tid ($).
FORMS - Trade: Tabs 5, 7.5 mg.
NOTES - Contraindicated in narrow-angle glaucoma, acute iritis & severe asthma. May potentiate beta-blockers.

triamcinolone (*Kenalog in Orabase*, ❧*Oracort*) ▶L ♀C ▶? $
ADULT - Using finger, apply about 1/2 cm of paste to oral lesion and a thin film will develop. Apply paste bid-tid, ideally pc & qhs.
PEDS - Not approved in children.
FORMS - Generic/Trade: 0.1% oral paste, 5 g tubes.
NOTES - Re-evaluate cause if lesion has not healed in 7 days.

ENT: Nasal Preparations

NOTE: For ALL nasal sprays except saline, oxymetazoline, & phenylephrine, tell patients to prime pump before 1st use and shake well before each subsequent use. For nasal steroids, decrease to the lowest effective dose for maintenance therapy.

azelastine (*Astelin*) ▶L ♀C ▶? $$$
ADULT - Allergic/vasomotor rhinitis: 2 sprays/nostril bid.
PEDS - Allergic rhinitis: ≥12 yo: Use adult dose. ≥5 yo: 1 spray/nostril bid. Vasomotor rhinitis ≥12 yo: Use adult dose.

FORMS - Trade: Nasal spray, 100 sprays/bottle.

beclomethasone (*Vancenase, Vancenase AQ Double Strength, Beconase AQ*) ▶L ♀C ▶? $$$

ADULT - Allergic rhinitis/nasal polyp prophylaxis: Vancenase: 1 spray in each nostril bid-qid. Beconase AQ: 1-2 spray(s) in each nostril bid. Vancenase AQ Double Strength: 1-2 spray(s) in each nostril qd.

PEDS - Allergic rhinitis/nasal polyp prophylaxis: Vancenase: >12 yo: adult dose. 6-12 yo: 1 spray in each nostril tid. Beconase AQ: >6 yo 1-2 spray(s) in each nostril bid. Vancenase AQ Double Strength: >6 yo: 1-2 spray(s) in each nostril qd.

FORMS - Trade: Nasal inhalation aerosol (Vancenase) 42 mcg/spray, 80 & 200 sprays/bottle. Nasal aqueous suspension (Beconase AQ) 42 mcg/spray, 200 sprays/bottle. Nasal aqueous suspension double strength (Vancenase AQ Double Strength) 84 mcg/spray, 120 sprays/bottle.

NOTES - AQ (aqueous) formulation may cause less stinging.

budesonide (*Rhinocort, Rhinocort Aqua*) ▶L ♀C ▶? $$$

ADULT - Allergic rhinitis: 2 sprays per nostril bid or 4 sprays per nostril qd (Rhinocort). 1-4 sprays per nostril qd (Rhinocort Aqua).

PEDS - Allergic rhinitis ≥6 yo: 2 sprays per nostril bid or 4 sprays per nostril qd (Rhinocort). 1-2 sprays per nostril qd (Rhinocort Aqua).

FORMS - Trade: (Rhinocort): Nasal inhaler 200 sprays/bottle. (Rhinocort Aqua): Nasal inhaler 120 sprays/bottle.

NOTES - CYP3A4 inhibitors such as ketoconazole, erythromycin, ritonavir, etc significantly increase systemic concentrations, possibly causing adrenal suppression.

cromolyn (*NasalCrom, BenaMist, Children's NasalCrom*) ▶LK ♀B ▶+ $

ADULT - Allergic rhinitis: 1 spray per nostril tid-qid up to 6 times/day.

PEDS - Allergic rhinitis ≥2 yo: Use adult dose.

FORMS - OTC: Generic/Trade: Nasal inhaler 200 sprays/bottle. Trade: Children's Nasal-Crom w/special "child-friendly" applicator. 100 sprays/bottle.

NOTES - Therapeutic effects may not be seen for 1-2 weeks.

flunisolide (*Nasalide, Nasarel, ✿Rhinalar*) ▶L ♀C ▶? $$

ADULT - Allergic rhinitis: 2 sprays per nostril bid, may increase to tid. Max 8 sprays/nostril/day.

PEDS - Allergic rhinitis 6-14 yo: 1 spray per nostril tid or 2 sprays per nostril bid. Max 4 sprays/nostril/day.

FORMS - Generic/Trade: Nasal soln 0.025%, 200 sprays/bottle. Nasalide with pump unit. Nasarel with meter pump & nasal adapter.

fluticasone (*Flonase*) ▶L ♀C ▶? $$$

ADULT - Allergic rhinitis: 2 sprays per nostril qd or 1 spray per nostril bid, decrease to 1 spray per nostril qd when appropriate. Seasonal allergic rhinitis alternative: 2 sprays per nostril prn.

PEDS - Allergic rhinitis: >4 yo: 1-2 sprays per nostril qd. Max 2 sprays/nostril/day. Seasonal allergic rhinitis alternative: >12 yo: 2 sprays per nostril qd prn.

FORMS - Trade: Nasal spray 0.05%, 120 sprays/bottle.

NOTES - CYP3A4 inhibitors such as ketoconazole, erythromycin, ritonavir, etc significantly increase systemic concentrations, possibly causing adrenal suppression.

ipratropium (*Atrovent Nasal Spray*) ▶L ♀B ▶? $$

ADULT - Rhinorrhea due to allergic/non-allergic rhinitis: 2 sprays (0.03%) per nostril bid-tid or 2 sprays (0.06%) per nostril qid. Rhinorrhea due to common cold: 2 sprays (0.06%) per nostril tid-qid.

PEDS - Rhinorrhea due to allergic/non-allergic rhinitis ≥6 yo: Use adult dose (0.03%) or ≥5 yo: Use adult dose (0.06%). Rhinorrhea due to common cold ≥5 yo: 2 sprays (0.06%) per nostril tid.

UNAPPROVED ADULT - Vasomotor rhinitis: 2 sprays (0.06%) in each nostril tid-qid.

FORMS - Generic/Trade: Nasal spray 0.03%, 345 sprays/bottle & 0.06%, 165 sprays/bottle.

levocabastine (*✿Livostin Nasal Spray*) ▶L (but minimal absorption) ♀C ▶- ?

ADULT - Canada only. Allergic rhinitis: 2 sprays per nostril bid; increase prn to 2 sprays per nostril tid-qid.

PEDS - Not approved in children <12 yo.

FORMS - Trade: nasal spray 0.5mg/ml, plastic bottles of 15ml. Each spray delivers 50 mcg.

NOTES - Nasal spray is devoid of CNS effects. Safety/efficacy in patients >65 yo has not been established.

mometasone (*Nasonex*) ▶L ♀C ▶? $$$

ADULT - Allergic rhinitis: 2 sprays per nostril qd.

PEDS - Allergic rhinitis ≥12 yo: Use adult dose. 2-11 yo: 1 spray per nostril qd.

FORMS - Trade: Nasal spray, 120 sprays/bottle.

oxymetazoline (*Afrin, Dristan 12 Hr Nasal,*

Nostrilla) ▶L ♀C ▶? $
ADULT - Nasal congestion: 2-3 sprays or drops (0.05%) per nostril bid x 3 days.
PEDS - Nasal congestion ≥6 yo: 2-3 sprays or drops (0.05%) per nostril bid x 3 days. 2-5 yo: 2-3 drops (0.025%) per nostril bid x 3 days.
FORMS - OTC: Generic/Trade: Nasal spray 0.05%, 15 & 30 ml bottles. Nose drops 0.025% & 0.05%, 20 ml w/dropper.
NOTES - Overuse (>3-5 days) may lead to rebound congestion. If this occurs, taper to use in one nostril only, alternating sides, then discontinue. Substituting an oral decongestant or nasal steroid may also be useful.

phenylephrine (*Neo-Synephrine, Sinex, Nostril*) ▶L ♀C ▶? $
ADULT - Nasal congestion: 2-3 sprays or drops (0.25 or 0.5%) per nostril q4h prn x 3 days. Use 1% soln for severe congestion.
PEDS - Nasal congestion: >12 yo: Use adult dose. 6-12 yo: 2-3 drops or sprays (0.25%) per nostril q4h prn x 3 days. 1-5 yo: 2-3 drops (0.125% or 0.16%) per nostril q4h prn x 3 days. 6-11 mo: 1-2 drops (0.125% or 0.16%) per nostril q4h prn x 3 days.
FORMS - OTC: Trade: Nasal drops 0.125, 0.16%. Generic/Trade: Nasal spray/drops 0.25, 0.5, 1%.
NOTES - Overuse (>3-5 days) may lead to rebound congestion. If this occurs, taper to use in one nostril only, alternating sides, then discontinue. Substituting an oral decongestant or na-

sal steroid may also be useful.
saline nasal spray (*SeaMist, Pretz, NaSal, Ocean, ♣HydraSense*) ▶Not metabolized ♀A ▶+ $
ADULT - Nasal dryness: 1-3 sprays per nostril prn.
PEDS - Nasal dryness: 1-3 drops per nostril prn.
FORMS - Generic/Trade: Nasal spray 0.4,0.5, 0.6,0.65,0.75%. Nasal drops 0.4,0.65,0.75%.
NOTES - May be prepared at home by combining: 1/4 teaspoon salt with 8 ounces (1 cup) warm water. Add 1/4 teaspoon baking soda (optional) and put in spray bottle, ear syringe, or any container with a small spout. Discard after one week.

triamcinolone (*Nasacort, Nasacort AQ, Nasacort HFA, Tri-Nasal*) ▶L ♀C ▶- $$
ADULT - Allergic rhinitis: Nasacort, Tri-Nasal: Start 2 sprays per nostril qd, may increase to 2 sprays/nostril bid. Max 4 sprays/nostril/day. Nasacort AQ: 2 sprays per nostril qd.
PEDS - Allergic rhinitis: ≥12 yo: Use adult dose. 6-12 yo: 1-2 sprays per nostril qd (Nasacort & Nasacort AQ).
FORMS - Trade: Nasal inhaler 55 mcg/spray, 100 sprays/bottle (Nasacort). Nasal spray, 55 mcg/spray, 120 sprays/bottle (Nasacort AQ). Nasal spray 50 mcg/spray, 120 sprays/bottle (Tri-Nasal).
NOTES - AQ (aqueous) formulation may cause less stinging. Decrease to lowest effective dose after allergy symptom improvement.

ENT: Other

montelukast (*Singulair*) ▶L ♀B ▶? $$$
ADULT - Allergic rhinitis: 10 mg PO q pm.
PEDS - Allergic rhinitis: 6-14 yo: 5 mg PO q pm. 2-5 yo: 4 mg (chew tab or oral granules) PO q pm.
UNAPPROVED PEDS - Allergic rhinitis 12-23 months: 4 mg (oral granules) PO q pm.
FORMS - Trade: Tabs 4, 5 mg (chew cherry flavored) & 10 mg. Oral granules 4 mg packet, 30/box.
NOTES - Chew tabs contain phenylalanine. Oral granules may be mixed with a spoonful of applesauce, carrots, rice or ice cream (use within 15 minutes if mixed with food). Levels decreased by phenobarbital & rifampin. Dyspepsia may occur.

GASTROENTEROLOGY: Antidiarrheals

bismuth subsalicylate (*Pepto-Bismol, Kaopectate*) ▶K ♀D ▶? $
WARNING - Avoid in children and teenagers with chickenpox or flu due to possible association with Reye's syndrome.
ADULT - Diarrhea: 2 tabs or 30 ml (262 mg/15 ml) PO q 30 min-60 min up to 8 doses/day.
PEDS - Diarrhea: 100 mg/kg/day divided into 5

doses. Age 3-6 yo: 1/3 tab or 5 ml (262 mg/15 ml) every 30 min-60 min prn up to 8 doses/day. 6-9 yo: 2/3 tab or 10 ml (262 mg/15 ml) every 30 min-1 hr prn up to 8 doses/day. 9-12 yo: 1 tab or 15 ml (262 mg/15 ml) every 30 min-1 hr prn up to 8 doses/day.
UNAPPROVED ADULT - Prevention of traveler's diarrhea: 2.1 g/day or 2 tab qid before

meals and qhs. Has been used as part of a multi-drug regimen for Helicobacter pylori.

UNAPPROVED PEDS - Chronic infantile diarrhea: Age 2-24 mo: 2.5 ml (262 mg/15 ml) PO q4h. 24-48 mo: 5 ml (262 mg/15 ml) q4h. 48-70 mo: 10 ml (262 mg/15 ml) q4h.

FORMS - OTC Generic/Trade: chew tab 262 mg, susp 87 mg/5 ml (Kaopectate Children's Liquid), 262 & 524 mg/15 ml. Generic only: susp 130 mg/15 ml. Trade only: caplets 262 mg (Pepto-Bismol).

NOTES - Use with caution if already taking salicylates or warfarin, or in children recovering from chickenpox or flu. Decreases absorption of tetracycline. May darken stools or tongue.

***Imodium Advanced* (loperamide + simethicone)** ►L 9B ►+ $

ADULT - Diarrhea: 2 caplets PO initially, then 1 caplet PO after each unformed stool to a maximum of 4 caplets/24 h.

PEDS - Diarrhea: 1 caplet PO initially, then ½ caplet PO after each unformed stool to a max of 2 caplets/day (if 6-8 yo or 48-59 lbs) or 3 caplets/day (if 9-11 yo or 60-95 lbs).

FORMS - OTC: Trade: caplet 2 mg loperamide/125 mg simethicone.

NOTES - Not for pseudomembranous colitis, toxigenic bacterial diarrhea, or most childhood diarrhea (difficult to exclude toxigenic).

***Lomotil* (diphenoxylate + atropine)** ►L 9C ►- ©V $

ADULT - Diarrhea: 2 tabs or 10 ml PO qid.

PEDS - Diarrhea: 0.3-0.4 mg diphenoxylate/kg/ 24h in 4 divided dose. Age <2 yo: not recommended. 2 yo: 1.5-3 ml PO qid; 3 yo: 2-3 ml PO qid; 4 yo: 2-4 ml PO qid; 5 yo: 2.5-4.5 ml PO qid; 6-8 yo: 2.5-5 ml PO qid; 9-12 yo: 3.5-5 ml PO qid.

FORMS - Generic/Trade: solution 2.5 mg diphenoxylate + 0.025 mg atropine per 5 ml, tab 2.5 mg diphenoxylate + 0.025 mg atropine per tab.

NOTES - Give with food to decrease GI upset. May cause atropinism in children, esp with Down syndrome, even at recommended doses. Can cause delayed toxicity. Has been reported to cause severe respiratory depression, coma, brain damage, death after overdose in children. Naltrexone reverses toxicity. Do not use for pseudomembranous colitis, toxigenic bacterial diarrhea, or most childhood diarrhea (difficult to exclude toxigenic).

loperamide (*Imodium, Imodium AD*, ♣*Loperacap, Diarr-eze*) ►L 9B ►+ $

ADULT - Diarrhea: 4 mg PO initially, then 2 mg after each unformed stool to max 16 mg/day.

PEDS - Diarrhea (first day): Age 2-5 yo (13-20 kg): 1 mg PO tid. 6-8 yo (20-30 kg): 2 mg PO bid. 9-12 yo (>30 kg): 2 mg PO tid. After first day, give 1 mg/10 kg PO after each loose stool; daily dose not to exceed daily dose of first day.

UNAPPROVED ADULT - Chronic diarrhea or ileostomy drainage : 4 mg initially then 2 mg after each stool until symptoms are controlled, then reduce dose for maintenance treatment, average adult maintenance dose 4-8 mg daily as a single dose or in divided doses.

UNAPPROVED PEDS - Chronic diarrhea: limited information. Average doses of 0.08-0.24 mg/kg/day PO in 2-3 divided doses.

FORMS - Generic/Trade: cap 2 mg, tab 2 mg. OTC generic/trade: liquid 1 mg/5 ml.

NOTES - Not for pseudomembranous colitis, toxigenic bacterial diarrhea, or most childhood diarrhea (difficult to exclude toxigenic).

***Motofen* (difenoxin + atropine)** ►L 9C ►- ©IV $

ADULT - Diarrhea: 2 tabs PO initially, then 1 after each loose stool q3-4 h prn. Maximum of 8 tabs/24h.

PEDS - Not approved in children. Contraindicated in children <2 yo.

FORMS - Trade only: tab difenoxin 1 mg + atropine 0.025 mg.

NOTES - Do not use for pseudomembranous colitis, toxigenic bacterial diarrhea, or most childhood diarrhea (difficult to exclude toxigenic). May cause atropinism in children, esp with Down's syndrome, even at recommended doses. Can cause delayed toxicity. Has been reported to cause severe respiratory depression, coma, brain damage, death after overdose in children. Difenoxin is the primary metabolite of diphenoxylate.

opium (opium tincture, paregoric) ►L 9B (D with long-term use) ►? ©II (opium tincture), III (paregoric) $

ADULT - Diarrhea: 5-10 ml paregoric PO qd-qid or 0.3-0.6 ml PO opium tincture qid.

PEDS - Diarrhea: 0.25-0.5 ml/kg paregoric PO qd-qid or 0.005-0.01 ml/kg PO opium tincture q3-4h, max 6 doses/day.

FORMS - Trade: opium tincture 10% (deodorized opium tincture, 10 mg morphine equivalent per mL). Generic: paregoric (camphorated opium tincture, 2 mg morphine equiv./5 ml).

NOTES - Opium tincture contains 25 times more morphine than paregoric. Do not use for pseudomembranous colitis, toxigenic bacterial diarrhea, or most childhood diarrhea.

GASTROENTEROLOGY: Antiemetics – 5-HT3 Receptor Antagonists

dolasetron (*Anzemet*) ▶LK ♀B ▶? $$$
ADULT - Prevention of N/V with chemo: 1.8 mg/kg up to 100 mg IV/PO single dose 30 min (IV) or 60 min (PO) before chemo. Prevention/treatment of post-op N/V: 12.5 mg IV as a single dose 15 minutes before end of anesthesia or as soon as N/V starts. Alternative for prevention 100 mg PO 2 h before surgery.
PEDS - Prevention of N/V with chemo in children 2-16 yo: 1.8 mg/kg up to 100 mg IV/PO single dose 30 min (IV) or 60 min (PO) before chemo. Prevention/treatment of post-op N/V in children 2-16 yo: 0.35 mg/kg IV as single dose 15 minutes before end of anesthesia or as soon as N/V starts. Max 12.5 mg. Prevention alternative 1.2 mg/kg PO to max of 100 mg 2 h before surgery.
UNAPPROVED ADULT - N/V due to radiotherapy: 40 mg IV as a single dose. Alternatively, 0.3 mg/kg IV as a single dose.
FORMS - Trade only: tab 50,100 mg.
NOTES - Use caution in patients who have or may develop prolongation of QT interval (i.e. hypokalemia, hypomagnesemia, concomitant antiarrhythmic therapy, cumulative high-dose anthracycline therapy).

granisetron (*Kytril*) ▶L ♀B ▶? $$$
ADULT - Prevention of N/V with chemo: 10 mcg/kg over 5 min IV 30 mins prior to chemo. Oral: 1 mg PO bid x 1 day only. Radiation-induced N/V: 2 mg PO 1 hr before first irradiation fraction of each day. Prevention/treatment post-op N/V: 1 mg IV.
PEDS - Children 2-16 yo: Prevention of N/V with chemo: 10 mcg/kg IV 30 minutes prior to chemo. Oral form not approved in children.
FORMS - Trade only: tab 1 mg, oral soln 2 mg/ 10 ml.

ondansetron (*Zofran*) ▶L ♀B ▶? $$$
ADULT - Prevention of N/V with chemo: 32 mg IV as a single dose over 15 min, or 0.15 mg/kg

IV 30 minutes prior to chemo and repeated at 4 and 8 hrs after first dose. Alternatively, 8 mg PO 30 min before moderately emetogenic chemo and 8 h later. Can be given q12h for 1-2 days after completion of chemo. For single-day highly emetogenic chemo, 24 mg PO 30 min before chemo. Prevention of post-op nausea: 4 mg IV over 2-5 min or 4 mg IM or 16 mg PO 1 hr before anesthesia. Prevention of N/V associated with radiotherapy: 8 mg PO tid.
PEDS - Prevention of N/V with chemo: IV: Age >4 yo: 0.15 mg/kg 30 minutes prior to chemo and repeated at 4 and 8 hrs after first dose. PO: Children 4-11 yo: 4 mg 30 minutes prior to chemo and repeated at 4 and 8 hrs after first dose. Can be given q8h for 1-2 days after completion of chemo. Children ≥12 yo: 8 mg PO 30 min before chemo and 8 h later. Prevention of post-op N/V: 2-12 yo: 0.1 mg/kg IV over 2-5 min x 1 if ≤40kg; 4 mg IV over 2-5 min x 1 if >40 kg.
UNAPPROVED ADULT - Has been used in hyperemesis associated with pregnancy.
UNAPPROVED PEDS - <4 yo based on BSA: <0.3 m^2: 1 mg PO tid. 0.3-0.6 m^2: 2 mg PO tid. 0.6-1 m^2: 3 mg PO tid. >1 m^2: 4 mg PO tid.
FORMS - Trade only: tab 4,8,24 mg, orally disintegrating tab 4, 8 mg, solution 4 mg/5 ml.
NOTES - Most common adverse effects - headache, fever, constipation, diarrhea. No experience using ondansetron in post-op nausea in children. Maximum oral dose in patients with severe liver disease is 8 mg/day. PO peds dosing from Ped Drug Handbook 2003-04.

palonosetron (*Aloxi*) ▶L ♀B ▶? $$$$$
ADULT - Prevention of N/V with chemo: 0.25 mg IV over 30 seconds, 30 minutes prior to chemo.
PEDS - Not approved in children.
NOTES - Caution with cardiac conduction delay propensity, especially prolonged QTc.

GASTROENTEROLOGY: Antiemetics – Other

aprepitant (*Emend*) ▶L ♀B ▶? $$$$$
ADULT - Prevention of N/V with chemo, in combination with dexamethasone and ondansetron: 125 mg PO on day 1 (1 h prior to chemo), then 80 mg PO qam on days 2 & 3.
PEDS - Not approved in children.
FORMS - Trade only: cap 80, 125 mg.
NOTES - Use caution with other medications

metabolized by CYP3A4 hepatic enzyme system. Contraindicated with pimozide. May decrease efficacy of oral contraceptives; women should use alternate/back-up method. Monitor INR in patients receiving warfarin.

Diclectin (doxylamine + pyridoxine) ▶LK ♀A ▶? $
ADULT - Canada only. Nausea / vomiting in

pregnancy. 2 tabs PO qhs. May add 1 tab in am and 1 tab in afternoon, if needed.

PEDS - Not approved in children.

FORMS - Trade: delayed-release tab doxylamine 10 mg + pyridoxine 10 mg.

dimenhydrinate (*Dramamine*, ✦*Gravol*) ▶LK ♀B ▶- $

ADULT - Nausea: 50-100 mg/dose PO/IM/IV q4-6h prn. Maximum PO dose 400 mg/24h, maximum IM dose 300 mg/24h.

PEDS - Nausea: Age <2 yo: not recommended. 2-6 yo: 12.5-25 mg PO q6-8h or 5 mg/kg/24h divided q6h. Max daily PO dose: 75 mg/24h. Children 6-12 yo: 25-50 mg PO q6-8h. Max daily PO doses150 mg/24h.

FORMS - OTC: Generic/Trade: tab/cap 50 mg. Trade only: chew tab 50 mg.

NOTES - May cause drowsiness. Use with caution in conditions which may be aggravated by anticholinergic effects (i.e. prostatic hypertrophy, asthma, narrow-angle glaucoma).

doxylamine (*Unisom Nighttime Sleep Aid, others*) ▶L ♀A ▶? $

PEDS - Not approved in children.

UNAPPROVED ADULT - Nausea and vomiting associated with pregnancy: 12.5 mg PO bid; often used in combination with pyridoxine.

FORMS - OTC Trade/Generic: tab 25 mg.

dronabinol (*Marinol*) ▶L ♀C ▶- ©III $$$$$

ADULT - Nausea with chemo: 5 mg/m² 1-3 h before chemo then 5 mg/m²/dose q2-4h after chemo for 4-6 doses/day. Dose can be increased to max 15 mg/m². Anorexia associated with AIDS: Initially 2.5 mg PO bid before lunch and dinner. Maximum 20 mg/day.

PEDS - Not approved in children.

UNAPPROVED PEDS - Nausea with chemo: 5 mg/m² 1-3 h before chemo then 5 mg/m²/dose q2-4h after chemo for 4-6 doses/day. Dose can be increased to max 15 mg/m².

FORMS - Trade only: cap 2.5,5,10 mg.

NOTES - Additive CNS effects with alcohol, sedatives, hypnotics, psychomimetics. Additive cardiac effects with amphetamines, antihistamines, anticholinergic medications, tricyclic antidepressants.

droperidol (*Inapsine*) ▶L ♀C ▶? $

WARNING - Cases of fatal QT prolongation and /or torsades de pointes have occurred in patients receiving droperidol at or below recommended doses (some without risk factors for QT prolongation). Reserve for non-response to other treatments, and perform 12-lead ECG prior to administration and continue ECG monitoring 2-3 hours after treatment. Use with ex-

treme caution (if at all) if prolonged baseline QT.

ADULT - Antiemetic premedication: 0.625-2.5 mg IV or 2.5 mg IM then 1.25 mg prn.

PEDS - Preop: Age 2-12 yo: 0.088-0.165 mg/kg IV. Post-op antiemetic: 0.01-0.03 mg/kg/dose IV q 6-8h prn. Usual dose 0.05-0.06 mg/kg/ dose; maximum of 0.1 mg/kg.

UNAPPROVED ADULT - Chemo-induced nausea: 2.5-5 mg IV/IM q 3-4h prn.

UNAPPROVED PEDS - Chemo-induced nausea: 0.05-0.06 mg/kg/dose IV/IM q 4-6h prn.

NOTES - Has no analgesic or amnestic effects. Consider lower doses in geriatric, debilitated, or high-risk patients such as those receiving other CNS depressants. May cause hypotension or tachycardia, extrapyramidal reactions, drowsiness.

meclizine (*Antivert, Bonine, Medivert, Meclicot, Meni-D,* ✦*Bonamine*) ▶L ♀B ▶? $

ADULT - Motion sickness: 25-50 mg PO 1 hr before travel. May repeat q24h prn.

PEDS - Not approved in children.

FORMS - Rx/OTC/Generic/Trade: Tabs 12.5, 25 mg. chew Tabs 25 mg. Rx/Trade only: Tabs 30, 50 mg. Caps 25 mg.

NOTES - May cause dizziness and drowsiness.

metoclopramide (*Reglan,* ✦*Maxeran*) ▶K ♀B ▶? $$

ADULT - Gastroesophageal reflux: 10-15 mg PO qid 30 min before meals and qhs. Diabetic gastric stasis: 10 mg PO/IV/IM 30 min before meals and bedtime. Prevention of chemo-induced emesis: 1-2 mg/kg 30 min before chemo and then q2h for 2 doses then q3h for 3 doses prn. Prevention of post-op nausea: 10-20 mg IM/IV near end of surgical procedure, may repeat q3-4 h prn. Intubation of small intestine: 10 mg IV. Radiographic exam of upper GI tract: 10 mg IV.

PEDS - Intubation of small intestine: Age <6 yo: 0.1 mg/kg IV. 6-14 yo: 2.5-5 mg IV. Radiographic exam of upper GI tract: Age <6 yo: 0.1 mg/kg IV; 6-14 yo: 2.5-5 mg IV.

UNAPPROVED ADULT - Prevention/treatment of chemo-induced emesis: 3 mg/kg over 1h followed by continuous IV infusion of 0.5 mg/kg/h for 12h. To improve patient response to ergotamine, analgesics and sedatives in migraines: 10 mg PO 5-10 min before ergotamine/analgesic/sedative.

UNAPPROVED PEDS - Gastroesophageal reflux: 0.4-0.8 mg/kg/day in 4 divided doses. Prevention of chemo-induced emesis: 1-2 mg/kg 30 min before chemo and then q3h prn, maxi-

mum of 5 doses/day or 5-10 mg/kg/day.
FORMS - Generic/Trade: tabs 5,10 mg, liquid 5 mg/5 ml.
NOTES - If extrapyramidal reactions occur (especially with high IV doses) give diphenhydramine IM/IV. Adjust dose in renal dysfunction. May cause drowsiness, agitation, seizures, hallucinations, galactorrhea, constipation, diarrhea. Increases cyclosporine and ethanol absorption. Do not use if bowel perforation or mechanical obstruction present. Levodopa decreases metoclopramide effects. Tardive dyskinesia in <1% with long-term use.

phosphorated carbohydrates (*Emetrol*) ▶L ♀A ▶+ $
ADULT - Nausea: 15-30 ml PO q15min until nausea subsides or up to 5 doses.
PEDS - Nausea: 2-12 yo: 5-10 ml q15min until nausea subsides or up to 5 doses.
UNAPPROVED ADULT - Morning sickness: 15-30 ml PO upon rising, repeat q3h prn. Motion sickness or nausea due to drug therapy or anesthesia: 15 ml/dose.
UNAPPROVED PEDS - Regurgitation in infants: 5-10 ml PO 10-15 min prior to each feeding. Motion sickness or nausea due to drug therapy or anesthesia: 5 ml/dose.
FORMS - OTC Generic/Trade: Solution containing dextrose, fructose, and phosphoric acid.
NOTES - Do not dilute. Do not ingest fluids before or for 15 min after dose. Monitor blood glucose in diabetic patients.

prochlorperazine (*Compazine*, ✤*Stemetil*) ▶LK ♀C ▶? $
ADULT - Nausea and vomiting: 5-10 mg PO/IM tid-qid max 40 mg/day; 15-30 mg PO qd or 10 mg PO q12h of sustained release or 15 mg PO qam of sustained release; 25 mg PR q12h; 5-10 mg IV over at least 2 min q3-4h prn max 40 mg/day; 5-10 mg IM q3-4h prn max 40 mg/day.
PEDS - Nausea and vomiting: Age <2 yo or <10 kg: not recommended. >2 yo: 0.4 mg/kg/day PO/PR in 3-4 divided doses; 0.1-0.15 mg/kg/dose IM; IV not recommended.
UNAPPROVED ADULT - Migraine: 10 mg IV/IM or 25 mg PR single dose for acute headache.
UNAPPROVED PEDS - N/V during surgery: 5-10 mg IM 1-2 hr before anesthesia induction, may repeat in 30 min; 5-10 mg IV 15-30 min before anesthesia induction, may repeat once.
FORMS - Generic/Trade: tabs 5,10,25 mg, supp 25 mg. Trade only: extended release caps (Compazine Spansules) 10,15,30 mg, supp 2.5,5 mg, liquid 5 mg/5 ml.

NOTES - May cause extrapyramidal reactions, hypotension (with IV), arrhythmias, sedation, seizures, gynecomastia, dry mouth, constipation, urinary retention, leukopenia, thrombocytopenia.

promethazine (*Phenergan*) ▶LK ♀C ▶- $
ADULT - Nausea and vomiting: 12.5-25 mg q4-6h PO/IM/PR prn. Motion sickness: 25 mg PO/PR 30-60 min prior to departure and q12h prn.
PEDS - Nausea and vomiting: 0.25-1 mg/kg/dose PO/IM/PR q4-6h prn. Motion sickness: 0.5 mg/kg PO 30-60 min prior to departure and q12h prn. Max 25 mg/dose.
UNAPPROVED ADULT - Nausea and vomiting: 12.5-25 mg IV q4h prn.
UNAPPROVED PEDS - Nausea and vomiting: 0.25-0.5 mg/kg/dose IV q4h prn.
FORMS - Generic/Trade: tab 25,50 mg, syrup 6.25 mg/5 ml, supp 50 mg. Trade only: tab 12.5 mg, syrup 25 mg/5 ml, supp 12.5,25 mg.
NOTES - May cause sedation, extrapyramidal reactions (esp. with high IV doses), hypotension with rapid IV administration, anticholinergic side effects, eg, dry mouth, blurred vision.

scopolamine (*Transderm-Scop*, ✤*Transderm-V*) ▶L ♀C ▶+ $
ADULT - Motion sickness: 1 disc behind ear at least 4h before travel and q3 days prn. Prevention of post-op N/V: Apply patch behind ear 4 h before surgery, remove 24 h after surgery.
PEDS - Not approved in children <12 yo.
UNAPPROVED PEDS - Pre-op and antiemetic: 6 mcg/kg/dose IM/IV/SC (max dose 0.3 mg/dose). May repeat q6-8h. Has been used in severe drooling.
FORMS - Trade only: topical disc 1.5 mg/72h, box of 4.
NOTES - Dry mouth common. Also causes drowsiness, blurred vision.

thiethylperazine (*Torecan*) ▶L ♀? ▶? $
ADULT - N/V: 10 mg PO/IM 1-3 times/day.
PEDS - Not approved in children.
FORMS - Trade only: tab 10 mg.

trimethobenzamide (*Tigan*) ▶LK ♀C but + ▶? $
ADULT - Nausea and vomiting: 250 mg PO q6-8h, 200 mg PR/IM q6-8h.
PEDS - N/V: Children <13.6kg (except neonates): 100 mg PR q6-8h. Children 13.6-40.9 kg: 100-200 mg PO/PR q6-8h.
FORMS - Trade/generic: cap 300 mg. Generic: cap 250 mg, supp 100,200 mg.
NOTES - Not for IV use. May cause sedation.

GASTROENTEROLOGY: Antiulcer – Antacids

Alka-Seltzer (aspirin + citrate + bicarbonate) ▶LK ♀? (- 3rd trimester) ▶? $
ADULT - Relief of upset stomach: 2 regular strength tablets in 4 oz. water q4h PO prn, maximum 8 tablets (<60 yo) or 4 tablets (>60 yo) in 24h or 2 extra-strength tablets in 4 oz. water q6h PO prn, maximum 7 tablets (<60 yo) or 4 tablets (>60 yo) in 24h.
PEDS - Not approved in children.
FORMS - OTC Trade: regular strength, original: ASA 325 mg + citric acid 1000 mg + sodium bicarbonate 1916 mg. Regular strength lemon lime and other: 325 mg + 1000 mg + 1700 mg. Extra-strength: 500 mg + 1000 mg + 1985 mg. Not all forms of Alka Seltzer contain aspirin (eg, Alka Seltzer Heartburn Relief).
NOTES - Avoid ASA-containing forms in children and teenagers due to risk of Reye's syndrome.

aluminum hydroxide (Alternagel, Amphojel, Alu-Tab, Alu-Cap) ▶K ♀+ (? 1st trimester) ▶? $
ADULT - Hyperphosphatemia in chronic renal failure (short term treatment only to avoid aluminum accumulation): 30-60 ml PO with meals. Upset stomach, indigestion: 5-10 ml or 1-2 tabs PO 6 times/day, between meals & qhs prn.
PEDS - Not approved in children.
UNAPPROVED ADULT - Hyperphosphatemia in chronic renal failure (short term treatment only to avoid aluminum accumulation): 30-60 ml PO with meals. Symptomatic reflux: 15-30 ml PO q30-60 min. For long-term management of reflux disease: 15-30 ml PO 1 and 3 h after meals and qhs prn. Peptic ulcer disease: 15-45 ml or 1-3 tab PO 1 and 3h after meals and qhs. Prophylaxis against GI bleeding (titrate dose to maintain gastric pH >3.5): 30-60 ml or 2-4 tab PO q1-2h.
UNAPPROVED PEDS - Peptic ulcer disease: 5-15 ml PO 1 and 3h after meals and qhs. Prophylaxis against GI bleeding (titrate dose to maintain gastric pH >3.5): Neonates 0.5-1 ml/kg/dose PO q4h. Infants 2-5 ml PO q1-2h. Child: 5-15 ml PO q1-2h.
FORMS - OTC Generic/Trade: cap 475 mg, susp 320, 600, 40/5 ml.
NOTES - For concentrated suspensions, use ½ the recommended dose. May cause constipation. Avoid administration with tetracyclines, digoxin, iron, isoniazid, buffered/enteric aspirin, diazepam, fluoroquinolones.

calcium carbonate (Tums, Mylanta Children's, Titralac, Rolaids Calcium Rich, Surpass) ▶K ♀+ (? 1st trimester) ▶? $
ADULT - Antacid: 1000-3000 mg (2-4 tab) PO q2h prn or 1-2 pieces gum chewed prn, max 7000 mg/day.
PEDS - Safe dosing above the RDA has not been established.
UNAPPROVED PEDS - Hypocalcemia: 20-65 mg/kg/day elem Ca PO in 4 divided doses.
FORMS - OTC Generic/Trade: tabs 500, ,600, 650,750, 1000 mg, susp 1250 mg/5 ml, gum (Surpass) 300, 450 mg.
NOTES - May cause constipation. Avoid concomitant administration with tetracyclines, fluoroquinolones.

Citrocarbonate (bicarbonate + citrate) ▶K ♀? ▶? $
ADULT - 1-2 teaspoonfuls in cold water PO 15 minutes to 2 hours after meals prn.
PEDS - 6-12 yo: ¼-1/2 teaspoonful in cold water PO after meals prn.
FORMS - OTC Trade: sodium bicarbonate 0.78 g + sodium citrate anhydrous 1.82 g in each 1 teaspoonful dissolved in water.
NOTES - Chronic use may cause metabolic alkalosis. Contains sodium.

Gaviscon (aluminum hydroxide + magnesium carbonate) ▶K ♀? ▶? $
ADULT - 2-4 tabs or 15-30 ml (regular strength) or 10 ml (extra strength) PO qid prn.
PEDS - Not approved in children.
UNAPPROVED PEDS - Peptic ulcer disease: 5-15 ml PO after meals and qhs.
FORMS - OTC Trade: Tab: regular strength (Al hydroxide 80 mg + Mg trisilicate 20 mg), extra strength (Al hydroxide 160 mg + Mg carbonate 105 mg). Liquid: regular strength (Al hydroxide 95 mg + Mg carbonate 358 mg per 15 ml), extra strength (Al hydroxide 508 mg + Mg carbonate 475 mg per 30 ml)
NOTES - Contains alginic acid or sodium alginate which is considered an "inactive" ingredient. Alginic acid forms foam barrier which floats in stomach to minimize esophageal contact with acid. Chronic use may cause metabolic alkalosis. Contains sodium.

Maalox (aluminum hydroxide + magnesium hydroxide) ▶K ♀+ (? 1st trimester) ▶? $
ADULT - Heartburn/indigestion: 10-20 ml or 1-4 tab PO qid, after meals and qhs and prn.
PEDS - Not approved in children.
UNAPPROVED ADULT - Peptic ulcer disease: 15-45 ml PO 1 & 3h after meals & qhs. Symp-

tomatic reflux: 15-30 ml PO q30-60 min prn. For long-term management of reflux disease: 15-30 ml PO 1 and 3 h after meals & qhs prn. Prophylaxis against GI bleeding (titrate dose to maintain gastric pH >3.5): 30-60 ml PO q1-2h.

UNAPPROVED PEDS - Peptic ulcer disease: 5-15 ml PO 1 and 3h after meals and qhs. Prophylaxis against GI bleeding to maintain gastric pH >3.5): Neonates 1 ml/kg/dose PO q4h. Infants 2-5 ml PO q1-2h. Child: 5-15 ml PO q1-2h.

FORMS - OTC Generic/Trade: chew tabs, susp.

NOTES - Maalox Extra Strength and Maalox TC are more concentrated than Maalox. Maalox Plus has added simethicone. May cause constipation or diarrhea. Avoid concomitant administration with tetracyclines, digoxin, iron, isoniazid, buffered/enteric aspirin, diazepam, fluoroquinolones. Avoid chronic use in patients with renal dysfunction due to potential for magnesium accumulation.

magaldrate (Riopan) ▶K ♀+ (? 1st trimester) ▶? $

ADULT - Relief of upset stomach: 5-10 ml between meals and qhs and prn.

PEDS - Not approved in children.

UNAPPROVED PEDS - Peptic ulcer disease: 5-10 ml PO 1 and 3h after meals and qhs.

FORMS - OTC Generic/Trade: susp 540 mg/5 ml. (Riopan Plus available as susp 540, 1080 mg/5 ml, chew tab 480, 1080).

NOTES - Riopan Plus has added simethicone. Avoid concomitant administration with tetracyclines, fluoroquinolones, digoxin, iron, isoniazid, buffered/enteric aspirin, diazepam. Avoid chronic use in patients with renal failure.

Mylanta suspension (aluminum hydroxide + magnesium hydroxide + simethicone) ▶K ♀+ (? 1st trimester) ▶? $

ADULT - Heartburn/indigestion: 10-45 ml or 2-4 tab PO qid, after meals and qhs and prn.

PEDS - Safe dosing has not been established.

UNAPPROVED ADULT - Peptic ulcer disease: 15-45 ml PO 1 and 3h after meals and qhs. Symptomatic reflux: 15-30 ml PO q30-60 min. For long-term management of reflux: 15-30 ml PO 1 and 3 h postprandially and qhs prn.

UNAPPROVED PEDS - Peptic ulcer disease: 5-15 ml PO 1 and 3h after meals and qhs.

FORMS - OTC Generic/Trade: Liquid, double strength liquid, tab, double strength tab.

NOTES - Mylanta Gelcaps contain calcium carbonate and magnesium hydroxide. May cause constipation or diarrhea. Avoid concomitant administration with tetracyclines, fluoroquinolones, digoxin, iron, isoniazid, buffered/enteric aspirin, diazepam. Avoid in renal dysfunction.

Rolaids (calcium carbonate + magnesium hydroxide) ▶K ♀? ▶? $

ADULT - 2-4 tabs PO q1h prn, max 12 tabs/day (regular strength) or 10 tabs/day (extra-strength).

PEDS - Not approved in children.

FORMS - OTC Trade: Tab: regular strength (Ca carbonate 550 mg, Mg hydroxide 110 mg), extra-strength (Ca carbonate 675 mg, Mg hydroxide 135 mg).

NOTES - Chronic use may cause metabolic alkalosis.

GASTROENTEROLOGY: Antiulcer – H2 Antagonists

cimetidine (_Tagamet, Tagamet HB_, ♥_Peptol_) ▶LK ♀B ▶+ $$$

ADULT - Treatment of duodenal or gastric ulcer: 800 mg PO qhs or 300 mg PO qid with meals and qhs or 400 mg PO bid. Prevention of duodenal ulcer: 400 mg PO qhs. Erosive esophagitis: 800 mg PO bid or 400 mg PO qid. Heartburn: (OTC product only approved for this indication) 200 mg PO prn max 400 mg/day. Hypersecretory conditions: 300 mg PO qid with meals and qhs. Patients unable to take oral medications: 300 mg IV/IM q6-8h or 37.5 mg/h continuous IV infusion. Prevention of upper GI bleeding in critically ill patients: 50 mg/h continuous infusion.

PEDS - Not approved in children.

UNAPPROVED ADULT - Prevention of aspira-

tion pneumonitis during surgery: 400-600 mg PO or 300 mg IV 60-90 min prior to anesthesia. Has been used as adjunctive therapy with H1 antagonist for severe allergic reactions.

UNAPPROVED PEDS - Treatment of duodenal or gastric ulcers, erosive esophagitis, hypersecretory conditions: Neonates: 5-10 mg/kg/day PO/IV/IM divided q 8-12h. Infants: 10-20 mg/kg/day PO/IV/IM divided q6h. Children: 20-40 mg/kg/day PO/IV/IM divided q6h. Chronic viral warts in children: 25-40 mg/kg/day PO in divided doses.

FORMS - Generic/Trade: tab 200,300,400,800 mg, liquid 300 mg/5 ml. OTC, trade only: tab 100 mg, susp 200 mg/20 ml.

NOTES - May cause dizziness, drowsiness, headache, diarrhea, nausea. Decreased absorption of ketoconazole, itraconazole. Increased levels of carbamazepine, cyclosporine, diazepam, labetalol, lidocaine, theophylline, phenytoin, procainamide, quinidine, propranolol, tricyclic antidepressants, valproic acid, warfarin. Stagger doses of cimetidine and antacids. Decrease dose with CrCl <30 ml/min.

famotidine (*Pepcid, Pepcid RPD, Pepcid AC, Maximum Strength Pepcid AC*) ▶LK ♀B ▶? $$$$

ADULT - Treatment of duodenal ulcer: 40 mg PO qhs or 20 mg PO bid. Maintenance of duodenal ulcer: 20 mg PO qhs. Treatment of gastric ulcer: 40 mg PO qhs. GERD: 20 mg PO bid. Treatment or prevention of heartburn: (OTC product only approved for this indication) 10-20 mg PO prn. Hypersecretory conditions: 20 mg PO q6h. Patients unable to take oral medications: 20 mg IV q12h.

PEDS - Not approved in children.

UNAPPROVED ADULT - Prevention of aspiration pneumonitis during surgery: 40 mg PO/IM prior to anesthesia. Upper GI bleeding: 20 mg IV q12h. Has been used as adjunctive therapy with H1 antagonist for severe allergic reactions.

UNAPPROVED PEDS - Treatment of duodenal or gastric ulcers, GERD, hypersecretory conditions: 0.6-0.8 mg/kg/day IV in 2-3 divided doses or 1-1.2 mg/kg/day PO in 2-3 divided doses, maximum 40 mg/day. GERD: <3 mo: 0.5 mg/kg PO qd; 3-12 months: 0.5 mg/kg PO bid; 1-16 yo:1 mg/kg/day PO divided bid.

FORMS - Generic/Trade: tab 10 mg (OTC, Pepcid AC Acid Controller), 20 (Rx and OTC, Maximum Strength Pepcid AC), 30, 40 mg. Trade only: orally disintegrating tab (Pepcid RPD) 20, 40 mg, suspension 40 mg/5 ml.

NOTES - May cause dizziness, headache, constipation, diarrhea. Decreased absorption of ketoconazole, itraconazole. Adjust dose in patients with CrCl <60 ml/min.

nizatidine (*Axid, Axid AR*) ▶K ♀B ▶? $$$$

ADULT - Treatment of duodenal or gastric ulcer: 300 mg PO qhs or 150 mg PO bid. Maintenance of duodenal ulcer: 150 mg PO qhs. GERD: 150 mg PO bid. Treatment or prevention of heartburn: (OTC product only approved for this indication) 75 mg prn, max 150 mg/day.

PEDS - Age ≥12 yo: Esophagitis, GERD: 150 mg PO bid.

UNAPPROVED ADULT - Has been used as adjunctive therapy with H1 antagonist for severe allergic reactions.

UNAPPROVED PEDS - 6 mos-11 yo (limited data): 6-10 mg/kg/day PO in 2 divided doses.

FORMS - Trade only: tabs 75 mg (OTC, Axid AR), oral solution 15 mg/mL (480 mL). Generic/Trade: cap 150,300 mg.

NOTES - May cause dizziness, headache, constipation, diarrhea. Decreased absorption of ketoconazole, itraconazole. Adjust dose in patients with CrCl <80 ml/min.

***Pepcid Complete* (famotidine + calcium carbonate + magnesium hydroxide)** ▶LK ♀B ▶? $

ADULT - Treatment of heartburn: 1 tab PO prn. Max 2 tabs/day.

PEDS - Not approved in children.

FORMS - OTC: Trade only: chew tab famotidine 10 mg with calcium carbonate 800 mg & magnesium hydroxide 165 mg.

ranitidine (*Zantac, Zantac 25, Zantac 75, Peptic Relief*) ▶K ♀B ▶? $$$$

ADULT - Treatment of duodenal ulcer: 150 mg PO bid or 300 mg qhs. Treatment of gastric ulcer or GERD: 150 mg PO bid. Maintenance of duodenal or gastric ulcer: 150 mg PO qhs. Treatment of erosive esophagitis: 150 mg PO qid. Maintenance of erosive esophagitis: 150 mg PO bid. Treatment of heartburn: (OTC product only approved for this indication) 75 mg PO prn, max 150 mg/day. Hypersecretory conditions: 150 mg PO bid. Patients unable to take oral meds: 50 mg IV/IM q6-8h or 6.25 mg/h continuous IV infusion.

PEDS - Children 1 month - 16 years: Treatment of duodenal or gastric ulcers: 2-4 mg/kg/24h PO divided bid (max 300 mg) or 2-4 mg/kg/day IV divided q6-8h. GERD, erosive esophagitis: 5-10 mg/kg/24h PO divided bid or 2-4 mg/kg/day IV divided q6-8h. Maintenance of duodenal or gastric ulcers: 2-4 mg/kg/24h PO qd (max 150 mg).

UNAPPROVED ADULT - Prevention of upper GI bleeding in critically ill patients: 6.25 mg/h continuous IV infusion (150 mg/d). Has been used as adjunctive therapy with H1 antagonist for severe allergic reactions.

UNAPPROVED PEDS - Treatment of duodenal or gastric ulcers, GERD, hypersecretory conditions: Neonates: 2-4 mg/kg/24h PO divided q12h or 2 mg/kg/24h IV divided q12h. Infants and children: 2-4 mg/kg/24h IV/IM divided q12h or 0.1-0.2 mg/kg/h continuous IV infusion. Premature and term infants <2 weeks of age: 2 mg/kg/day PO divided q12h. 1.5 mg/kg IV x1 then 12 h later 1.5-2 mg/kg/day IV divided q12h. Continuous infusion 1.5 mg/kg x1 then 0.04-0.08 mg/kg/h infusion.

FORMS - Generic/Trade: tabs 75 mg (OTC, Zantac 75), 150,300 mg, syrup 75 mg/5 ml. Trade only: effervescent tab 25, 150 mg, caps 150,300 mg, granules 150 mg.

NOTES - May cause dizziness, sedation, headache, drowsiness, rash, nausea, constipation, diarrhea. Variable effects on warfarin, decreased absorption of ketoconazole, itraconazole. Dissolve granules and effervescent tablets in water. Stagger doses of ranitidine and antacids. Adjust dose in patients with CrCl <50 ml/min.

GASTROENTEROLOGY: Antiulcer – Helicobacter pylori Treatment

***Helidac* (bismuth subsalicylate + metronidazole + tetracycline)** ▶LK ♀D ▶- $$$$

ADULT - Active duodenal ulcer associated with Helicobacter pylori: 1 dose (2 bismuth subsalicylate Tabs, 1 metronidazole tab and 1 tetracycline cap) PO qid, at meals and qhs for 2 weeks with an H2 antagonist.

PEDS - Not approved in children.

UNAPPROVED ADULT - Active duodenal ulcer associated with Helicobacter pylori: Same dose as in "adult", but substitute proton pump inhibitor for H2 antagonist.

FORMS - Trade only: Each dose: bismuth subsalicylate 524 (2x262 mg) + metronidazole 250 mg + tetracycline 500 mg.

NOTES - Tetracycline decreases effectiveness of oral contraceptives; use another form of contraception during therapy. Avoid alcohol. May cause photosensitivity, darkening of tongue and stools, nausea.

***PrevPac* (lansoprazole + amoxicillin + clarithromycin, ♣*Hp-Pac*)** ▶LK ♀C ▶? $$$$$

ADULT - Active duodenal ulcer associated with H. pylori: 1 dose PO bid x 10-14 days.

PEDS - Not approved in children.

FORMS - Trade only: lansoprazole 30 mg x 2 + amoxicillin 1 g (2x500 mg) x 2, clarithromycin 500 mg x 2.

NOTES - See components.

HELICOBACTER PYLORI THERAPY

- Triple therapy PO x 7-14 days: clarithromycin 500 mg bid + amoxicillin 1 g bid (or metronidazole 500 mg bid) + a proton pump inhibitor*
- Quadruple therapy PO x 14 days: bismuth subsalicylate 525 mg (or 30 mL) tid-qid + metronidazole 500 mg tid-qid + tetracycline 500 mg tid-qid + a proton pump inhibitor* or a H$_2$ blocker[†]

*PPI's esomeprazole 40 mg qd, lansoprazole 30 mg bid, omeprazole 20 mg bid, pantoprazole 40 mg bid, rabeprazole 20 mg bid.

[†]H$_2$ blockers cimetidine 400 mg bid, famotidine 20 mg bid, nizatidine 150 mg bid, ranitidine 150 mg bid.

Adapted from *The Medical Letter Treatment Guidelines* 2004:10.

GASTROENTEROLOGY: Antiulcer – Other

***Bellergal-S* (phenobarbital + belladonna + ergotamine, ♣*Bellergal Spacetabs*)** ▶LK ♀X ▶- $$

WARNING - Serious or life-threatening peripheral ischemia has been noted with ergotamine component when used with cytochrome P450 3A4 inhibitors such as ritonavir, nelfinavir, indinavir, erythromycin, clarithromycin, ketoconazole, and itraconazole.

ADULT - Hypermotility/hypersecretion: 1 tab bid.

PEDS - Not approved in children.

FORMS - Generic/Trade: tab phenobarbital 40 mg, ergotamine 0.6 mg, belladonna 0.2 mg.

NOTES - May decrease INR in patients receiving warfarin. Variable effect on phenytoin levels. May cause sedation especially with alcohol, phenothiazines, opioids, or tricyclic antidepressants. Additive anticholinergic effects with tricyclic antidepressants.

***dicyclomine* (*Bentyl, Bentylol, Antispas*)** ▶LK ♀B ▶- $$

ADULT - Treatment of functional bowel/irritable bowel syndrome (irritable colon, spastic colon, mucous colon): Initiate with 20 mg PO qid and increase to 40 mg PO qid, if tolerated. Patients who are unable to take oral medications: 20 mg IM q6h.

PEDS - Not approved in children.

UNAPPROVED PEDS - Treatment of functional / irritable bowel syndrome: Infants >6 months: 5 mg PO tid-qid. Children: 10 mg PO tid-qid.

FORMS - Generic/Trade: tab 20 mg, cap 10 mg, syrup 10 mg/5 ml. Generic only: cap 20 mg.

NOTES - Although some use lower doses (i.e., 10-20 mg PO qid), the only adult oral dose proven to be effective is 160 mg/day.

Donnatal **(phenobarbital + atropine + hyoscyamine + scopolamine)** ▶LK ♀C ▶- $

ADULT - Adjunctive therapy of irritable bowel syndrome or adjunctive treatment of duodenal ulcers: 1-2 tabs/caps or 5-10 ml PO tid-qid or 1 extended release tab PO q8-12h.

PEDS - Adjunctive therapy of irritable bowel syndrome: 0.1 ml/kg/dose PO q4h, maximum dose 5 ml. Adjunctive treatment of duodenal ulcers: 0.1 ml/kg/dose q4h. Alternative dosing regimen: Weight 4.5kg: 0.5 ml PO q4h or 0.75 ml PO q6h; 9.1kg: 1 ml PO q4h or 1.5 ml PO q6h; 13.6kg: 1.5 ml PO q4h or 2 ml PO q6h; 22.7kg: 2.5 ml PO q4h or 3.75 ml PO q6h; 34kg: 3.75 ml PO q4h or 5 ml PO q6h; 45.5kg: 5 ml PO q4h or 7.5 ml PO q6h.

FORMS - Generic/Trade: Phenobarbital 16.2 mg + hyoscyamine 0.1 mg + atropine 0.02 mg + scopolamine 6.5 mcg in each tab, cap or 5 ml. Each extended release tab has phenobarbital 48.6 mg + hyoscyamine 0.3111 mg + atropine 0.0582 mg + scopolamine 0.0195 mg.

NOTES - The FDA has classified Donnatal as "possibly effective" for treatment of irritable bowel syndrome and duodenal ulcer. Heat stroke may occur in hot weather. Can cause anticholinergic side effects; use caution in narrow-angle glaucoma, BPH, etc.

GI cocktail (green goddess) ▶LK ♀See individual ▶See individual $

ADULT - See components

PEDS - Not approved in children.

UNAPPROVED ADULT - Acute GI upset: mixture of Maalox/Mylanta 30 ml + viscous lidocaine (2%) 10 ml + Donnatal 10 ml administered PO in a single dose.

NOTES - Avoid repeat dosing due to risk of lidocaine toxicity.

hyoscyamine (*Levsin, NuLev*) ▶LK ♀C ▶- $

ADULT - Control gastric secretion, GI hypermotility, irritable bowel syndrome, and others: 0.125-0.25 mg PO/SL q4h prn, maximum 1.5 mg/24h; 0.375-0.75 mg PO q12h of sustained release preparations.

PEDS - Control gastric secretion, GI hypermotility, irritable bowel syndrome, and others: Initial oral dose by weight for children <2 yo: 12.5 mcg (2.3 kg), 16.7 mcg (3.4 kg), 20.8 mcg (5 kg), 25 mcg (7 kg), 31.3-33.3 mcg (10 kg), and 45.8 mcg (15 kg). Doses can be repeated q4h prn, but maximum daily dose is six times initial dose. Initial oral dose by weight for children 2-12 yo: 31.3-33.3 mcg (10kg), 62.5 mcg (20kg), 93.8 mcg (40kg), and 125 mcg (50kg). Doses may be repeated q4h, but maximum daily dose

should not exceed 750 mcg.

FORMS - Generic/Trade: tab 0.125,0.15 mg, SL tab 0.125 mg, solution 0.125 mg/ml. Trade only: extended release tab/cap 0.375 mg, orally disintegrating tab 0.125 mg (NuLev), elixir 0.125 mg/5 ml.

NOTES - May cause drowsiness, dizziness, blurred vision. Can cause anticholinergic side effects so use caution in narrow-angle glaucoma, BPH, etc.

mepenzolate (*Cantil*) ▶LK ♀B ▶? ?

ADULT - Approved, not yet marketed. Adjunctive therapy in peptic ulcer disease: 25-50 mg PO qid, with meals and qhs.

PEDS - Not approved in children.

FORMS - Trade only: tab: 25 mg.

NOTES - Contraindicated in glaucoma, obstructive uropathy, paralytic ileus, toxic megacolon, myasthenia gravis.

misoprostol (*Cytotec*) ▶LK ♀X ▶- $$$$

WARNING - Contraindicated in pregnant women because of its abortifacient properties. Do not use in women of child-bearing potential unless patient requires NSAID and is at high risk of complications from gastric ulcer. If misoprostol is used in such patients, they must receive oral and written warnings, have a negative serum pregnancy test within 2 weeks before starting therapy, begin therapy on 2nd or 3rd day of next normal menstrual period and use effective contraceptive measures.

ADULT - Prevention of NSAID-induced gastric ulcers: 200 mcg PO qid. If not tolerated, use 100 mcg PO qid.

PEDS - Not approved in children.

UNAPPROVED ADULT - Treatment of duodenal ulcers: 100 mcg PO qid. Prevention of NSAID-induced gastric ulcers: 200 mcg PO bid-tid.

UNAPPROVED PEDS - Improvement in fat absorption in cystic fibrosis in children 8 - 16 yo: 100 mcg PO qid.

FORMS - Trade/generic: tab 100,200 mcg.

NOTES - Many practitioners start at 100 mcg PO qid and increase to 200 mcg PO qid, if tolerated. Take with food. May cause diarrhea (13-40%) and abdominal pain (7-20%).

propantheline (*Pro-Banthine*, ♣*Propanthel*) ▶LK ♀C ▶- $$$

ADULT - Adjunctive therapy in peptic ulcer disease: 7.5-15 mg PO 30 min before meals and qhs.

PEDS - Not approved in children.

UNAPPROVED ADULT - Irritable bowel, pancreatitis, urinary bladder spasms: 7.5-15 mg

PO qid.

UNAPPROVED PEDS - Antisecretory effects: 1.5 mg/kg/day PO in 3-4 divided doses. Antispasmodic effects: 2-3 mg/kg/day PO divided q4-6h and qhs.

FORMS - Generic/Trade: tab 15 mg. Trade only: tab 7.5 mg.

NOTES - For elderly adults and those with small stature use 7.5 mg dose. May cause constipation, dry mucous membranes.

simethicone (*Mylicon, Gas-X, Phazyme*, ♣*Ovol*) ▶Not absorbed ♀C but + ▶? $

ADULT - Excessive gas in GI tract: 40-160 mg PO after meals and qhs prn, max 500 mg/day.

PEDS - Excessive gas in GI tract: <2 yo: 20 mg PO qid prn, maximum of 240 mg/d. Children 2-12 yo: 40 mg PO qid prn.

UNAPPROVED PEDS - Although used to treat infant colic (in approved dose for gas), several studies suggest no benefit.

FORMS - OTC: Generic/Trade: tab 60,95 mg, chew tab 40,80,125 mg, cap 125 mg, drops 40 mg/0.6 ml.

NOTES - For administration to infants, may mix dose in 30 ml of liquid. chew Tabs should be chewed thoroughly.

sucralfate (*Carafate*, ♣*Sulcrate*) ▶Not absorbed ♀B ▶? $$$

ADULT - Duodenal ulcer: 1g PO qid, 1h before meals and qhs. Maintenance therapy of duodenal ulcer: 1g PO bid.

PEDS - Not approved in children.

UNAPPROVED ADULT - Gastric ulcer, reflux esophagitis, NSAID-induced GI symptoms, stress ulcer prophylaxis: 1g PO qid 1h before meals & qhs. Oral and esophageal ulcers due to radiation/chemo/sclerotherapy: (suspension only) 5-10 ml swish and spit /swallow qid.

UNAPPROVED PEDS - Reflux esophagitis, gastric or duodenal ulcer, stress ulcer prophylaxis: 40-80 mg/kg/day PO divided q6h. Alternative dosing: children <6 yo: 500 mg PO qid, children >6 yo: 1g PO qid.

FORMS - Generic/Trade: tab 1 g. Trade only: susp 1 g/10 ml.

NOTES - May cause constipation. May reduce the absorption of cimetidine, ciprofloxacin, digoxin, ketoconazole, itraconazole, norfloxacin, phenytoin, ranitidine, tetracycline, theophylline and warfarin; separate doses by at least 2 hours. Antacids should be separated by at least 30 minutes.

GASTROENTEROLOGY: Antiulcer – Proton Pump Inhibitors

esomeprazole (*Nexium*) ▶L ♀B ▶? $$$$

ADULT - Erosive esophagitis: 20-40 mg PO bid x 4-8 weeks. Maintenance of erosive esophagitis: 20 mg PO qd. GERD: 20 mg PO qd x 4 weeks. H pylori eradication: 40 mg PO qd with amoxicillin 1000 mg PO bid & clarithromycin 500 mg PO bid x 10 days.

PEDS - Not approved in children.

FORMS - Trade only: delayed-release cap 20, 40 mg.

NOTES - May decrease absorption of ketoconazole, itraconazole, digoxin, iron, and ampicillin. Capsule can be opened and mixed in applesauce, but pellets should not be chewed or crushed.

lansoprazole (*Prevacid, Prevacid Napra-Pac*) ▶L ♀B ▶? $$$$

ADULT - Erosive esophagitis: 30 mg PO qd or 30 mg IV qd x 7 days or until taking PO. Maintenance therapy following healing of erosive esophagitis: 15 mg PO qd. NSAID-induced gastric ulcer: 30 mg PO qd x 8 weeks (treatment), 15 mg PO qd for up to 12 weeks (prevention). GERD: 15 mg PO qd. Duodenal ulcer treatment and maintenance: 15 mg PO qd. Gastric ulcer: 30 mg PO qd. Part of a multidrug regimen for H. pylori: 30 mg PO bid with amoxicillin 1000 mg PO bid & clarithromycin 500 mg PO bid x 10-14 days (see table) or 30 mg PO tid with amoxicillin 1000 mg PO tid x 14 days. Hypersecretory conditions: 60 mg PO qd.

PEDS - Erosive esophagitis and GERD (1-11 yo) ≤30 kg: 15 mg PO qd x up to 12 weeks. >30 kg: 30 mg PO qd x up to 12 weeks. Nonerosive GERD (12-17 yo): 15 mg PO qd x up to 8 weeks. GERD with erosive esophagitis (12-17 yo): 30 mg PO qd x up to 8 weeks.

FORMS - Trade only: cap 15,30 mg. Susp 15,30 mg packets. Orally disintegrating tab 15,30 mg. Prevacid NapraPac: 7 lansoprazole 15 mg caps packaged with 14 naproxen tabs 375 mg or 500 mg.

NOTES - Take before meals. Avoid concomitant administration with sucralfate. May decrease absorption of ketoconazole, itraconazole, ampicillin, digoxin and iron.

omeprazole (*Prilosec, Zegerid, Rapinex*, ♣*Losec*) ▶L ♀C ▶? $$$$

ADULT - GERD: 20 mg PO qd. Maintenance therapy following healing of erosive esophagitis: 20 mg PO qd. Duodenal ulcer: 20 mg PO qd. Heartburn (OTC): 20 mg PO qd x 14 days.

Gastric ulcer: 40 mg PO qd. Hypersecretory conditions: 60 mg PO qd. Part of a multidrug regimen for H pylori eradication: 20 mg PO bid with amoxicillin 1000 mg PO bid & clarithromycin 500 mg PO bid x 10 days, with additional 18 days of omeprazole 20 mg PO qd if ulcer present (see table). Or 40 mg PO qd with clarithromycin 500 mg PO tid x 14 days, with additional 14 days of omeprazole 20 mg PO qd if ulcer present.
PEDS - GERD (2-16 yo) <20 kg: 10 mg PO qd. ≥20 kg: 20 mg PO qd.
UNAPPROVED PEDS - Gastric or duodenal ulcers, hypersecretory states: 0.7-3.3 mg/kg/dose PO qd. GERD: 1 mg/kg/day PO qd or bid.
FORMS - Trade/generic: cap 10, 20 mg. OTC: 20 mg. Trade only: cap 40 mg, powder for suspension 20 mg (Zegerid), oral suspension 20 mg (Rapinex).
NOTES - Take before meals. Caps contain enteric-coated granules; do not chew. Caps may be opened and administered in acidic liquid (i.e. apple juice). Powder for suspension (Zegerid) mixed with 30 mL (2 tablespoons) water and consumed immediately. May increase levels of diazepam, warfarin, and phenytoin. May decrease absorption of ketoconazole, itraconazole, iron, ampicillin, and digoxin. Avoid administration with sucralfate.
pantoprazole (*Protonix*, ♣*Pantoloc*) ▶L ♀B ▶? $$$

ADULT - GERD: 40 mg PO qd for 8-16 weeks, or 40 mg IV qd x 7-10 days until taking PO. Maintenance therapy following healing of erosive esophagitis: 40 mg PO qd. Zollinger-Ellison syndrome: 80 mg IV q8-12h x 6 days until taking PO.
PEDS - Not approved in children.
UNAPPROVED ADULT - Has been studied as part of various multidrug regimens for H pylori eradication. Decreases peptic ulcer rebleeding after hemostasis: 80 mg IV bolus, then 8 mg/h continuous IV infusion x 3 days, followed by oral therapy (or 40 mg IV q12h for 4-7 days if unable to tolerate PO).
FORMS - Trade only: tab 40 mg.
NOTES - May decrease absorption of ketoconazole, itraconazole, digoxin, iron, and ampicillin. Can increase INR when used with warfarin.
rabeprazole (*Aciphex*, ♣*Pariet*) ▶L ♀B ▶? $$$$

ADULT - GERD: 20 mg PO qd x 8-16 weeks. Duodenal ulcers: 20 mg PO qd x 4 weeks. Zollinger-Ellison syndrome: 60 mg PO qd, may increase up to 100 mg qd or 60 mg bid. Part of a multidrug regimen for H. pylori eradication: 20 mg PO bid, with amoxicillin 1000 mg PO bid & clarithromycin 500 mg PO bid x 7 days.
PEDS - Not approved in children.
FORMS - Trade only: tab 20 mg.
NOTES - May decrease absorption of ketoconazole, itraconazole, digoxin, iron, ampicillin.

GASTROENTEROLOGY: Laxatives

bisacodyl (*Correctol, Dulcolax, Feen-a-Mint*) ▶L ♀+ ▶? $
ADULT - Constipation/colonic evacuation prior to a procedure: 10-15 mg PO qd prn, 10 mg PR qd prn.
PEDS - Constipation/colonic evacuation prior to a procedure: 0.3 mg/kg/d PO qd prn. Children <2 yo: 5 mg PR prn. 2-11 yo: 5-10 mg PR prn. >11 yo: 10 mg PR prn.
FORMS - OTC Generic/Trade: tab 5 mg, supp 10 mg.
NOTES - Oral tablet has onset of 6-10 h. Onset of action of suppository is approximately 15-60 min. Do not chew Tabs, swallow whole. Do not give within 1h of antacids or dairy products. Chronic use of stimulant laxatives may be habit forming.
cascara ▶L ♀C ▶+ $
ADULT - Constipation: 325 mg PO qhs prn or 5 ml/day of aromatic fluid extract PO qhs prn.
PEDS - Constipation: Infants: 1.25 ml/day of

aromatic fluid extract PO qd prn. Children 2-11 yo: 2.5 ml/day of aromatic fluid extract PO qd prn.
FORMS - OTC Generic: tab 325 mg, liquid aromatic fluid extract.
NOTES - Cascara sagrada fluid extract is 5 times more potent than cascara sagrada aromatic fluid extract. Chronic use of stimulant laxatives may be habit forming.
castor oil (*Purge, Fleet Flavored Castor Oil*) ▶Not absorbed ♀- ▶? $
ADULT - Constipation: 15 ml PO qd prn. Colonic evacuation prior to procedure: 15-30 ml of castor oil or 30-60 ml emulsified castor oil PO as a single dose 16h prior to procedure.
PEDS - Colonic evacuation prior to procedure: Children <2 yo: 1-5 ml of castor oil or 5-15 ml emulsified castor oil PO as a single dose 16h prior to procedure. 2-11 yo: 5-15 ml of castor oil or 7.5-30 ml of emulsified castor oil PO as a single dose 16h prior to procedure.

FORMS - OTC Generic/Trade: liquid 30,60,120, 480 ml, emulsified susp 45,60,90,120 ml.

NOTES - Emulsions somewhat mask the bad taste. Onset of action approximately 2-6h. Do not give at bedtime. Chill or administer with juice to improve taste.

docusate calcium (*Surfak*) ▶L ♀+ ▶? $
ADULT - Constipation: 240 mg PO qd.
PEDS - Safe dosing has not been established.
FORMS - OTC Generic/Trade: cap 240 mg.
NOTES - Takes 1-3 days to notably soften stools.

docusate sodium (*Colace*) ▶L ♀+ ▶? $
ADULT - Constipation: 50-500 mg/day PO in 1-4 divided doses.
PEDS - Constipation: Children <3 yo: 10-40 mg/day PO in 1-4 divided doses. 3-6 yo: 20-60 mg/day PO in 1-4 divided doses. 6-12 yo: 40-150 mg/day PO in 1-4 divided doses.
UNAPPROVED ADULT - Constipation: Can be given as a retention enema: Mix 50-100 mg docusate liquid with saline or oil retention enema for rectal use.
FORMS - OTC Generic/Trade: cap 50,100, 250 mg, tab 50,100 mg, liquid 10 & 50 mg/5 ml, syrup 16.75 & 20 mg/5 ml.
NOTES - Takes 1-3 days to notably soften stools. Use higher doses initially. Liquids (not syrups) should be mixed with juice, milk or formula to mask bitter taste.

glycerin ▶Not absorbed ♀C ▶? $
ADULT - Constipation: 1 adult supp PR prn.
PEDS - Constipation: Neonates: 0.5 ml/kg/dose PR prn. Children <6 yo: 1 infant supp or 2-5 ml rectal solution as an enema PR prn. Children ≥6 yo: 1 adult supp or 5-15 ml of rectal solution as enema PR prn.
FORMS - OTC Generic/Trade: supp infant & adult, solution (Fleet Babylax) 4 ml/applicator.

lactulose (*Chronulac, Cephulac, Kristalose*) ▶Not absorbed ♀B ▶? $$
ADULT - Constipation: 15-30 ml (syrup) or 10-20 g (powder for oral solution) PO qd. Evacuation of barium following barium procedures: 5-10 ml (syrup) PO bid. Acute hepatic encephalopathy: 30-45 ml syrup/dose PO q1h until laxative effect observed or 300 ml in 700 ml water or saline PR as a retention enema q4-6h. Prevention of encephalopathy: 30-45 ml syrup PO tid-qid.
PEDS - Prevention or treatment of encephalopathy: Infants: 2.5-10 ml/day (syrup) PO in 3-4 divided doses. Children/adolescents: 40-90 ml/day (syrup) PO in 3-4 divided doses.
UNAPPROVED ADULT - Restoration of bowel

movements in hemorrhoidectomy patients: 15 ml syrup PO bid on day before surgery and for 5 days following surgery.
UNAPPROVED PEDS - Constipation: 7.5 ml syrup PO qd, after breakfast.
FORMS - Generic/Trade: syrup 10 g/15 ml. Trade only (Kristalose): 10, 20 g packets for oral solution.
NOTES - May be mixed in water, juice or milk to improve palatability. Packets for oral solution should be mixed in 4 oz of water. Titrate dose to produce 2-3 soft stools/day.

magnesium citrate (❋ *Citro-Mag*) ▶K♀+▶? $
ADULT - Evacuate bowel prior to procedure: 150-300 ml PO divided qd-bid.
PEDS - Evacuate bowel prior to procedure: Children <6 yo: 2-4 ml/kg/24h PO divided qd-bid. Children 6-12 yo: 100-150 ml/24h PO divided qd-bid.
FORMS - OTC Generic: solution 300 ml/bottle.
NOTES - Use caution with impaired renal function. May decrease absorption of phenytoin, ciprofloxacin, benzodiazepines, and glyburide. May cause additive CNS depression with CNS depressants. Chill to improve palatability.

magnesium hydroxide (*Milk of Magnesia*) ▶K ♀+ ▶? $
ADULT - Laxative: 30-60 ml PO as a single dose or divided doses. Antacid: 5-15 ml/dose PO qid prn or 622-1244 mg PO qid prn.
PEDS - Laxative: Age <2 yo: 0.5 ml/kg PO as a single dose. 2-5 yo: 5-15 ml/day PO as a single dose or in divided doses. 6-11 yo: 15-30 ml PO in a single dose or in divided doses. Antacid (children >12yo): 2.5-5 ml/dose PO qid prn.
FORMS - OTC Generic/Trade: liquid 400 & 800 (concentrated) mg/5 ml, chew tab 311 mg.
NOTES - Milk of magnesia concentrated liquid contains 800 mg/5 ml, so use half of the dose. Use caution with impaired renal function.

methylcellulose (*Citrucel*) ▶Not absorbed ♀+ ▶? $
ADULT - Laxative: 1 heaping tablespoon in 8 ounces cold water PO qd-tid.
PEDS - Laxative: Age 6-12 yo: 1½ heaping teaspoons in 4 ounces cold water qd-tid PO prn.
FORMS - OTC Trade only: Packets, multiple use canisters.
NOTES - Must be taken with water to avoid esophageal obstruction or choking.

mineral oil (*Agoral, Kondremul, Fleet Mineral Oil Enema*, ❋ *Lansoyl*) ▶Not absorbed ♀C ▶? $
ADULT - Laxative: 15-45 ml PO in a single dose or in divided doses, 60-150 ml PR.

PEDS - Laxative: Children 6-11 yo: 5-15 ml PO in a single dose or in divided doses. Children 2-11 yo: 30-60 ml PR.

FORMS - OTC Generic/Trade: plain mineral oil, mineral oil emulsion (Agoral, Kondremul).

NOTES - Use with caution in young children due to concerns for aspiration pneumonitis. Although usual directions for plain mineral oil are to administer at bedtime, this increases risk of lipid pneumonitis. Mineral oil emulsions may be administered with meals.

***Peri-Colace* (docusate + casanthranol)** ▶L ♀C ▶? $

ADULT - Constipation: 1-2 cap or 15-30 ml PO qhs prn.

PEDS - Constipation: 5-15 ml PO qhs prn.

FORMS - OTC Generic/Trade: cap 100 mg docusate + 30 mg casanthranol/cap, syrup 60 mg docusate + 30 mg casanthranolol/15 ml.

NOTES - Dilute syrup in 6-8 oz. of juice, milk or infant formula to prevent throat irritation. Chronic use of stimulant laxatives (casanthranol) may be habit forming.

polycarbophil (*FiberCon, Fiberall, Konsyl Fiber, Equalactin*) ▶Not absorbed ♀+ ▶? $

ADULT - Laxative: 1 g PO qid prn.

PEDS - Laxative: Children 3-5 yo: 500 mg PO qd-bid prn. ≥6 yo: 500 mg PO qd-tid prn.

UNAPPROVED ADULT - Diarrhea: 1 g PO q30min prn. Max daily dose 6 g.

UNAPPROVED PEDS - Diarrhea: Children 3-5 yo: 500 mg PO q30min prn. Max daily dose 1.5 g. >6 yo: 500 mg PO qd-tid or prn. Max daily dose 3 g.

FORMS - OTC Generic/Trade: tab 500,625 mg, chew tab 500,1000 mg.

NOTES - When used as a laxative, take dose with at least 8 ounces of fluid. Do not administer concomitantly with tetracycline; separate by at least 2 hours.

polyethylene glycol (*MiraLax, GlycoLax*) ▶Not absorbed ♀C ▶? $

ADULT - Constipation: 17 g (1 heaping tablespoon) in 4-8 oz water, juice, soda, coffee, or tea PO qd.

PEDS - Not approved in children.

UNAPPROVED PEDS - Constipation: 0.8 g/kg/day PO in 2 divided doses.

FORMS - Trade only: powder for oral solution.

NOTES - Takes 2-4 days to produce bowel movement. Indicated for up to 14 days.

polyethylene glycol with electrolytes (*Go-Lytely, Colyte, TriLyte, NuLytely, Half-Lytely and Bisacodyl Tablet Kit, ✦Klean -Prep, Lyteprep, Electropeg, Peg-Lyte*) ▶Not absorbed ♀C ▶? $

ADULT - Bowel cleansing prior to GI exam: 240 ml PO every 10 min or 20-30 ml/min NG until 4L are consumed or rectal effluent is clear.

PEDS - Bowel prep, >6 months (NuLYTELY, TriLyte): 25 mL/kg/hour PO/NG, until rectal effluent is clear, maximum 4L.

UNAPPROVED ADULT - Chronic constipation: 125-500 ml/day PO qd-bid.

UNAPPROVED PEDS - Bowel cleansing prior to GI examination: 25-40 ml/kg/h PO/NG for 4-10 h or until rectal effluent is clear or 20-30 ml/min NG until 4L are consumed or rectal effluent is clear. Acute iron overdoses: children <3 yo: 0.5 L/h.

FORMS - Generic/Trade: powder for oral soln. Available as a kit of 2L bottle of polyethylene glycol with electrolytes and 4 bisacodyl tabs 5 mg (HalfLytely and Bisacodyl Tablet Kit).

NOTES - Solid food should not be given within 2 h of solution. Effects should occur within 1-2 hours. Chilling improves palatability.

psyllium (*Metamucil, Fiberall, Konsyl, Hydrocil, ✦Prodium Plain*) ▶Not absorbed ♀+ ▶? $

ADULT - Laxative: 1 rounded tsp in liquid, 1 packet in liquid or 1 wafer with liquid PO qd-tid.

PEDS - Laxative (children 6-11yo): ½-1 rounded tsp in liquid, ½-1 packet in liquid or 1 wafer with liquid PO qd-tid.

UNAPPROVED ADULT - Reduction in cholesterol: 1 rounded tsp in liquid, 1 packet in liquid or 1-2 wafers with liquid PO tid. Prevention of GI side effects with orlistat: 6 g in liquid with each orlistat dose or 12 g in liquid qhs.

FORMS - OTC: Generic/Trade: powder, granules, wafers, including various flavors and various amounts of psyllium.

NOTES - Powders and granules must be mixed with liquid prior to ingestion. Start with 1 dose/day and gradually increase to minimize gas and bloating. Can bind with warfarin, digoxin, potassium-sparing diuretics, salicylates, tetracycline and nitrofurantoin; space at least 3 h apart.

senna (*Senokot, SenokotXTRA, Ex-Lax, Fletcher's Castoria, ✦Glysennid*) ▶L ♀C ▶+ $

ADULT - Laxative or evacuation of the colon for bowel or rectal examinations: 1 tsp granules in water or 10-15 ml or 2 tabs PO qhs. Max daily dose 4 tsp of granules, 30 ml of syrup, 8 tabs or 2 supp.

PEDS - Laxative: 10-20 mg/kg/dose PO qhs. Alternative regimen: 1 mo-2 yo: 1.25-2.5 ml syrup PO qhs, max 5 ml/day; 2-5yo: 2.5-3.75 ml syrup PO qhs, max 7.5 ml/day; 6-12 yo: 5-7.5 ml syrup PO qhs, max 15 ml/day.

FORMS - OTC Generic/Trade (All dosing is based on sennosides content; 1 mg sennosides = 21.7 mg standardized senna concentrate): granules 15 mg/tsp, syrup 8.8 mg/5 ml, liquid 3 mg/ml (Fletcher's Castoria), tab 8.6, 15, 17, 25 mg , chewable tab 15 mg.

NOTES - Effects occur 6-24 h after oral administration. Use caution in renal dysfunction. Chronic use of stimulant laxatives may be habit forming.

Senokot-S (senna + docusate) ▶L ♀C ▶+ $

ADULT - 2 tabs PO qd, maximum 4 tabs bid.

PEDS - 6-12 yo: 1 tab PO qd, max 2 tabs bid. 2-6 yo: ½ tab PO qd, max 1 tab bid.

FORMS - OTC Trade: tab 8.6 mg senna concentrate/50 mg docusate.

NOTES - Effects occur 6-24 h after oral administration. Use caution in renal dysfunction. Chronic use of stimulant laxatives may be habit forming.

sodium phosphate (*Fleet enema, Fleet Phospho-Soda, Visicol, ♥Enemol*) ▶Not absorbed ♀C ▶? $

ADULT - 1 adult or pediatric enema PR or 20-30 ml of oral soln PO prn (max 45 ml/24 h). Visi-col: Evening before colonoscopy: 3 tabs with 8 oz clear liquid q15 min until 20 tabs are consumed. Day of colonoscopy: starting 3-5 h before procedure, 3 tabs with 8 oz clear liquid q15 min until 20 tabs are consumed.

PEDS - Laxative: 1 pediatric enema (67.5 ml) PR prn or 5-9 yo: 5 ml of oral solution PO prn. 10-12 yo: 10 ml of oral solution PO prn.

UNAPPROVED ADULT - Visicol: Evening before colonoscopy: 3 tabs with 8 oz clear liquid q15 min until 20 tabs are consumed. Day of colonoscopy: starting 3-5 h before procedure, 3 tabs with 8 oz clear liquid q15 min until 8-12 tabs are consumed.

FORMS - OTC Trade only: pediatric & adult enema, oral solution. Visicol tab (trade $$): 1.5 g.

NOTES - Taking the last 2 doses of Visicol with ginger ale appears to minimize residue. Excessive doses (>45 ml/24 h) of oral products may lead to serious electrolyte disturbances. Use with caution in severe renal impairment.

sorbitol ▶Not absorbed ♀+ ▶? $

ADULT - Laxative: 30-150 ml (of 70% solution) PO or 120 ml (of 25-30% solution) PR.

PEDS - Laxative: Children 2-11 yo: 2 ml/kg (of 70% solution) PO or 30-60 ml (of 25-30% solution) PR.

FORMS - Generic: solution 70%.

GASTROENTEROLOGY: Other GI Agents

alosetron (*Lotronex*) ▶L ♀B ▶? $$$$

WARNING - Can cause severe constipation & ischemic colitis. Can be prescribed only by drug company authorized clinicians using special sticker and written informed consent.

ADULT - Diarrhea-predominant irritable bowel syndrome in women who have failed conventional therapy: 1 mg PO qd for 4 weeks; may increase to 1 mg PO bid. Discontinue if symptoms not controlled in 4 weeks on 1 mg PO bid.

PEDS - Not approved in children.

FORMS - Tablets 0.5, 1 mg.

alpha-galactosidase (*Beano*) ▶Minimal absorption ♀? ▶? $

ADULT - 5 drops per ½ cup gassy food, 3 tabs PO (chew, swallow or crumble) or 15 drops per typical meal.

PEDS - Not approved in children <12 yo.

FORMS - Trade: drops 150 GalU/5 drops, tab 150 GalU.

NOTES - Beano produces 2-6 grams of carbohydrates for every 100 grams of food treated by Beano; may increase glucose levels.

balsalazide (*Colazal*) ▶Minimal absorption ♀B ▶? $$$$$

ADULT - Ulcerative colitis: 2.25 g PO tid x 8-12 weeks.

PEDS - Not approved in children.

FORMS - Trade: cap 750 mg.

NOTES - Contraindicated in salicylate allergy.

budesonide (*Entocort EC*) ▶L ♀C ▶? $$$$$

ADULT - Mild-moderate Crohn's: 9 mg PO qd x 8 weeks. May repeat 8 week course for recurring episodes.

PEDS - Not approved in children.

UNAPPROVED PEDS - Mild-moderate Crohn's and ≥9 yo: 0.45 mg/kg up to 9 mg PO qd x 8-12 weeks.

FORMS - Trade: cap 3 mg.

NOTES - May taper dose to 6 mg for 2 weeks prior to discontinuation.

cisapride (*Propulsid*, ♥*Prepulsid*) ▶LK ♀C ▶? $

WARNING - Available only through limited-access protocol through manufacturer. Can cause potentially fatal cardiac arrhythmias. Many drug and disease interactions.

ADULT - 10 mg PO qid, at least 15 min before

meals and qhs. Some patients may require 20 mg PO qid. Max 80 mg/day.

PEDS - Not approved in children.

UNAPPROVED PEDS - Gastroesophageal reflux disease: 0.2-0.3 mg/kg/dose PO tid-qid.

FORMS - Trade: Tab 10,20 mg, susp 1 mg/1 ml.

domperidone (✤*Motilium*) ▶L, gut wall ♀C ▶- $

ADULT - Canada only. Upper GI motility disorders associated with chronic and subacute gastritis and diabetic gastroparesis: 10 mg PO 3-4 times daily, 15-30 minutes before meals, and at bedtime if needed. May increase to maximum of 20 mg 3-4 times daily in severe/recalcitrant cases. N/V associated with dopamine agonist antiparkinsonian agents: 20 mg PO 3-4 times daily.

PEDS - Not approved in children.

FORMS - Rx:Trade / generic: tabs 10 mg.

NOTES - Contraindicated whenever GI stimulation may be dangerous, eg, GI hemorrhage, mechanical obstruction, perforation. Use cautiously with CYP 3A4 inhibitors (azole antifungals, macrolide antibiotics, HIV protease inhibitors, nefazodone). May accelerate absorption of drugs from small bowel while slowing absorption of drugs from stomach, particularly sustained release/enteric-coated preparations.

glycopyrrolate (*Robinul, Robinul Forte*) ▶K ♀B ▶? $$$

ADULT - Drooling: 0.1 mg/kg PO bid-tid, max 8 mg/day. Pre-op/intraoperative respiratory antisecretory: 0.1 mg IV/IM prn.

PEDS - Not approved in children.

UNAPPROVED PEDS - Drooling: 0.04-0.1 mg/kg PO tid-qid, max 8 mg/day. Pre-op/intraoperative respiratory antisecretory: 0.004-0.01 mg/kg IV/IM prn, max 0.2 mg/dose or 0.8 mg/24h.

FORMS - Trade: tab 1, 2 mg.

infliximab (*Remicade*) ▶Serum ♀B ▶? $$$$$

WARNING - Serious, life-threatening infections, including sepsis & disseminated TB have been reported. Evaluate patients for latent TB, and treat if necessary, prior to initiation of infliximab. May worsen heart failure; monitor signs /symptoms of CHF. Hypersensitivity reactions may occur.

ADULT - Moderately to severely active Crohn's disease or fistulizing disease: 5 mg/kg IV infusion at 0, 2, and 6 weeks, then every 8 weeks. See entry in analgesics section for rheumatoid arthritis dosing.

PEDS - Not approved in children.

UNAPPROVED PEDS - Moderately to severely active Crohn's disease or fistulizing disease: 5 mg/kg IV infusion. May repeat up to 3 times in 12 weeks.

NOTES - Up to 16% patients experience adverse effects, eg, headache, nausea, infections, abdominal pain, fever. Dose is infused over ≥2 hours.

lactase (*Lactaid*) ▶Not absorbed ♀+ ▶+ $

ADULT - Swallow or chew 3 caplets (Original strength), 2 caplets (Extra strength), 1 caplet (Ultra) with first bite of dairy foods. Adjust dose based on response.

PEDS - Titrate dose based on response.

FORMS - OTC Trade/generic: caplets, chew tab.

Librax (clidinium + chlordiazepoxide) ▶K ♀D ▶- $

ADULT - Irritable bowel syndrome: 1 cap PO tid-qid.

PEDS - Not approved in children.

FORMS - Generic/Trade: cap clidinium 2.5 mg + chlordiazepoxide 5 mg.

NOTES - May cause drowsiness. After prolonged use, gradually taper to avoid withdrawal symptoms.

mercaptopurine (6-MP, *Purinethol*) ▶L ♀D ▶? $$$

ADULT - See oncology section

PEDS - Not approved in children.

UNAPPROVED ADULT - Inflammatory bowel disease: Start at 50 mg PO qd, titrate to response. Typical dose range 0.5-1.5 mg/kg qd.

UNAPPROVED PEDS - 1.5 mg/kg PO qd.

FORMS - Generic/Trade: tab 50 mg.

NOTES - May cause severe toxicity including hepatitis in up to 10% of patients. Consider folate supplementation.

mesalamine (5-aminosalicylic acid, 5-ASA, *Asacol, Pentasa, Rowasa, Canasa, ✤Mesasal, Salofalk*) ▶Gut ♀B ▶? $$$$

ADULT - Ulcerative colitis: Tab: 800-1600 mg PO tid. Cap: 1 g PO qid. Rowasa supp: 500 mg PR retained for 1-3h or longer bid. Canasa supp: 500 mg PR bid-tid. Susp: 4 g (60 ml) PR retained for 8h qhs. Maintenance of ulcerative colitis: 1600 mg/day PO in divided doses.

PEDS - Not approved in children.

UNAPPROVED ADULT - Active Crohn's: 0.4-4.8 g/day PO in divided doses. Maintenance of remission of Crohn's: 2.4 g/day in divided doses.

UNAPPROVED PEDS - Tab: 50 mg/kg/day PO divided q6-12h. Cap: 50 mg/kg/day PO divided q8-12h.

FORMS - Trade only: delayed release tab 400 mg (Asacol), controlled release cap 250 mg

(Pentasa), supp 500 mg (Rowasa), rectal susp 4 g/60 ml (Rowasa), rectal supp 400 mg (Canasa).

NOTES - Avoid in salicylate sensitivity. May decrease digoxin levels. May discolor urine yellow-brown. Most common adverse effects include headache, abdominal pain, fever, rash.

neomycin (*Mycifradin*) ▶Minimally absorbed ♀D ▶? $$$

ADULT - Suppression of intestinal bacteria (given with erythromycin): 1 g PO at 19h, 18h and 9h prior to procedure (i.e. 1 pm, 2 pm, 11 pm on prior day). Alternative regimen 1 g PO q1h for 4 doses then 1 g PO q4h for 5 doses. Hepatic encephalopathy: 4-12 g/day PO divided q6h. Diarrhea caused by enteropathogenic E. coli: 3 g/day PO divided q6h.

PEDS - Suppression of intestinal bacteria (given with erythromycin): 25 mg/kg PO at 19h, 18h and 9h prior to procedure (i.e. 1 pm, 2 pm, 11 pm on prior day). Alternative regimen 90 mg/kg/day PO divided q4h for 2-3 days. Hepatic encephalopathy: 50-100 mg/kg/day PO divided q6-8h. Diarrhea caused by enteropathogenic E. coli: 50 mg/kg/day PO divided q6h.

FORMS - Generic/Trade: tab 500 mg, solution 125 mg/5 ml.

NOTES - Increased INR with warfarin, decreased levels of digoxin, methotrexate.

octreotide (*Sandostatin, Sandostatin LAR*) ▶LK ♀B ▶? $$$$$

ADULT - Diarrhea associated with carcinoid tumors: 100-600 mcg/day SC/IV in 2-4 divided doses or 20 mg IM (Sandostatin LAR) q4 weeks x 2 months. Adjust dose based on response. Diarrhea associated with vasoactive intestinal peptide-secreting tumors: 200-300 mcg/day SC/IV in 2-4 divided doses or 20 mg IM (Sandostatin LAR) q4 weeks x 2 months. Adjust dose based on response.

PEDS - Not approved in children.

UNAPPROVED ADULT - Variceal bleeding: Bolus 50-100 mcg IV followed by 25-50 mcg/h continuous IV infusion. AIDS diarrhea: 100-500 mcg SC tid. Irritable bowel syndrome: 100 mcg as a single dose to 125 mcg SC bid. GI and pancreatic fistulas: 50-200 mcg SC/IV q8h. Other uses.

UNAPPROVED PEDS - Diarrhea: initially 1-10 mcg/kg SC/IV q12h.

FORMS - Trade only: vials for injection 0.05,0.1, 0.2,0.5,1 mg, long-acting injectable suspension (Sandostatin LAR) 10 mg, 20 mg, 30 mg.

NOTES - For the treatment of variceal bleeding, most studies treat for 3-5 days. Individualize dose based on response. Dosage reduction often necessary in elderly. May cause hypoglycemia, hyperglycemia, hypothyroidism, cardiac arrhythmias. Sandostatin LAR only indicated for patients who are stabilized on Sandostatin.

olsalazine (*Dipentum*) ▶L ♀C ▶- $$$$

ADULT - Maintenance of remission of ulcerative colitis in patients intolerant to sulfasalazine: 500 mg PO bid.

PEDS - Not approved in children.

UNAPPROVED ADULT - Crohn's: 1.5-3 g/day PO in divided doses.

FORMS - Trade only: cap 250 mg.

NOTES - Diarrhea in up to 17%. Avoid in salicylate sensitivity.

orlistat (*Xenical*) ▶Gut ♀B ▶? $$$$

ADULT - Weight loss, weight management: 120 mg PO tid with meals or up to 1 h after meals.

PEDS - Children 12-16 yo: 120 mg PO tid with meals. Not approved in children <12 yo.

FORMS - Trade only: cap 120 mg.

NOTES - May cause fatty stools, fecal urgency, flatus with discharge and oily spotting in >20% of patients. GI adverse effects greater when taken with high fat diet.

pancreatin (*Creon, Donnazyme, Ku-Zyme*, ♣*Entozyme*) ▶Gut ♀C ▶? $$$

ADULT - Enzyme replacement (initial dose): 8,000-24,000 units lipase (1-2 cap/tab) PO with meals and snacks.

PEDS - Enzyme replacement (initial dose): <1 yo: 2,000 units lipase PO with meals. 1-6 yo: 4,000-8,000 units lipase PO with meals, 4,000 units lipase with snacks. 7-12 yo: 4,000-12,000 units lipase PO with meals and snacks.

FORMS - Tab, cap with varying amounts of pancreatin, lipase, amylase and protease.

NOTES - Titrate dose to stool fat content. Products are not interchangeable. Avoid concomitant calcium carbonate and magnesium hydroxide since these may affect the enteric coating. Do not crush/chew microspheres or tabs. Possible association of colonic strictures and high doses of lipase (>16,000 units/kg/meal) in pediatric patients.

pancrelipase (*Viokase, Pancrease, Cotazym, Ku-Zyme HP*) ▶Gut ♀C ▶? $$$

ADULT - Enzyme replacement (initial dose): 4,000-33,000 units lipase (1-3 cap/tab) PO with meals and snacks.

PEDS - Enzyme replacement (initial dose): 6 mo -1 yo: 2,000 units lipase or 1/8 tsp PO with feedings. 1-6 yo: 4,000-8,000 units lipase PO with meals, 4,000 units lipase with snacks. 7-12 yo: 4,000-12,000 units lipase PO w/ meals/

snacks.

FORMS - Tab, cap, powder with varying amounts of lipase, amylase and protease.

NOTES - Titrate dose to stool fat content. Products are not interchangeable. Avoid concomitant calcium carbonate and magnesium hydroxide since these may affect the enteric coating. Do not crush/chew microspheres or tabs. Possible association of colonic strictures and high doses of lipase (>16,000 units/kg/meal) in pediatric patients.

pinaverium (✿ *Dicetel*) ▶? ♀C ▶- $$-$$$

ADULT - Canada only. Irritable bowel syndrome: 50 mg PO tid, may increase to maximum of 100 mg tid.

PEDS - Not for children.

FORMS - Trade: tabs 50, 100 mg.

NOTES - Take with a full glass of water during meal or snack.

secretin (*SecreMax, ChiRhoClin*) ▶Serum ♀C ▶? $$$$$

ADULT - Stimulation of pancreatic secretions, to aid in diagnosis of exocrine pancreas dysfunction: Test dose 0.2 mcg IV. If tolerated, 0.2 mcg/kg IV over 1 minute. Stimulation of gastrin to aid in diagnosis of gastrinoma: Test dose 0.2 mcg IV. If tolerated, 0.4 mcg/kg IV over 1 minute. Identification of ampulla of Vater and accessory papilla during ERCP: 0.2 mcg/kg IV over 1 minute.

PEDS - Not approved in children.

NOTES - Previously known as Secreflo. Contraindicated in acute pancreatitis.

sibutramine (*Meridia*) ▶L ♀C ▶- ©IV $$$

ADULT - Weight loss: 10 mg PO qd; can increase to 15 mg qd after 4 weeks.

PEDS - Not approved in children.

FORMS - Trade only: cap 5,10,15 mg.

NOTES - Monitor BP and heart rate. Use for up to 1 year. Avoid concurrent use of SSRIs, MAO inhibitors, sumatriptan, ergotamine and other serotonin agents to avoid development of serotonin syndrome.

sulfasalazine (*Azulfidine, Azulfidine EN-tabs*, ✿ *Salazopyrin, Salazopyrin EN*) ▶K ♀- ▶? $$

ADULT - Ulcerative colitis: Initially, 500-1000 mg PO qid. Maintenance: 500 mg PO qid.

PEDS - Ulcerative colitis, >2yo: Initially 30-60 mg/kg/day PO divided into 3-6 doses. Maximum 75 mg/kg/day. Maintenance: 30 mg/kg/day PO divided qid.

FORMS - Generic/Trade: tab 500 mg.

NOTES - Contraindicated in children <2 yo. Avoid with hepatic or renal dysfunction, intesti-

nal or urinary obstruction, porphyria, sulfonamide or salicylate sensitivity. Monitor CBCs & LFTs. Beware of hypersensitivity, marrow suppression, renal & liver damage, irreversible neuromuscular & CNS changes, fibrosing alveolitis, oligospermia & infertility, and photosensitivity. May decrease folic acid, digoxin, cyclosporine & iron levels. May turn body fluids, contact lenses, or skin orange-yellow. Enteric coated (Azulfidine EN, Salazopyrin EN) tabs may cause fewer GI adverse effects.

tegaserod (*Zelnorm*) ▶stomach/L ♀B ▶? $$$$

WARNING - Severe diarrhea leading to hypovolemia, hypotension and syncope has been reported, as has ischemic colitis and other forms of intestinal ischemia. Discontinue immediately if hypotension, syncope, or symptoms of intestinal ischemia (eg, rectal bleeding, bloody diarrhea or new or worsening abdominal pain). Do not restart if ischemic colitis is diagnosed.

ADULT - Constipation-predominant irritable bowel syndrome in women: 6 mg PO bid before meals for 4-6 weeks. May repeat for an additional 4-6 weeks.

PEDS - Not approved in children.

UNAPPROVED ADULT - Chronic constipation in women <65 yo: 6 mg PO bid.

FORMS - Trade: tabs 2, 6 mg.

trimebutine (✿ *Modulon*) ▶? ♀C ▶? $$

ADULT - Canada only. Irritable bowel syndrome: Up to 600 mg/day PO in divided doses (usually 200 mg tid before meals).

PEDS - Not indicated for use in children <12 yo.

FORMS - Rx:Trade: tabs 100, 200 mg.

ursodiol (*Actigall, Ursofalk, URSO*) ▶Bile ♀B ▶? $$$$

ADULT - Radiolucent gallstone dissolution (Actigall): 8-10 mg/kg/day PO divided in 2-3 doses. Prevention of gallstones associated with rapid weight loss (Actigall): 300 mg PO bid. Primary biliary cirrhosis (URSO): 13-15 mg/kg/day PO divided in 2-4 doses.

PEDS - Not approved in children.

UNAPPROVED ADULT - Cholestasis of pregnancy: 300-600 mg PO bid.

UNAPPROVED PEDS - Biliary atresia: 10-15 mg/kg/day PO divided tid. Cystic fibrosis with liver disease: 30 mg/kg/day PO divided bid. TPN-induced cholestasis: 30 mg/kg/day PO divided tid.

FORMS - Trade/generic: cap 300 mg. Trade only: Tab 250, 500 mg (URSO).

NOTES - Gallstone dissolution requires months of therapy. Complete dissolution does not occur in all patients and 5-year recurrence up to 50%. Does not dissolve calcified cholesterol stones, radiopaque stones or radiolucent bile pigment stones. Avoid concomitant antacids, cholestyramine, colestipol, estrogen, oral contraceptives.

vasopressin (*Pitressin*, ADH, ✛*Pressyn AR*) ▶LK ♀C ▶? $$$$$
ADULT - See endocrine section.
PEDS - Not approved in children.

UNAPPROVED ADULT - Bleeding esophageal varices: 0.2-0.4 units/min initially (max 0.9 units /min).
UNAPPROVED PEDS - Bleeding esophageal varices: 0.002-0.005 units/kg/min initially (max 0.01 units/kg/min).
NOTES - Carbamazepine and chlorpropamide potentiate vasopressin. Use with caution in coronary artery disease. May cause tissue necrosis with extravasation.

HEMATOLOGY: Anticoagulants – Heparin, LMW Heparins, & Fondaparinux

NOTE: See cardiology section for antiplatelet drugs & thrombolytics. Contraindicated in active major bleeding. Avoid spinal punctures or neuraxial anesthesia before/during treatment due to risk of spinal/epidural hematomas. Risk of bleeding increased by oral anticoagulants, ASA, dipyridamole, dextran, glycoprotein IIb/IIIA inhibitors, NSAIDs (including ketorolac), ticlopidine, clopidogrel, and thrombolytics. Monitor platelets, Hb, stool for occult blood.

dalteparin (*Fragmin*) ▶KL ♀B ▶+ $$$$
ADULT - DVT prophylaxis, abdominal surgery: 2,500 units SC 1-2 h preop and qd postop x 5-10 days. DVT prophylaxis, abdominal surgery in patients with malignancy: 5,000 units SC evening before surgery and qd postop x 5-10 days. Alternatively, 2,500 units SC 1-2 h preop and 12 h later, then 5,000 units SC qd x 5-10 days. DVT prophylaxis, hip replacement: Give SC for up to 14 days. Preop start regimens: 2,500 units 2 h preop and 4-8h postop, then 5,000 units qd starting ≥6h after second dose. Alternatively, 5,000 units 10-14 h preop, 4-8h postop, then qd (approximately 24h between doses). Postop start regimen: 2,500 units 4-8h postop, then 5,000 units qd starting ≥6h after first dose. Unstable angina or non-Q-wave MI: 120 units/kg up to 10,000 units SC q12h with aspirin (75-165 mg/day PO) until clinically stable. DVT prophylaxis, acute medical illness with restricted mobility: 5,000 units SC qd x 12-14 days.
PEDS - Not approved in children.
UNAPPROVED ADULT - Therapeutic anticoagulation: 200 units/kg SC qd or 100-120 units/kg SC bid. DVT prophylaxis, medical conditions: 2,500 units SC qd. Venous thromboembolism in pregnancy. Prevention: 5,000 units SC qd. Treatment: 200 units/kg SC qd. To avoid unwanted anticoagulation during delivery, stop LMWH 24 h before elective induction of labor. Prevention of recurrent thrombosis in

cancer: 200 units/kg SC qd x 1 month, then ~150 units/kg (rounded to nearest commercially available syringe dose) qd x 5 months.
FORMS - Trade: Single-dose syringes 2,500 & 5,000 anti-Xa units/0.2 ml, 7500 anti-Xa/0.3 ml, 10,000 anti-Xa units/1 ml; multi-dose vial 10,000 units/ml, 9.5 ml and 25,000 units/ml, 3.8 ml.
NOTES - Contraindicated in heparin or pork allergy, history of heparin-induced thrombocytopenia. Not for treatment of unstable angina/non-Q-wave MI in patients receiving regional anesthesia. Use caution and consider monitoring anti-Xa levels if obese, underweight, pregnant, or renal/liver failure.

enoxaparin (*Lovenox*) ▶KL ♀B ▶+ $$$$$
ADULT - DVT prophylaxis, hip/knee replacement: 30 mg SC q12h starting 12-24 h postop for ≤14 days. Alternative for hip replacement: 40 mg SC qd starting 12 h preop. After hip replacement may continue 40 mg SC qd x 3 weeks. DVT prophylaxis, abdominal surgery: 40 mg SC qd starting 2 h preop for ≤12 days. DVT prophylaxis, acute medical illness with restricted mobility: 40 mg SC qd for ≤14 days. Outpatient treatment of DVT without pulmonary embolus: 1 mg/kg SC q12h. Inpatient treatment of DVT with/without pulmonary embolus: 1 mg/kg SC q12h or 1.5 mg/kg SC q24h. Give at the same time each day. Continue enoxaparin for ≥5 days and until therapeutic oral anticoagulation established. Unstable angina or non-Q-wave MI: 1 mg/kg SC q12h with aspirin (100-325 mg PO qd) for ≥2 days and until clinically stable. Can give 30 mg IV bolus before first SC dose in unstable angina. Dose adjustment in severe renal impairment (<30 ml/min): DVT prophylaxis in abdominal surgery, hip/knee replacement, and in medical patients during acute illness: 30 mg SC qd. Unstable angina or non-Q wave MI: 1 mg/kg SC qd. Inpatient DVT therapy with/without pulm em-

bolus: 1 mg/kg SC qd. Outpatient DVT therapy without pulmonary embolus: 1 mg/kg SC qd.

PEDS - Not approved in children.

UNAPPROVED ADULT - Prevention of venous thromboembolism. After major trauma: 30 mg SC q12h starting 12-36 h postinjury if hemostatically stable. Acute spinal cord injury: 30 mg SC q12h. Recurrent thromboembolism: 40 mg SC qd. Venous thromboembolism in pregnancy. Prevention: 40 mg SC qd. Treatment: 1 mg/kg SC q12h. To avoid unwanted anticoagulation during delivery, stop LMWH 24 h before elective induction of labor.

UNAPPROVED PEDS - Therapeutic anticoagulation: Age <2 mo: 1.5 mg/kg/dose SC q12h. Age >2 mo: 1 mg/kg/dose SC q12h titrated to anti-Xa level of 0.5-1.0 units/ml. DVT prophylaxis: Age <2 mo: 0.75 mg/kg/dose q12h. Age >2 mo: 0.5 mg/kg/dose q12h.

FORMS - Trade: Multi-dose vial 300 mg; Syringes 30,40 mg; graduated syringes 60,80, 100,120,150 mg. Concentration is 100 mg/mL except for 120,150 mg which are 150 mg/mL. Avoid multi-dose vial formulation in pregnancy, as it contains benzyl alcohol which can cross placenta.

NOTES - Contraindicated in patients with heparin or pork allergy, history of heparin-induced thrombocytopenia. Not recommended for thromboprophylaxis of prosthetic heart valves, especially during pregnancy, due to reports of valve thrombosis (maternal & fetal deaths reported). Congenital anomalies linked to enoxaparin use during pregnancy; causality unclear. Use caution and consider monitoring anti-Xa levels if obese, underweight, renal dysfunction, or abnormal coagulation/bleeding.

fondaparinux (*Arixtra*) ▶K ♀B ▶? $$$$$

ADULT - DVT prophylaxis, hip/knee replacement or hip fracture surgery: 2.5 mg SC qd starting 6-8 h postop (giving earlier increases risk of bleeding). Usual duration is 5-9 days (max 11 days); extend prophylaxis up to 24 additional days (max 32 days) in hip fracture surgery. DVT / PE treatment based on weight: 5 mg (if <50 kg), 7.5 mg (if 50-100 kg), 10 mg (if >100 kg) SC qd for ≥5 days & therapeutic oral anticoagulation.

PEDS - Not approved in children.

FORMS - Trade: Pre-filled syringes 2.5 mg/0.5 mL, 5 mg/0.4 mL,7.5 mg/0.6 mL,10 mg/0.8 mL.

NOTES - Can cause thrombocytopenia. Risk of major bleeding increased in elderly. Contraindicated if CrCl <30 mL/minute or body weight <50 kg due to increased bleeding risk. Caution

advised if CrCl 30-50 mL/minute. Monitor renal function in all; discontinue if severely impaired or labile. Protamine ineffective for reversing anticoagulant effect. Store at room temperature.

heparin (*♥Hepalean*) ▶Reticuloendothelial system ♀C but + ▶+ $

ADULT - Venous thrombosis/pulmonary embolus treatment: Load 80 units/kg IV, then mix 25,000 units in 250 ml D5W (100 units/ml) and infuse at 18 units/kg/h. Adjust based on coagulation testing (PTT). DVT prophylaxis: 5000 units SC q8-12h. Adjusted-dose for prevention of venous thromboembolism: 3,500 units SC q8h initially. Adjust up/ down by 500 units/dose to maintain mid-interval PTT at high normal value. Low-dose for prevention of thromboembolism in pregnancy: 5,000-10,000 units SC q12h. Treatment of thromboembolism in pregnancy: 80 units/kg IV load, then infuse ≥30,000 units/24h with dose titrated to achieve full anticoagulation for ≥5 days. Then adjusted-dose prophylaxis with ≥10,000 units SC q8-12h to achieve PTT of 1.5-2.5 x control. To avoid unwanted anticoagulation during delivery, stop adjusted-dose heparin 24 h before elective induction of labor.

PEDS - Venous thrombosis/pulmonary embolus treatment: Load 50 units/kg IV, then 25 units/ kg/h infusion.

UNAPPROVED ADULT - Adjunct to thrombolytics for acute MI. For use with alteplase, reteplase, or tenecteplase: 5,000 unit IV load, then infuse 1,000 units/h. Or 60 units/kg IV load (max 4,000 units), then infuse 12 units/kg/ h (max 1,000 units/h). Maintain for ≥48 h. If high risk of thromboembolism, continue heparin IV or SC (initial SC dose ~17,500 units q12h), LMWH, or warfarin. If not high risk of thromboembolism, continue heparin 7,500-12,500 units SC q12h until ambulatory. For use with streptokinase: 12,500 units SC q12h x 48 h. IV heparin only for patients receiving streptokinase/ anistreplase who are at high risk for systemic/ venous thromboembolism. Do not start heparin until ≥4 h after start of streptokinase/ anistreplase and APTT <70 s. After 48 h, consider continuing heparin 17,500 units SC q12h, LMWH SC, or warfarin. Anticoagulation for acute MI not treated with thrombolytics: 75 units/kg IV load, then infuse 1,000-1,200 units/h. Unstable angina/non ST-elevation MI: 60-70 units/kg IV load (max 5000 units), then infuse 12-15 units/kg/h (max 1000 units) for 2-5 days (Goal APTT is 1.5-2.5 x control). Goal APTT for all other regimens is 1.5-2 x control

(50-70 seconds).

UNAPPROVED PEDS - Venous thrombosis/pulmonary embolus treatment: Load 75 units/kg IV over 10 minutes, then 28 units/kg/h if age <1 yo, 20 units/kg/h if age >1 yo.

FORMS - Generic: 1000, 2500, 5000, 7500, 10,000, 20,000 units/ml in various vial and syringe sizes.

NOTES - Beware of heparin-induced thrombocytopenia (HIT; immune-mediated thrombocytopenia associated with thrombotic events), elevated LFTs, hyperkalemia/ hypoaldosteronism. HIT can occur up to 3 weeks after heparin discontinued. Osteoporosis with long-term use. Bleeding risk increased by high dose; concomitant thrombolytic or platelet GPIIb/IIIa receptor inhibitor; recent surgery, trauma, or invasive procedure; concomitant hemostatic defect. Monitor platelets, hemoglobin, stool for occult blood.

tinzaparin (*Innohep*) ▶K ♀B ▶+ $$$$$

ADULT - DVT with/without pulmonary embolus: 175 units/kg SC qd for ≥6 days & until adequate anticoagulation with warfarin.

PEDS - Not approved in children.

UNAPPROVED ADULT - DVT prophylaxis. Moderate-risk general surgery: 3,500 units SC given 2 h preop and qd postop. Orthopedic surgery: 75 units/kg SC qd starting 12-24h postop or 4,500 units SC given 12h preop and qd postop.

FORMS - Trade: 20,000 anti-Xa units/ml, 2 ml multi-dose vial.

NOTES - Contraindicated if history of heparin-induced thrombocytopenia, or allergy to heparin, pork, sulfites, or benzyl alcohol. Can cause thrombocytopenia, priapism (rare), increased AST/ALT. Tinzaparin may slightly prolong PT; draw blood for INR just before giving tinzaparin. Use caution and consider monitoring anti-Xa levels if obese, underweight, pregnant, or renal dysfunction.

WEIGHT-BASED HEPARIN DOSING FOR DVT/PE*

Initial dose: 80 units/kg IV bolus, then 18 units/kg/h. Check PTT in 6 h.

PTT <35 seconds (<1.2 x control): 80 units/kg IV bolus, then ↑ infusion rate by 4 units/kg/h.

PTT 35-45 seconds (1.2-1.5 x control): 40 units/kg IV bolus, then ↑ infusion by 2 units/kg/h.

PTT 46-70 seconds (1.5-2.3 x control): No change.

PTT 71-90 seconds (2.3-3 x control): ↓ infusion rate by 2 units/kg/h.

PTT >90 seconds (>3 x control): Hold infusion for 1 h, then ↓ infusion rate by 3 units/kg/h.

*DVT= Deep venous thrombosis. PE = Pulmonary embolus. Note: Reagent-specific target PTT may differ; use institutional nomogram when appropriate. Adjusted dosing may be appropriate in obesity. Consider establishing a max bolus dose and max initial infusion rate or use an adjusted body weight in obesity. PTT = Activated partial thromboplastin time. Monitor PTT q6h during first 24h of therapy and 6h after each heparin dosage adjustment. The frequency of PTT monitoring can be reduced to q morning when PTT is stable within therapeutic range. Check platelet count between days 3 to 5. Can begin warfarin on first day of heparin; continue heparin for at least ≥4 to 5 days of combined therapy. Adapted from *Ann Intern Med* 1993;119:874; *Chest* 2001:119:69S, and *Circulation* 2001; 103:2994.

HEMATOLOGY: Anticoagulants – Other

argatroban ▶L ♀B ▶- $$$$$

ADULT - Prevention/treatment of thrombosis in heparin-induced thrombocytopenia: Start 2 mcg/kg/min IV infusion. Get PTT at baseline and 2 h after starting infusion. Adjust dose (up to 10 mcg/kg/min) until PTT is 1.5-3 times baseline (but not >100 seconds). Also approved for use during percutaneous coronary intervention in those with or at risk for heparin-induced thrombocytopenia; see package insert for dosing.

PEDS - Not approved in children.

NOTES - Argatroban prolongs INR with warfarin; see package insert for guidance when considering concurrent therapy. Dosage reduction recommended in liver dysfunction.

bivalirudin (*Angiomax*) ▶proteolysis/K ♀B ▶? $$$$$

ADULT - Anticoagulation in patients with unstable angina undergoing PTCA: 1 mg/kg IV bolus just prior to PTCA, then infuse 2.5 mg/kg/h for 4 h. Can additionally infuse 0.2 mg/kg/h for up to 20 h more. Intended for use with aspirin 300-325 mg PO qd.

PEDS - Not approved in children.

UNAPPROVED ADULT - Percutaneous coronary intervention: 0.75 mg/kg IV bolus prior to intervention, then 1.75 mg/kg/hr for duration of procedure (with provisional Gp IIb/IIIa inhibition). Additional bolus of 0.3 mg/kg if activated clotting time <225 sec. Anticoagulation with streptokinase thrombolysis in ST elevation MI & known heparin-induced thrombocytopenia: 0.25 mg/kg bolus followed by 0.5 mg/kg/hr for first 12 hours, then 0.25 mg/kg/hr for subsequent 36 hours (consider dose reduction if PTT >75 seconds within first 12 hours).

NOTES - Former trade name Hirulog. Contraindicated in active major bleeding. Monitor activated clotting time and consider reduced dose if CrCl <60 ml/min.

lepirudin (*Refludan*) ▶K ♀B ▶? $$$$$

ADULT - Anticoagulation in heparin-induced thrombocytopenia (HIT) and associated thromboembolic disease: Bolus 0.4 mg/kg up to 44 mg IV over 15-20 seconds, then infuse 0.15 mg/kg/h up to 16.5 mg/h x 2-10 days. Adjust dose to maintain APTT ratio of 1.5-2.5.

PEDS - Not approved in children.

UNAPPROVED ADULT - Adjunct to thrombolytics for acute MI in patients with HIT: 0.1 mg/kg IV bolus, then infuse 0.15 mg/h.

NOTES - Dosage adjustment for renal impairment: Bolus 0.2 mg/kg IV followed by 0.075 mg/kg/h for CrCl 45-60 ml/min, 0.045 mg/kg/h for CrCl 30-44 ml/min, 0.0225 mg/kg/h for CrCl 15-29 ml/min. Hemodialysis/CrCl <15 ml/min: Bolus 0.1 mg/kg IV qod if APTT ratio <1.5. Severe anaphylactic reactions resulting in death have been reported upon initial or re-exposure.

warfarin (*Coumadin, Jantoven*) ▶L ♀X ▶+ $

WARNING - Many important drug interactions that increase/decrease INR, see table.

ADULT - Oral anticoagulation for prophylaxis/ treatment of DVT/PE, thromboembolic complications associated with A-fib +/- cardiac valve replacement, or to decrease post-MI risk of death, recurrent MI, stroke: Start 2-5 mg PO qd x 3-4 days, then adjust dose to PT/INR. Consider initial dose <5 mg/day if elderly, malnourished, liver disease, or high bleeding risk. Target INR of 2-3 for most indications, 2.5-3.5 for mechanical heart valves. See table for specific target INRs and duration of anticoagulation.

PEDS - Not approved in children.

UNAPPROVED ADULT - Outpatient anticoagulation treatment of acute DVT/PE: Start 10 mg PO qd (with ≥5 days of LMWH/heparin) until target INR (2.0 to 3.0) reached. See table for target INRs and duration of anticoagulation for specific indications.

FORMS - Generic/Trade: Tabs 1, 2, 2.5, 3, 4, 5, 6, 7.5, 10 mg.

NOTES - Tissue necrosis in protein C or S deficiency. Many important drug interactions that increase/decrease INR, see table. Warfarin onset of action is within 24 hours, peak effect delayed by 3-4 days. Most patients can begin warfarin at the same time as heparin/LMWH. Continue heparin/LMWH treatment for thrombosis until the INR has been in the therapeutic range for ≥4 days. See phytonadione (vitamin K) entry for management of abnormally high INRs.

ximelagatran (*Exanta*) ▶? ♀? ▶? ?

ADULT - New drug; dosing not finalized at press time.

PEDS - Not approved in children.

UNAPPROVED ADULT - Prevention of recurrent DVT/PE: 36 mg PO bid x 6 months. DVT/PE prophylaxis following total knee replacement: 36 mg PO bid beginning a.m. following surgery. Secondary prophylaxis in DVT/PE following 6 months warfarin treatment: 24 mg PO bid. Post-MI: 24 mg PO bid x 6 months (plus 160 mg daily aspirin). Stroke prevention in high-risk A-fib: 36 mg PO bid.

NOTES - Prodrug converted to melagatran (active form). Monitor LFT's closely during therapy.

THERAPEUTIC GOALS FOR ANTICOAGULATION

INR Range*	Indication
2.0-3.0	Atrial fibrillation, deep venous thrombosis, pulmonary embolism, bioprosthetic heart valve, mechanical prosthetic heart valve: aortic position, bileaflet or tilting disk with normal sinus rhythm and normal left atrium
2.5-3.5	Mechanical prosthetic heart valve: (1) mitral position, (2) aortic position with atrial fibrillation, (3) caged ball or caged disk

Adapted from: *Chest* suppl 2001; 119: 9S, 225S; see this manuscript for additional information, other indications.

*Aim for an INR in the middle of the INR range (e.g. 2.5 for range of 2-3 and 3.0 for range of 2.5-3.5)

WARFARIN – SELECTED DRUG INTERACTIONS

Assume possible interactions with any new medication. When starting/stopping a medication, the INR should be checked weekly for ≥2-3 weeks and dose adjusted accordingly, especially in patients with intensive anticoagulation (INR 2.5-3.5). Similarly monitor if significant change in diet (including supplements) or illness resulting in decreased oral intake.

Increased anticoagulant effect of warfarin and increased risk of bleeding

- *Monitor INR when agents below started, stopped, or dosage changed.*

acetaminophen ≥2 g/d for ≥3-4 d	delavirdine	glucagon	neomycin (PO for >1-2 days)	rofecoxib
allopurinol	efavirenz	glyburide	olsalazine	sertraline
amiodarone*	fenofibrate	ifosfamide	omeprazole	tamoxifen
amprenavir	fluconazole	isoniazid	penicillin, high-	tetracyclines
cefazolin	**fluoroquinolones**	itraconazole	dose IV	tramadol
cefoxitin	fluorouracil	ketoconazole	pentoxifylline	tricyclic antide-
ceftriaxone	fluoxetine	leflunomide	phenytoin (acute)	pressants
celecoxib	flutamide	levamisole	propafenone	valproate
cisapride	fluvoxamine	levothyroxine#	propoxyphene	valdecoxib
corticosteroids	fosphenytoin	miconazole, in-	quinidine	voriconazole
	(acute)	travaginal	quinine	vitamin E
cyclophosphamide	gemcitabine	modafinil		zileuton

- *Consider alternative to agents below, or monitor INR when started, stopped, or dosage changed.*

cimetidine†, **macrolides‡**, nalidixic acid, paroxetine, ranitidine, **statins§**, **sulfonamides**, zafirlukast

- *Avoid unless benefit justifies risk; monitor INR when started, stopped, or dosage changed.*

aspirin¶, clofibrate, danazol , disulfiram , gemfibrozil , metronidazole, **NSAIDs¶**, sulfinpyrazone

- *Avoid agents below; benefits do not justify risks*

anabolic steroids	danshen (Chinese herb)	fish oil	ginkgo
cefoperazone, cefotetan	dong quai (Chinese herb)	garlic supplements	testosterone

Decreased anticoagulant effect of warfarin and increased risk of thrombosis

- *Monitor INR when agents below started, stopped, or dosage changed.*

American ginseng	dicloxacillin	mercapto-	panax ginseng	rifabutin
aminoglutethimide	efavirenz	purine	phenytoin (chronic,	rifapentine
aprepitant	fosphenytoin	mesalamine	consider alternative)	ritonavir
azathioprine	(chronic, consi-	methimazole#	primidone	St John's wort
carbamazepine	der alternative)	mitotane	propylthiouracil#	vitamin C, high-
coenzyme Q-10	griseofulvin	nafcillin	raloxifene	dose

- *Use alternative to agents below. Or give at different times of day and monitor INR when agent started, stopped, dose/dosing schedule changed.*

cholestyramine   colestipol (likely lower risk than cholestyramine)   sucralfate

- *Avoid unless benefit justifies risk. If used, monitor INR when started, stopped, or form changed.*

oral contraceptives (do not necessarily ↓INR, but may induce hypercoagulability), barbiturates, rifampin

*Interaction may be delayed; monitor INR for several weeks after starting & several months after stopping amiodarone. May need to decrease warfarin dose by 33% to 50%.

† Famotidine, nizatidine are alternatives.

‡ Azithromycin appears to have lower risk of interaction than clarithromycin or erythromycin.

§ Pravastatin appears to have lower risk of interaction.

Hyperthyroidism/thyroid replacement increases metabolism of clotting factors, increasing response to warfarin therapy and increased bleed risk (typically requires lowering warfarin dose).

¶ Does not necessarily increase INR , but increases bleeding risk. Check INR frequently and monitor for GI bleeding. COX-2 inhibitors (celecoxib, rofecoxib) may be preferred (less GI toxicity, no effect on platelet aggregation), but INR monitoring still recommended.

Table adapted from: www.coumadin.com, *Am Fam Phys* 1999;59:635, *Chest* 2001; 114: 11S; *Hansten and Horn's Drug Interactions Analysis and Management.* Ann Intern Med 2004;141:23.

HEMATOLOGY: Other

See endocrine section for vitamins and minerals.

aminocaproic acid (*Amicar*) ▶K ♀D ▶? $$

ADULT - To improve hemostasis when fibrinolysis contributes to bleeding: 4-5 g IV/PO over 1h, then 1 g/h x 8h or until bleeding controlled.

PEDS - Not approved in children.

UNAPPROVED ADULT - Prevention of recurrent subarachnoid hemorrhage: 6 g IV/PO q4h (6 doses/day). Reduction of postop bleeding after cardiopulmonary bypass: 5 g IV, then 1 g/h x 6-8 h.

UNAPPROVED PEDS - To improve hemostasis when fibrinolysis contributes to bleeding: 100 mg/kg or 3 g/m^2 IV infusion during first h, then continuous infusion of 33.3 mg/kg/h or 1 g/m^2/h. Max dose of 18 g/m^2/day. IV prep contains benzyl alcohol - do not use in newborns.

FORMS - Generic/Trade: Syrup or oral soln 250 mg/ml, tabs 500 mg.

NOTES - Contraindicated in active intravascular clotting. Do not use in DIC without heparin. Can cause intrarenal thrombosis, hyperkalemia. Skeletal muscle vasodilation, necrosis with prolonged use - monitor CPK. Use with estrogen/oral contraceptives can cause hypercoagulability. Rapid IV administration can cause hypotension, bradycardia, arrhythmia.

anagrelide (*Agrylin*) ▶LK ♀C ▶? $$$$$

ADULT - Thrombocythemia due to myeloproliferative disorders (including essential thrombocythemia): Start 0.5 mg PO qid or 1 mg PO bid, then after 1 week adjust to lowest effective dose that maintains platelets <600,000 mcL. Max 10 mg/day or 2.5 mg as a single dose.

PEDS - Not approved in children.

FORMS - Trade: Caps, 0.5,1 mg.

NOTES - Use with caution in patients with heart disease. May cause vasodilation, tachycardia, palpitations, CHF. Ensure women maintain effective contraception while on this drug.

aprotinin (*Trasylol*) ▶lysosomal enzymes & K ♀B ▶? $$$$$

WARNING - Anaphylaxis can occur even with test dose. Risk low in previously unexposed patients. Risk high with reexposure ≤6 months after first dose; use special precautions.

ADULT - To reduce blood loss during CABG: 1 ml IV test dose ≥10 min before loading dose. Regimen A: 200 ml loading dose, then 200 ml pump prime dose, then 50 ml/h. Regimen B: 100 ml loading dose, then 100 ml pump prime dose, then 25 ml/h. Pick regimen based on bleeding risk.

PEDS - Safety and efficacy not established.

NOTES - Hypotension with rapid administration. Prolongation of activated clotting time (ACT) by aprotinin may overestimate heparin anticoagulation. Effect of aprotinin on ACT may vary by ACT formulation. Determine dose of protamine to reverse heparin based on heparin dose rather than ACT value.

darbepoetin (*Aranesp, NESP*) ▶cellular sialidases, L ♀C ▶? $$$$$

ADULT - Anemia of chronic renal failure: 0.45 mcg/kg IV/SC q weekly, or SC q 2 weeks for some patients. Monitor Hb weekly until stable, then at least monthly. Increase dose by 25% if Hb increases by <1 g/dL over 1 month; reduce by 25% if Hb increases by >1 g/dL over 2 weeks, or is approaching 12 g/dL and still increasing. Increase dose at intervals of at least 1 month. Target Hb not to exceed 12 g/dL. Weekly dose conversion to darbepoetin (D) from erythropoietin (E): 6.25 mcg D for <2,500 units E; 12.5 mcg D for 2,500-4,999 units E; 25 mcg D for 5,000-10,999 units E; 40 mcg D for 11,000-17,999 units E; 60 mcg D for 18,000-33,999 units E; 100 mcg D for 34,000-89,999 units E; 200 mcg D for ≥90,000 units E. Give D once weekly for patients taking E 2-3 times weekly; give D once every 2 weeks for patients taking E once weekly. Maintenance dose may be lower in predialysis patients than dialysis patients. Anemia in cancer chemo patients: 2.25 mcg/kg SC q week initially. Max 4.5 mcg/kg/dose. Reduce dose if Hb >12 g/dL; hold if >13 g/dL.

PEDS - Not approved in children.

UNAPPROVED ADULT - Chemotherapy-induced anemia 3 mcg/kg SC q2 weeks

FORMS - Trade: Single-dose vials 25, 40, 60, 100, 200, 300, 500 mcg/1 ml. Additionally 150 mcg/0.75 ml. Prefilled syringes: 60, 100, 150, 200, 300, 500 mcg.

NOTES - Contraindicated in uncontrolled HTN. Higher Hb and/or too rapid increase in Hb may cause cardiovascular events & seizures. May exacerbate HTN; monitor & control BP. Evaluate iron stores before and during treatment. Most patients eventually require iron supplements. Consider other causes of anemia if no response. Use only one dose per vial/syringe; discard any unused portion. Do not shake. Protect from light.

desmopressin (*DDAVP, Stimate,* ✽*Octo-*

stim) ▶LK ♀B ▶? $$$$$
ADULT - Hemophilia A, von Willebrand's disease: 0.3 mcg/kg IV over 15-30 min; 300 mcg intranasally if ≥50 kg (1 spray in each nostril), 150 mcg intranasally if <50 kg (single spray in 1 nostril).
PEDS - Hemophilia A, von Willebrand's disease (age ≥3 mo for IV, age ≥11 mo - 12 yo for nasal spray): 0.3 mcg/kg IV over 15-30 min; 300 mcg intranasally if ≥50 kg (1 spray in each nostril), 150 mcg intranasally if <50 kg (single spray in 1 nostril).
UNAPPROVED ADULT - Uremic bleeding: 0.3 mcg/kg IV single dose or q12h (onset 1-2h; duration 6-8h after single dose). Intranasal is 20 mcg/day (onset 24-72 h; duration 14 days during 14-day course).
FORMS - Trade: Stimate nasal spray 150 mcg/0.1 ml (1 spray), 2.5 ml bottle (25 sprays). Generic/Trade (DDAVP nasal spray): 10 mcg/0.1 ml (1 spray), 5 ml bottle (50 sprays). Note difference in concentration of nasal solutions.
NOTES - Anaphylaxis reported with both IV and intranasal forms. Avoid excessive fluid intake to prevent water intoxication/hyponatremia. Do not give if type IIB von Willebrand's disease. Changes in nasal mucosa may impair absorption of nasal spray. Refrigerate nasal spray - stable for 3 weeks at room temperature. 10 mcg = 40 units desmopressin.

erythropoietin (*Epogen, Procrit, epoetin, ✚Eprex*) ▶L ♀C ▶? $$$$$
ADULT - Anemia of chronic renal failure: Initial dose 50-100 units/kg IV/SC 3 times/week. Target Hct: 30-36%. Reduce dose if Hct increases by >4 points in 2 weeks or is reaching target & is still increasing. Zidovudine-induced anemia in HIV-infected patients: 100-300 units/kg IV/SC 3 times/week. Hold and reduce dose if Hct ≥40%. Anemia in cancer chemo patients when Hgb falls to near 10 g/dL: 150-300 units/kg SC 3 times/week or 40,000 units SC once/week. Nonresponse is defined as <1-2 g/dL rise in Hgb after 6-8 weeks therapy, despite dose titration. Dose should be titrated to maintain Hb at or near 12 g/dL. Hold and reduce dose if Hct ≥40%. Reduction of allogeneic blood transfusion in surgical patients: 300 units/kg/day SC 10 days preop, on the day of surgery, and 4 days postop. Or 600 units/kg SC once weekly starting 21 days preop and ending on day of surgery (4 doses).
PEDS - Not approved in children.
UNAPPROVED ADULT - Reduce need for transfusion in critically ill: 40,000 units SC q week x 3-4 doses.
UNAPPROVED PEDS - Anemia of chronic renal failure: Initial dose 50-100 units/kg IV/SC 3 times/week. Zidovudine-induced anemia in HIV-infected patients: 100 units/kg SC 3 times/week; max of 300 units/kg/dose.
FORMS - Trade: Single-dose 1 ml vials 2,000, 3,000, 4,000, 10,000, 40,000 units/ml. Multidose vials 10,000 units/ml 2 ml & 20,000 units/ml 1 ml.
NOTES - Contraindicated in uncontrolled HTN. Not for immediate correction of anemia. Higher Hb and/or too rapid increase in Hb can cause cardiovascular events & seizures. May exacerbate HTN; monitor, control BP in chronic renal failure. Monitor Hct twice weekly in chronic renal failure, once weekly in HIV-infection and cancer until stable. Evaluate iron stores before and during treatment. Most patients eventually require iron supplements. Consider other causes of anemia if no response. Rare cases of pure red cell aplasia reported. Single-dose vials contain no preservatives. Use one dose per vial; do not re-enter vial. Discard unused portion.

factor VIIa (*NovoSeven, ✚Niastase*) ▶L ♀C ▶? $$$$$
ADULT, PEDS - Hemophilia A or B: individualize factor VIIa dose.
UNAPPROVED ADULT - Reversal of excessive warfarin anticoagulation (INR >10): 15-20 mcg/kg IV over 3-5 min.
FORMS - Trade: 1200, 2400, 4800 mcg/vial.
NOTES - Contraindicated with hypersensitivity to mouse, hamster or bovine proteins. Patients with DIC, advanced atherosclerotic disease, crush injury or septicemia may be at increase thrombotic risk. If DIC or thrombosis confirmed, reduce dose or stop treatment depending on symptoms.

factor VIII (*Advate, Hemofil M, Monoclate P, Monarc-M*) ▶L ♀C ▶? $$$$$
ADULT, PEDS - Hemophilia A: individualize factor VIII dose.
FORMS - Specific formulation usually chosen by specialist in Hemophilia Treatment Center. Advate is only current recombinant formulation of factor VIII.
NOTES - Risk of HIV/hepatitis transmission varies by product; no such risk with recombinant product. Reduced response with development of factor VIII inhibitors. Hemolysis with large/repeated doses in those with A, B, AB blood.

factor IX (*Benefix, Mononine, ✚Immunine*

VH) ▶L ♀C ▶? $$$$$
ADULT, PEDS - Hemophilia B: individualize factor IX dose.
FORMS - Specific formulation usually chosen by specialist in Hemophilia Treatment Center.
NOTES - Risk of HIV/hepatitis transmission varies by product. Products that contain factors II, VII, & X may cause thrombosis in at-risk patients. Stop infusion if signs of DIC.

filgrastim (G-CSF, Neupogen) ▶L ♀C ▶? $$$$$
ADULT - Reduction of febrile neutropenia after chemo for non-myeloid malignancies: 5 mcg/kg/day SC/IV for ≤2 weeks until post-nadir ANC is ≥10,000/mm3. Can increase by 5 mcg/kg/day with each cycle prn.
PEDS - Reduction of febrile neutropenia after chemo for non-myeloid malignancies: 5 mcg/kg/day SC/IV.
UNAPPROVED ADULT - AIDS: 0.3-3.6 mcg/kg/day.
FORMS - Trade: Single-dose vials 300 mcg/1 ml, 480 mcg/1.6 ml. Single-dose syringes 300 mcg/0.5 ml, 480 mcg/0.8 ml.
NOTES - Allergic-type reactions, bone pain, cutaneous vasculitis. Do not give within 24 h before/after cytotoxic chemotherapy. Store in refrigerator; use within 24 h when kept at room temperature.

oprelvekin (Neumega) ▶K ♀C ▶? $$$$$
ADULT - Prevention of severe thrombocytopenia after chemo for nonmyeloid malignancies: 50 mcg/kg SC qd starting 6-24 h after chemo and continuing until post-nadir platelet count is ≥50,000 cells/mcL.
PEDS - Not approved in children. Safe and effective dose not established. Papilledema with 100 mcg/kg; 50 mcg/kg ineffective.
FORMS - Trade: 5 mg single-dose vials.
NOTES - Fluid retention - monitor fluid and electrolyte balance. Transient atrial arrhythmias, visual blurring, papilledema.

pegfilgrastim (Neulasta) ▶Plasma ♀C ▶? $$$$$
WARNING - Do not use if <45 kg.
ADULT - To reduce febrile neutropenia after chemo for non-myeloid malignancies: 6 mg SC once each chemo cycle.
PEDS - Not approved in children.
FORMS - Trade: Single-dose syringes 6 mg/0.6 ml.
NOTES - Bone pain common. Do not give <14 days before or 24 h after cytotoxic chemo. Store in refrigerator. Stable at room temperature for ≤48 h. Protect from light

protamine ▶Plasma ♀C ▶? $
ADULT - Heparin overdose: 1 mg antagonizes ~100 units heparin. Give IV over 10 minutes in doses of not >50 mg.
PEDS - Not approved in children.
UNAPPROVED ADULT - Low molecular weight heparin overdose: 1 mg protamine per 100 anti-Xa units of dalteparin or tinzaparin. Give additional 0.5 mg protamine per 100 anti-Xa units of tinzaparin if PTT remains prolonged 2-4 h after first infusion of protamine. 1 mg protamine per 1 mg enoxaparin.
UNAPPROVED PEDS - Heparin overdose: <30 min since last heparin dose, give 1 mg protamine per 100 units of heparin received; 30-60 min since last heparin dose, give 0.5-0.75 mg protamine per 100 units of heparin received; 60-120 min since last heparin dose, give 0.375-0.5 mg protamine per 100 units of heparin; >120 min since last heparin dose, give 0.25-0.375 mg protamine per 100 units of heparin.
NOTES - Severe hypotension/anaphylactoid reaction with too rapid administration. Allergic reactions in patients with fish allergy, previous exposure to protamine (including insulin). Risk of allergy unclear in infertile/vasectomized men with anti-protamine antibodies. Additional doses of protamine may be required in some situations (neutralization of SC heparin, heparin rebound after cardiac surgery). Monitor APTT to confirm heparin neutralization.

sargramostim (GM-CSF, Leukine) ▶L ♀C ▶? $$$$$
ADULT - Specialized dosing for leukemia, bone marrow transplantation.
PEDS - Not approved in children.

tranexamic acid (Cyklokapron) ▶K ♀B ▶- $$$
ADULT - Prophylaxis/reduction of bleeding during tooth extraction in hemophilia patients: 10 mg/kg IV immediately before surgery, then 25 mg/kg PO 3-4 times/day for 2-8 days following surgery. Additional regimens include: 10 mg/kg IV 3-4 times/day if intolerant of oral therapies or 25 mg/kg PO 3-4 times/day beginning 1 day before surgery.
PEDS - Not approved in children.
FORMS - 500 mg tablets, 100 mg/ml ampules.
NOTES - Dose adjustment in renal impairment-Creat 1.36-2.83 mg/dL: 10 mg/kg IV bid or 15 mg/kg PO bid. Creat 2.83-5.66 mg/dL: 10 mg/kg IV qd or 15 mg/kg PO qd. Creat >5.66 mg/dL: 10 mg/kg IV q48h or 5 mg/kg IV q24h; 15 mg/kg PO q48h or 7.5 mg/kg PO q24h.

HERBAL & ALTERNATIVE THERAPIES

NOTE: For all, FORMS are not by prescription. In the US, herbal and alternative therapy products are regulated as dietary supplements, not drugs. Premarketing evaluation and FDA approval are not required unless specific therapeutic claims are made. Since these products are not required to demonstrate efficacy, it is unclear whether many of them have health benefits. In addition, there may be considerable variability in content from lot to lot or between products. See www.tarascon.com/herbals for evidence-based efficacy ratings used by the Tarascon editorial staff.

aloe vera (*acemannan, burn plant*) ▶LK ♀oral- topical +? ▶oral- topical +? $
UNAPPROVED ADULT - Topical: Efficacy unclear for seborrheic dermatitis, psoriasis, genital herpes, partial-thickness skin burns. Does not appear effective for radiation-induced skin injury. Do not apply to surgical incisions; impaired healing reported. Oral: Efficacy unclear for type 2 diabetes. Efficacy of acemannan (Carrisyn; constituent with immunomodulatory activity) unclear for AIDS.
UNAPPROVED PEDS - Not for use in children.
NOTES - OTC laxatives containing aloe were removed from the US market in 2002 due to concerns about increased risk of colon cancer. Concomitant topical application may increase absorption of topical hydrocortisone.

androstenedione (*andro*) ▶L, peripheral conversion to estrogens & androgens ♀- ▶- $
UNAPPROVED ADULT - Marketed as anabolic steroid to enhance athletic performance. Advise patients against use because of potential for androgenic and estrogenic side effects.
UNAPPROVED PEDS - Not for use in children.
NOTES - In March 204, FDA warned manufacturers to stop marketing androstenedione as dietary supplement. Also banned by many athletic associations. In theory, chronic use may increase risk of hormone-related cancers (prostate, breast, ovarian). Increase in androgen levels could exacerbate hyperlipidemia.

aristolochic acid (*Aristolochia, Asarum, Bragantia*) ▶? ♀- ▶- $
ADULT - Do not use. Was promoted for weight loss.
PEDS - Do not use.
NOTES - Banned by FDA; linked to nephrotoxicity and cancer. May be present as an adulterant in other Chinese herbal products like Akebia, Clematis, Stephania, and others. Rule out aristolochic acid nephrotoxicity in cases of unexplained renal failure. List of Internet products that may contain aristolochic acid available at http://potency.berkeley.edu/text/FDAAristolochicAcidLetter.pdf

arnica (*Arnica montana, leopard's bane, wolf's bane*) ▶? ♀- ▶- $
UNAPPROVED ADULT - Toxic if taken by mouth. Topical preparations promoted for treatment of skin wounds, bruises, aches, and sprains; but insufficient data to assess efficacy. Do not use on open wounds.
UNAPPROVED PEDS - Not for use in children.
NOTES - Repeated topical application can cause skin reactions.

artichoke leaf extract (*Cynara-SL, Cynara scolymus*) ▶? ♀? ▶? $
UNAPPROVED ADULT - May reduce total cholesterol, but clinical significance is unclear. Cynara-SL is promoted as digestive aid (possibly effective for dyspepsia) at a dose of 1-2 caps PO daily.
UNAPPROVED PEDS - Not for use in children.
NOTES - Advise against use by patients with bile duct obstruction or gallstones. Artichoke leaf is an ingredient in CholesTame and Digestive Formula.

astragalus (*Astragalus membranaceus, huang qi, vetch*) ▶? ♀? ▶? $
UNAPPROVED ADULT - Used in combination with other herbs in traditional Chinese medicine, but efficacy unclear for CHD, CHF, viral infections, upper respiratory tract infections, and as adjunct to cancer chemotherapy.
UNAPPROVED PEDS - Not for use in children.
NOTES - Not used for >3 weeks without close follow-up in traditional Chinese medicine. In theory, may enhance activity of drugs for diabetes, hypertension, and anticoagulation.

bilberry (*Vaccinium myrtillus, huckleberry, Tegens, VMA extract*) ▶Bile, K ♀- ▶- $
UNAPPROVED ADULT - Cataracts (efficacy unclear): 80-160 mg PO bid-tid of 25% anthocyanosides extract. Insufficient data to evaluate efficacy for macular degeneration. Does not appear effective for improving night vision.
UNAPPROVED PEDS - Not for use in children.
NOTES - High doses may impair platelet aggregation, affect clotting time, cause GI distress.

bitter melon (*Momordica charantia, karela*) ▶? ♀- ▶- $$
UNAPPROVED ADULT - Possibly effective for type 2 diabetes. Dose unclear; juice may be

more potent than dried fruit powder.

UNAPPROVED PEDS - Not for use in children. Two cases of hypoglycemic coma in children ingesting bitter melon tea.

bitter orange (*Citrus aurantium, Seville orange, Acutrim Natural AM, Dexatrim Natural Ephedrine Free*) ▶K ♀- ▶- $

UNAPPROVED ADULT - Similar to ephedra; safety and efficacy not established.

UNAPPROVED PEDS - Not for use in children.

NOTES - Contains synephrine, a sympathomimetic similar to phenylephrine. Do not use within 14 days of an MAOI. Juice inhibits CYP 3A4 metabolism of felodipine and midazolam. May also inhibit dextromethorphan metabolism.

black cohosh (*Cimicifuga racemosa, Remifemin, Menofem*) ▶? ♀- ▶- $

UNAPPROVED ADULT - Menopausal symptoms (possibly effective): 20 mg PO bid of Remifemin for ≤6 months. Onset may be delayed for 4-12 weeks. Does not appear effective for symptoms induced by breast cancer treatment (conflicting data). North American Menopause Society considers black cohosh + lifestyle changes an option for relief of mild symptoms.

UNAPPROVED PEDS - Not for use in children.

NOTES - Unclear if estrogenic effects. Potential for endometrial stimulation unclear; some experts recommend monitoring with vaginal ultrasound if long-term use.

chamomile (*Matricaria recutita - German chamomile, Anthemis nobilis - Roman chamomile*) ▶? ♀? ▶? $

UNAPPROVED ADULT - Promoted as a sedative or anxiolytic, to relieve GI distress, for skin infections or inflammation, many other indications. Efficacy unclear for any indication. Does not appear to reduce mucositis caused by 5-fluorouracil or radiation.

UNAPPROVED PEDS - Not for use in children.

NOTES - Theoretical concern (no clinical evidence) for interactions due to increased sedation, increased risk of bleeding (contains coumarin derivatives), delayed GI absorption of other drugs (due to antispasmodic effect).

chaparral (*Larrea divaricata, creosote bush*) ▶? ♀- ▶- $

UNAPPROVED ADULT - Do not use. Promoted as cancer cure.

UNAPPROVED PEDS - Not for use in children.

NOTES - Reports of irreversible liver damage in humans.

chasteberry (*Vitex agnus castus fruit extract, Femaprin*) ▶? ♀- ▶- $

UNAPPROVED ADULT - Premenstrual syndrome (possibly effective): 20 mg PO qd of extract ZE 440 (ratio 6-12:1; standardized for casticin).

UNAPPROVED PEDS - Not for use in children.

NOTES - Liquid formulations may contain alcohol. Avoid concomitant dopamine antagonists such as haloperidol or metoclopramide.

chondroitin ▶K ♀? ▶? $

UNAPPROVED ADULT - Osteoarthritis: (possibly effective): 200-400 mg PO bid-tid or 1200 mg PO qd. Onset of action may be several months.

UNAPPROVED PEDS - Not for use in children.

NOTES - No evidence for greater benefit of glucosamine-chondroitin formulations over glucosamine or chondroitin alone. Chondroitin content not standardized and known to vary. Labeled dose of Cosamin DS contains more than the tolerable upper limit of manganese; avoid. Some products made from bovine cartilage. Case report of increased INR with warfarin in patient taking chondroitin + glucosamine.

coenzyme Q10 (*CoQ-10, ubiquinone*) ▶Bile ♀- ▶- $

UNAPPROVED ADULT - Heart failure (efficacy unclear): 100 mg/day PO divided bid-tid. Parkinson's disease ($$$$): 1200 mg/day PO divided qid at meals and hs slowed progression of early disease in phase II study; benefit greater with 1200 mg/day than ≤600 mg/day. Study for progression of Huntington's disease was inconclusive. Efficacy unclear for improving athletic performance. Appears ineffective for diabetes. Promoted to prevent statin myopathy, but insufficient evidence to evaluate efficacy.

UNAPPROVED PEDS - Not for use in children.

NOTES - May decrease INR with warfarin. Effects may be inhibited by beta blockers.

comfrey (*Symphytum officinale*) ▶? ♀- ▶- $

UNAPPROVED ADULT - Do not use, even externally (application on broken skin could lead to systemic absorption). Topical use promoted for bruises, burns and sprains.

UNAPPROVED PEDS - Do not use, even externally (application on broken skin could lead to systemic absorption). Topical use promoted for bruises, burns and sprains.

NOTES - Reports of fatal hepatic veno-occlusive disease in humans. Contains pyrrolizidine alkaloids. FDA banned comfrey products from US market in July 2001.

cranberry (*Cranactin, Vaccinium macrocarpon*) ▶? ♀? ▶? $

UNAPPROVED ADULT - Prevention of UTI (possibly effective): 300 mL/day PO cranberry juice cocktail; 1-6 caps PO (hard gelatin caps with 300-400 mg concentrated cranberry juice extract) bid with water 1 h before meals or 2 h after. Insufficient data to assess efficacy for treatment of UTI. Should not be a substitute for antibiotics in acute UTI.

UNAPPROVED PEDS - Insufficient data to assess efficacy for prevention/treatment of UTI. Should not be a substitute for antibiotics in acute UTI.

NOTES - Reports of increased/ decreased INR with warfarin; patients taking warfarin should avoid/ limit cranberry juice. ~100 calories/6 oz of cranberry juice cocktail. Advise diabetics that some products have high sugar content. Not a substitute for antibiotics to treat UTI.

creatine ▶LK ♀- ▶- $

UNAPPROVED ADULT - Promoted to enhance athletic performance. No benefit for endurance exercise, but modest benefit for intense anaerobic tasks lasting <30 seconds. Usually taken as loading dose of 20 g/day PO x 5 days, then 2-5 g/day.

UNAPPROVED PEDS - Not for use in children.

NOTES - Caffeine may antagonize benefit on short exercise. Creatine is metabolized to creatinine; could increase serum creatinine despite normal renal function.

dehydroepiandrosterone (*DHEA, Aslera, Fidelin, Prasterone*) ▶Peripheral conversion to estrogens and androgens ♀- ▶- $

UNAPPROVED ADULT - No convincing evidence that DHEA slows aging or improves cognition in elderly. Rx product (Aslera) in development for treatment of women with chronic lupus. To improve well-being in women with adrenal insufficiency (effective): 50 mg PO qd.

UNAPPROVED PEDS - Not for use in children.

NOTES - In theory, chronic use may increase risk of hormone-related cancers (prostate, breast, ovarian).

dong quai (*Angelica sinensis*) ▶? ♀- ▶- $

UNAPPROVED ADULT - Appears ineffective for postmenopausal symptoms; North American Menopause Society recommends against use. Used with other herbs for treatment and prevention of dysmenorrhea, TIA, stroke, PVD, and cardiovascular conditions in traditional Chinese medicine.

UNAPPROVED PEDS - Not for use in children.

NOTES - Increased risk of bleeding with warfarin with/without increase in INR; avoid concurrent use.

echinacea (*E. purpurea, E. angustifolia, E. pallida*, cone flower, EchinaGuard, Echi-

nacin Madaus) ▶? ♀- ▶- $

UNAPPROVED ADULT - Promoted as immune stimulant. Efficacy unclear for prevention or treatment of upper respiratory infections.

UNAPPROVED PEDS - Not for use in children. Appears ineffective for treatment of upper respiratory tract infections in children. A formulation combining echinacea, vitamin C, and propolis (Chizukit; not available in US) appears effective for preventing respiratory infections.

NOTES - Could interact with immunosuppressants due to immunomodulating effects. Some experts limit use to ≤8 weeks and recommend against use in patients with autoimmune disorders. Rare allergic reactions including anaphylaxis. Photosensitivity possible. May inhibit CYP 450 1A2.

elderberry (*Sambucas nigra, Rubini, Sambucol, Sinupret*) ▶? ♀- ▶- $

UNAPPROVED ADULT - Efficacy unclear for influenza, sinusitis, and bronchitis.

UNAPPROVED PEDS - Not for use in children.

NOTES - Sinupret and Sanbucol also contain other ingredients. Eating uncooked elderberries may cause nausea or cyanide toxicity.

ephedra (*Ephedra sinica*, ma huang, Metabolife 356, Biolean, Ripped Fuel, Xenadrine) ▶K ♀- ▶- $

UNAPPROVED ADULT - Little evidence of efficacy, other than modest short-term weight loss. In Feb 2004, FDA banned ephedra supplements, with all products to be removed from shelves by April 5, 2004.

UNAPPROVED PEDS - Not for use in children.

NOTES - In Feb 2004, FDA banned ephedra supplements, with all products to be removed from shelves by April 5, 2004. Contains ephedrine and pseudoephedrine. Linked to CVA, MI, sudden death, HTN, palpitations, tachycardia, seizures. Risk of serious reactions may increase with dose, strenuous exercise, or concomitant use of other stimulants like caffeine (as in Biolean & Dexatrim Results). Metabolife 356 can prolong QT interval and increase systolic blood pressure. Country mallow (Sida cordifolia) contains ephedrine.

evening primrose oil (*Oenothera biennis*) ▶? ♀? ▶? $

UNAPPROVED ADULT - Appears ineffective for premenstrual syndrome, postmenopausal symptoms, atopic dermatitis.

UNAPPROVED PEDS - Not for use in children.

fenugreek (*Trigonelle foenum-graecum*) ▶? ♀- ▶? $$

UNAPPROVED ADULT - Efficacy unclear for

diabetes or hyperlipidemia. Insufficient data to evaluate efficacy as galactagogue.

UNAPPROVED PEDS - Not for use in children.

NOTES - Case report of increased INR with warfarin possibly related to fenugreek. Can cause maple syrup-like body odor. Fiber content could decrease GI absorption of some drugs.

feverfew (Chrysanthemum parthenium, Migra-Lief, MigraSpray, Tanacetum parthenium L.) ▶? ♀- ▶- $

UNAPPROVED ADULT - Prevention of migraine (possibly effective): 50-100 mg extract PO daily; 2-3 fresh leaves PO daily; 50-125 mg freeze-dried leaf PO daily. Take either leaf form with or after meals. Benefit of alcoholic extract questioned. May take 1-2 months to begin working. Inadequate data to evaluate efficacy for acute migraine. Efficacy unclear for rheumatoid arthritis.

UNAPPROVED PEDS - Not for use in children.

NOTES - May cause uterine contractions; avoid during pregnancy. Migra-Lief contains riboflavin and magnesium. MigraSpray contains only homeopathic amount of feverfew.

garcinia (Garcinia cambogia, Citri Lean) ▶? ♀- ▶- $

UNAPPROVED ADULT - Appears ineffective for weight loss.

UNAPPROVED PEDS - Not for use in children.

NOTES - Contains hydroxycitric acid which may inhibit lipogenesis.

garlic supplements (Allium sativum, Kwai, Kyolic) ▶LK ♀- ▶- $

UNAPPROVED ADULT - Modest reduction in lipids in short-term studies, but long-term benefit in hyperlipidemia unclear. Small reduction in BP, but efficacy in HTN unclear. Does not appear effective for diabetes.

UNAPPROVED PEDS - Not for use in children.

NOTES - Cytochrome P450 3A4 inducer. Significantly decreases saquinavir levels; may also interact with other protease inhibitors. May increase bleeding risk with warfarin with/without increase in INR.

ginger (Zingiber officinale) ▶? ♀? ▶? $

UNAPPROVED ADULT - Prevention of motion sickness (efficacy unclear): 500-1000 mg powdered rhizome PO single dose 1 h before exposure. American College of Obstetrics and Gynecology considers ginger 250 mg PO qid a nonpharmacologic option for N/V of pregnancy. Some experts advise pregnant women to limit dose to usual dietary amount (≤1 g/day). Efficacy unclear for postop N/V (conflicting study results). Efficacy unclear for relief of osteoarthritis pain.

UNAPPROVED PEDS - Not for use in children.

NOTES - High doses (12-14 g) may increase bleeding risk with warfarin with/without increase in INR.

ginkgo biloba (EGb 761, Ginkgold, Ginkoba, Quanterra Mental Sharpness) ▶K ♀- ▶- $

UNAPPROVED ADULT - Dementia (modest benefit for mild to moderate disease): 40 mg PO tid of standardized extract containing 24% ginkgo flavone glycosides and 6% terpene lactones. Improvement may be delayed for up to 4 weeks. Does not appear to improve memory in elderly with normal cognitive function. Unclear efficacy for prevention of acute altitude sickness. Limited benefit in intermittent claudication. ArginMax (also contains L-arginine and other ingredients) promoted for SSRI-induced sexual dysfunction.

UNAPPROVED PEDS - Not for use in children.

NOTES - May cause seizures; avoid using with drugs that lower the seizure threshold (antipsychotics, antidepressants, cholinesterase inhibitors, decongestants, sedating antihistamines, systemic corticosteroids). May have antiplatelet activity; avoid in patients taking warfarin. Case reports of bleeding in patients also taking rofecoxib, warfarin, or aspirin.

ginseng - American (Panax quinquefolius L.) ▶K ♀- ▶- $

UNAPPROVED ADULT - Reduction of postprandial glucose in type 2 diabetes (possibly effective): 3 g ground root caps PO taken with or up to 2h before meal.

UNAPPROVED PEDS - Not for use in children.

NOTES - Ginseng content varies widely and some products are mislabeled or adulterated with caffeine. American, Asian, and Siberian ginseng are often confused/ misidentified. Decreased INR with warfarin.

ginseng - Asian (Panax ginseng, Ginsana, Ginsai, G115, Korean red ginseng) ▶? ♀- ▶- $

UNAPPROVED ADULT - Promoted to improve vitality and well-being: 200 mg PO qd. Ginsana: 2 caps PO qd or 1 cap PO bid. Ginsana Sport: 1 cap PO qd. Efficacy unclear for improving physical or psychomotor performance, diabetes, herpes simplex infections, cognitive or immune function, postmenopausal hot flashes (American College of Obstetrics and Gynecologists and North American Menopause Society recommend against use).

UNAPPROVED PEDS - Not for use in children.

NOTES - Some formulations may contain up to 34% alcohol. Ginsana Gold also contains vitamins and minerals. Reports of an interaction with the MAOI, phenelzine. Decreased INR with warfarin. Ginseng content varies widely and some products are mislabeled or adulterated with caffeine. American, Asian, and Siberian ginseng are often confused/misidentified. Can cause false elevation of digoxin immunoassay.

glucosamine (*Aflexa, Cosamin DS, Dona, Flextend, Promotion*) ▶? ♀- ▶- $

UNAPPROVED ADULT - Osteoarthritis (effective for decreasing pain and joint space narrowing in knee OA): 500 mg PO tid. Dona (crystalline glucosamine sulfate): 1 packet (1500 mg) dissolved in glass of water PO qd.

UNAPPROVED PEDS - Not for use in children.

NOTES - Use cautiously or avoid in patients with shellfish allergy. No evidence that formulations with chondroitin have benefit over glucosamine alone. Case report of increased INR with warfarin in patient taking chondroitin + glucosamine.

goldenseal (*Hydrastis canadensis*) ▶? ♀- ▶- $

UNAPPROVED ADULT - Often used in attempts to achieve false-negative urine test for illicit drug use (efficacy unclear). Often combined with echinacea in cold remedies; but insufficient data to assess efficacy of goldenseal for the common cold or URIs.

UNAPPROVED PEDS - Not for use in children.

NOTES - Alkaloids in goldenseal with antibacterial activity not well-absorbed orally. Oral use contraindicated in pregnancy (may cause uterine contractions), newborns (may cause kernicterus), and hypertension (high doses may cause peripheral vasoconstriction). Adding goldenseal directly to urine turns it brown.

grapeseed extract (*Vitus vinifera L., procyanidolic oligomers, PCO*) ▶? ♀? ▶? $

UNAPPROVED ADULT - Small clinical trials suggest benefit in chronic venous insufficiency. No benefit in single study of seasonal allergic rhinitis.

UNAPPROVED PEDS - Not for use in children.

NOTES - Pine bark (pycnogenol) and grapeseed extract are often confused; they both contain oligomeric proanthocyanidins.

guggulipid (*Commiphora mukul extract, guggul*) ▶? ♀- ▶- $$

UNAPPROVED ADULT - Efficacy unclear for treatment of hyperlipidemia. Data is conflicting.

A randomized controlled trial conducted in US with 1000 mg or 2000 mg PO tid reported no change in cholesterol, triglycerides, or HDL, and a small increase in LDL. Earlier studies of weaker design conducted in India reported reductions in total cholesterol of up to 27%.

UNAPPROVED PEDS - Not for use in children.

NOTES - May decrease levels of propranolol and diltiazem.

hawthorn (*Crataegus laevigata, monogyna, oxyacantha, standardized extract WS 1442 - Crataegutt novo, HeartCare*) ▶? ♀- ▶- $

UNAPPROVED ADULT - Symptomatic improvement of mild CHF (NYHA I-II; possibly effective): 80 mg PO bid to 160 mg PO tid of standardized extract (19% oligomeric procyanidins; WS 1442; HeartCare 80 mg tabs); doses as high as 900-1800 mg/day have been studied.

UNAPPROVED PEDS - Not for use in children.

NOTES - Unclear whether hawthorn and digoxin should be used together; mechanisms of action may be similar.

horse chestnut seed extract (*Aesculus hippocastanum, HCE50, Venastat*) ▶? ♀- ▶- $

UNAPPROVED ADULT - Chronic venous insufficiency (effective): 1 cap Venastat PO bid with water before meals. Response within 1 month. Venastat is 16% aescin in standardized extract.

UNAPPROVED PEDS - Not for use in children.

NOTES - Venastat does not contain aesculin, a toxin in horse chestnuts.

kava (*Piper methysticum, One-a-day Bedtime & Rest, Sleep-Tite*) ▶K ♀- ▶- $

UNAPPROVED ADULT - Promoted as anxiolytic (possibly effective) or sedative; recommend against use due to hepatotoxicity.

UNAPPROVED PEDS - Not for use in children.

NOTES - Reports of severe hepatotoxicity leading to liver transplantation. May potentiate CNS effects of benzodiazepines and other sedatives, including alcohol. Reversible yellow skin discoloration with long-term use.

kombucha tea (*Manchurian or Kargasok tea*) ▶? ♀- ▶- $

UNAPPROVED ADULT - Promoted for many indications, but no scientific evidence to support benefit for any condition. FDA advises caution due to a case of fatal acidosis.

UNAPPROVED PEDS - Not for use in children.

NOTES - Culture of bacteria and yeast that is very acidic after preparation. Tea is made by steeping mushroom culture in tea and sugar for ~1 week. Tea may contain alcohol, ethyl acetate, acetic acid, and lactate.

licorice (*Glycyrrhiza glabra, Glycyrrhiza uralensis*) ▶Bile ♀- ▶- $

UNAPPROVED ADULT - Insufficient data to assess efficacy for postmenopausal vasomotor symptoms.

UNAPPROVED PEDS - Not for use in children.

NOTES - Diuretics or stimulant laxatives could potentiate licorice-induced hypokalemia. In the US, "licorice" candy usually does not contain licorice. Deglycyrrhizinated licorice does not have mineralocorticoid effects.

melatonin (*N-acetyl-5-methoxytryptamine*) ▶L ♀- ▶- $

ADULT - To reduce jet lag after flights across >5 time zones (effective; especially traveling East; may also help for 2-4 times zones): 0.5-5 mg PO qhs (10 pm to midnight) x 3-6 nights starting on day of arrival. Faster onset and better sleep quality with 5 mg over 0.5 mg, but no greater benefit with >5 mg. No benefit with use before departure or slow-release formulations. Do not take earlier in day (may cause drowsiness and delay adaptation to local time). Orphan drug for treatment of circadian rhythm-related sleep disorders in blind patients with no light perception.

PEDS - Not usually for use in children. Orphan drug treatment of circadian rhythm-related sleep disorders in blind patients with no light perception.

NOTES - High melatonin levels linked to nocturnal asthma; some experts advise patients with nocturnal asthma to avoid melatonin supplements until more data available.

methylsulfomethane (*MSM, dimethyl sulfone, crystalline DMSO2*) ▶? ♀- ▶- $

UNAPPROVED ADULT - Insufficient data to assess efficacy of oral and topical MSM for arthritis pain.

UNAPPROVED PEDS - Not for use in children.

NOTES - Can cause nausea, diarrhea, headache. DMSO metabolite promoted as a source of sulfur without odor.

milk thistle (*Silybum marianum, Legalon, silymarin, Thisylin*) ▶LK ♀- ▶- $

UNAPPROVED ADULT - Hepatic cirrhosis (possibly effective): 100-200 mg PO tid of standardized extract with 70-80% silymarin. Efficacy unclear in chronic hepatitis C. Used in Europe to treat Amanita mushroom poisoning.

UNAPPROVED PEDS - Not for use in children.

NOTES - May inhibit cytochrome P450 2C9 and

3A4; but no effect on pharmacokinetics of indinavir in human studies. May decrease blood glucose in patients with cirrhosis and diabetes.

nettle root (*stinging nettle, Urtica dioica radix*) ▶? ♀- ▶- $

UNAPPROVED ADULT - Efficacy unclear for treatment of BPH.

UNAPPROVED PEDS - Not for use in children.

NOTES - Lead contamination led to recall of some lots of Nature's Way nettle caps.

noni (*Morinda citrifolia*) ▶? ♀? ▶- $$$

UNAPPROVED ADULT - Promoted for many medical disorders; but insufficient data to assess efficacy.

UNAPPROVED PEDS - Not for use in children.

NOTES - Potassium concentration comparable to orange juice. Hyperkalemia reported in a patient with chronic renal failure.

probiotics (*Acidophilus, Bifidobacteria, Lactobacillus, Bacid, Culturelle, Intesti-Flora, Kala, Lactinex, LiveBac, Power-Dophilus, Primadophilus, Probiotica*) ▶? ♀+ ▶+ $

UNAPPROVED ADULT - Culturelle. Prevention of antibiotic-induced diarrhea (efficacy unclear): 1 cap PO bid during and for 1 week after antibiotic therapy. Give 2 h before/after antibiotic so culture isn't killed. Prevention of travelers' diarrhea (efficacy unclear): 1 cap PO bid from 2-3 days before until end of trip. Probiotica: 1 chew tab PO qd. Efficacy of probiotics unclear for irritable bowel syndrome, or prevention of bacterial vaginosis or vaginal candidiasis. Dose of other products may vary; check label.

UNAPPROVED PEDS - Early use of Lactobacillus (10-100 billion CFU PO within first 48 h) may reduce duration of acute infectious diarrhea due to rotavirus and other pathogens (possibly effective). Culturelle: 1 cap PO qd. Can open & mix contents into cool drink, baby food, or apple sauce. Probiotica, ≥2 yo. 1 chew tab PO qd. Dose of other products may vary; check label.

FORMS -- Culturelle contains Lactobacillus GG 10 billion cells/cap. Probiotica contains Lactobacillus reuteri 100 million cells/chew tab.

NOTES - Use cautiously in immunosuppressed patients; acquired infection possible. Microbial type and content varies by product. If yogurt is used, pick products with a label that says "Live and active cultures".

pycnogenol (*French maritime pine tree bark*) ▶L ♀? ▶? $

UNAPPROVED ADULT - Promoted for many

medical disorders, but insufficient data to assess efficacy. Data is limited to small studies in chronic venous insufficiency, sperm dysfunction, melasma, and ADHD.

UNAPPROVED PEDS - Not for use in children.

NOTES - Pycnogenol is the trade name of a commercial product in the UK and the scientific name for a group of flavonoids called flavan-3-ol derivatives.

pygeum africanum (*African plum tree, Prostata, Prostatonin, Provol*) ▶? ♀- ▶- $

UNAPPROVED ADULT - Benign prostatic hypertrophy (may have modest efficacy): 50-100 mg PO bid or 100 mg PO qd of standardized extract containing 14% triterpenes. Prostatonin (also contains Urtica dioica): 1 cap PO bid with meals; up to 6 weeks for full response. Prostata also contains saw palmetto and other ingredients.

UNAPPROVED PEDS - Not for use in children.

NOTES - Appears well-tolerated. Self-treatment could delay diagnosis of prostate cancer.

red clover isoflavone extract (*Trifolium pratense, trefoil, Promensil, Rimostil, Supplifem, Trinovin*) ▶Gut, L, K ♀- ▶- $$

UNAPPROVED ADULT - Promensil (1 tab PO qd-bid with meals) marketed for menopausal symptoms; Rimostil (1 tab PO qd) for bone & cholesterol health, and to promote health & well-being after menopause; Trinovin (1 tab PO qd) for maintaining prostate health & urinary function in men. Conflicting evidence of efficacy for postmenopausal vasomotor symptoms. Does not appear effective overall, but may have modest benefit for severe symptoms. Efficacy unclear for prevention of osteoporosis & treatment of hyperlipidemia in postmenopausal women, and for BPH sx in men.

UNAPPROVED PEDS - Not for use in children.

Isoflavone content (genistein, daidzein, biochanin, formononetin) is 40 mg/tab in Promensil and Trinovin, 57 mg/tab in Rimostil.

NOTES - Does not appear to stimulate endometrium. Effect on breast cancer risk is unclear; some experts recommend against use of isoflavone supplements by women with breast cancer. H2 blockers, proton pump inhibitors, and antibiotics may decrease metabolic activation of isoflavones in GI tract. Ingesting large amounts of red clover can cause bleeding in cattle; bleeding risk of supplements in humans is theoretical. Supplifem contains soy and red clover extract (51 mg isoflavones/caplet).

s-adenosylmethionine (*Flexium, SAM-e, sammy*) ▶L ♀? ▶? $$$

UNAPPROVED ADULT - Depression (possibly effective): 400-1600 mg/day PO. Osteoarthritis (possibly effective): 400-1200 mg/day PO. Flexium (labeled for joint health): 200 mg bid or 400 mg PO qd on empty stomach. Onset of response in OA in 2-4 weeks.

UNAPPROVED PEDS - Not for use in children.

NOTES - Serotonin syndrome possible with SSRI. Do not use within 2 weeks of an MAOI or in bipolar disorder.

Saint John's wort (*Alterra, Hypericum perforatum, Kira, Movana, One-a-day Tension & Mood, LI-160, St John's wort*) ▶L ♀- ▶- $

UNAPPROVED ADULT - Short-term treatment of mild depression (effective): 300 mg PO tid of standardized extract (0.3% hypericin). May be ineffective for moderate major depression.

UNAPPROVED PEDS - Not for use in children.

NOTES - Photosensitivity possible with >1800 mg/day. Inducer of hepatic cytochrome P450 3A4, 2C19, and 1A2, and P-glycoprotein. May decrease efficacy of drugs with hepatic metabolism including alprazolam, cyclosporine, methadone, non-nucleoside reverse transcriptase inhibitors, omeprazole, oral contraceptives, protease inhibitors, statins. May need increased dose of digoxin, theophylline, tricyclic antidepressants. Decreased INR with warfarin. Administration with SSRIs, nefazodone, triptans may cause serotonin syndrome. Do not use within 14 days of monoamine oxidase inhibitors.

saw palmetto (*Serenoa repens, One-a-day Prostate Health, Prostata, Quanterra*) ▶? ♀- ▶- $

UNAPPROVED ADULT - BPH (effective): 160 mg PO bid or 320 mg PO qd of standardized liposterolic extract. Relieves symptoms, but little effect on prostate volume. Response reported in 1-2 months. Take with food. Prostata also contains Pygeum africanum and other ingredients. Brewed teas may not be effective.

UNAPPROVED PEDS - Not for use in children.

NOTES - Symptomatic improvement appears comparable to finasteride with better tolerability. Not for use by women of child-bearing potential. Does not interfere with PSA test. Self-treatment could delay diagnosis of prostate cancer.

shark cartilage (*BeneFin, Cancenex, Cartilade*) ▶? ♀- ▶- $$$$$

UNAPPROVED ADULT - Efficacy unclear for palliative care of advanced cancer. Neovastat (AE-941), a derivative of shark cartilage, is in phase III clinical trials for renal cell carcinoma and non-small cell lung cancer.

UNAPPROVED PEDS - Not for use in children.

silver - colloidal (*mild & strong silver protein, silver ion*) ▶? ♀- ▶- $

UNAPPROVED ADULT - The FDA does not recognize OTC colloidal silver products as safe or effective for any use.

UNAPPROVED PEDS - Not for use in children. May come as silver chloride, cyanide, iodide, oxide, or phosphate.

NOTES - Silver accumulates in skin (leads to grey tint), conjunctiva, and internal organs with chronic use.

soy (*Genisoy, Healthy Woman, Novasoy, Phytosoya, Supplifem, Supro*) ▶Gut, L, K ♀+ for food, ? for supplements ▶+ for food, ? for supplements $

UNAPPROVED ADULT - Cardiovascular risk reduction: ≥25 g/day soy protein (50 mg/day isoflavones) PO. Hypercholesterolemia: ~50 g/day soy protein PO reduces LDL cholesterol by ~13%; efficacy unclear for isoflavone supplements. Postmenopausal vasomotor symptoms (conflicting evidence; modest benefit possible): 20-60 g/day soy protein PO (40-80 mg/day isoflavones). North American Menopause Society considers dietary isoflavones + lifestyle changes an option for relief of mild symptoms. Efficacy unclear for prevention of osteoporosis.

UNAPPROVED PEDS - Soy foods are regarded as safe for children.

NOTES - Effect on breast cancer risk is unclear; some experts recommend against use of isoflavone or phytoestrogen supplements by women with endometrial or breast cancer (esp estrogen receptor-positive tumor or receiving tamoxifen). Case report of decreased INR with ingestion of soy milk by patient taking warfarin. Report of decreased levothyroxine absorption with soy protein. Soy milk contains soy + red clover extract (51 mg isoflavones/caplet).

stevia (*Stevia rebaudiana*) ▶L ♀? ▶? $

UNAPPROVED ADULT - Leaves traditionally used as a sweetener, but not enough safety data for FDA approval as such. Efficacy unclear for treatment of type 2 diabetes or HTN.

UNAPPROVED PEDS - Not for use in children.

NOTES - Stevia available as dietary supplement, but not approved by the FDA as sweetener in the US.

tea tree oil (*melaleuca oil*) ▶? ♀- ▶- $

UNAPPROVED ADULT - Not for oral use; CNS toxicity reported. Efficacy unclear for onychomycosis, tinea pedis, acne vulgaris.

UNAPPROVED PEDS - Not for use in children.

valerian (*Valeriana officinalis, Alluna, One -a-day Bedtime & Rest, Sleep-Tite*) ▶? ♀- ▶- $

UNAPPROVED ADULT - Insomnia (possibly effective): 400-900 mg of standardized extract PO 30 minutes before bedtime. Response reported in 2-4 weeks. Alluna (valerian + hops): 2 tabs PO 1 h before bedtime. Some products have unpleasant smell.

UNAPPROVED PEDS - Not for use in children.

NOTES - Do not combine with CNS depressants. Withdrawal symptoms reported after long-term use.

wild yam (*Dioscorea villosa*) ▶L ♀? ▶? $

UNAPPROVED ADULT - Ineffective as topical "natural progestin".

UNAPPROVED PEDS - Not for use in children.

yohimbe (*Corynanthe yohimbe, Pausinystalia yohimbe, Potent V*) ▶L ♀- ▶- $

UNAPPROVED ADULT - Nonprescription yohimbe promoted for impotence and as aphrodisiac, but these products rarely contain much yohimbine (active constituent). FDA considers yohimbe bark in herbal remedies an unsafe herb. Yohimbine HCl is available in US as a prescription drug.

UNAPPROVED PEDS - Not for use in children.

FORMS - Yohimbine is the primary alkaloid in the bark of the yohimbe tree. Yohimbine HCl is a prescription drug in the US; yohimbe bark is available without prescription. Yohimbe bark (not by prescription) and prescription yohimbine HCl are not interchangeable.

NOTES - Can cause CNS stimulation. High doses of yohimbine have MAOI activity and can increase blood pressure. Avoid in patients with hypotension, diabetes, heart, liver or kidney disease. Reports of renal failure, seizures, death in patients taking products containing yohimbe.

IMMUNOLOGY: Immunizations

NOTE: For vaccine info see CDC www.cdc.gov.

BCG vaccine (*Tice BCG*, ♣*Pacis*) ▶Immune system ♀C ▶? $$$$

ADULT - 0.2-0.3 ml percutaneously (using 1 ml sterile water for reconstitution).

PEDS - Age >1 month: use adult dose. Age <1 month: Decrease concentration by 50% using

2 ml sterile water for reconstitution, then 0.2-0.3 ml percutaneously. May revaccinate with full dose (adult dose) after 1 yo if necessary.

Comvax (haemophilus b + hepatitis B vaccine) ▶Immune system ♀C ▶? $$$

ADULT - Do not use in adults.

PEDS - Infants born of HBsAg (-) mothers: 0.5 ml IM x 3 doses at 2, 4, and 12-15 months.

NOTES - Combination is made of PedvaxHIB (haemophilus b vaccine) + Recombivax HB (hepatitis B vaccine). For infants >8 weeks of age.

diphtheria tetanus & acellular pertussis vaccine (DTaP, Tripedia, Infanrix, Daptacel, ♥Tripacel, Adacel) ▶Immune system ♀C ▶- $

ADULT - Do not use in adults.

PEDS - Check immunization history: DTaP is preferred for all DTP doses. Give first dose of 0.5 ml IM at approximately 2 months, second dose at 4 months, third dose at 6 months, fourth dose at 15-18 months, and fifth dose (booster) at 4-6 yo.

NOTES - Do not immunize persons ≥7 yo with pertussis vaccine. When feasible, use same brand for first 3 doses. Do not give if prior DTP vaccination caused anaphylaxis or encephalopathy within 7 days. Avoid Tripedia in thimerosal allergic patients.

diphtheria-tetanus toxoid (Td, DT, ♥D2T5) ▶Immune system ♀C ▶? $

ADULT - Age ≥7 yo: 0.5 ml IM, second dose 4-8 weeks later, and third dose 6-12 months later. Give 0.5 ml booster dose at 10 year intervals. Use adult formulation (Td) for adults and children ≥7 years of age.

PEDS - Age 6 weeks- 6 yo: 0.5 ml IM , second dose 4-8 weeks later, and third dose 6-12 months later using DT for pediatric use. If immunization of infants begins in the first year of life using DT rather than DTP (i.e. pertussis is contraindicated), give three 0.5 ml doses 4- 8 weeks apart, followed by a fourth dose 6- 12 months later.

FORMS - Injection DT (pediatric: 6 weeks- 6 yo). Td (adult and children: ≥7 years).

NOTES - DTaP is preferred for most children <7 years of age. Td is preferred for adults and children ≥7 yo. Avoid in thimerosal allergy.

haemophilus b vaccine (ActHIB, HibTITER, PedvaxHIB) ▶Immune system ♀C ▶? $

PEDS - Doses vary depending on formulation used and age at first dose. ActHIB/ OmniHIB/ HibTITER: 2- 6 months- 0.5 ml IM x 3 doses at two month intervals. 7- 11 months- 0.5 ml IM x

2 doses at two month intervals. 12- 14 months- 0.5 ml IM x 1 dose. A single 0.5 ml IM (booster) dose is given to children ≥15 months old, and at least 2 months after the previous injection. 15- 60 months: 0.5 ml IM x 1 dose (no booster). PedvaxHIB: 2- 14 months- 0.5 ml IM x 2 doses at two month intervals. If the 2 doses are given before 12 months of age, a third 0.5 ml IM (booster) dose is given at least 2 months after the second dose. 15- 60 months- 0.5 ml IM x 1 dose (no booster).

UNAPPROVED ADULT - Asplenia, prior to elective splenectomy, or immunodeficiency: 0.5 ml IM x 1 dose of any Hib conjugate vaccine.

UNAPPROVED PEDS - Asplenia, prior to elective splenectomy, or immunodeficiency age ≥5 yo: 0.5 ml IM x 1 dose of any Hib vaccine.

NOTES - Not for IV use. No data on interchangeability between brands; AAP & ACIP recommend use of any product in children >12-15 months of age.

hepatitis A vaccine (Havrix, Vaqta, ♥Avaxim) ▶Immune system ♀C ▶+ $$$

ADULT - Havrix ≥18 yo: 1 ml (1440 ELU) IM, then 1 ml (1440 ELU) IM booster dose 6- 12 months later. Vaqta ≥18 yo: 1 ml (50 U) IM, then 1 ml (50 U) IM booster 6 months later.

PEDS - Havrix 2-18 yo: 0.5 ml (720 ELU) IM x 1 dose, then 0.5 ml (720 ELU) IM booster 6-12 months after first dose. Vaqta 2-18 yo: 0.5 ml (25 U) IM x 1 dose, then 0.5 ml (25 U) IM booster 6- 18 months later.

FORMS - Single dose vial (specify peds, adult).

NOTES - Do not inject IV, SC, or ID. Brands may be used interchangeably. Need for boosters is unclear. Post-exposure prophylaxis with hepatitis A vaccine alone is not recommended. Should be given 4 weeks prior to travel to endemic area. May be given at the same time as immune globulin, but preferably at different site.

hepatitis B vaccine (Engerix-B, Recombivax HB) ▶Immune system ♀C ▶+ $$$

ADULT - Engerix-B ≥20 yo: 1 ml (20 mcg) IM, repeat in 1 and 6 months. Hemodialysis: Give 2.0 ml (40 mcg) IM, repeat in 1, 2, & 6 months. Give 2.0 ml (40 mcg) IM booster when antibody levels <10 mIU/ml. Recombivax HB: 1 ml (10 mcg) IM, repeat in 1 and 6 months. Hemodialysis: 1 ml (40 mcg) IM, repeat in 1 & 6 months. Give 1 ml (40 mcg) IM booster when antibody levels <10 mIU/ml.

PEDS - Specialized dosing based on age and maternal HBsAg status. Infants of hepatitis B negative and positive mothers, children, adolescents <20 years: Engerix-B 10 mcg (0.5 ml) IM 0,1,6 months. Recombivax 5 mcg (0.5 ml) IM 0,1,6 months. In adolescents 11-15 year, a 2-dose schedule can be used (Recombivax HB 10 mcg (1.0 ml) IM 0, 4-6 months).

NOTES - Infants born to hepatitis B positive mothers should also receive hepatitis B immune globulin and hepatitis B vaccine within 12 hours of birth. Not for IV or ID use. May interchange products. Recombivax HB Dialysis Formulation is intended for adults only. Avoid if yeast allergy. Adult formulations contain thimerosal; avoid if allergy.

influenza vaccine (*Fluzone, Fluvirin, FluMist, ✦Fluviral*) ▶Immune system ♀C ▶+ $

ADULT - 0.5 ml IM single dose once yearly. Healthy adults ages 18-49 yo: 1 dose (0.5 mL) intranasally once yearly (FluMist).

PEDS - Age 6- 35 months: 0.25 ml IM, repeat dose ≥4 weeks. Age 3- 8 yo: 0.5 ml IM, repeat dose ≥4 weeks. Age 9- 12 yo: 0.5 ml IM once yearly. Healthy children 5-17 yo: 1 dose (0.5 mL) intranasally (FluMist), repeat dose in 2 months in children 5-8 yo receiving for first time. When using the intramuscular formulations, use only the split virus vaccine (i.e. subvirion or purified surface antigen) in children 6 months- 8 yo. Give repeat dose only in previously unvaccinated children.

NOTES - Avoid in Guillain-Barre Syndrome, chicken egg allergy, ASA therapy. Avoid intramuscular formulations if thimerosal allergy. Optimal administration October to November. Since FluMist is a live vaccine, do not use in patients with immune deficiencies (e.g., HIV, malignancy, etc.) or who may have altered immune status (e.g., taking systemic corticosteroids, chemotherapy, radiation, etc.).

Japanese encephalitis vaccine (*JE-Vax*) ▶Immune system ♀C ▶? $$$$$

ADULT - 1 ml SC x 3 doses on days 0, 7, and 30.

PEDS - Age ≥3 yo: 1.0 ml SC x 3 doses on days 0, 7, and 30. Age 1-3 yo: 0.5 ml SC x 3 doses on days 0, 7, and 30.

NOTES - Give at least 10 days before travel to endemic areas. An abbreviated schedule on days 0, 7, and 14 can be given if time constraints. A booster dose may be given after 2 years. Avoid in thimerosal allergy.

measles mumps & rubella vaccine (*M-M-R II, ✦Priorix*) ▶Immune system ♀C ▶+ $$

ADULT - 0.5 ml (1 vial) SC.

PEDS - 12-15 months of age: 0.5 ml (1 vial) SC. Revaccinate prior to elementary and/or middle

school according to local health guidelines. If measles outbreak, may immunize infants 6-12 months old with 0.5 ml SC; then start 2 dose regimen between 12-15 months of age.

NOTES - Do not inject IV. Contraindicated in pregnancy. Advise women to avoid pregnancy for 4 weeks following vaccination. Live virus, contraindicated in immunocompromised patients. Avoid if allergic to neomycin; caution in patients with egg allergies.

meningococcal polysaccharide vaccine (*Menomune-A/C/Y/W-135, ✦Menjugate*) ▶Immune system ♀C ▶? $$$

ADULT - 0.5 ml SC.

PEDS - Age ≥2 yo: 0.5 ml SC.

UNAPPROVED PEDS - Age 3-18 months: 0.5 ml SC x 2 doses separated by 3 months

NOTES - Give 2 weeks before elective splenectomy or travel to endemic areas. May consider revaccination q3-5 yrs in high risk patients. Do not inject IV. Contraindicated in pregnancy. Consider vaccinating first-year college students living in dormitories. Avoid in thimerosal allergy.

Pediarix (DTaP + hepatitis B + polio) ▶Immune system ♀C ▶? $$$

PEDS - 0.5 ml at 2, 4, 6 months IM.

NOTES - Do not administer before 6 weeks of age.

plague vaccine (*Plague vaccine*) ▶Immune system ♀C ▶+ $

ADULT - Age 18-61 yo: 1 ml IM x 1 dose, then 0.2 ml IM 1-3 months after the 1st injection, then 0.2 ml IM 5-6 months after the 2nd injection.

PEDS - Not approved in children.

NOTES - Up to 3 booster doses (0.2 ml) may be administered at 6 month intervals in high risk patients. Jet injector gun may be used for IM administration.

pneumococcal 23-valent vaccine (*Pneumovax, ✦Pneumo 23*) ▶Immune system ♀C ▶+ $

ADULT - 0.5 ml IM/SC. Routine revaccination in immunocompetent patients is not recommended. Consider revaccination once in patients ≥65 yo (if <65 yo at initial vaccination) or at high risk of developing serious pneumococcal infection if >5 years from initial vaccine.

PEDS - ≥2 yo: 0.5 ml IM/SC. Consider revaccination once in patients at high risk of developing serious pneumococcal infection after 3-5 yo from initial vaccine in patients that would be ≤10 yo at revaccination.

ADULT IMMUNIZATION SCHEDULE*

Tetanus, diphtheria (Td): For all ages, 1 dose booster every 10 years. *Influenza*:1 yearly dose if ≥50 years old. If <50 years, then 1 yearly dose if healthcare worker, chronic underlying illness, or household contact of person with chronic underlying illness. Intranasal vaccine indicated for healthy adults <50 years. *Pneumococcal* (polysaccharide): 1 dose if ≥65 years old. If <65 years, consider immunizing if chronic underlying illness, nursing home resident, or Native American. Consider revaccination 5 years later if high risk or if ≥65 years and received primary dose before age 65. *Hepatitis A*: For all ages with clotting factor disorders, chronic liver disease, or exposure risk (travel to endemic areas, IV drug use, men having sex with men), 2 doses (0, 6-12 months). *Hepatitis B*: For all ages with medical (hemodialysis, clotting factor recipients), occupational (healthcare or public safety workers with blood exposure), behavioral (IV drug use, multiple sex partners, recent sexually transmitted disease, men having sex with men) or other (household/sex contacts of those with chronic HBV infections, clients/staff of developmentally disabled, >6 month travel to high risk areas, inmates of correctional facilitites) indications , 3 doses (0, 1-2, 4-6 months). *Measles, mumps, rubella (MMR)*: If <50 years old and immunity in doubt, see www.cdc.gov. *Varicella*: For all ages if immunity in doubt, 2 doses separated by 8 weeks, see www.cdc.gov. *Meningococcal* (polysaccharide): For all ages if medical (complement deficiency, anatomic or functional asplenia) or other (travel to endemic regions, consider for college dormitory residents) indications, 1 dose. Consider revaccination in 3-5 years if high-risk.

*2004 schedule from the CDC, ACIP, & AAFP, see CDC website (www.cdc.gov).

CHILDHOOD IMMUNIZATION SCHEDULE*						Months				Years	
Age	Birth	1	2	4	6	12	15	18	24	4-6	11-12
Hepatitis B	HB-1		HB-2			HB-3					
DTP†			DTP	DTP	DTP		DTP			DTP	Td
H influenza b			Hib	Hib	Hib	Hib					
Pneumococci			PCV	PCV	PCV	PCV					
Polio§			IPV	IPV		IPV				IPV	
MMR						MMR				MMR	
Varicella						Varicella					
Influenza						Influenza‡					
Hepatitis A¶										HA (some areas)	

*2004 schedule from the CDC, ACIP, AAP, & AAFP, see CDC website (www.cdc.gov). †Acellular form preferred for all DTP doses. §Inactivated form (IPV) preferred for all doses in the US. ‡Also annually immunize older children (and contacts) with risk factors such as asthma, cardiac disease, sickle cell diseases, HIV, diabetes. Live-attenuated influenza (nasal formulation) only for healthy children ≥5 yo. ¶HA series recommended for selected high-risk areas, consult local public health authorities.

NOTES - Do not give IV or ID. May be given in conjunction with influenza virus vaccine at different site. OK for high risk children ≥2 yo who received Prevnar series already to provide additional serotype coverage. Avoid in thimerosal allergy.

pneumococcal 7-valent conjugate vaccine (*Prevnar*) ▶Immune system ♀C ▶? $$$
ADULT - Not approved in adults.
PEDS - 0.5 ml IM x 3 doses 6-8 weeks apart starting at 2-6 months of age, followed by a 4th dose of 0.5 ml IM at 12-15 months. For previously unvaccinated older infants and children age 7-11 months: 0.5 ml x 2 doses 6-8 weeks apart, followed by a 3rd dose of 0.5 ml at 12-15 months. Age 12-23 months: 0.5 ml x 2 doses

6-8 weeks apart. Age 2-9 yo: 0.5 ml x 1 dose; give 2nd dose 4 weeks later in immunocompromised or chronically ill children.
NOTES - For IM use only; do not inject IV. Shake suspension vigorously prior to administration.

poliovirus vaccine (*Orimune, IPOL*) ▶Immune system ♀C ▶? $$
ADULT - Not generally recommended. Previously unvaccinated adults at increased risk of exposure should receive a complete primary immunization series of 3 doses of IPV (two doses at intervals of 4-8 weeks; a third dose at 6-12 months after the second dose). Accelerated schedules are available. Travelers to endemic areas who have received primary immu-

nization should receive a single booster (IPV) in adulthood.

PEDS - An all-IPV schedule is now recommended: 0.5 ml IM or SC (IPV, IPOL) at 2 months of age. Second dose at 4 months, third dose at 6- 18 months, and fourth dose at 4- 6 yo. OPV (Orimune) may be used in special circumstances.

NOTES - Orimune = Sabin; IPOL = inactivated.

rabies vaccine (*RabAvert, Imovax Rabies, BioRab, Rabies Vaccine Adsorbed*) ▶Immune system ♀C ▶? $$$$$

ADULT - Post-exposure prophylaxis: Give rabies immune globulin (20 IU/ kg) immediately after exposure, then give rabies vaccine 1 ml IM in deltoid region on days 0, 3, 7, 14, and 28. If patients have received pre-exposure immunization, give 1 ml IM rabies vaccine on days 0 and 3 only without rabies immune globulin. Pre-exposure immunization: 1 ml IM rabies vaccine on days 0, 7, and between days 21-28. Or 0.1 ml ID on days 0, 7, and between days 21-28. (Imovax Rabies I.D. vaccine formula only). Repeat q2-5 years based on antibody titer.

PEDS - Same as adults.

NOTES - Do not use ID preparation for post-exposure prophylaxis.

smallpox vaccine (*Dryvax*) ▶Immune system ♀C ▶- ?

ADULT - Prevention of smallpox or monkeypox: Specialized administration using a bifurcated needle SC x 1.

PEDS - >1 yo: Specialized administration using a bifurcated needle SC x 1.

NOTES - Contraindicated in polymyxin, neomycin, tetracycline, or streptomycin allergy. Avoid in those (or household contacts of those) with eczema or a history of eczema, those with a rash due to other causes (eg, burns, zoster, impetigo, psoriasis), immunocompromise, or pregnancy. Persons with known cardiac disease or 3+ risk factors for cardiac disease should not be vaccinated as response team members in the pre-event smallpox vaccination program.

tetanus toxoid ▶Immune system ♀C ▶+ $

WARNING - Td is preferred in adults and children ≥7 yo. DTP is preferred in children <7 yo. Use fluid tetanus toxoid in assessing cell-mediated immunity only.

ADULT - 0.5 ml IM (adsorbed) x 2 doses 4-8 wks apart. Give third dose 6-12 months after 2nd injection. Give booster q10 yrs. Assess cell-mediated immunity: 0.1 ml of 1:100 diluted

skin-test reagent or 0.02 ml of 1: 10 diluted skin-test reagent injected intradermally.

PEDS - 0.5 ml IM (adsorbed) x 2 doses 4-8 wks apart. Give third dose 6-12 months after 2nd injection. Give booster q10 years.

NOTES - Tetanus toxoid is currently in short supply. Delay routine Td boosters in adolescents and adults until supply is available. May use tetanus toxoid fluid for active immunization in patients hypersensitive to the aluminum adjuvant of the adsorbed formulation: 0.5 ml IM or SC x 3 doses at 4- 8 week intervals. Give fourth dose 6-12 months after third injection. Give booster dose q10 years. Avoid in thimerosal allergy

TriHibit (*haemophilus b + DTaP*) ▶Immune system ♀C ▶- $$

PEDS - For 4th dose only, 15-18 mos: 0.5 ml IM.

NOTES - Tripedia (DTaP) is used to reconstitute ActHIB (Haemophilus b) to make TriHIBit and will appear whitish in color. Use within 30 min. Avoid in thimerosal allergy.

Twinrix (*hepatitis A inactivated + hepatitis B recombinant vaccines*) ▶Immune system ♀C ▶) $$$

ADULT - ≥18 yo: 1 ml IM in deltoid only, repeat in 1 & 6 months.

PEDS - Not approved in children.

NOTES - Not for IV or ID use. 1 ml = 720 ELU inactivated hepatitis A + 20 mcg hepatitis B surface antigen.

typhoid vaccine (*Vivotif Berna, Typhim Vi, Typhoid Vaccine*) ▶Immune system ♀C ▶? $$

ADULT - Typhim Vi: 0.5 ml IM x 1 dose given at least 2 weeks prior to potential exposure. May consider revaccination q2 yrs in high risk patients. Typhoid Vaccine, USP: 0.5 ml SC x 2 doses separated by 4 weeks. May consider revaccination q3 yrs in high risk patients. Vivotif Berna: One cap 1 hr before a meal with cold or lukewarm drink qod x 4 doses to be completed at least 1 week prior to potential exposure. May consider revaccination q5 yrs in high-risk patients.

PEDS - age ≥6 yo: Typhim Vi- same as adult dose. Age ≥10 yo: Typhoid Vaccine, USP- same as adult dose; age <10 yo: 0.25 ml SC x 2 doses separated by 4 weeks. Age ≥2 yo: Vivotif Berna- same as adult dose.

FORMS - Trade only: Caps

NOTES - Recommended for travel to endemic areas. Typhoid vaccine, USP has more adverse reactions, but is no more effective than

Typhim Vi or Vivotif Berna. Oral vaccine, Vivotif Berna, may be inactivated by antibiotics, including antimalarials.

varicella vaccine (*Varivax*) ▶Immune system ♀C ▶+ $$$
ADULT - 0.5 ml SC. Repeat 4- 8 weeks later.
PEDS - age 1- 12 yo: 0.5 ml SC x 1 dose. Age ≥13 yo: same as adult dose. Not recommended for infants <1 yo.
UNAPPROVED PEDS - Postexposure prophylaxis: 0.5 ml SC within 3-5 days of exposure.
NOTES - Do not inject IV. Following vaccination avoid pregnancy for 3 months and ASA / sali-

cylates for 6 weeks. The need for booster doses is not defined. This live vaccine is contraindicated in immunocompromised. Vaccine is stored in freezer; thawed vaccine must be used within 30 minutes.

yellow fever vaccine (*YF-Vax*) ▶Immune system ♀C ▶+ $$$
ADULT - 0.5 ml SC
PEDS - age 6 months-3 yo: 0.5 ml SC into the thigh; Age ≥3 yo: 0.5 ml SC into the deltoid.
NOTES - Approval by state and/or federal authorities required to obtain vaccine. A booster dose (0.5 ml) may be administered q10 years.

TETANUS WOUND MANAGEMENT (www.cdc.gov)	Uncertain or <3 prior tetanus immunizations	≥3 prior tetanus immunizations
Non tetanus prone wound, ie, clean & minor	Td (DT if <7 yo)	Td if >10 years since last dose
Tetanus prone wound, eg, dirt, contamination, punctures, crush components	Td (DT if <7 yo), tetanus immune globulin 250 units IM at site other than Td.	Td if >5 years since last dose

IMMUNOLOGY: Immunoglobulins

NOTE: Adult IM injections should be given in the deltoid region; injection in the gluteal region may result in suboptimal response.

antivenin - crotalidae immune Fab ovine polyvalent (*CroFab*) ▶? ♀C ▶? $$$$$
ADULT - Rattlesnake envenomation: Give 4-6 vials IV infusion over 60 minutes, <6 h of bite if possible. Administer 4-6 additional vials if no initial control of envenomation syndrome, then 2 vials q6h for up to 18 h (3 doses) after initial control has been established.
PEDS - Same as adults, although specific studies in children have not been conducted.
NOTES - Contraindicated in allergy to papaya or papain. Start IV infusion slowly over the first 10 minutes at 25-50 ml/hr and observe for allergic reaction, then increase to full rate of 250 ml/hr.

antivenin - crotalidae polyvalent ▶L ♀C ▶? $$$$$
ADULT - Pit viper envenomation: minimal envenomation: 20- 40 ml (2- 4 vials) IV infusion; moderate envenomation: 50- 90 ml (5- 9 vials) IV infusion; severe envenomation: ≥100- 150 ml (10- 15 vials) IV infusion. Administer within 4 h of bite, less effective after 8 hours, and of questionable value after 12 hours. May give additional 10- 50 ml (1- 5 vials) IV infusion based on clinical assessment and response to initial dose.
PEDS - Larger relative doses of antivenin are

needed in children and small adults because of small volume of body fluid to dilute the venom. The dose is not based on weight.
NOTES - Test first for sensitivity to horse serum. Serum sickness may occur 5-24 days after dose. IV route is preferred. May give IM.

antivenin - latrodectus mactans ▶L ♀C ▶? $$
ADULT, PEDS - Specialized dosing for black widow spider toxicity; consult poison center.
NOTES - Test first for horse serum sensitivity. Serum sickness may occur 5-24 days after dose.

botulism immune globulin (*BabyBIG*) ▶L ♀? ▶? ?
ADULT - Not approved in >1 yo.
PEDS - Infant botulism <1 yo: 1 mL (50 mg)/kg IV.

hepatitis B immune globulin (*H-BIG, Bay-Hep B, NABI-HB*) ▶L ♀C ▶? $$$
ADULT - Post-exposure prophylaxis (i.e. needlestick, ocular, mucosal exposure): 0.06 ml/kg IM (usual dose 3- 5 ml) within 24 h of exposure. Initiate hepatitis B vaccine series within 7 days. Consider a second dose of hepatitis B immune globulin (HBIG) one month later if patient refuses hepatitis B vaccine series. Post-exposure prophylaxis (i.e. sexual exposure): 0.06 ml/kg IM within 14d of sexual contact. Initiate hepatitis B vaccine series.
PEDS - Prophylaxis of infants born to HBsAg (+)

mothers: 0.5 ml IM within 12 h of birth. Initiate hepatitis B vaccine series within 7 days. If hepatitis B vaccine series is refused, repeat HBIG dose at 3 and 6 months. Household exposure <12 months of age: 0.5 ml IM within 14d of exposure. Initiate hep B vaccine series.

NOTES - HBIG may be administered at the same time or up to 1 month prior to hepatitis B vaccine without impairing the active immune response from hepatitis B vaccine.

immune globulin - intramuscular (*Baygam*) ▶L ♀C ▶? $$$$

ADULT - Hepatitis A post-exposure prophylaxis (ie, household or institutional contacts): 0.02 ml /kg IM within 2 weeks of exposure. Hepatitis A pre-exposure prophylaxis (ie, travel to endemic area): <3 months length of stay = 0.02 ml/kg IM. >3 months length of stay = 0.06 ml/kg IM and repeat q4-6 months. Measles: 0.2-0.25 ml/ kg IM within 6 days of exposure, max 15 ml. Varicella zoster (if VZIG unavailable): 0.6-1.2 ml/kg IM. Rubella exposure in pregnant, susceptible women: 0.55 ml/kg IM. Immunoglobulin deficiency: 0.66 ml/kg IM every 3-4 weeks.

PEDS - Not approved in children.

UNAPPROVED PEDS - Measles: 0.2-0.25 ml/kg IM within 6 days of exposure. In susceptible immunocompromised children use 0.5 ml/kg IM (max 15 ml) immediately after exposure. Varicella zoster (if VZIG unavailable): 0.6-1.2 ml/kg IM.

NOTES - Human derived product, increased infection risk. Hepatitis A vaccine preferred over immune globulin for persons >2 years old who plan to travel to high risk areas repeatedly or for long periods of time.

immune globulin - intravenous (*Gamimune, Polygam, Panglobulin, Octagam, Flebogamma, Sandoglobulin, Gammagard, Gammar, Gamunex, Iveegam, Venoglobulin*) ▶L ♀C ▶? $$$$$

ADULT - Idiopathic thrombocytopenic purpura (induction): 400 mg/kg IV qd x 5 days (or 1 g/kg IV qd for 1-2 days). Bone marrow transplant (>20 yo): 500 mg/kg IV qd, given 7 and 2 days before transplant, and then weekly until 90 days post transplant. Primary humoral immunodeficiency: 200-300 mg/kg IV each month; increase as needed to max 400-800 mg/kg/month. B-cell chronic lymphocytic leukemia: specialized dosing.

PEDS - Pediatric HIV: 400 mg/kg IV q28 days. Idiopathic thrombocytopenic purpura (induction): 400 mg/kg IV qd x 5 days (or 1 g/kg IV qd for 1-2 days). Kawasaki Syndrome (acute): 400

mg/kg IV qd x 4 days (or 2 g/kg IV x 1 over 10 hours). Primary humoral immunodeficiency: 200-300 mg/kg IV each month; increase as needed to max 400-800 mg/kg/month.

UNAPPROVED ADULT - First-line therapy in Guillain-Barre´ syndrome, chronic inflammatory demyelinating polyneuropathy, multifocal motor neuropathy; second-line therapy in stiff-person syndrome, dermatomyositis, myasthenia gravis, and Lambert-Eaton myasthenic syndrome: Various dosing regimens have been used; a common one is Myasthenia gravis (induction): 400 mg/kg IV qd x 5 days (total 2 g/kg).

UNAPPROVED PEDS - Myasthenia gravis (induction): 400 mg/kg IV qd x 5 days. Other dosing regimens have been used.

NOTES - Indications and doses vary by product. Follow LFTs, renal function, vital signs, and urine output closely. Contraindicated in IgA deficiency. Use caution (and lower infusion rates) if risk factors for thrombosis, CHF, or renal insufficiency. Use slower infusion rates for initial doses. Consider pretreatment with acetaminophen and/or diphenhydramine to minimize some infusion-related adverse effects. Human-derived product, increased infection risk.

lymphocyte immune globulin human (*Atgam*) ▶L ♀C ▶? $$$$$

ADULT - Renal allograft recipients: 10-30 mg/kg IV qd. Delaying onset of allograft rejection: 15 mg/kg IV qd x 14 days, then qod x 14 days. Treatment of renal transplant rejection: 10-15 mg/kg IV x 14 days. Aplastic anemia: 10-20 mg/kg IV qd x 8-14 days, then qod, as needed, up to 21 total doses.

PEDS - Limited experience. Has been safely administered to a limited number of children with renal transplant and aplastic anemia at doses comparable to adults.

NOTES - Doses should be administered over ≥4 hours.

rabies immune globulin human (*Imogam, BayRab*) ▶L ♀C ▶? $$$$$

ADULT - Post-exposure prophylaxis: 20 units/ kg (0.133 ml/kg), with as much as possible infiltrated around the bite and the rest given IM. Give as soon as possible after exposure. Administer with the first dose of vaccine, but in a different extremity.

PEDS - Not approved in children.

UNAPPROVED PEDS - Use adult dosing.

NOTES - Do not repeat dose once rabies vaccine series begins. Do not give to patients who have been completely immunized with rabies vaccine. Do not administer IV.

RHO immune globulin (*RhoGAM, MICRho-GAM, BayRho-D, BayRho-D Mini Dose, WinRho SDF, Rhophylac*) ►L ♀C ▶? $$$$
ADULT - Prevention of hemolytic disease of the newborn if mother Rh- and baby is or might be Rh+: 300 mcg vial IM to mother at 28 weeks gestation followed by a 2nd dose ≤72 hours of delivery. (See OB/GYN section for more detailed dosing.) Rh-incompatible transfusion: specialized dosing. Immune thrombocytopenic purpura (ITP), nonsplenectomized (WinRho): 250 units/kg/dose (50 mcg/kg/dose) IV x 1 if hemoglobin >10 g/dL or 125-200 units/kg/dose (25-40 mcg/kg/dose) IV x 1 if hemoglobin <10 g/dL. Additional doses of 125-300 units/kg/dose (25-60 mcg/kg/dose) IV may be given as determined by patient's response.
PEDS - Immune thrombocytopenic purpura (ITP), nonsplenectomized (WinRho): 250 units/kg/dose (50 mcg/kg/dose) IV x 1 if hemoglobin >10g/dL or 125-200 units/kg/dose (25-40 mcg/kg/dose) IV x 1 if hemoglobin <10 g/dL. Additional doses of 125-300 units/kg/dose (25-60 mcg/kg/dose) IV may be given as determined by patient's response.
NOTES - Do not give IV. If the dose required is ≥2 vials, may inject as divided doses at different injection sites or divide the total dose and inject at intervals within 72 hours.

RSV immune globulin (*RespiGam*) ►Plasma ♀C ▶? $$$$$
PEDS - RSV prophylaxis in children <24 months: 1.5 ml/kg/hr x 15 minutes. Increase rate as clinical condition permits to 3 ml/kg/hr x 15 minutes, then to a maximum rate of 6 ml/kg/hr. Max total dose/ month is 750 mg/kg.
NOTES - May cause fluid overload; monitor vital signs frequently during IV infusion. RSV season is typically November-April.

tetanus immune globulin (*BayTet*) ►L ♀C ▶? $$$$
ADULT - See tetanus wound management table. Post-exposure prophylaxis in tetanus prone wounds in patients ≥7 years of age: if <3 doses of tetanus vaccine have been administered or if history is uncertain, give 250 units IM x 1 dose along with dT. If ≥3 doses of tetanus vaccine have been administered in the past, do not give tetanus immune globulin. Tetanus treatment: 3000-6000 units IM in combination with other therapies.
PEDS - <7 yo: 4 units/ kg IM or 250 units IM. Initiate tetanus toxoid vaccine (DTP or DT).
NOTES - Do not give tetanus immune globulin for clean, minor wounds. May be given at the same time as tetanus toxoid active immunization. Do not inject IV.

varicella-zoster immune globulin (*VZIG*) ►L ♀C ▶? $$$$$
ADULT, PEDS - Specialized dosing for post-exposure prophylaxis.

IMMUNOLOGY: Immunosuppression

basiliximab (*Simulect*) ►Plasma ♀B ▶? $$$$$
ADULT, PEDS - Specialized dosing for organ transplantation.

cyclosporine (*Sandimmune, Neoral, Gengraf*) ►L ♀C ▶- $$$$$
ADULT - Specialized dosing for organ transplantation, rheumatoid arthritis, and psoriasis.
PEDS - Not approved in children.
UNAPPROVED ADULT - Specialized dosing for autoimmune eye disorders, vasculitis, inflammatory myopathies, Behcet's disease, psoriatic arthritis.
UNAPPROVED PEDS - Specialized dosing for organ transplantation.
FORMS - Generic/Trade: microemulsion Caps 25, 100 mg. Generic/Trade: Caps (Sandimmune) 25,100 mg. Solution (Sandimmune) 100 mg/ml. Microemulsion solution (Neoral, Gengraf) 100 mg/ml.
NOTES - Monitor cyclosporine blood concentrations closely. Many drug interactions including atorvastatin, lovastatin, rosuvastatin, simvastatin Reduce dose in renal dysfunction. Monitor blood pressure and renal function closely. Monitor patients closely when switching from Sandimmune to microemulsion formulations.

daclizumab (*Zenapax*) ►L ♀C ▶? $$$$$
ADULT - Specialized dosing for organ transplantation.
PEDS - Not approved in children.
UNAPPROVED PEDS - Specialized dosing for organ transplantation.

mycophenolate mofetil (*Cellcept*) ▶? ♀C ▶? $$$$$
ADULT - Specialized dosing for organ transplantation.
PEDS - Not approved in children.
UNAPPROVED ADULT - Lupus nephritis: 1000 mg PO bid.
UNAPPROVED PEDS - Specialized dosing for organ transplantation.
FORMS - Trade only: Caps 250 mg. Tabs 500

mg. Oral suspension 200 mg/ml.
sirolimus (*Rapamune*) ▶L ♀C ▶- $$$$$
WARNING - Combination of sirolimus plus cyclosporine or tacrolimus is associated with hepatic artery thrombosis in liver transplant patients. Combination with tacrolimus and corticosteroids in lung transplant patients may cause bronchial anastomotic dehiscence. Avoid with strong inhibitors of CYP3A4 and/or P-glycoprotein (ketoconazole, voriconazole, itraconazole, erythromycin, telithromycin, clarithromycin) or strong inducers CYP3A4 and/or P-glycoprotein (rifampin, rifabutin).
ADULT - Specialized dosing for organ transplantation.
PEDS - Not approved in children.

UNAPPROVED PEDS - Specialized dosing for organ transplantation.
FORMS - Trade: oral solution 1 mg/ml. Tablet 1, 2, 5 mg.
tacrolimus (*Prograf, FK 506*) ▶L ♀C ▶- $$$$$
ADULT, PEDS - Specialized dosing for organ transplantation.
UNAPPROVED ADULT - Rheumatoid arthritis (approved in Canada), active vasculitis, systemic lupus erythematosus nephritis & vasculitis.
FORMS - Trade only: Caps 1,5 mg.
NOTES - Reduce dose in renal dysfunction. Monitor blood pressure and renal function closely.

IMMUNOLOGY: Other

tuberculin PPD (*Aplisol, Tubersol, Mantoux, PPD*) ▶L ♀C ▶+ $
ADULT - 5 TU (0.1 ml) intradermally.
PEDS - Same as adult dose. AAP recommends screening at 12 months, 4- 6 yo, and 14- 16 yo.

NOTES - Avoid SC injection. Read 48- 72 h after intradermal injection. Repeat testing in patients with known prior positive PPD may cause scarring at injection site.

MOTOR FUNCTION BY NERVE ROOTS

Level	Motor function
C4	Spontaneous breathing
C5	Shoulder shrug / deltoid
C6	Biceps / wrist extension
C7	Triceps / wrist flexion
C8/T1	finger flexion
T1-T12	Intercostal / abd muscles

Level	Motor function
T12	cremasteric reflex
L1/L2	hip flexion
L2/L3/L4	hip adduction / quads
L5	great toe dorsiflexion
S1/S2	foot plantarflexion
S2-S4	rectal tone

LUMBOSACRAL NERVE ROOT COMPRESSION	Root	Motor	Sensory	Reflex
	L4	quadriceps	medial foot	knee-jerk
	L5	dorsiflexors	dorsum of foot	medial hamstring
	S1	plantarflexors	lateral foot	ankle-jerk

NEUROLOGY: Alzheimer's Disease – Cholinesterase Inhibitors

NOTE: Avoid concurrent anticholinergic agents. Use caution in asthma/COPD. No known adverse drug interactions when cholinesterase inhibitors are co-administered with memantine.
donepezil (*Aricept*) ▶LK ♀C ▶? $$$$
ADULT - Alzheimer's disease: Start 5 mg PO qhs. May increase to 10 mg qhs in 4-6 weeks.
PEDS - Not approved in children.
FORMS - Trade: Tabs 5, 10 mg.
NOTES - Some clinicians start with 5 mg PO qod to minimize GI side effects.

galantamine (*Reminyl*) ▶LK ♀B ▶? $$$$
ADULT - Alzheimer's disease: Start 4 mg PO bid with meals; increase to 8 mg bid after 4 weeks. May increase to 12 mg PO bid after another 4 weeks. Usual dose is 16-24 mg/day.
PEDS - Not approved in children.
FORMS - Trade: Tabs 4, 8, 12 mg. Oral solution 4 mg/ml.
NOTES - Do not exceed 16 mg/day with renal or hepatic impairment. Use caution with CYP3A4 and CYP2D6 inhibitors (eg, cimetidine, ranitidine, ketoconazole, erythromycin, paroxetine).

rivastigmine (*Exelon*) ▶K ♀B ▶? $$$$
ADULT - Alzheimer's disease: Start 1.5 mg PO bid with food. Increase to 3 mg bid after 2 weeks. Usual effective dose is 6-12 mg/day. Max 12 mg/day.
PEDS - Not approved in children.
FORMS - Trade: Caps 1.5, 3, 4.5, 6 mg. Oral solution 2 mg/ml.
NOTES - Restart treatment with the lowest daily dose (ie, 1.5 mg bid) if discontinued for several days to reduce the risk of severe vomiting.

tacrine (*Cognex*) ▶L ♀C ▶? $$$$
ADULT - Alzheimer's disease: Start 10 mg PO qid for 4 weeks, then increase to 20 mg qid. Titrate to higher doses q4 weeks as tolerated. Max 160 mg/day.
PEDS - Not approved in children.
FORMS - Trade: Caps 10, 20, 30, 40 mg.
NOTES - Hepatotoxicity may occur. Monitor LFTs q2 weeks x 16 weeks, then q3 months.

NEUROLOGY: Alzheimer's Disease – NMDA Receptor Antagonists

memantine (*Namenda*) ▶KL ♀B ▶? $$$$
ADULT - Alzheimer's disease (moderate to severe): Start 5 mg PO qd. Increase by 5 mg/day at weekly intervals to max 20 mg/day. Doses >5 mg/day should be divided bid.
PEDS - Not approved in children.
FORMS - Trade: Tabs 5, 10 mg
NOTES - No known drug interactions with acetylcholinesterase inhibitors.

GLASGOW COMA SCALE		
	Verbal Activity	*Motor Activity*
		6. Obeys commands
Eye Opening	5. Oriented	5. Localizes pain
4. Spontaneous	4. Confused	4. Withdraws to pain
3. To command	3. Inappropriate	3. Flexion to pain
2. To pain	2. Incomprehensible	2. Extension to pain
1. None	1. None	1. None

NEUROLOGY: Anticonvulsants

NOTE: Avoid rapid discontinuation of anticonvulsants, since this can precipitate seizures or other withdrawal symptoms.

carbamazepine (*Tegretol, Tegretol XR, Carbatrol, Epitol*) ▶LK ♀D ▶+ $
WARNING - Risk of aplastic anemia and agranulocytosis. Monitor CBC at baseline and periodically.
ADULT - Epilepsy: Start 200 mg PO bid. Increase by 200 mg/day at weekly intervals divided tid-qid (regular release), bid (extended-release), or qid (suspension) to max 1,600 mg/day. Trigeminal neuralgia: Start 100 mg PO bid or 50 mg PO qid (suspension); increase by 200 mg/day until pain relief. Max 1,200 mg/day.
PEDS - Epilepsy, age >12 yo: Start 200 mg PO bid or 100 mg PO qid (suspension); increase by 200 mg/day at weekly intervals divided tid-qid (regular release), bid (extended-release), or qid (suspension) to max 1,000 mg/day (age 12-15 yo) or 1,200 mg/day (age >15 yo). Epilepsy age 6-12 yo: Start 100 mg PO bid or 50 mg PO qid (suspension); increase by 100 mg/day at weekly intervals divided tid-qid (regular release), bid (extended-release), or qid (suspension) to max 1,000 mg/day. Epilepsy age <6 yo: Start 10-20 mg/kg/day PO divided bid-tid or qid (suspension). Increase weekly prn. Max 35 mg/kg/day.
UNAPPROVED ADULT - Neuropathic pain: Start 100 mg PO bid; usual effective dose is 200 mg PO bid-qid. Max 1,200 mg/day.
FORMS - Trade: Tabs 200 mg (Tegretol, Epitol). Chew tabs 100 mg (Tegretol, Epitol). Susp 100 mg/5 ml (Tegretol). extended-release tabs 100, 200, 400 mg (Tegretol XR). extended-release caps 200, 300 mg. Generic: Tabs 200 mg. Chew tabs 100, 200 mg. Susp 100 mg/5 ml.
NOTES - Usual therapeutic range = 4-12 mcg/ml. Stevens-Johnson Syndrome, hepatitis, aplastic anemia, and hyponatremia may occur. Monitor CBC and LFTs. Many drug interactions. Should not be used for absence or atypical absence seizures.

clobazam (*Frisium*) ▶L ♀X (first trimester) D (2nd/3rd trimesters) ▶- $
WARNING - Use cautiously in the elderly; may accumulate and lead to side effects such as

psychomotor impairment.

ADULT - Canada only. Epilepsy, adjunctive: Start 5-15 mg PO qd. Gradually increase prn to max 80 mg qd.

PEDS - Canada only. Epilepsy, adjunctive, <2 yo: Start 0.5-1 mg/kg PO qd. 2-16 yo: Start 5 mg PO qd; may increase prn to max 40 mg qd.

FORMS - Generic/Trade: Tabs 10 mg.

NOTES - Reduce dose in hepatic or renal dysfunction. Drug interactions with enzyme-inducing anticonvulsants such as carbamazepine and phenytoin; may need to adjust levels.

clonazepam (*Klonopin*, ♣*Clonapam*, *Rivotril*) ▶LK ♀D ▶- ⊙IV $$$

ADULT - Akinetic or myoclonic seizures: Start 0.5 mg PO tid. Increase by 0.5-1 mg q3 days prn. Max 20 mg/day.

PEDS - Akinetic or myoclonic seizures, Lennox-Gastaut syndrome (petit mal variant), or absence seizures (≤10 yo or ≤30 kg): 0.01-0.03 mg/kg/day PO divided bid-tid. Increase by 0.25-0.5 mg q3 days prn. Max 0.1- 0.2 mg/kg/day divided tid.

UNAPPROVED ADULT - Neuralgias: 2-4 mg PO qd. Restless legs syndrome: Start 0.25 mg PO qhs. Max 2 mg qhs. REM sleep behavior disorder: 1-2 mg PO qhs.

FORMS - Generic/Trade: Tabs 0.5, 1, 2 mg. Trade: Orally disintegrating tabs (Klonopin Wafers) 0.125, 0.25, 0.5, 1, 2 mg. (Orally disintegrating tablets approved for panic disorder only.)

NOTES - Usual therapeutic range = 20-80 ng/ml. Contraindicated in hepatic failure or acute narrow angle glaucoma.

diazepam (*Valium*, *Diastat*, ♣*Vivol*, *E Pam*) ▶LK ♀D ▶- ⊙IV $

ADULT - Status epilepticus: 5-10 mg IV. Repeat q10-15 minutes prn to max 30 mg. Epilepsy, adjunctive therapy: 2-10 mg PO bid-qid. Increased seizure activity: 0.2-0.5 mg/kg PR (rectal gel) to max 20 mg/day. Muscle spasm: 2-10 mg PO tid-qid. Alcohol withdrawal: 10 mg PO tid-qid x 24 hrs then 5 mg PO tid-qid prn.

PEDS - Status epilepticus, age 1 m to 5 yo: 0.2-0.5 mg IV slowly q2-5 minutes to max 5 mg. Status epilepticus, >5 yo: 1 mg IV slowly q2-5 minutes to max 10 mg. Repeat q2-4 hours prn. Epilepsy, adjunctive therapy, age >6 months: 1-2.5 mg PO tid-qid; gradually increase to max 30 mg/day. Increased seizure activity (rectal gel, age >2 yo): 0.5 mg/kg PR (2-5 yo), 0.3 mg/kg PR (6-11 yo), or 0.2 mg/kg PR (>12 yo). Max 20 mg. May repeat in 4-12 hours prn.

UNAPPROVED ADULT - Restless legs syn-

drome: 0.5-4.0 mg PO qhs. Loading dose strategy for alcohol withdrawal: 10-20 mg PO or 10 mg slow IV in closely monitored setting, then repeat similar or lower doses q1-2 hr prn until sedated. Further doses should be unnecessary due to long half-life.

FORMS - Generic/Trade: Tabs 2, 5, 10 mg. Solution 5 mg/ 5 ml. Trade only: concentrated solution (Intensol) 5 mg/ml. Rectal gel (Diastat) 2.5, 5, 10, 15, 20 mg.

NOTES - Respiratory and CNS depression may occur. Risk of venous thrombosis and vascular impairment (IV only). Use lower doses, slower titration in geriatric or debilitated patients.

ethosuximide (*Zarontin*) ▶LK ♀C ▶+ $$$$

ADULT - Absence seizures: 500 mg PO qd or divided bid. Increase by 250 mg/day q4-7 days prn. Max 1.5 g/day.

PEDS - Absence seizures: age 3-6 yo: start 250 mg PO qd or divided bid. Max 500 mg/day. Age >6 yo: start 500 mg PO qd or divided bid. Increase by 250 mg q 4-7 days prn. Usual dose 20 mg/kg/day. Max 1.5 g/day.

UNAPPROVED PEDS - Absence seizures: age <3 yo: start 15 mg/kg/day divided bid. Increase q4-7d prn. Usual dose 15-40 mg/kg/day divided bid. Max 500 mg/day.

FORMS - Generic/Trade: Caps 250 mg. Syrup 250 mg/5 ml.

NOTES - Usual therapeutic range = 40-100 mcg/ml. Monitor CBC for blood dyscrasias. Use caution in hepatic and renal impairment.

felbamate (*Felbatol*) ▶KL ♀C ▶- $$$$

WARNING - Aplastic anemia and fatal hepatic failure have occurred.

ADULT - Severe, refractory epilepsy: Start 400 mg PO tid. Increase by 600 mg/day q2 weeks to max 3,600 mg/day.

PEDS - Lennox-Gastaut syndrome, adjunctive therapy, age 2- 14 yo: Start 15 mg/kg/day PO in 3-4 divided doses. Increase by 15 mg/kg/day at weekly intervals to max 45 mg/kg/day.

FORMS - Trade: Tabs 400, 600 mg. Susp 600 mg/5 ml.

NOTES - Use only after discussing the risks and obtaining written informed consent. Many drug interactions.

fosphenytoin (*Cerebyx*) ▶L ♀D ▶+ $$$$$

ADULT - Status epilepticus: Load 15-20 mg "phenytoin equivalents" (PE) per kg IV no faster than 100-150 mg PE/minute. Non-emergent loading dose: 10-20 mg PE/kg IM/IV at rate ≤150 mg/minute. Maintenance: 4-6 mg PE/kg/day.

PEDS - Not approved in children.

UNAPPROVED PEDS - Status epilepticus: 15-20 mg PE/kg IV at a rate <2 mg PE/kg/min.

NOTES - Fosphenytoin is dosed in "phenytoin equivalents" (PE). Use beyond 5 days has not been systematically studied. Usual therapeutic range = 10- 20 mcg/ml in patients with normal hepatorenal function. Monitor ECG & vital signs continuously during and after infusion. Contraindicated in patients with cardiac conduction block. Many drug interactions. Renal/hepatic disease may change protein binding and levels. Low albumin levels may increase free fraction.

gabapentin (Neurontin) ▶K ♀C ▶? $$$$

ADULT - Partial seizures, adjunctive therapy: Start 300 mg PO qhs. Increase gradually to usual effective dose of 300-600 mg PO tid. Max 3,600 mg/day. Postherpetic neuralgia: Start 300 mg PO on day 1. Increase to 300 mg bid on day 2, and to 300 mg tid on day 3. Max 1,800 mg/day divided tid.

PEDS - Partial seizures, adjunctive therapy, 3-12 yo: Start 10-15 mg/kg/day PO divided tid. Titrate over 3 days to usual effective dose of 25-40 mg/kg/day divided tid. Max 50 mg/kg/day. Use adult dosing in patients >12 yo.

UNAPPROVED ADULT - Partial seizures, initial monotherapy: Titrate as above. Usual effective dose is 900-1,800 mg/day. Neuropathic pain: 300 mg PO tid, max 3,600 mg/day in 3-4 divided doses. Migraine prophylaxis: Start 300 mg PO qd; then gradually increase to 1,200-2,400 mg/day in 3-4 divided doses. Restless legs syndrome: Start 300 mg PO qhs. Max 3,600 mg/day divided tid.

FORMS - Generic: Caps 100, 300, 400 mg. Trade: Caps 100, 300, 400 mg. Tabs 600, 800 mg (scored). Soln 50 mg/ml.

NOTES - Decrease dose in renal impairment (CrCl <60 mL/min); table in package insert. Discontinue gradually over ≥1 week.

lamotrigine (Lamictal, Lamictal CD) ▶LK ♀C ▶- $$$$

WARNING - Potentially life-threatening rashes (eg, Stevens-Johnson Syndrome) have been reported in 0.3% of adults and 0.8% of children, usually within 2-8 weeks of initiation; discontinue at first sign of rash. Drug interaction with valproate; see adjusted dosing guidelines.

ADULT - Partial seizures or Lennox Gastaut syndrome, adjunctive therapy with an enzyme-inducing anticonvulsant (age >12 yo): Start 50 mg PO qd x 2 weeks, then 50 mg PO bid x 2 weeks. Increase by 100 mg/day q1-2 weeks to usual maintenance dose of 150-250 mg PO bid. Partial seizures, conversion to monotherapy from adjunctive therapy with a single enzyme-inducing anticonvulsant (age ≥16 yo): Use above guidelines to gradually increase the dose to 250 mg PO bid; then taper the enzyme-inducing anticonvulsant by 20% a week over 4 weeks. Partial seizures or Lennox-Gastaut syndrome, adjunctive therapy with valproate (age >12 yo): Start 25 mg PO qod x 2 weeks, then 25 mg PO qd x 2 weeks. Increase by 25-50 mg/day q1-2 weeks to usual maintenance dose of 100-400 mg/day given qd or divided bid. Partial seizures, conversion to monotherapy from adjunctive therapy with valproate (age ≥16 yo): Use above guidelines to gradually increase the dose to 200 mg/day PO given qd or divided bid; then decrease valproate weekly by ≤500 mg/day to an initial goal of 500 mg/day. After 1 week at these doses, increase lamotrigine to 300 mg/day and decrease valproate to 250 mg/day divided bid. A week later, discontinue valproate; then increase lamotrigine weekly by 100 mg/day to usual maintenance dose of 500 mg/day. See psychiatry section for bipolar disorder dosing.

PEDS - Partial seizures or Lennox-Gastaut syndrome, adjunctive therapy with an enzyme-inducing anticonvulsant, age 2-12 yo: Start 0.6 mg/kg/day PO divided bid x 2 weeks, then 1.2 mg/kg/day PO divided bid x 2 weeks. Increase q1-2 weeks by 1.2 mg/kg/day (rounded down to nearest whole tablet) to usual maintenance dose of 5-15 mg/kg/day. Max 400 mg/day. Age >12 yo: use adult dosing. Partial seizures or Lennox-Gastaut syndrome, adjunctive therapy with valproate, age 2-12 yo: Start 0.15 mg/kg/day PO (given qd or divided bid) x 2 weeks, then 0.3 mg/kg/day PO (given qd or divided bid) x 2 weeks. Increase q1-2 weeks by 0.3 mg/kg/day (rounded down to nearest whole tablet) to usual maintenance dose of 1-5 mg/kg/day. Max 200 mg/day. Age >12 yo: use adult dosing.

UNAPPROVED ADULT - Initial monotherapy for partial seizures: Start 25 mg PO qd. Usual maintenance dose is 100-300 mg/day divided bid. Max 500 mg/day.

UNAPPROVED PEDS - Initial monotherapy for partial seizures: Start 0.5 mg/kg/day given qd or divided bid. Max 10 mg/kg/day. Newly-diagnosed absence seizures: Titrate as above. Usual effective dose is 2-15 mg/kg/day.

FORMS - Trade: Tabs 25, 100, 150, 200 mg. Chewable dispersible tabs (Lamictal CD) 2, 5, 25 mg (2 mg chew tab not available in pharmacies; obtain through manufacturer representative, or by calling 1-888-825-5249).

NOTES - Drug interactions with valproate and enzyme-inducing antiepileptic drugs (ie, carbamazepine, phenobarbital, phenytoin, primidone); may need to adjust dose. May increase carbamazepine toxicity.

levetiracetam (*Keppra*) ▶K ♀C ▶? $$$$$
ADULT - Partial seizures, adjunctive therapy: Start 500 mg PO bid. Increase by 500 mg bid q2 weeks prn. Max 3,000 mg/day.
PEDS - Not approved in children.
FORMS - Trade: Tabs 250, 500, 750 mg. Oral solution 100 mg/ml.
NOTES - Drug interactions unlikely. Decrease dose in renal dysfunction (CrCl <80 mL/min). Emotional lability and depression may occur.

lorazepam (*Ativan*) ▶LK ♀D ▶- ©IV $$$
ADULT - See psychiatry section
PEDS - Not approved in children.
UNAPPROVED ADULT - Status epilepticus: 0.05-0.1 mg/kg IV over 2-5 minutes, or 4 mg IV. May repeat in 5-15 minutes. Max 8 mg /12 hours.
UNAPPROVED PEDS - Status epilepticus: 0.05-0.1 mg/kg IV over 2-5 minutes. May repeat 0.05 mg/kg x 1 in 10-15 minutes. Do not exceed 4 mg as single dose.

methsuximide (*Celontin*) ▶L ♀C ▶? $$$
ADULT - Refractory absence seizures: Start 300 mg PO qd; increase weekly by 300 mg/day. Max 1,200 mg/day.
PEDS - Refractory absence seizures: Start 10-15 mg/kg PO in 3-4 divided doses; increase weekly prn. Max 30 mg/kg/day.
FORMS - Trade: Caps 150, 300 mg.
NOTES - Monitor CBC, UA and LFTs.

oxcarbazepine (*Trileptal*) ▶LK ♀C ▶- $$$$
ADULT - Partial seizures, monotherapy: Start 300 mg PO bid. Increase by 300 mg/day q3 days to usual effective dose of 1,200 mg/day. Max 2,400 mg/day. Partial seizures, adjunctive: Start 300 mg PO bid. Increase by 600 mg/day at weekly intervals to usual effective dose of 1,200 mg/day. Max 2,400 mg/day.
PEDS - Partial seizures, adjunctive (4-16 yo): Start 8-10 mg/kg/day divided bid (max starting dose 600 mg/day). Titrate to usual effective dose of 900 mg/day (20-29 kg children), 1,200 mg/day (29.1-39 kg children), or 1,800 mg/day (>39 kg children). Partial seizures, initial monotherapy (4-16 yo): Start 8-10 mg/kg/day divided BID. Increase by 5 mg/kg/day q3 days. Partial seizures, conversion to monotherapy (4-16 yo): Start 8-10 mg/kg/day divided BID. Increase at

weekly intervals by ≤10 mg/kg/day. See PI for recommended daily dose when used as monotherapy (based on patient's weight).
FORMS - Trade: Tabs 150, 300, 600 mg. Oral suspension 300 mg/5 ml.
NOTES - Monitor sodium in high risk patients for possible hyponatremia. Decrease initial dose by one-half in renal dysfunction (CrCl <30 ml/min). Inhibits CYP 2C19 and induces CYP 3A4/5. Interactions with other antiepileptic drugs, oral contraceptives, and dihydropyridine calcium channel blockers.

phenobarbital (*Luminal*) ▶L ♀D ▶- ©IV $
ADULT - Epilepsy: 100-300 mg/day PO divided qd-tid. Status epilepticus: 20 mg/kg IV at rate ≤60 mg/min.
PEDS - Epilepsy: 3-5 mg/kg/day PO divided bid-tid. Status epilepticus: 20 mg/kg IV at rate ≤60 mg/min.
UNAPPROVED ADULT - Status epilepticus: may give up to a total dose of 30 mg/kg IV.
UNAPPROVED PEDS - Status epilepticus: 15-20 mg/kg IV load; may give additional 5 mg/kg doses q15-30 minutes to total dose of 30 mg/kg. Epilepsy: 3-5 mg/kg/day divided qd-bid (neonates), 5-6 mg/kg/day divided qd-bid (infants), 6-8 mg/kg/day divided qd-bid (age 1-5 yo), 4-6 mg/kg/day divided qd-bid (age 6-12 yo), or 1-3 mg/kg/day divided qd-bid (age >12 yo).
FORMS - Generic/Trade: Tabs 15, 16, 30, 32, 60, 65, 100 mg. Elixir 20 mg/5 ml.
NOTES - Usual therapeutic range = 15- 40 mcg/ml. Monitor cardiopulmonary function closely when administering IV. Decrease dose in renal or hepatic dysfunction. Many drug interactions.

phenytoin (*Dilantin, Phenytek*) ▶L ♀D ▶+ $
ADULT - Status epilepticus: 10-15 mg/kg IV at rate ≤50 mg/ min, then 100 mg IV/PO q6-8h. Epilepsy, oral loading dose: 400 mg PO initially, then 300 mg in 2 hours and 4 hours. Maintenance dose: 300 mg/day PO given qd (extended release) or divided tid (standard release).
PEDS - Epilepsy, age >6 yo: 5 mg/kg/day PO divided bid-tid, to max 300 mg/day. Status epilepticus: 15-20 mg/kg IV at ≤1 mg/kg/min.
FORMS - Generic/Trade: Extended-release caps 100 mg (Dilantin). Suspension 125 mg/5 ml. Trade only: Extended-release caps 30 mg (Dilantin), 200, 300 mg (Phenytek). Chew tabs 50 mg. Generic: Prompt-release caps 100 mg.
NOTES - Usual therapeutic range 10-20 mcg/ml. Monitor ECG and vital signs when administering IV. Many drug interactions. Monitor lev-

els closely when switching between forms (free acid vs. sodium salt). The free fraction may be increased in patients with low albumin levels. IV loading doses of 15-20 mg/kg have also been recommended. May need to reduce loading dose if patient already on phenytoin.

primidone (*Mysoline*) ▶LK ♀D ▶- $

ADULT - Epilepsy: Start 100-125 mg PO qhs. Increase over 10 days to usual maintenance dose of 250 mg PO tid-qid. Max 2 g/day.

PEDS - Epilepsy <8 yo: Start 50 mg PO qhs. Increase over 10 days to usual maintenance dose of 125-250 mg tid or 10-25 mg/kg/day.

UNAPPROVED ADULT - Essential tremor: 250 mg PO tid.

FORMS - Generic/Trade: Tabs 50, 250 mg.

NOTES - Usual therapeutic range = 5- 12 mcg/ml. Metabolized to phenobarbital.

tiagabine (*Gabitril*) ▶L ♀C ▶? $$$$

ADULT - Partial seizures, adjunctive therapy: Start 4 mg PO qd. Increase by 4-8 mg q week prn to max 56 mg/day divided bid-qid.

PEDS - Partial seizures, adjunctive therapy (12-18 yo): Start 4 mg PO qd. Increase by 4 mg q1-2 weeks prn to max 32 mg/day divided bid-qid.

FORMS - Trade: Tabs 2, 4, 12, 16 mg.

NOTES - Take with food. Dosing is for patients on enzyme-inducing anticonvulsants such as carbamazepine, phenobarbital, phenytoin, or primidone. Reduce dosage in patients who are not taking enzyme-inducing medications, and in those with liver dysfunction.

topiramate (*Topamax*) ▶K ♀C ▶? $$$$$

ADULT - Partial seizures, primary generalized tonic-clonic seizures, or Lennox Gastaut Syndrome, adjunctive therapy: Start 25-50 mg qhs. Increase weekly by 25-50 mg/day to usual effective dose of 200 mg PO bid. Doses >400 mg/day not shown to be more effective. Migraine prophylaxis: Start 25 mg PO qhs week 1, then 25 mg bid week 2, 25 mg q am and 50 mg q pm week 3, then 50 mg bid week 4 and thereafter.

PEDS - Partial seizures, primary generalized tonic-clonic seizures, or Lennox-Gastaut Syndrome, adjunctive therapy (2-16 yo): Start 1-3 mg/kg (max 25 mg) PO qhs. Increase by 1-3 mg/kg/day q 1-2 weeks to usual effective dose of 5-9 mg/kg/day divided bid.

UNAPPROVED ADULT - Partial seizures, monotherapy and bipolar disorder: Start 25-50 mg PO qd. Titrate prn to max 400 mg/day. Migraine prophylaxis: Start 25 mg PO qd. Titrate to 100-200 mg/day divided bid.

FORMS - Trade only: Tabs 25, 100, 200 mg. Sprinkle Caps 15, 25 mg.

NOTES - Give ½ usual adult dose to patients with renal impairment (CrCl <70 ml/ min). Confusion, nephrolithiasis, glaucoma, and weight loss may occur. Risk of oligohidrosis and hyperthermia, particularly in children; use caution in warm ambient temperatures and/or with vigorous physical activity. Hyperchloremic, non-anion gap metabolic acidosis may occur; monitor serum bicarbonate and either reduce dose or taper off entirely if this occurs. Max dose tested was 1,600 mg/day.

valproic acid (*Depakene, Depakote, Depakote ER, Depacon, divalproex, ✚Epiject, Epival, Deproic*) ▶L ♀D ▶+ $$$$

WARNING - Fatal hepatic failure has occurred; monitor LFTs during first 6 months of treatment. Life-threatening cases of pancreatitis have been reported after initial or prolonged use. Evaluate for abdominal pain, N/V, and/or anorexia. Discontinue if pancreatitis occurs.

ADULT - Epilepsy: 10-15 mg/kg/day PO or IV infusion over 60 min (≤20 mg/min) divided bid to qid (standard release or IV) or qd (Depakote ER). Increase dose by 5-10 mg/kg/day at weekly intervals to max 60 mg/kg/day. Migraine prophylaxis: Start 250 mg PO bid (Depakote) or 500 mg PO qd (Depakote ER) x 1 week, then 1000 mg/day PO given bid (Depakote) or qd (Depakote ER). Max 1,000 mg/day.

PEDS - Seizures >2 yo: 10- 15 mg/kg/day PO or IV infusion over 60 minutes (rate ≤20 mg/min). Increase dose by 5-10 mg/kg/day at weekly intervals to max 60 mg/kg/day. Divide doses >250 mg/day into bid-qid; may give qd (Depakote ER) if >10 yo.

UNAPPROVED ADULT - Preliminary evidence to support IV use in refractory status epilepticus; optimal dose unclear.

UNAPPROVED PEDS - Preliminary evidence to support IV use in refractory status epilepticus (age >2 yo); optimal dose unclear.

FORMS - Trade only: Tabs, delayed release (Depakote, divalproex sodium) 125, 250, 500 mg. Tabs, extended release (Depakote ER) 250, 500 mg. Caps, sprinkle (Depakote) 125 mg. Generic/Trade: Syrup (Depakene, valproic acid) 250 mg/5 ml. Caps (Depakene) 250 mg.

NOTES - Contraindicated in urea cycle disorders or hepatic dysfunction. Usual therapeutic trough = 50-100 mcg/ml. Depakote and Depakote ER are not interchangeable. Depakote ER is ~10% less bioavailable than Depakote. Depakote releases divalproex sodium over 8-12h (qd-qid dosing); Depakote ER releases divalproex sodium over 18-24h (qd dosing). Many drug interactions. Patients receiving other anticonvulsants may require higher doses of valproic acid. Reduce dose in the elderly. Hyperammonemia, GI irritation, or thrombocytopenia may occur.

zonisamide (*Zonegran*) ▶LK ♀C ▶? $$$$
ADULT - Partial seizures, adjunctive: Start 100 mg PO qd. Increase to 200 mg PO qd after two weeks. May increase q2 weeks prn to 300-400 mg qd (or divided bid). Max 600 mg/day.
PEDS - Not approved in children.

FORMS - Trade: Caps 25, 50, 100 mg.
NOTES - This is a sulfonamide; avoid in those allergic. Fatalities and severe reactions including Stevens-Johnson syndrome, toxic epidermal necrolysis, fulminant hepatic necrosis, and blood dyscrasias have occurred with sulfonamides. Clearance is affected by CYP3A4 inhibitors or inducers such as phenytoin, carbamazepine, phenobarbital, and valproic acid. Nephrolithiasis may occur. Oligohidrosis and hyperthermia may occur, and are more common in children. Patients with renal disease may require slower dose titration.

DERMATOMES

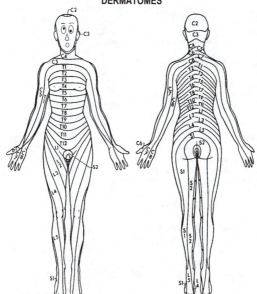

NEUROLOGY: Migraine Therapy – Triptans (5-HT1 Receptor Agonists)

NOTE: 5-HT1 agonists may cause vasospasm. Avoid use in ischemic or vasospastic heart disease, cerebrovascular syndromes, peripheral arterial disease, uncontrolled HTN, and hemiplegic or basilar migraine. Do not use within 24 hours of ergots or other triptans. Increased risk of serotonin syndrome if used with SSRIs.

almotriptan (*Axert*) ▶LK ♀C ▶? $
ADULT - Migraine treatment: 6.25-12.5 mg PO.
May repeat in 2 hours prn. Max 25 mg/day.
PEDS - Not approved in children.
FORMS - Trade: Tabs 6.25, 12.5 mg.
NOTES - MAOIs inhibit almotriptan metabolism; use together only with extreme caution. Use lower doses (6.25 mg) in renal and/or hepatic dysfunction.

eletriptan (*Relpax*) ▶LK ♀C ▶? $
ADULT - Migraine treatment: 20-40 mg PO at

onset. May repeat in >2 hours prn. Max 40 mg/dose or 80 mg/day.

PEDS - Not approved in children.

FORMS - Trade: Tabs 20 mg, 40 mg

NOTES - Do not use within 72 hours of potent CYP3A4 inhibitors such as ketoconazole, itraconazole, nefazodone, troleandomycin, clarithromycin, ritonavir, or nelfinavir.

frovatriptan (*Frova*) ▶LK ♀C ▶? $

ADULT - Migraine treatment: 2.5 mg PO. May repeat in 2 hours prn. Max 7.5 mg/24 hours.

PEDS - Not approved in children.

FORMS - Trade: Tabs 2.5 mg.

naratriptan (*Amerge*) ▶KL ♀C ▶? $$

ADULT - Migraine treatment: 1-2.5 mg PO. May repeat in 4 hours prn. Max 5 mg/24 hours.

PEDS - Not approved in children.

FORMS - Trade: Tabs 1, 2.5 mg.

NOTES - Contraindicated in severe renal or hepatic impairment.

rizatriptan (*Maxalt, Maxalt MLT*) ▶LK ♀C ▶? $$

ADULT - Migraine treatment: 5-10 mg PO; May repeat in 2 hours prn. Max 30 mg/24 hours.

PEDS - Not approved in children.

FORMS - Trade: Tabs 5, 10 mg. Orally disintegrating tabs (MLT) 5, 10 mg.

NOTES - Should not be combined with MAOIs. MLT form dissolves on tongue without liquids.

sumatriptan (*Imitrex*) ▶K ♀C ▶+ $$

ADULT - Migraine treatment: 6 mg SC. May repeat after 1 hour prn. Max 12 mg/24 hours.

Tablets: 25-50 mg PO. May repeat q2h prn with 25-100 mg doses. Max 200 mg/24 hours. Intranasal spray: 5-20 mg. May repeat q2h prn. Max 40 mg/24 hours. Cluster headache treatment: 6 mg SC. May repeat in >1h prn. Max 12 mg/24 hours. Consider starting oral dosing with 50 mg, since this appears to be more effective than 25 mg. Tablets may be used q2h prn if HA returns after initial SC injection to max 100 mg/24 hours.

PEDS - Not approved in children.

FORMS - Trade: Tabs 25, 50, 100 mg. Nasal spray 5, 20 mg/ spray. Injection 6 mg/0.5 ml.

NOTES - Should not be combined with MAOIs. Avoid IM/IV route.

zolmitriptan (*Zomig, Zomig ZMT*) ▶L ♀C ▶? $$

ADULT - Migraine treatment: Tabs: 1.25-2.5 mg PO q2h. Max 10 mg/24 hours. Orally disintegrating tabs (ZMT): 2.5 mg PO. May repeat in 2 hours prn. Max 10 mg/24 hours. Nasal spray: 5 mg (1 spray) in one nostril. May repeat in 2 hours prn. Max 10 mg/24 hours.

PEDS - Not approved in children.

FORMS - Trade: Tabs 2.5, 5 mg. Orally disintegrating tabs $$$ (ZMT) 2.5, 5 mg. Nasal spray 5 mg/spray.

NOTES - Risk of vasospastic complications. Should not be combined with MAOIs. Use lower doses (<2.5 mg) in hepatic dysfunction. May break 2.5 mg tabs in half.

NEUROLOGY: Migraine Therapy – Other

***Cafergot* (ergotamine + caffeine)** ▶L ♀X▶- $

WARNING - Contraindicated with concomitant use of potent CYP 3A4 inhibitors (e.g., macrolides, protease inhibitors) due to risk of serious / life-threatening peripheral ischemia. Ergots have been associated with potentially life-threatening fibrotic complications.

ADULT - Migraine and cluster headache treatment: 2 tabs PO at onset, then 1 tab q30 minutes prn to max 6 tabs/attack or 10 tabs/week. Suppositories: 1 suppository PR at onset; may repeat in 1 hour prn. Max 2 suppositories/attack or 5/week.

PEDS - Not approved in children.

UNAPPROVED PEDS - Migraine treatment: 1 tab PO at onset, then 1 tab q 30 minutes prn to max 3 tabs/attack.

FORMS - Trade: Tabs 1 mg ergotamine/100 mg caffeine. The tablet form of this product is available as Wigraine. Suppositories 2 mg ergotamine/100 mg caffeine.

NOTES - Contraindicated in sepsis, CAD, peripheral arterial disease, HTN, impaired hepatic or renal function, malnutrition, severe pruritus.

dihydroergotamine (*D.H.E. 45, Migranal*) ▶L ♀X ▶- $$

WARNING - Contraindicated with concomitant use of potent CYP 3A4 inhibitors (e.g., macrolides, protease inhibitors) due to risk of serious / life-threatening peripheral ischemia. Ergots have been associated with potentially life-threatening fibrotic complications.

ADULT - Migraine treatment: Solution (DHE 45): 1 mg IV/IM/SC; may repeat q1h prn to max of 2 mg (IV) or 3 mg (IM/SC) per 24 hours. Nasal spray (Migranal): 1 spray (0.5 mg) in each nostril; may repeat in 15 min prn to max 6 sprays (3 mg)/ 24 hours or 8 sprays (4 mg)/week.

PEDS - Not approved in children.

FORMS - Trade: Nasal spray 0.5 mg/spray.

Self-injecting solution: 1 mg/ml.

NOTES - Contraindicated in basilar or hemiplegic migraine, sepsis, ischemic or vasospastic cardiac disease, peripheral vascular disease, vascular surgery, impaired hepatic or renal function, or uncontrolled HTN. Avoid concurrent ergotamine, methysergide, or triptan use.

Excedrin Migraine **(acetaminophen + aspirin + caffeine)** ▶LK ♀D ▶? $

ADULT - Migraine treatment: 2 tabs PO q6h. Max 8 tabs/day.

PEDS - Not approved in children.

FORMS - OTC/Generic/Trade: Tabs acetaminophen 250 mg/ aspirin 250 mg/ caffeine 65 mg.

NOTES - Avoid concomitant use of other acetaminophen-containing products.

flunarizine (✚ *Sibelium***)** ▶L ♀C ▶- $$

ADULT - Canada only. Migraine prophylaxis: 10 mg PO qhs. If side effects, then 5 mg qhs. Safety of long-term use (>4 months) has not been established.

PEDS - Not approved in children.

FORMS - Generic/Trade: Caps 5 mg

NOTES - Gradual onset of benefit, over 6-8 weeks. Not for acute therapy. Contraindicated if history of depression or extrapyramidal disorders.

Midrin **(isometheptene + dichloralphenazone + acetaminophen)** ▶L ♀? ▶? ©IV $

ADULT - Tension and vascular headache treatment: 1-2 caps PO q4h, to max of 8 caps/day. Migraine treatment: 2 caps PO x 1, then 1 cap q1h prn to max of 5 caps/12 hours.

PEDS - Not approved in children.

FORMS - Generic/Trade: Caps 65 mg isometheptene/100 mg dichloralphenazone/325 mg acetaminophen.

NOTES - FDA has classified Midrin as "possibly" effective for migraine treatment. Contraindicated in glaucoma, severe renal disease, heart disease, hepatic disease, or concurrent MAOI use. Use caution in HTN, peripheral arterial disease, or recent MI.

rofecoxib (*Vioxx***)** ▶Plasma ♀C (D in 3rd trimester) ▶? $$$

ADULT - Migraine treatment: Start 25 mg PO qd. Max 50 mg PO qd. Avoid chronic daily use. See entry in analgesics section for other uses.

PEDS - Not approved in children.

FORMS - Trade: Tabs 12.5, 25 & 50 mg. Suspension 12.5 mg/5 ml and 25 mg/5ml.

NOTES - Contraindicated in aspirin-sensitive asthma. Use caution in hepatic or renal dysfunction, dehydration, or peptic ulcer disease. Reduce dose in hepatic dysfunction. Drug interactions with warfarin, theophylline, and rifampin – may need to adjust dosing. May diminish the antihypertensive effects of ACE inhibitors. Not a sulfonamide – may be used in sulfa allergy. Use of 50 mg >5 days/month for migraine treatment has not been studied.

valproic acid (*Depakene, Depakote, Depakote ER***, ✚***Epiject, Epival, Deproic***)** ▶L ♀D ▶+ $$

WARNING - Fatal hepatic failure has occurred; monitor LFTs during first 6 months. Life-threatening cases of pancreatitis have been reported after initial or prolonged use. Evaluate for abdominal pain, N/V, and/or anorexia. Discontinue if pancreatitis is diagnosed.

ADULT - Migraine prophylaxis: Start 250 mg PO bid (Depakote), or 500 mg PO qd (Depakote ER) x 1 week, then 1,000 mg/day PO given bid (Depakote) or qd (Depakote ER). Max 1,000 mg/day.

PEDS - Not approved for migraine prophylaxis.

FORMS - Trade: Tabs, delayed release (Depakote) 125, 250, 500 mg. Tabs, extended release (Depakote ER) 500 mg. Caps, sprinkle (Depakote) 125 mg. Generic/Trade: Syrup (Depakene) 250 mg/ 5 ml. Caps (Depakene) 250 mg.

NOTES - Contraindicated in hepatic dysfunction & urea cycle disorders. Many drug interactions. Reduce dose in elderly. Hyperammonemia, GI irritation, or thrombocytopenia may occur. Depakene (valproic acid), Depakote (divalproex sodium).

NEUROLOGY: Multiple Sclerosis

glatiramer (*Copaxone***)** ▶Serum ♀B ▶? $$$$$

ADULT - Multiple sclerosis (relapsing-remitting): 20 mg SC qd.

PEDS - Not approved in children.

FORMS - Trade: Injection 20 mg single dose vial.

NOTES - Do not inject IV.

interferon beta-1A (*Avonex, Rebif***)** ▶L ♀C ▶? $$$$$

ADULT - Multiple sclerosis (relapsing forms): Avonex- 30 mcg (6 million units) IM q week. Rebif- start 8.8 mcg SC three times weekly; titrate over 4 weeks to maintenance dose of 44 mcg three times weekly over 4 weeks.

PEDS - Not approved in children.

FORMS - Trade: Avonex: Injection 33 mcg (6.6

million units) single dose vial. Rebif: Starter kit 20 or 44 mcg pre-filled syringes.

NOTES - Use caution in patients with depression, seizure disorders, or cardiac disease. Follow LFTs and CBC. Avonex: indicated for the first attack of MS. Rebif: give same dose 3 days each week, with at least 48 hours between doses.

interferon beta-1B (Betaseron) ▶L ♀C ▶? $$$$$

ADULT - Multiple sclerosis (relapsing-remitting): Start 0.0625 mg SC qod; titrate over six weeks to 0.25 mg (8 million units) SC qod.

PEDS - Not approved in children.

FORMS - Trade: Injection 0.3 mg (9.6 million units) single dose vial.

NOTES - Use caution in patients with depression. Product can be stored at room temp until reconstituted, then refrigerate and use within 3 hours.

NEUROLOGY: Parkinsonian Agents – Anticholinergics

benztropine mesylate (Cogentin, ✦Bensylate) ▶LK ♀C ▶? $

ADULT - Parkinsonism: 0.5- 2 mg/day PO/IM/IV. Increase in 0.5 mg increments at weekly intervals to max 6 mg/day. May divide doses qd-qid. Drug-induced extrapyramidal disorders: 1-4 mg PO/IM/IV qd-bid.

PEDS - Not approved in children.

UNAPPROVED PEDS - Parkinsonism (>3 yo): 0.02-0.05 mg/kg/dose qd-bid. Use caution; potential for undesired anticholinergic effects.

FORMS - Generic/Trade: Tabs 0.5, 1, 2 mg.

NOTES - Contraindicated in narrow-angle glaucoma.

biperiden (Akineton) ▶LK ♀C ▶? $$

ADULT - Parkinsonism: 2 mg PO tid-qid. Titrate to max of 16 mg/day. Drug-induced extrapyramidal disorders: 2 mg PO qd-tid to max of 8 mg/24 hours.

PEDS - Not approved in children.

FORMS - Trade: Tabs 2 mg

NOTES - Contraindicated in narrow angle glaucoma, bowel obstruction, and megacolon.

procyclidine (Kemadrin) ▶LK ♀C ▶? $$$

ADULT - Parkinsonism: Start 2.5-5 mg PO tid; may add qhs dose. Usual max 20 mg/day. Drug-induced extrapyramidal side effects: 2.5-5 mg PO tid.

PEDS - Not approved in children.

FORMS - Trade: Tabs 5 mg.

NOTES - Contraindicated in narrow angle glaucoma.

trihexyphenidyl (Artane) ▶LK ♀C ▶? $

ADULT - Parkinsonism: 1 mg PO qd. Increase by 2 mg/day at 3-5 day intervals to max 6-10 mg/day. Divide doses tid with meals. Max 15 mg/day.

PEDS - Not approved in children.

FORMS - Generic/Trade: Tabs 2, 5 mg. Elixir 2 mg/ 5 ml.

NEUROLOGY: Parkinsonian Agents – COMT Inhibitors

entacapone (Comtan) ▶L ♀C ▶? $$$$

ADULT - Parkinsonism, adjunctive: Start 200 mg PO with each dose of carbidopa/levodopa. Max 8 tabs/day (1,600 mg).

PEDS - Not approved in children.

FORMS - Trade: Tabs 200 mg.

NOTES - Adjunct to carbidopa/levodopa in patients who have end-of-dose "wearing off." Has no antiparkinsonian effect on its own. Avoid concomitant use of non-selective MAOIs. Use caution in hepatobiliary dysfunction. Avoid rapid withdrawal, which may precipitate neuroleptic malignant syndrome.

tolcapone (Tasmar) ▶LK ♀C ▶? $$$$

WARNING - Fatal hepatic failure has occurred. Use only in patients on carbidopa-levodopa who fail alternative therapies and provide written informed consent. Monitor LFTs at baseline

and q2 weeks. Discontinue if LFT elevation or if no clinical benefit after 3 weeks of therapy.

ADULT - Parkinsonism, adjunctive: Start 100 mg PO tid. Increase to 200 mg PO tid only if expected benefit is justified. Max 600 mg/day. Must be taken concurrently with carbidopa/levodopa.

PEDS - Not approved in children.

FORMS - Trade: Tabs 100, 200 mg.

NOTES - Adjunct to carbidopa-levodopa in patients who have refractory end-of-dose "wearing off." Has no antiparkinsonian effect on its own. Contraindicated in hepatic dysfunction. Monitor LFTs. Avoid concomitant use of non-selective MAOIs. Avoid rapid withdrawal, which may precipitate neuroleptic malignant syndrome. Informed consent forms are available from the manufacturer (www.tasmar.com).

NEUROLOGY: Parkinsonian Agents – Dopaminergic Agents & Combinations

NOTE: Dopaminergic medications may cause hallucinations, particularly when used in combination. Avoid rapid discontinuation, which may precipitate neuroleptic malignant syndrome.

amantadine (*Symmetrel*, ♣*Endantadine*) ▶K ♀C ▶- $

ADULT - Parkinsonism: 100 mg PO bid. Max 400 mg/day. Drug-induced extrapyramidal disorders: 100 mg PO bid. Max 300 mg/day.

PEDS - See antimicrobials section for influenza use. No approved neuro indications in children.

FORMS - Trade only: Tabs 100 mg. Generic: Caps 100 mg. Generic/Trade: Syrup 50 mg/5 ml.

NOTES - Decrease dose in CHF, peripheral edema, orthostatic hypotension, impaired renal function, seizure disorders, or age >65 years.

apomorphine (*Apokyn*) ▶L ♀C ▶? ?

WARNING - Never administer IV due to risk of severe adverse effects including pulmonary embolism.

ADULT - Acute, intermittent treatment of hypomobility ("off episodes") in Parkinson's disease: Start 0.2 ml SC prn. May increase dose by 0.1 ml every few days as tolerated. Max 0.6 ml/dose or 2 ml/day. Monitor for orthostatic hypotension after initial dose and with dose escalation. Potent emetic - pretreat with trimethobenzamide 300 mg PO tid (or domperidone 20 mg PO tid) starting three days prior to use; continue this for ≥2 months before weaning.

PEDS - Not approved in children.

FORMS - Trade only: Cartridges (for injector pen, 10 mg/ml) 3 ml. Ampules (10 mg/ml) 2 ml.

NOTES - Write doses exclusively in ml rather than mg to avoid errors. Most effective when administered at (or just prior to) the onset of an "off" episode. Avoid concomitant use of 5HT3 antagonists (eg, ondansetron, granisetron, dolasetron, palonosetron, alosetron), which may precipitate severe hypotension and loss of consciousness. Inform patients that the dosing pen is labeled in ml (not mg), and that it is possible to dial in a dose of medication even if the cartridge does not contain sufficient drug. Rotate injection sites. Restart at 0.2 ml/day if treatment is interrupted for ≥1 week. Adjust dosing in hepatic impairment. Reduce starting dose to 0.1 ml in patients with mild or moderate renal failure. Contains sulfites; avoid in sulfa allergy.

bromocriptine (*Parlodel*) ▶L ♀B ▶- $$$$

ADULT - Parkinson's disease: Start 1.25 mg PO bid. Increase by 2.5 mg/day q14-28 days to usual effective dose of 10- 40 mg/day. Max 100 mg/day.

PEDS - Not approved in children.

UNAPPROVED ADULT - Neuroleptic malignant syndrome: 2.5- 5 mg PO 2-6 times/day.

FORMS - Generic/Trade: Tabs 2.5 mg. Caps 5 mg.

NOTES - Adverse effects include N/V, dizziness, hypotension, and erythromelalgia. Take with food to minimize dizziness and nausea. Ergots have been associated with potentially life-threatening fibrotic complications.

carbidopa (*Lodosyn*) ▶LK ♀C ▶? $$$

ADULT - Parkinson's Disease, adjunct to carbidopa/levodopa: start 25 mg PO qd with first daily dose of carbidopa/levodopa. May give an additional 12.5 mg (with later doses of carbidopa/levodopa 10/100 mg) or 12.5-25 mg (with later doses of carbidopa/levodopa 25/100 or 25/250 mg) as needed. Max 200 mg/day.

PEDS - Not approved in children.

FORMS - Trade: Tabs 25 mg.

NOTES - Adjunct to carbidopa/levodopa to reduce peripheral side-effects such as nausea and orthostatic hypotension. Also increases the CNS availability of levodopa. Reduce the dosage of levodopa and monitor for CNS side-effects such as dyskinesias and hallucinations when initiating therapy.

carbidopa-levodopa (*Atamet, Sinemet, Sinemet CR*) ▶L ♀C ▶- $$$

ADULT - Parkinsonism: Standard release: start 1 tab (25/100 mg; alternatively 10/100 mg) PO tid. Increase by 1 tab/day q 1-2 days prn. Use 1 tab (25/250 mg) PO tid-qid when higher levodopa doses are needed. Sustained release: Start 1 tab (50/200 mg) PO bid; separate doses by ≥4 hrs. Increase as needed at intervals ≥3 days. Typical max dose is 1,600-2,000 mg/day of levodopa.

PEDS - Not approved in children.

UNAPPROVED ADULT - Restless legs syndrome: start 1/2 tab (25/100 mg) PO qhs; increase q3-4d to max of 50/200 mg (two 25/100 tabs) qhs. If symptoms recur during the night, then a combination of standard release (25/100 mg, 1-2 tabs qhs) and sustained release (25/100 or 50/200 mg qhs) tablets may be used.

FORMS - Generic/Trade: Tabs (carbidopa/levodopa) 10/100, 25/100, 25/250 mg. Tabs, sustained release (Sinemet CR, carbidopa-levodopa ER) 25/100, 50/200 mg.

NOTES - Motor fluctuations and dyskinesias may occur. Provide at least 70-100 mg/day carbidopa to reduce the risk of N/V. Extended release formulations have a lower bioavailability than conventional preparations. Do not use within two weeks of a nonselective MAOI. When used for restless legs syndrome, may precipitate rebound (recurrence of symptoms during the night) or augmentation (earlier daily onset of symptoms).

pergolide (*Permax*) ▶K ♀B ▶? $$$$$

ADULT - Parkinsonism: Start 0.05 mg PO qd x 2 days. Increase by 0.1-0.15 mg/day q3 days x 12 days. After that, increase by 0.25 mg/day q3 days to response. Usual effective dose is 1 mg tid. Max 5 mg/day.

PEDS - Not approved in children.

UNAPPROVED ADULT - Restless legs syndrome: 0.025 mg PO qd (taken 2 hours before bedtime) or bid (taken in the late afternoon and 1 hour before bedtime). Increase to max 0.5 mg/day in divided doses.

FORMS - Generic/Trade: Tabs 0.05, 0.25, 1 mg.

NOTES - Sleep attacks, syncope, and/or hypotension may occur. Titrate slowly. Ergots have been associated with potentially life-threatening fibrotic complications.

pramipexole (*Mirapex*) ▶K ♀C ▶? $$$$

ADULT - Parkinsonism: Start 0.125 mg PO tid x 1 week, then 0.25 mg x 1 week; after that, increase by 0.75 mg/week divided tid. Usual effective dose is 0.5-1.5 mg PO tid.

PEDS - Not approved in children.

UNAPPROVED ADULT - Restless legs syndrome: start 0.125 mg PO qhs. Increase q7d to max 1.5 mg/day divided bid-tid.

FORMS - Trade: Tabs 0.125,0.25,0.5,1,1.5 mg.

NOTES - Decrease dose in renal impairment. Sleep attacks, syncope, and/or hypotension may occur. Titrate slowly.

ropinirole (*Requip*) ▶L ♀C ▶? $$$

ADULT - Parkinsonism: Start 0.25 mg PO tid. Increase by 0.25 mg/dose at weekly intervals

to 1 mg PO tid. Max 24 mg/day.

PEDS - Not approved in children.

UNAPPROVED ADULT - Restless legs syndrome (limited data): Start 0.25 mg PO qhs and gradually increase as needed. Max 3 mg/day divided bid-tid.

FORMS - Trade: Tabs 0.25, 0.5, 1, 2, 4, 5 mg.

NOTES - Sleep attacks, syncope, and/or hypotension may occur. Titrate slowly.

selegiline (*Eldepryl, Atapryl, Carbex, Selpak*) ▶LK ♀C ▶? $$$

ADULT - Parkinsonism: 5 mg PO q am and q noon. Max 10 mg/day.

PEDS - Not approved in children.

FORMS - Generic/Trade: Caps 5 mg. Tabs 5 mg.

NOTES - Adjunct to carbidopa/levodopa. Should not be used in combination with meperidine or other opioids. Do not exceed max recommended dose; risk of non-selective MAO inhibition.

***Stalevo* (carbidopa + levodopa + entacapone) ▶L ♀C ▶- $$$$**

ADULT - Parkinson's disease (conversion from carbidopa-levodopa +/- entacapone): Start Stalevo tablet that contains the same amount of carbidopa-levodopa. Titrate to desired response. May need to lower the dose of levodopa in patients not already taking entacapone. Max dose 1,600 mg/day of entacapone or 1,600-2,000 mg/day of levodopa.

PEDS - Not approved in children.

FORMS - Trade: Tabs (carbidopa/levodopa/entacapone): 12.5/50/200 mg, 25/100/200 mg, 37.5/150/200 mg.

NOTES - Patients who are not currently taking entacapone may benefit from titration of the individual components of this medication before conversion to this fixed-dose preparation. Avoid concomitant use of non-selective MAOIs. Use caution in hepatobiliary dysfunction. Motor fluctuations and dyskinesias may occur. Should not be used in patients with undiagnosed skin lesions or a history of melanoma.

NEUROLOGY: Other Agents

***Aggrenox* (aspirin + dipyridamole) ▶LK ♀D ▶? $$$**

ADULT - Stroke risk reduction: one cap PO bid.

PEDS - Not approved in children.

FORMS - Trade: Caps 25 mg aspirin/ 200 mg extended-release dipyridamole.

alteplase (*tpa, t-PA, Activase*, ✚*Activase rt-PA*) ▶L ♀C ▶? $$$$$

ADULT - Acute ischemic stroke within 3 hours of symptom onset: 0.9 mg/kg (max 90 mg). Give 10% of total dose as an IV bolus over 1 minute, and the remainder as an IV infusion over 60 minutes.

PEDS - Not approved in children.

NOTES - Multiple important exclusion criteria.

dexamethasone (*Decadron*, ✚*Dexasone*)

▶L ♀C ▶- $$$

ADULT - Cerebral edema: 10-20 mg IV/IM load, then 4 mg IV/IM q6h or 1-3 mg PO tid.

PEDS - Not approved in children.

UNAPPROVED ADULT - Cerebral edema: 1-2 mg/kg PO/IV/IM load, followed by 1-1.5 mg/kg/day divided q4-6h; max 16 mg/day. Bacterial meningitis (controversial): 0.15 mg/kg IV q6h x 2-4 days; start 10-15 minutes before the first dose of antibiotic.

UNAPPROVED PEDS - Bacterial meningitis (controversial): 0.15 mg/kg IV q6h x 2-4 days; start 10-15 minutes before the first dose of antibiotic.

FORMS - Generic/Trade: Tabs 0.25, 0.5, 0.75, 1.0, 1.5, 2, 4, 6 mg. Elixir/ solution 0.5 mg/5 ml. Trade only: Solution concentrate 0.5 mg/ 0.5 ml (Intensol)

NOTES - Contraindicated in systemic fungal infections. Adjust dose with concomitant use of CYP 3A4 inhibitors such as ketoconazole and macrolide antibiotics. Avoid prolonged use in children due to risk of bone growth retardation.

edrophonium (Tensilon, Enlon, Reversol) ▶Plasma ♀C ▶? $

ADULT - Evaluation for myasthenia gravis: 2 mg IV over 15-30 seconds (test dose), then 8 mg IV after 45 seconds. Reversal of neuromuscular blockade: 10 mg IV over 30-45 seconds; repeat prn to max 40 mg.

PEDS - Evaluation for myasthenia gravis, weight ≤34 kg: 1 mg IV (test dose), then 1 mg IV q30-45 seconds to max 5 mg. Weight >34 kg: 2 mg IV (test dose), then 2 mg IV q30- 45 seconds to max 10 mg.

UNAPPROVED ADULT - Reversal of non-depolarizing neuromuscular blocking agents: 0.5-1.0 mg/kg IV together with atropine 0.007-0.014 mg/kg.

NOTES - Not for maintenance therapy of myasthenia gravis because of short duration of action (5-10 minutes). May give IM. Monitor cardiac function. Atropine should be readily available in case of cholinergic reaction. Contraindicated in mechanical urinary or intestinal obstruction. Effective for reversal of neuromuscular blockade by curare, tubocurarine, gallamine triethiodide, or dimethyl-tubocurarine only.

mannitol (Osmitrol, Resectisol) ▶K ♀C ▶? $$$

ADULT - Intracranial HTN: 0.25-2 g/kg IV over 30-60 minutes as a 15, 20, or 25% solution.

PEDS - Not approved in children.

UNAPPROVED ADULT - Increased ICP/Head trauma: 0.25-1 g/kg IV push over 20 minutes.

Repeat q4-6h prn.

UNAPPROVED PEDS - Increased ICP/Cerebral edema: 0.25-1 g/kg/dose IV push over 20-30 minutes, then 0.25-0.5 g/kg/dose IV q4-6h prn.

NOTES - Monitor fluid and electrolyte balance and cardiac function. Filter IV solutions with concentrations ≥20%; crystals may be present.

meclizine (Antivert, Bonine, Medivert, Meclicot, Meni-D, ✦Bonamine) ▶L ♀B ▶? $

ADULT - Motion sickness: 25-50 mg PO 1 hour prior to travel, then 25-50 mg PO qd.

PEDS - Not approved in children.

UNAPPROVED ADULT - Vertigo: 25 mg PO qd-qid prn.

FORMS - Rx/OTC/Generic/Trade: Tabs 12.5, 25 mg. Chew tabs 25 mg. Rx/Trade only: Tabs 30, 50 mg. Caps 25 mg.

NOTES - FDA classifies meclizine as "possibly effective" for vertigo. May cause dizziness and drowsiness.

methylprednisolone (Solu-Medrol, Medrol, Depo-Medrol) ▶L ♀C ▶- $$$$$

ADULT - Multiple sclerosis flare: 200 mg PO/IV qd x 1 week followed by 80 mg PO qd x 1 month.

PEDS - Not approved in children.

UNAPPROVED ADULT - Optic neuritis: 1 g IV daily (or in divided doses) x 3 days, then PO prednisone 1 mg/kg/day x 11 days (followed by a 3-day taper). Multiple sclerosis flare: 1 g IV daily (or in divided doses) x 3-5 days. May follow with PO prednisone 1 mg/kg/day for 14 days, then taper off. Spinal cord injury: 30 mg/kg IV over 15 minutes, followed in 45 minutes by 5.4 mg/kg/h IV infusion for 23 hours (if initiated within 3 hours of injury) or for 47 hours (if initiated 3-8h after injury).

UNAPPROVED PEDS - Spinal cord injury: 30 mg/kg IV over 15 minutes, followed in 45 minutes by 5.4 mg/kg/hour IV infusion x 23 hours.

NOTES - Other dosing regimens have been used for MS and optic neuritis. Avoid initial treatment of optic neuritis with oral steroids, as it may increase the risk of new episodes.

neostigmine (Prostigmin) ▶L ♀C ▶? $$$

ADULT - Myasthenia gravis: 15-375 mg/day PO in divided doses, or 0.5 mg IM/SC when oral therapy is not possible. Reversal of non-depolarizing neuromuscular blocking agents: 0.5-2.0 mg slow IV (preceded by atropine 0.6-1.2 mg or glycopyrrolate 0.2-0.6 mg); repeat prn to max 5 mg.

PEDS - Not approved in children.

UNAPPROVED PEDS - Myasthenia gravis: 7.5-15 mg PO tid-qid; or 0.03 mg/kg IM q2-4h. Re-

versal of non-depolarizing neuromuscular blocking agents: 0.025-0.08 mg/kg/dose slow IV, preceded by either atropine (0.4 mg for each mg of neostigmine) or glycopyrrolate (0.2 mg for each mg of neostigmine).
FORMS - Trade: Tabs 15 mg.
NOTES - Oral route preferred when possible.

nimodipine (*Nimotop*) ▶L ♀C ▶- $$$$$
ADULT - Subarachnoid hemorrhage: 60 mg PO q4h for 21 days.
PEDS - Not approved in children.
FORMS - Trade: Caps 30 mg.
NOTES - Begin therapy within 96 hours. Give 1 hour before or 2 hours after meals. May give cap contents SL or via NG tube. Decrease dose in hepatic dysfunction.

oxybate (*Xyrem, GHB, gamma hydroxybutyrate*) ▶L ♀B ▶? ©III $$$$$
WARNING - CNS depressant with abuse potential; avoid concurrent alcohol or sedative use.
ADULT - Cataplexy associated with narcolepsy: 2.25 g PO qhs. Repeat in 2.5-4 hours. May increase by 1.5 g/day at >2 week intervals to max 9 g/day. Dilute each dose in 60 ml water.
PEDS - Not approved in children.
FORMS - Trade: Solution 180 ml (500 mg/ml) supplied with measuring device and child-proof dosing cups.
NOTES - Available only through the Xyrem Success Program centralized pharmacy (1-866-

997-3688). Adjust dose in hepatic dysfunction. Prepare doses just prior to bedtime, and use within 24 hours. May need an alarm to signal second dose.

pyridostigmine (*Mestinon, Regonal*) ▶Plasma, K ♀C ▶+ $$$
ADULT - Myasthenia gravis: Start 60 mg PO tid. Gradually increase to usual dose of 200 mg PO tid. Or give 180 mg PO qd-bid (extended release). Max 1,500 mg/day. May give 2 mg IM or slow IV injection q2-3h.
PEDS - Not approved in children.
UNAPPROVED PEDS - Myasthenia gravis, neonates: 5 mg PO q4-6h or 0.05- 0.15 mg/kg IM/IV q4-6h. Myasthenia gravis, children: 7 mg/kg/day PO in 5-6 divided doses, or 0.05-0.15 mg/kg/dose IM/IV q4-6h. Max 10 mg IM/IV single dose.
FORMS - Trade: Tabs 60 mg. Extended release tabs 180 mg. Syrup 60 mg/5 ml.
NOTES - Give injection at 1/30th of oral dose when oral therapy is not possible.

riluzole (*Rilutek*) ▶LK ♀C ▶- $$$$$
ADULT - Amyotrophic lateral sclerosis: 50 mg PO q12h.
PEDS - Not approved in children.
FORMS - Trade: Tabs 50 mg.
NOTES - Take 1 hour before or 2 hours after meals. Monitor LFTs.

OB/GYN: Estrogens

NOTE: See also Vaginal Preparations, Hormone Replacement Combinations. Unopposed estrogens increase the risk of endometrial cancer in postmenopausal women. Malignancy should be ruled out in cases of persistent or recurrent abnormal vaginal bleeding. In women with an intact uterus, a progestin may be administered daily throughout the month or for the last 10-12 days of the month. Do not use during pregnancy. May increase the risk of DVT/PE, gallbladder disease. Interactions with oral anticoagulants, certain anticonvulsants, rifampin, barbiturates, corticosteroids & St. John's wort. Estrogens should not be used in the prevention of cardiovascular disease. In the Women's Health Initiative, the use of conjugated estrogens (Premarin) caused an increase in the risk of CVA & PE. Additionally, the combination with medroxyprogesterone increased the risk of breast cancer and MI. Estrogens should be prescribed at the lowest effective doses and for the shortest durations. Patients should be counseled regarding the risks/benefits of HRT.

esterified estrogens (*Menest*) ▶L ♀X ▶- $
ADULT - Moderate to severe menopausal vasomotor symptoms: 1.25 mg PO qd. Atrophic vaginitis: 0.3 to 1.25 mg PO qd. Female hypogonadism: 2.5 - 7.5 mg PO qd in divided doses for 20 days followed by a 10-day rest period. Repeat until bleeding occurs. Bilateral oophorectomy & ovarian failure: 1.25 mg PO qd. Prevention of postmenopausal osteoporosis: 0.3 - 1.25 mg PO qd.
PEDS - Not approved in children.
FORMS - Trade: Tabs 0.3, 0.625, 1.25, 2.5 mg.
NOTES - Typical HRT regimen consists of a daily estrogen dose with a progestin added either daily or for the last 10-12 cycle days.

estradiol (*Estrace, Estradiol, Gynodiol*) ▶L ♀X ▶- $
ADULT - Moderate to severe menopausal vasomotor symptoms & atrophic vaginitis, female hypogonadism, bilateral oophorectomy & ovarian failure: 1-2 mg PO qd. Prevention of postmenopausal osteoporosis: 0.5 mg PO qd.

PEDS - Not approved in children.

FORMS - Generic/Trade: Tabs, micronized 0.5, 1, 2 mg, scored. Trade only: 1.5 mg (Gynodiol).

NOTES - Typical HRT regimen consists of a daily estrogen dose with a progestin added either daily or for the last 10-12 cycle days.

estradiol cypionate (*Depo-Estradiol*) ▶L ♀X ▶- $

ADULT - Moderate to severe menopausal vasomotor symptoms: 1-5 mg IM q3-4 weeks. Female hypogonadism: 1.5-2 mg IM q month.

PEDS - Not approved in children.

estradiol gel (*Estrogel*) ▶L ♀X ▶- $

ADULT - Moderate to severe menopausal vasomotor symptoms & atrophic vaginitis: Thinly apply contents of one complete pump depression or applicatorful (1.25 g) to one entire arm, from wrist to shoulder. Allow to dry completely before dressing. Wash both hands thoroughly after application.

PEDS - Not approved in children.

FORMS - Trade: Gel 0.06% in non-aerosol, metered-dose pump with 64 1.25 g doses or in tube, 80 g (64 doses) with applicator.

NOTES - Depress the pump twice to prime. Typical HRT regimen consists of a daily estrogen dose with a progestin added either daily or for the last 10-12 days of the cycle.

estradiol topical emulsion (*Estrasorb*) ▶L ♀X ▶- $$

ADULT - Moderate to severe menopausal vasomotor symptoms: Apply entire contents of one pouch each to left and right legs (spread over thighs & calves) qam. Rub for 3 minutes until entirely absorbed. Allow to dry completely before dressing. Wash both hands thoroughly after application. Daily dose=two 1.74 g pouches.

PEDS - Not approved in children.

FORMS - Trade: Topical emulsion, 56 pouches/carton.

NOTES - Typical HRT regimen consists of a daily estrogen dose with a progestin added either daily or for the last 10-12 cycle days. Concomitant sunscreen may increase absorption.

estradiol transdermal system (*Alora, Climara, Esclim, Estraderm, FemPatch, Menostar, Vivelle, Vivelle Dot, ✚Estradot, Oesclim*) ▶L ♀X ▶- $$

ADULT - Moderate to severe menopausal vasomotor symptoms & atrophic vaginitis, female hypogonadism, bilateral oophorectomy & primary ovarian failure: initiate with 0.025 - 0.05 mg/day patch once or twice weekly, depending on the product (see FORMS). Prevention of postmenopausal osteoporosis: 0.025-0.1 mg/day patch.

PEDS - Not approved in children.

FORMS - Trade: Transdermal patches doses in mg/day: Climara (q week) 0.025,0.0375, 0.05, 0.06, 0.075, 0.1. FemPatch (q week) 0.025. Esclim (twice/week) 0.025, 0.0375, 0.05, 0.075, 0.1. Vivelle, Vivelle Dot (twice/week) 0.025, 0.0375, 0.05, 0.075, 0.1. Estraderm (twice/week) 0.05, & 0.1. Alora (twice/week) 0.025, 0.05, 0.075, 0.1. Generic: Estradiol transdermal patches: (q week) 0.05 & 0.1.

NOTES - Rotate application sites, avoid the waistline. Transdermal may be preferable if high triglycerides & chronic liver disease.

estradiol valerate (*Delestrogen*) ▶L ♀X ▶- $

ADULT - Moderate to severe menopausal vasomotor symptoms & atrophic vaginitis: 10-20 mg IM q4 weeks. Female hypogonadism, bilateral oophorectomy & ovarian failure: 10-20 mg IM q4 weeks.

PEDS - Not approved in children.

estrogens conjugated (*Premarin, C.E.S., Congest*) ▶L ♀X ▶- $$

ADULT - Moderate to severe menopausal vasomotor symptoms, atrophic vaginitis, & urethritis: 0.3-1.25 mg PO qd. Female hypogonadism: 2.5-7.5 mg PO qd in divided doses x 20 days, followed by a 10-day rest period. Bilateral oophorectomy & premature ovarian failure: 1.25 mg PO qd. Prevention of postmenopausal osteoporosis: 0.625 mg PO qd. Abnormal uterine bleeding: 25 mg IV/IM. Repeat in 6-12 hours if needed.

PEDS - Not approved in children.

UNAPPROVED ADULT - Prevention of postmenopausal osteoporosis: 0.3 mg PO qd. Normalizing bleeding time in patients with AV malformations or underlying renal impairment: 30-70 mg IV/PO qd until bleeding time normalized.

FORMS - Trade: Tabs 0.3, 0.45, 0.625, 0.9, 1.25, 2.5 mg.

NOTES - Typical HRT regimen consists of a daily estrogen dose with a progestin either daily or for the last 10-12 days of the cycle.

estrogens synthetic conjugated A (*Cenestin*) ▶L ♀X ▶- $$

ADULT - Moderate to severe menopausal vasomotor symptoms: 0.3-1.25 mg PO qd.

PEDS - Not approved in children.

FORMS - Trade: Tabs 0.3, 0.45, 0.625, 0.9, 1.25 mg.

NOTES - Typical HRT regimen consists of a daily estrogen dose with a progestin either daily or for the last 10-12 cycle days. The difference between synthetic conjugated estrogens A and B is the additional component of delta-8,9-dehydroestrone sulfate in the B prep. The clinical significance of this is unknown.

estrogens synthetic conjugated B (Enjuvia) ▶L ♀X ▶- $$

ADULT - Moderate to severe menopausal vasomotor symptoms: 0.625-1.25 mg PO qd.

PEDS - Not approved in children.

FORMS - Trade: Tabs 0.625 & 1.25 mg.

NOTES - Typical HRT regimen consists of a daily estrogen dose with a progestin either daily or for the last 10-12 cycle days. The difference between synthetic conjugated estrogens A and B is the additional component of delta-

8,9-dehydroestrone sulfate in the B prep. The clinical significance of this is unknown.

estropipate (Ogen, Ortho-Est) ▶L ♀X ▶- $

ADULT - Moderate to severe menopausal vasomotor symptoms, vulvar & vaginal atrophy: 0.625-5 mg PO qd. Female hypogonadism, bilateral oophorectomy, or ovarian failure: 1.25-7.5 mg PO qd. Prevention of osteoporosis: 0.625 mg PO qd.

PEDS - Not approved in children.

FORMS - Generic/Trade: Tabs 0.625, 1.25, 2.5, 5 mg.

NOTES - Typical HRT regimen consists of a daily estrogen dose with a progestin either daily or for the last 10-12 days of the cycle.

OB/GYN: GnRH Agents

NOTE: Anaphylaxis has occurred with synthetic GnRH agents.

cetrorelix acetate (Cetrotide) ▶Plasma ♀X ▶- $$$$$

ADULT - Infertility: Multiple dose regimen: 0.25 mg SC qd during the early to mid follicular phase. Continue treatment qd until the day of hCG administration. Single dose regimen: 3 mg SC x 1 usually on stimulation day 7.

PEDS - Not approved in children.

FORMS - Trade: Injection 0.25 mg in 1 & 7-dose kits. 3 mg in 1 dose kit.

NOTES - Best sites for SC self-injection are on the abdomen around the navel. Storage in original carton: 0.25 mg refrigerated (36-46F); 3 mg room temperature (77F). Contraindicated with severe renal impairment.

ganirelix (Follistim-Antagon Kit, ✦Orgalutran) ▶Plasma ♀X ▶? $$$$$

ADULT - Infertility: 250 mcg SC qd during the early to mid follicular phase. Continue treatment qd until the day of hCG administration.

PEDS - Not approved in children.

FORMS - Trade: Injection 250 mcg/0.5 ml in pre-filled, disposable syringes with 3 vials follitropin beta.

NOTES - Best sites for SC self-injection are on the abdomen around the navel or upper thigh. Store at room temperature (77F) for up to 3 months. Protect from light. Packaging contains natural rubber latex which may cause allergic reactions.

goserelin (Zoladex) ▶LK ♀X ▶- $$$$$

ADULT - Endometriosis: 3.6 mg implant SC q 28 days or 10.8 mg implant q12 weeks x 6 months. Palliative treatment of breast cancer: 3.6 mg implant SC q28 days indefinitely. En-

dometrial thinning prior to ablation for dysfunctional uterine bleeding: 3.6 mg SC 4 weeks prior to surgery or 3.6 mg SC q4 weeks x 2 with surgery 2-4 weeks after last dose.

PEDS - Not approved in children.

NOTES - Transient increases in symptoms may occur with initiation of therapy in patients with breast cancer. Hypercalcemia may occur in patients with bone metastases. Vaginal bleeding may occur during the first 2 months of treatment & should stop spontaneously. Reliable contraception is recommended.

leuprolide (Lupron, Lupron Depot) ▶L ♀X ▶- $$$$$

ADULT - Endometriosis or uterine leiomyomata (fibroids): 3.75 mg IM q month or 11.25 mg IM q3 months for total therapy of 6 months (endometriosis) or 3 months (fibroids). Administer concurrent iron for fibroid-associated anemia.

PEDS - Central precocious puberty: Injection: 50 mcg/kg/day SC. Increase by 10 mcg/kg/day until total down regulation. Depot-Ped: 0.3 mg/kg q4 weeks IM (minimum dose 7.5 mg). Increase by 3.75 mg q4 weeks until adequate down regulation.

NOTES - A fractional dose of the 3-month depot preparation is not equivalent to the same dose of the monthly formulation. Rotate the injection site periodically.

nafarelin (Synarel) ▶L ♀X ▶- $$$$$

ADULT - Endometriosis: 200 mcg spray into one nostril q am & the other nostril q pm. May be increased to one 200 mcg spray into each nostril bid. Duration of treatment: 6 months.

PEDS - Central precocious puberty: 2 sprays into each nostril bid for a total of 1600 mcg/day. May be increased to 1800 mcg/day.

Allow 30 seconds to elapse between sprays. FORMS - Trade: Nasal soln 2 mg/ml in 8 ml bottle (200 mcg per spray) about 80 sprays/bottle. NOTES - Ovarian cysts have occurred in the first 2 months of therapy. Symptoms of hypoestrogenism may occur. Elevations of phosphorus & eosinophils, and decreases in serum calcium & WBC counts have been documented.

DRUGS GENERALLY ACCEPTED AS SAFE IN PREGNANCY (selected)

Analgesics: acetaminophen, codeine*, meperidine*, methadone*. Antimicrobials: penicillins, cephalosporins, erythromycins (not estolate), azithromycin, nystatin, clotrimazole, metronidazole**, nitrofurantoin***, Nix. Antivirals: acyclovir, valacyclovir, famciclovir. CV: labetalol, methyldopa, hydralazine. Derm: erythromycin, clindamycin, benzoyl peroxide. Endo: insulin, liothyronine, levothyroxine. ENT: chlorpheniramine, diphenhydramine, dimenhydrinate, dextromethorphan, guaifenesin, nasal steroids, nasal cromolyn. GI: trimethobenzamide, antacids*, simethicone, cimetidine, famotidine, ranitidine, nizatidine, psyllium, metoclopramide, bisacodyl, docusate, doxylamine, meclizine. Psych: fluoxetine****, desipramine, doxepin. Pulmonary: short-acting inhaled beta-2 agonists, cromolyn, nedocromil, beclomethasone, budesonide, theophylline, prednisone**. Other - heparin.

*Except if used long-term or in high does at term **Except 1st trimester.
***Contraindicated at term and during labor and delivery. ****Except 3rd trimester.

OB/GYN: Hormone Replacement Combinations

NOTE: See also vaginal preparations and estrogens. Unopposed estrogens increase the risk of endometrial cancer in postmenopausal women. Malignancy should be ruled out in cases of persistent or recurrent abnormal vaginal bleeding. Do not use during pregnancy. May increase the risk of DVT/PE, gallbladder disease. Interactions with oral anticoagulants, phenytoin, rifampin, barbiturates, corticosteroids and St. John's wort. For preparations containing testosterone derivatives, observe women for signs of virilization and lipid abnormalities. In the Women's Health Initiative, the combination of conjugated estrogens and medroxyprogesterone (PremPro) caused an increase in the risk of breast cancer, MI, CVA, & DVT/PE and did not improve overall quality of life. Estrogen/progestin combinations should be prescribed at the lowest effective doses and for the shortest durations. Patients should be counseled regarding the risks/benefits of HRT.

Activella (estradiol + norethindrone) ▶L ♀X ▶- $$
ADULT - Moderate to severe menopausal vasomotor symptoms, vulvar & vaginal atrophy, prevention of postmenopausal osteoporosis: 1 tab PO qd.
PEDS - Not approved in children.
FORMS - Trade: Tab 1 mg estradiol/0.5 mg norethindrone acetate in calendar dial pack dispenser.

Climara Pro (estradiol + levonorgestrel) ▶L ♀X ▶- $$
ADULT - Moderate to severe menopausal vasomotor symptoms: 1 patch weekly.
PEDS - Not approved in children.
FORMS - Trade: Transdermal patch 0.045 estradiol/ 0.015 levonorgestrel in mg/day, 4 patches/box.
NOTES - Rotate application sites; avoid the waistline.

CombiPatch (estradiol + norethindrone, ✦*Estalis*) ▶L ♀X ▶- $$
ADULT - Moderate to severe menopausal vasomotor symptoms, vulvar & vaginal atrophy, female hypogonadism, bilateral oophorectomy, & ovarian failure, prevention of postmenopausal osteoporosis: 1 patch twice weekly.
PEDS - Not approved in children.
FORMS - Trade: Transdermal patch 0.05 estradiol/ 0.14 norethindrone & 0.05 estradiol/0.25 norethindrone in mg/day, 8 patches/box.
NOTES - Rotate application sites, avoid the waistline.

Estratest (esterified estrogens + methyltestosterone) ▶L ♀X ▶- $$
ADULT - Moderate to severe menopausal vasomotor symptoms: 1 tab PO qd.
PEDS - Not approved in children.
UNAPPROVED ADULT - Menopause-associated decrease in libido: 1 tab PO qd.
FORMS - Trade: Tabs 1.25 mg esterified estrogens / 2.5 mg methyltestosterone.
NOTES - Monitor LFTs and lipids.

***Estratest H.S.* (esterified estrogens + methyltestosterone)** ▶L ♀X ▶- $$

ADULT - Moderate to severe menopausal vasomotor symptoms: 1 tab PO qd.

PEDS - Not approved in children.

UNAPPROVED ADULT - Menopause-associated decrease in libido: 1 tab PO qd.

FORMS - Trade: Tabs 0.625 mg esterified estrogens / 1.25 mg methyltestosterone.

NOTES - HS = half-strength. Monitor LFTs and lipids.

FemHRT **(ethinyl estradiol + norethindrone)** ▶L ♀X ▶- $$

ADULT - Moderate to severe menopausal vasomotor symptoms, prevention of postmenopausal osteoporosis: 1 tab PO qd.

PEDS - Not approved in children.

FORMS - Trade: Tabs 5 mcg ethinyl estradiol / 1 mg norethindrone, 28/blister card.

Prefest **(estradiol + norgestimate)** ▶L ♀X ▶- $$

ADULT - Moderate to severe menopausal vasomotor symptoms, vulvar atrophy, atrophic vaginitis, prevention of postmenopausal osteoporosis: 1 pink tab PO qd x 3 days followed by 1 white tab PO qd x 3 days, sequentially throughout the month.

PEDS - Not approved in children.

FORMS - Trade: Tabs in 30-day blister packs 1 mg estradiol (15 pink) & 1 mg estadiol/0.09 mg norgestimate (15 white).

Premphase **(estrogens conjugated + medroxyprogesterone)** ▶L ♀X ▶- $$

ADULT - Moderate to severe menopausal vasomotor symptoms, vulvar/vaginal atrophy, & prevention of postmenopausal osteoporosis: 0.625 mg conjugated estrogens PO qd days 1-14 & 0.625 mg conjugated estrogens/5 mg medroxyprogesterone PO qd days 15-28.

PEDS - Not approved in children.

FORMS - Trade: Tabs in 28-day EZ-Dial dispensers: 0.625 mg conjugated estrogens (14) & 0.625 mg/5 mg conjugated estrogens/medroxyprogesterone (14).

Prempro **(estrogens conjugated + medroxyprogesterone, ♣*PremPlus*)** ▶L ♀X ▶- $$

WARNING - In the Women's Health Initiative, this combination caused an increase in the risk of breast cancer, MI, CVA, & DVT/PE. Estrogen/progestin combinations should be prescribed at the lowest effective doses and for the shortest durations. Patients should be counseled regarding the risks/benefits of HRT.

ADULT - Moderate to severe menopausal vasomotor symptoms, vulvar/vaginal atrophy, & prevention of postmenopausal osteoporosis: 1 PO qd.

PEDS - Not approved in children.

FORMS - Trade: Tabs in 28-day EZ-Dial dispensers: 0.625 mg/5 mg, 0.625 mg/2.5 mg, 0.45 mg/1.5 mg, or 0.3 mg/1.5 mg conjugated estrogens/medroxyprogesterone.

NOTES - Three strengths available, specify dose on Rx.

***Syntest D.S.* (esterified estrogens + methyltestosterone)** ▶L ♀X ▶- $$

ADULT - Moderate to severe menopausal vasomotor symptoms: 1 tab PO qd.

PEDS - Not approved in children.

UNAPPROVED ADULT - Menopause-associated decrease in libido: 1 tab PO qd.

FORMS - Trade: Tabs 1.25 mg esterified estrogens/2.5 mg methyltestosterone.

NOTES - Monitor LFTs and lipids.

***Syntest H.S.* (esterified estrogens + methyltestosterone)** ▶L ♀X ▶- $$

ADULT - Moderate to severe menopausal vasomotor symptoms: 1 tab PO qd.

PEDS - Not approved in children.

UNAPPROVED ADULT - Menopause-associated decrease in libido: 1 tab PO qd.

FORMS - Trade: Tabs 0.625 mg esterified estrogens/1.25 mg methyltestosterone.

NOTES - HS = half-strength. Monitor LFTs and lipids.

EMERGENCY CONTRACEPTION within 72 hours of unprotected sex: Take first dose ASAP, then identical dose 12h later. Each dose is either 2 pills of *Ovral* or *Ogestrel*, 4 pills of *Cryselle, Levlen, Levora, Lo/Ovral, Nordette, Tri-Levlen*, Triphasil*, Trivora*,* or *Low Ogestrel*, or 5 pills of *Alesse, Aviane, Lessina,* or *Levlite*. If vomiting occurs within 1 hour of taking either dose of medication, consider whether or not to repeat that dose and give an antiemetic 1h prior. *Preven* kit includes patient info booklet, urine pregnancy test, & blister pack of 4 tablets containing levonorgestrel 0.25mg & ethinyl estradiol 0.05mg. Each dose is 2 pills. *Plan B* kit contains two levonorgestrel 0.75mg tablets. Each dose is 1 pill. The progestin-only method causes less nausea & may be more effective. See www.not-2-late.com.
*Use 0.125 mg levonorgestrel/30 mcg ethinyl estradiol tabs.

ORAL CONTRACEPTIVES* ▶L ♀X *Monophasic*	Estrogen (mcg)	Progestin (mg)
Norinyl 1+50, Ortho-Novum 1/50, Necon 1/50	50 mestranol	1 norethindrone
Ovcon-50	50 ethinyl estradiol	
Demulen 1/50, Zovia 1/50E		1 ethynodiol
Ovral, Ogestrel		0.5 norgestrel
Norinyl 1+35, Ortho-Novum 1/35, Necon 1/35, Nortrel 1/35	35 ethinyl estradiol	1 norethindrone
Brevicon, Modicon, Necon 0.5/35, Nortrel 0.5/35		0.5 norethindrone
Ovcon-35		0.4 norethindrone
Previfem		0.18 norgestimate
Ortho-Cyclen, MonoNessa, Sprintec-28		0.25 norgestimate
Demulen 1/35, Zovia 1/35E		1 ethynodiol
Loestrin 21 1.5/30, Loestrin Fe 1.5/30, Junel 1.5/30, Junel 1.5/30 Fe, Microgestin 1.5/30	30 ethinyl estradiol	1.5 norethindrone
Cryselle, Lo/Ovral, Low-Ogestrel		0.3 norgestrel
Apri, Desogen, Ortho-Cept		0.15 desogestrel
Levlen, Levora, Nordette, Portia		0.15 levonorgestrel
Yasmin		3 drospirenone
Loestrin 21 1/20, Loestrin Fe 1/20, Junel 1/20, Junel Fe 1/20, Microgestin Fe 1/20	20 ethinyl estradiol	1 norethindrone
Alesse, Aviane, Lessina, Levlite		0.1 levonorgestrel
Progestin-only		
Micronor, Nor-Q.D., Camila, Errin, Jolivette, Nora-BE	none	0.35 norethindrone
Ovrette		0.075 norgestrel
Biphasic (estrogen & progestin contents vary)		
Kariva, Mircette	20/10 eth estrad	0.15/0 desogestrel
Ortho Novum 10/11, Necon 10/11	35 eth estradiol	0.5/1 norethindrone
Triphasic (estrogen & progestin contents vary)		
Cyclessa, Velivet	25 ethinyl estradiol	0.100/0.125/0.150 desogestrel
Ortho-Novum 7/7/7, Necon 7/7/7, Nortrel 7/7/7	35 ethinyl estradiol	0.5/0.75/1 norethindr
Tri-Norinyl		0.5/1/0.5 norethindr
Enpresse, Tri-Levlen, Triphasil, Trivora-28	30/40/30 ethinyl estradiol	0.5/0.75/0.125 levonorgestrel
Ortho Tri-Cyclen, Trinessa, Tri-Sprintec, Tri-Previfem	35 eth estradiol	0.18/0.215/0.25
Ortho Tri-Cyclen Lo	25 eth estradiol	norgestimate
Estrostep Fe	20/30/35 eth estr	1 norethindrone

*All: Not recommended in smokers. Increase risk of thromboembolism, stroke, MI, hepatic neoplasia & gallbladder disease. Nausea, breast tenderness, & breakthrough bleeding are common transient side effects. Effectiveness reduced by hepatic enzyme-inducing drugs such as certain anticonvulsants and barbiturates,rifampin, rifabutin, griseofulvin, & protease inhibitors. Coadministration with antibiotics or St. John's wort may decrease efficacy. Consider an additional form of birth control in above circumstances. See product insert for instructions on missing doses. Most available in 21 and 28 day packs. **Progestin only**: Must be taken at the same time every day. Because much of the literature regarding adverse effects associated with oral contraceptives pertains mainly to combination products containing estrogen and progestins, the extent to which progestin-only contraceptives cause these effects is unclear. No significant interaction has been found with broad-spectrum antibiotics. The effect of St. John's wort is unclear. No placebo days, start new pack immediately after finishing current one. Available in 28 day packs. Readers may find the following site useful: www.managingcontraception.com.

OB/GYN: Labor Induction / Cervical Ripening

NOTE: Fetal well-being should be documented prior to use.

dinoprostone (*PGE2, Prepidil, Cervidil, ✦Prostin E2*) ▶Lung ♀C ▶? $$$$

ADULT - Cervical ripening: Gel - one syringe via catheter placed into cervical canal below the internal os. May be repeated q6h to a max of 3 doses. Vaginal insert: place in posterior fornix.

PEDS - Not approved in children.

FORMS - Trade: Gel (Prepidil) 0.5 mg/3 g syringe. Vaginal insert (Cervidil) 10 mg.

NOTES - Patient should remain supine for 15 - 30 minutes after gel and 2 h after vaginal insert. For hospital use only. Monitor for uterine hyperstimulation & abnormal fetal heart rate. Caution with asthma or glaucoma. Contraindicated in prior C-section or major uterine surgery due to potential for uterine rupture.

misoprostol (*PGE1, Cytotec*) ▶LK ♀X ▶- $

WARNING - Contraindicated in desired early or preterm pregnancy due to its abortifacient property. Pregnant women should avoid contact/exposure to tabs. Uterine rupture reported with use for labor induction & medical abortion.

ADULT - Prevention of NSAID- (including aspirin) induced gastric ulcers.

PEDS - Not approved in children.

UNAPPROVED ADULT - Cervical ripening & labor induction: 25 mcg intravaginally q3-6h (or 50 mcg q6h). Medical abortion ≤49 days gestation: w/ mifepristone, see mifepristone; w/

methotrexate: 800 mcg intravaginally 5-7 days after 50 mg/m^2 PO or IM methotrexate. Preop cervical ripening in 1st trimester: 400 mcg intravaginally 3-4h before suction curettage. Missed abortion: 200 mcg q4h or 800 mcg x 1 intravaginally. Post-partum hemorrhage: 800 mcg PR x 1.

FORMS - Generic/Trade: Oral tabs 100 & 200 mcg.

NOTES - Contraindicated with prior C-section. Oral tabs can be inserted into the vagina for labor induction/cervical ripening. Monitor for uterine hyperstimulation & abnormal fetal heart rate. Risk factors for uterine rupture: prior uterine surgery & ≥5 previous pregnancies.

oxytocin (*Pitocin*) ▶LK ♀? ▶- $

WARNING - Not approved for elective labor induction, although widely used.

ADULT - Induction/stimulation of labor: 10 units in 1000 ml NS, 1-2 milliunits/min IV as a continuous infusion (6-12 mU/hr). Increase in increments of 1-2 milliunits/min q30 minutes until a contraction pattern is established, up to a max of 20 milliunits/min.

PEDS - Not approved in children.

NOTES - Use a pump to accurately control the infusion while patient is under continuous observation. Continuous fetal monitoring is required. Concurrent sympathomimetics may result in postpartum hypertension. Anaphylaxis and severe water intoxication have occurred.

OB/GYN: Ovulation Stimulants

NOTE: Potentially serious adverse effects include DVT/PE, ovarian hyperstimulation syndrome, adnexal torsion, ovarian enlargement & cysts, & febrile reactions.

choriogonadotropin alfa (*hCG, Ovidrel*) ▶L ♀X ▶? $$$

ADULT - Specialized dosing for ovulation induction.

PEDS - Not approved in children.

FORMS - Trade: Powder for injection or, pre-filled syringe 250 mcg.

NOTES - Best site for SC self-injection is on the abdomen below the navel. Beware of multiple pregnancy & multiple adverse effects. Store in original package & protect from light. Use immediately after reconstitution.

chorionic gonadotropin (*hCG, Pregnyl, Profasi*) ▶L ♀X ▶? $$

ADULT - Specialized dosing for ovulation induction.

PEDS - Not approved in children.

NOTES - Beware of multiple pregnancy & multiple adverse effects. For IM use only.

clomiphene (*Clomid, Serophene*) ▶L ♀D ▶? $$

ADULT - Specialized dosing for infertility.

PEDS - Not approved in children.

FORMS - Generic/Trade: Tabs 50 mg, scored.

NOTES - Beware of multiple pregnancy & multiple adverse effects.

follitropin alpha (*FSH, Gonal-F, Gonal-F RFF Pen*) ▶L ♀X ▶? $$$$$

ADULT - Specialized dosing for infertility.

PEDS - Not approved in children.

FORMS - Trade: Powder for injection, 37.5 IU, 75 IU, & 150 IU FSH activity. 450 & 1200 IU multi-dose vial. Pre-filled, multiple-dose pen, 300 IU, 450 IU, & 900 IU FSH activity with single-use disposable needles.

NOTES - Best site for SC self-injection is on the abdomen below the navel. Beware of multiple gestation pregnancy & multiple adverse effects. Store in original package & protect from light. Use immediately after reconstitution. Pen may be stored at room temperature for up to 1 month or expiration, whichever is first.

follintropin beta (FSH, Follistim, Follistim AQ) ►L ♀X ►? $$$$$

ADULT - Specialized dosing for infertility.

PEDS - Not approved in children.

FORMS - Trade: Powder for injection, 75 IU FSH activity. Cartridge, for use with the Follistim Pen, 300 IU & 600 IU.

NOTES - Best site for SC self-injection is on the abdomen below the navel. Beware of multiple pregnancy & multiple adverse effects. Store in original package & protect from light. Use powder for injection immediately after reconstitution. Cartridge may be stored for up to 28 days.

gonadotropins (menotropins, Pergonal, Repronex, FSH/LH, ✤Propasi HP) ►L ♀X ►? $$$$$

ADULT - Specialized dosing for infertility.

PEDS - Not approved in children.

FORMS - Trade: Powder or pellet for injection, 75 IU & 150 IU FSH activity.

NOTES - Best site for SC self-injection is on the abdomen below the navel. Beware of multiple pregnancy & numerous adverse effects. Use immediately after reconstitution.

urofollintropin (Bravelle, FSH, Fertinex) ►L ♀X ►? $$$$$

ADULT - Specialized dosing for infertility & polycystic ovary syndrome.

PEDS - Not approved in children.

FORMS - Trade: Powder or pellet for injection, 75 IU & 150 IU (FSH, Fertinex only) FSH activity.

NOTES - Best site for SC self-injection is on the abdomen below the navel. Beware of multiple pregnancy & numerous adverse effects. Use immediately after reconstitution.

OB/GYN: Progestins

NOTE: Do not use in pregnancy. DVT, PE, cerebrovascular disorders, & retinal thrombosis may occur. Effectiveness may be reduced by hepatic enzyme-inducing drugs such as certain anticonvulsants and barbiturates, rifampin, rifabutin, griseofulvin & protease inhibitors. The effects of St. John's wort-containing products on progestin only pills is currently unknown. In the Women's Health Initiative, the combination of conjugated estrogens and medroxyprogesterone (PremPro) caused a statistically significant increase in the risk of breast cancer, MI, CVA, & DVT/PE. Estrogen/progestin combinations should be prescribed at the lowest effective doses and for the shortest durations. Patients should be counseled regarding the risks/benefits of HRT.

hydroxyprogesterone caproate ►L ♀X ►? $

ADULT - Amenorrhea, dysfunctional uterine bleeding, metrorrhagia: 375 mg IM. Production of secretory endometrium and desquamation: 125-250 mg IM on 10th day of the cycle, repeat q7days until suppression no longer desired.

PEDS - Not approved in children.

UNAPPROVED ADULT - Endometrial hyperplasia: 500 mg IM weekly.

medroxyprogesterone (Provera, Amen) ►L ♀X ►+ $

WARNING - In the Women's Health Initiative,

the combination of conjugated estrogens and medroxyprogesterone (PremPro) caused a statistically significant increase in the risk of breast cancer, MI, CVA, & DVT/PE. Estrogen/progestin combinations should be prescribed at the lowest effective doses and for the shortest durations. Patients should be counseled regarding the risks/benefits of HRT.

ADULT - Secondary amenorrhea: 5-10 mg PO qd x 5-10 days. Abnormal uterine bleeding: 5-10 mg PO qd x 5-10 days beginning on the 16th or 21st day of the cycle (after estrogen priming). Withdrawal bleeding usually occurs 3-7 days after therapy ends.

PEDS - Not approved in children.

UNAPPROVED ADULT - Add to estrogen replacement therapy to prevent endometrial hyperplasia: 10 mg PO qd for 10-12 days of month, or 2.5-5 mg PO qd daily. Endometrial hyperplasia: 10-30 mg PO qd (long-term); 40-100 mg PO qd (short-term) or 500 mg IM twice/week.

FORMS - Generic/Trade: Tabs 2.5, 5, & 10 mg, scored.

NOTES - Breakthrough bleeding/spotting may occur. Amenorrhea usually after 6 months of continuous dosing.

medroxyprogesterone, injectable (Depo-Provera) ►L ♀X ►+ $$

ADULT - Contraception: 150 mg IM in deltoid or gluteus maximus q13 weeks.

PEDS - Not approved in children.

UNAPPROVED ADULT - Dysfunctional uterine bleeding: 150 mg IM in deltoid or gluteus maximus q13 weeks.

NOTES - Breakthrough bleeding/spotting may occur. Amenorrhea usually after 6 months. Weight gain is common. To be sure that the patient is not pregnant give this injection only during the first 5 days after the onset of a normal menstrual period or after a negative pregnancy test. May be given immediately post-pregnancy termination as well as postpartum, including breastfeeding women. May be given as often as 11 weeks apart. If the time between injections is >14 weeks, exclude pregnancy before administering. Bone loss may occur with prolonged administration.

megestrol (*Megace*) ▶L ♀D ▶? $$$$$

ADULT - AIDS anorexia: 800 mg (20 ml) suspension PO qd. Palliative treatment of advanced carcinoma of the breast: 40 mg (tabs) PO qid. Endometrial carcinoma: 40-320 mg/day (tabs) in divided doses.

PEDS - Not approved in children.

UNAPPROVED ADULT - Endometrial hyperplasia: 40-160 mg PO qd x 3-4 months. Cancer-associated anorexia/cachexia: 80-160 mg PO qid.

FORMS - Generic/Trade: Tabs 20 & 40 mg. Suspension 40 mg/ml in 237 ml.

NOTES - In HIV-infected women, breakthrough bleeding/spotting may occur.

norethindrone (*Aygestin*) ▶L ♀D ▶? $

ADULT - Amenorrhea, abnormal uterine bleeding: 2.5-10 mg PO qd x 5-10 days during the second half of the menstrual cycle. Endometriosis: 5 mg PO qd x 2 weeks. Increase by 2.5 mg q 2 weeks to 15 mg/day.

PEDS - Not approved in children.

FORMS - Generic/trade: Tabs 5 mg, scored.

progesterone in oil ▶L ♀X ▶? $

WARNING - Contraindicated in peanut allergy since some products contain peanut oil.

ADULT - Amenorrhea, uterine bleeding: 5-10 mg IM qd for 6-8 days.

PEDS - Not approved in children.

progesterone micronized (*Prometrium*) ▶L ♀B ▶+ $

WARNING - Contraindicated in patients allergic to peanuts since caps contain peanut oil.

ADULT - Hormone replacement therapy to prevent endometrial hyperplasia: 200 mg PO qhs 10-12 days per month. Secondary amenorrhea: 400 mg PO qhs x 10 days.

PEDS - Not approved in children.

UNAPPROVED ADULT - Hormone replacement therapy to prevent endometrial hyperplasia: 100 mg qhs daily.

FORMS - Trade: Caps 100 & 200 mg.

NOTES - Breast tenderness, dizziness, headache & abdominal cramping may occur.

OB/GYN: Selective Estrogen Receptor Modulators

raloxifene (*Evista*) ▶L ♀X ▶- $$$

WARNING - Do not use during pregnancy.

ADULT - Osteoporosis prevention/treatment: 60 mg PO qd.

PEDS - Not approved in children.

UNAPPROVED ADULT - Breast cancer prevention: 60-120 mg PO qd.

FORMS - Trade: Tabs 60 mg.

NOTES - Interactions with oral anticoagulants & cholestyramine. May increase risk of DVT/PE. Does not decrease (and may increase) hot

flashes. Leg cramps.

tamoxifen (*Nolvadex, Tamone*) ▶L ♀D ▶- $$$

WARNING - Uterine malignancies, CVA & PE, sometimes fatal. Do not use during pregnancy.

ADULT - Breast cancer prevention in high-risk women: 20 mg PO qd x 5 years.

PEDS - Not approved in children.

FORMS - Generic/Trade: Tabs 10 & 20 mg.

NOTES - Interacts with oral anticoagulants. Does not decrease hot flashes.

OB/GYN: Tocolytics

NOTE: Although tocolytics may prolong pregnancy, they have not been shown to improve perinatal or neonatal outcomes & can have adverse effects on women in preterm labor.

indomethacin (*Indocin, Indocid*) ▶L ♀? ▶- $

WARNING - Premature closure of the ductus arteriosus & fetal pulmonary hypertension have been reported. Oligohydramnios has been observed. There tends to be a higher rate of postpartum hemorrhage in women treated with

indomethacin for tocolysis.
ADULT - See analgesics section
PEDS - Not approved in children.
UNAPPROVED ADULT - Preterm labor: initial 50-100 mg PO/PR followed by 25 mg PO/PR q6-12h up to 48 hrs.
FORMS - Generic/Trade: Immediate release caps 25 & 50 mg. Trade: Oral suspension 25 mg/5 ml. Suppositories 50 mg.
NOTES - May be effective for stopping premature labor and delaying delivery, but conflicting data concerning the potential for complications in the mother and fetus may limit usage.

magnesium sulfate ▶K ♀A ▶+ $$
ADULT - Seizure prevention in pre-eclampsia or eclampsia: 4-6 g IV over 30 min, then 2 g IV per hour. 5 g in 250 ml D5W (20 mg/ml), 2 g = 100 ml/h. 4-5 g of a 50% soln IM q4h prn.
PEDS - Not approved in children.
UNAPPROVED ADULT - Premature labor: 6 g IV over 20 minutes, then 1-3 g/h titrated to decrease contractions.
NOTES - Concomitant use with terbutaline may lead to fatal pulmonary edema. Extreme caution in renal insufficiency. Hypermagnesemia may occur in the newborn if administered >24h. Watch for signs of magnesium intoxication including decreased respirations & reflexes. Symptomatic hypocalcemia has occurred. If needed, may reverse effects with calcium gluconate 1 g IV.

nifedipine (Procardia, Adalat, Procardia XL, Adalat CC, ♣Adalat XL) ▶L ♀C ▶+ $
WARNING - Excessive hypotension is possible.

ADULT - See cardiovascular section
PEDS - Not approved in children.
UNAPPROVED ADULT - Preterm labor: loading dose 10 mg PO q20-30 min if contractions persist up to 40 mg within the first hour. (SL or bite & swallow regimens result in SLIGHTLY earlier plasma concentrations but may cause more side effects). After contractions are controlled, maintenance dose: 10-20 mg PO q4-6h or 60-160 mg extended release PO qd. Duration of treatment has not been established.
FORMS - Generic/Trade: immediate release caps 10,20 mg. Ext'd release tab 30,60,90 mg.
NOTES - Vasodilation & flushing may occur frequently. Headache & nausea are possible, but usually transient. Hepatotoxicity has been reported and concomitant treatment with magnesium may result in neuromuscular blockade.

terbutaline (Brethine, Bricanyl) ▶L ♀B ▶+ $$$$$
ADULT - See pulmonary section
PEDS - Not approved in children.
UNAPPROVED ADULT - Preterm labor: 0.25 mg SC q30 min up to 1 mg in four hours. Infusion: 2.5-10 mcg/min IV, gradually increased to effective max doses of 17.5-30 mcg/min.
FORMS - Generic/Trade: Tabs 2.5, 5 mg (Brethine scored)
NOTES - Concomitant use with magnesium sulfate may lead to fatal pulmonary edema. Tachycardia, transient hyperglycemia, hypokalemia, arrhythmias, pulmonary edema, cerebral & cardiac ischemia & increased fetal heart rate may occur.

APGAR SCORE		0	1	2
	Heart rate	0. Absent	1. <100	2. >100
	Respirations	0. Absent	1. Slow/irreg	2. Good/crying
	Muscle tone	0. Limp	1. Some flexion	2. Active motion
	Reflex irritability	0. No response	1. Grimace	2. Cough/sneeze
	Color	0. Blue	1. Blue extremities	2. Pink

OB/GYN: Uterotonics

carboprost (Hemabate, 15-methyl-prostaglandin F2 alpha) ▶LK ♀C ▶? $$$
ADULT - Refractory postpartum uterine bleeding: 250 mcg deep IM. If necessary, may repeat at 15-90 minute intervals up to a total dose of 2 mg (8 doses).
PEDS - Not approved in children.
NOTES - Caution with asthma. Transient fever, HTN, nausea, bronchoconstriction & flushing. May augment oxytocics.

methylergonovine (Methergine) ▶LK ♀C ▶?

$
ADULT - To increase uterine contractions & decrease postpartum bleeding: 0.2 mg IM after delivery of the placenta, delivery of the anterior shoulder, or during the puerperium. Repeat q2-4h prn. 0.2 mg PO tid-qid in the puerperium for a max of 1 wk.
PEDS - Not approved in children.
FORMS - Trade: Tabs 0.2 mg.
NOTES - Contraindicated in pregnancy-induced hypertension/pre-eclampsia. Avoid IV route

due to risk of sudden HTN and stroke. If IV absolutely necessary, give slowly over no less than 1 min, monitor BP.

oxytocin (*Pitocin*) ▶LK ♀? ▶? $

WARNING - Not approved for elective labor induction, although widely used.

ADULT - Uterine contractions/postpartum bleed-

ing: 10 units IM after delivery of the placenta. 10-40 units in 1000 ml NS IV infusion, infuse 20-40 milliunits/minute.

PEDS - Not approved in children.

NOTES - Concurrent sympathomimetics may result in postpartum HTN. Anaphylaxis & severe water intoxication have occurred.

OB/GYN: Vaginal Preparations

NOTE: See also STD/vaginitis table in antimicrobial section. Many experts recommend 7 day antifungal therapy for pregnant women w/candida vaginitis. Many of these creams & suppositories are oil-based and may weaken latex condoms & diaphragms. Do not use latex products for 72 hrs after last dose.

boric acid ▶Not absorbed ♀? ▶- $

PEDS - Not approved in children.

UNAPPROVED ADULT - Resistant vulvovaginal candidiasis: 600 mg suppository intravaginally qhs x 2 weeks.

FORMS - No commercial preparation; must be compounded by pharmacist. Vaginal suppositories 600 mg in gelatin capsules.

NOTES - Reported use for azole-resistant non-albicans (C. glabrata) or recurrent albicans failing azole therapy. Do not use if abdominal pain, fever or foul-smelling vaginal discharge is present. Avoid vaginal intercourse during treatment.

butoconazole (*Gynazole, Mycelex-3*) ▶LK ♀C ▶? $(OTC)

ADULT - Local treatment of vulvovaginal candidiasis, nonpregnant patients: Mycelex 3: 1 applicatorful (~5g) intravaginally qhs x 3 days, up to 6 days, if necessary. Pregnant patients: (2nd & 3rd trimesters only) 1 applicatorful (~5g) intravaginally qhs x 6 days. Gynazole-1: 1 applicatorful (~5g) intravaginally qd x 1.

PEDS - Not approved in children.

FORMS - OTC: Trade (Mycelex 3): 2% vaginal cream in 5 g pre-filled applicators (3s) & 20 g tube with applicators. Rx: Trade (Gynazole-1): 2% vaginal cream in 5 g pre-filled applicator.

NOTES - Do not use if abdominal pain, fever or foul-smelling vaginal discharge is present. Since small amount may be absorbed from the vagina, use during the 1st trimester only when essential. During pregnancy, use of a vaginal applicator may be contraindicated & manual insertion may be preferred. Vulvar/vaginal burning may occur. Avoid vaginal intercourse during treatment.

clindamycin (*Cleocin, ♣Dalacin*) ▶L ♀- ▶+

$$

ADULT - Bacterial vaginosis: 1 applicatorful (~ 100 mg clindamycin phosphate in 5g cream) intravaginally qhs x 7 days, or one supp qhs x 3 days.

PEDS - Not approved in children.

FORMS - Trade: 2% vaginal cream in 40 g tube with 7 disposable applicators. Vag supp (Ovules) 100 mg (3) w/applicator.

NOTES - Not recommended during pregnancy despite B rating, as it does not prevent the adverse effects of bacterial vaginosis (eg, preterm birth, neonatal infection). Cervicitis, vaginitis, & vulvar irritation may occur. Avoid vaginal intercourse during treatment.

clotrimazole (*Mycelex 7, Gyne-Lotrimin, ♣Canesten, Clotrimaderm*) ▶LK ♀B ▶? $

ADULT - Local treatment of vulvovaginal candidiasis: 1 applicatorful 1% cream qhs x 7 days. 1 applicatorful 2% cream qhs x 3 days. 100 mg suppository intravaginally qhs x 7 days. 200 mg tablet qhs x 3 days. Topical cream for external symptoms bid x 7 days.

PEDS - Not approved in children.

FORMS - OTC: Generic/Trade: 1% vag cream with applicator (some pre-filled). 2% vaginal cream with applicator. Vaginal suppositories 100 mg (7) & 200 mg (3) with applicators. 1% topical cream in some combination packs.

NOTES - Do not use if abdominal pain, fever or foul-smelling vaginal discharge is present. Since small amounts of these drugs may be absorbed from the vagina, use during the 1st trimester only when essential. During pregnancy, use of a vaginal applicator may be contraindicated; manual insertion of tabs may be preferred. Skin rash, lower abdominal cramps, bloating, vulvar irritation may occur. Avoid vaginal intercourse during treatment.

estradiol acetate vaginal ring (*Femring*) ▶L ♀X ▶- $$

WARNING - Do not use during pregnancy. Unopposed estrogens increase the risk of endometrial cancer in postmenopausal women. Malignancy should be ruled out in cases of persis-

tent or recurrent abnormal vaginal bleeding. In women with an intact uterus, a progestin may be administered daily throughout the month or for the last 10-12 days of the month. In the Women's Health Initiative, the combination of conjugated estrogens and medroxyprogesterone (PremPro) caused an increase in the risk of breast cancer, MI, CVA, & DVT/PE. Estrogens should be prescribed at the lowest effective doses and for the shortest durations. Patients should be counseled regarding the risks/benefits of HRT.
ADULT - Menopausal atrophic vaginitis or vasomotor symptoms: insert ring into the vagina and replace after 90 days.
PEDS - Not approved in children.
FORMS - Trade: 0.05 mg/day and 0.1 mg/day.
NOTES - Should the ring fall out or be removed during the 90 day period, rinse in lukewarm water and re-insert.

estradiol vaginal ring (*Estring*) ▶L ♀X ▶- $$
WARNING - Do not use during pregnancy.
ADULT - Menopausal atrophic vaginitis: insert ring into upper 1/3 of the vaginal vault and replace after 90 days.
PEDS - Not approved in children.
FORMS - Trade: 2 mg ring single pack.
NOTES - Should the ring fall out or be removed during the 90 day period, rinse in lukewarm water and re-insert. Minimal systemic absorption, probable lower risk of adverse effects than systemic estrogens.

estradiol vaginal tab (*Vagifem*) ▶L ♀X ▶- $-$$
WARNING - Do not use during pregnancy.
ADULT - Menopausal atrophic vaginitis, initial: insert one tab vaginally qd x 2 weeks. Maintenance: one tab vaginally 2x/week.
PEDS - Not approved in children.
FORMS - Trade: Vaginal tab: 25 mcg in disposable single-use applicators, 8 & 18/pack.

estrogen cream (*Premarin, Estrace*) ▶L ♀X ▶? $$$$
WARNING - Unopposed estrogens increase the endometrial cancer risk in postmenopausal women. If an intact uterus, a progestin may be administered daily throughout the month or for the last 10-12 days of the month.
ADULT - Menopausal atrophic vaginitis: Premarin: 0.5-2 g intravaginally qd. Estrace: 2-4 g intravaginally qd for 1-2 weeks. Gradually reduce to a maintenance dose of 1 g 1-3 x/week.
PEDS - Not approved in children.
FORMS - Trade: Vaginal cream. Premarin: 0.625 mg conjugated estrogens/g in 42.5 g

with or w/o calibrated applicator. Estrace: 0.1 mg estradiol/g in 42.5 g w/calibrated applicator.
NOTES - Possibility of vaginal mucosa absorption. Uterine bleeding might be provoked by excessive use in menopausal women. Breast tenderness & vaginal discharge due to mucus hypersecretion may result from excessive estrogenic stimulation. Endometrial withdrawal bleeding may occur if use is discontinued.

metronidazole (*MetroGel-Vaginal*, ♣*Flagyl*) ▶LK ♀B ▶? $$$
ADULT - Bacterial vaginosis: 1 applicatorful (~ 5 g containing ~ 37.5 mg metronidazole) intravaginally qhs or bid x 5 days.
PEDS - Not approved in children.
FORMS - Trade: 0.75% gel in 70 g tube with applicator.
NOTES - Cure rate same with qhs and bid dosing. Vaginally applied metronidazole could be absorbed in sufficient amounts to produce systemic effects. Caution in patients with CNS diseases due to rare reports of seizures, neuropathy & numbness. Do not administer to patients who have taken disulfiram within the last 2 weeks. Interaction with ethanol. Caution with warfarin. Candida cervicitis & vaginitis, & vaginal, perineal or vulvar itching may occur. Avoid vaginal intercourse during treatment.

miconazole (*Monistat, Femizol-M, M-Zole, Micozole, Monazole*) ▶LK ♀+ ▶? $
ADULT - Local treatment of vulvovaginal candidiasis: 1 applicatorful 2% cream intravaginally qhs x 7 days or 4% cream qhs x 3 days. 100 mg supp intravaginally qhs x 7 days or 400 mg qhs x 3 days. Topical cream for external symptoms bid x 7 days.
PEDS - Not approved in children.
FORMS - OTC: Generic/Trade: 2% vaginal cream in 45 g with 1 applicator or 7 disposable applicators. Vaginal suppositories 100 mg (7) OTC: Trade: 400 mg (3) with applicator. 4% vaginal cream in 25 g tubes or 3 prefilled applicators. Some in combination packs with 2% miconazole cream for external use.
NOTES - Do not use if abdominal pain, fever or foul-smelling vaginal discharge is present. Since small amounts of these drugs may be absorbed from the vagina, use during the 1st trimester only when essential. During pregnancy, use of a vaginal applicator may be contraindicated; manual insertion of suppositories may be preferred. Vulvovaginal burning, itching, irritation & pelvic cramps may occur. Avoid vaginal intercourse during treatment. May increase warfarin effect.

***NuvaRing* (ethinyl estradiol + etonogestrel)** ▸L ♀X ▸- $$
WARNING - Not recommended in women >35 yo who smoke. Increase risk of thromboembolism, stroke, MI, hepatic neoplasia & gallbladder disease. Vaginitis, headache, nausea & weight gain are common side effects. Effectiveness is reduced by hepatic enzyme-inducing drugs such as certain anticonvulsants and barbiturates, rifampin, rifabutin, griseofulvin & protease inhibitors. Additionally, antibiotics or products that contain St John's wort may decrease efficacy. An additional form of birth control may be advisable.
ADULT - Contraception: 1 ring intravaginally x 3 weeks each month.
PEDS - Not approved in children.
FORMS - Trade: Flexible intravaginal ring, 15 mcg ethinyl estradiol/0.120 mg etonogestrel/day. 1 and 3 rings/box.
NOTES - Insert on day 5 of cycle or within 7 days of the last oral contraceptive pill. The ring must remain in place continuously for 3 weeks, including during intercourse. Remove for 1 week, then insert a new ring. May be used continuously for 4 weeks & replaced immediately to skip a withdrawal week. Store at room temperature. In case of accidental removal, reinsert ASAP after rinsing with cool to lukewarm water. If removal >3 hours, use back up method until ring in place for ≥7 days.

nystatin (*Mycostatin*, ♣*Nilstat, Nyaderm*) ▸Not metabolized ♀A ▸? $$
ADULT - Local treatment of vulvovaginal candidiasis: 100,000 units tab intravaginally qhs x 2 weeks.
PEDS - Not approved in children.
FORMS - Generic/Trade: Vaginal Tabs 100,000 units in 15s & 30s with or without applicator(s).
NOTES - Topical azole products more effective. Do not use if abdominal pain, fever or foul-smelling vaginal discharge is present. During pregnancy use of a vaginal applicator may be contraindicated, manual insertion of tabs may be preferred. Avoid vaginal intercourse during treatment.

progesterone gel (*Prochieve*) ▸Plasma ♀- ▸? $$$
ADULT - Secondary amenorrhea: 45 mg (4%) intravaginally every other day up to 6 doses. If no response, use 90 mg (8%) intravaginally every other day up to 6 doses. Specialized dosing for infertility.
PEDS - Not approved in children.
FORMS - Trade: 4 & 8% single-use, prefilled applicators.
NOTES - An increase in dose from the 4% gel can only be accomplished using the 8% gel; doubling the volume of 4% does not increase absorption.

terconazole (*Terazol*) ▸LK ♀C ▸- $$
ADULT - Local treatment of vulvovaginal candidiasis: 1 applicatorful 0.4% cream intravaginally qhs x 7 days. 1 applicatorful 0.8% cream intravaginally qhs x 3 days. 80 mg supp intravaginally qhs x 3 days.
PEDS - Not approved in children.
FORMS - Trade: Vaginal cream 0.4% in 45 g tube with applicator. Vaginal suppositories 80 mg (3) with applicator. Generic/trade: Vaginal cream 0.8% in 20 g tube with applicator.
NOTES - Do not use if abdominal pain, fever or foul-smelling vaginal discharge is present. Since small amounts of these drugs may be absorbed from the vagina, use during the 1st trimester only when essential. During pregnancy, use of a vaginal applicator may be contraindicated; manual insertion of suppositories may be preferred. Avoid vaginal intercourse during treatment. vulvovaginal irritation, burning, & pruritus most common.

tioconazole (*Monistat 1-Day, Vagistat-1*) ▸Not absorbed ♀C ▸- $
ADULT - Local treatment of vulvovaginal candidiasis: 1 applicatorful (~ 4.6 g) intravaginally qhs x 1.
PEDS - Not approved in children.
FORMS - OTC: Trade: Vaginal ointment: 6.5% (300 mg) in 4.6 g prefilled single-dose applicator.
NOTES - Do not use if abdominal pain, fever or foul-smelling vag discharge is present. Since small amounts of these drugs may be absorbed from the vagina, use during the 1st trimester only when essential. During pregnancy, use of a vaginal applicator may be contraindicated. Avoid vaginal intercourse during treatment. Vulvovaginal burning & itching may occur.

OB/GYN: Other

betamethasone sodium phosphate (*Celestone*) ▸L ♀C ▸- $$$
ADULT - Not approved for fetal lung maturation
PEDS - Not approved in children.
UNAPPROVED ADULT - Fetal lung maturation, maternal antepartum between 24 & 34 weeks

gestation: 12 mg IM q24h x 2 doses.

clonidine (Catapres, Catapres-TTS, ♥Dixirit) ▶LK ♀C ▶? $

ADULT - See cardiovascular section

PEDS - Not approved in children.

UNAPPROVED ADULT - Menopausal flushing: 0.1-0.4 mg/day PO divided bid-tid. Transdermal system applied weekly 0.1 mg/day.

FORMS - Generic/Trade: Tabs, non-scored 0.1, 0.2, 0.3 mg. Trade only: transdermal weekly patch 0.1 mg/day (TTS-1), 0.2 mg/day (TTS-2), 0.3 mg/day (TTS-3).

NOTES - Hypotension, sedation, and constipation may occur.

danazol (Danocrine, ♥Cyclomen) ▶L ♀X ▶- $$$$

ADULT - Endometriosis: Start 400 mg PO bid, then titrate downward to a dose sufficient to maintain amenorrhea x 3-6 months, up to 9 months. Fibrocystic breast disease: 100-200 mg PO bid x 4-6 months.

PEDS - Not approved in children.

UNAPPROVED ADULT - Menorrhagia: 100-400 mg PO qd x 3 months. Cyclical mastalgia: 100-200 mg PO bid x 4-6 months.

FORMS - Generic/Trade: Caps 50,100,200 mg.

NOTES - Contraindications: impaired hepatic, renal or cardiac function. Androgenic effects may not be reversible even after the drug is discontinued. May alter voice. Hepatic dysfunction has occurred. Insulin requirements may increase in diabetics. Prolongation of PT/INR has been reported with concomitant warfarin.

dexamethasone (Decadron) ▶L ♀C ▶- $

ADULT - Fetal lung maturation, maternal antepartum between 24 & 34 weeks gestation: 6 mg IM q12h x 4 doses.

PEDS - Not approved in children.

fluconazole (Diflucan) ▶K ♀C ▶- $

ADULT - Vaginal candidiasis: 150 mg PO x 1.

PEDS - Approved in children for oral, esophageal & systemic but not vaginal candidiasis.

FORMS - Trade: Tabs 50, 100, 150, & 200 mg; Suspension 10 mg/ml & 40 mg/ml.

NOTES - Headache, nausea, abdominal pain & diarrhea may occur. Single dose fluconazole exposure in the 1st trimester of pregnancy does not appear to increase the risk of congenital disorders.

levonorgestrel (Plan B) ▶L ♀X ▶- $

ADULT - Emergency contraception: 1 tab PO ASAP but within 72h of intercourse. 2nd tab 12h later.

PEDS - Not approved in children.

UNAPPROVED ADULT - 2 tabs (1.5 mg) PO ASAP but within 72h of intercourse (lesser efficacy at up to 120 hours).

FORMS - Trade: Kit contains two 0.75 mg tabs.

NOTES - Nausea uncommon, however, if vomiting occurs within 1h, initial dose must be given again. Consider adding an antiemetic. Patients should be instructed to then contact their healthcare providers. Can be used at any time during the menstrual cycle.

mifepristone (Mifeprex, RU-486) ▶L ♀X ▶? $$$$$

WARNING - Incomplete abortions may require surgical intervention. Patients need to be given info on where such services are available & what do in case of an emergency.

ADULT - Termination of pregnancy, up to 49 days: Day 1: 600 mg PO. Day 3: 400 mcg misoprostol (unless abortion confirmed). Day 14: confirmation of pregnancy termination.

PEDS - Not approved in children.

FORMS - Trade: Tabs 200 mg.

NOTES - Bleeding/spotting & cramping most common side effects. Contraindications: ectopic pregnancy, IUD use, adrenal insufficiency & long-term steroid use, use of anticoagulants, hemorrhagic disorders & porphyrias. CYP3A4 inducers may increase metabolism & lower levels. Available through physician offices only.

Ortho Evra (norelgestromin + ethinyl estradiol, ♥Evra) ▶L ♀X ▶- $$

WARNING - Not recommended in women >35 yo who smoke. Increased risk of thromboembolism, stroke, MI, hepatic neoplasia & gallbladder disease. Nausea, breast tenderness, & breakthrough bleeding are common transient side effects. Effectiveness is reduced by hepatic enzyme-inducing drugs such as certain anticonvulsants and barbiturates, rifampin, rifabutin, griseofulvin & protease inhibitors. Additionally, antibiotics or products that contain St John's wort may decrease efficacy. An additional form of birth control may be advisable.

ADULT - Contraception: 1 patch q week x 3 weeks, then 1 week patch-free.

PEDS - Not approved in children.

FORMS - Trade: Transdermal patch: 150 mcg norelgestromin + 20 mcg ethinyl estradiol/day. 1 and 3 patches/box.

NOTES - May be less effective in women ≥90 kg (198 lbs). Apply new patch on the same day each week. Do not exceed 7 days between patches. Rotate application sites, avoid the waistline. Do not use earlier than 4 weeks postpartum if not breastfeeding.

Premesis-Rx (B6 + folic acid + B12 + cal-

cium carbonate) ▶L ♀A ▶+ $

ADULT - Treatment of pregnancy-induced nausea: 1 tab PO qd.

PEDS - Unapproved in children.

FORMS - Trade: Tabs 75 mg vitamin B6 (pyridoxine), sustained-release, 12 mcg vitamin B12 (cyanocobalamin), 1 mg folic acid, and 200 mg calcium carbonate.

NOTES - May be taken in conjunction with prenatal vitamins.

Preven (levonorgestrel + ethinyl estradiol) ▶L ♀X ▶- $

ADULT - Emergency contraception: 2 tabs PO ASAP but within 72h of intercourse. 2 tabs 12h later.

PEDS - Not approved in children.

FORMS - Trade: Kit contains patient info booklet, pregnancy test, & 4 tabs 0.25mg levonorgestrel/50 mcg ethinyl estradiol.

NOTES - Consider adding antiemetic regimen. If vomiting occurs within 1h, initial dose must be given again. Patients should be instructed to then contact their healthcare providers. Can be used at any time during the menstrual cycle.

RHO immune globulin (RhoGAM, BayRho-D, WinRho SDF, MICRhoGAM, BayRho-D Mini Dose) ▶L ♀C ▶? $$$$

ADULT - Prevention of hemolytic disease of the newborn if mother Rh- and baby is or might be Rh+: 300 mcg vial IM to mother at 28 weeks gestation followed by a 2nd dose ≤72 hours of delivery. Doses >1 vial may be needed if large fetal-maternal hemorrhage occurs during delivery (see complete prescribing information to determine dose). Following amniocentesis, miscarriage, abortion, or ectopic pregnancy ≥13 weeks gestation: 1 vial (300 mcg) IM. <12 weeks gestation: 1 vial (50 mcg) microdose IM.

PEDS - See entry in Immunology section.

NOTES - Do not give IV. One 300 mcg vial prevents maternal sensitization to the Rh factor if the fetomaternal hemorrhage is less than 15 ml fetal RBCs (30 ml of whole blood). When the fetomaternal hemorrhage exceeds this (as estimated by Kleihauer-Betke testing), administer more than one 300 mcg vial.

Women's Tylenol Menstrual Relief (acetaminophen + pamabrom) ▶LK ♀B ▶+ $

ADULT - Menstrual cramps: 2 caplets PO q4-6h.

PEDS - >12 yo: use adult dose.

FORMS - OTC: Caplets 500 mg acetaminophen/25 mg pamabrom (diuretic).

NOTES - Hepatotoxicity with chronic use, especially in alcoholics.

ONCOLOGY

Alkylating agents: altretamine (*Hexalen*), busulfan (*Myleran, Busulfex*), carmustine (*BCNU, BiCNU, Gliadel*), chlorambucil (*Leukeran*), cyclophosphamide (*Cytoxan, Neosar, ✦Procytox*), dacarbazine (*DTIC-Dome*), ifosfamide (*Ifex*), lomustine (*CeeNu, CCNU*), mechlorethamine (*Mustargen*), melphalan (*Alkeran*), procarbazine (*Matulane, ✦Natulan*), streptozocin (*Zanosar*), temozolomide (*Temodar, ✦Temodal*), thiotepa (*Thioplex*). **Antibiotics:** bleomycin (*Blenoxane*), dactinomycin (*Cosmegen*), daunorubicin (*DaunoXome, Cerubidine*), doxorubicin liposomal (*Doxil, ✦Caelyx*), doxorubicin non-liposomal (*Adriamycin, Rubex*), epirubicin (*Ellence, ✦Pharmorubicin*), idarubicin (*Idamycin*), mitomycin (*Mutamycin, Mitomycin-C*), mitoxantrone (*Novantrone*), plicamycin (*mithramycin, Mithracin*), valrubicin (*Valstar, ✦Valtaxin*). **Antimetabolites:** azacitidine (*Vidaza*), capecitabine (*Xeloda*), cladribine (*Leustatin, chlorodeoxyadenosine*), cytarabine (*Cytosar-U, Tarabine, Depo-Cyt, AraC*), floxuridine (*FUDR*), fludarabine (*Fludara*), fluorouracil (*Adrucil, 5-FU*), gemcitabine (*Gemzar*), hydroxyurea (*Hydrea, Droxia*), mercaptopurine (*6-MP, Purinethol*), methotrexate (*Rheumatrex, Trexall*), pemetrexed (*Alimta*), pentostatin (*Nipent*), thioguanine (*✦Lanvis*). **Cytoprotective Agents:** amifostine (*Ethyol*), dexrazoxane (*Zinecard*), mesna (*Mesnex, ✦Uromitexan*). **Hormones:** abarelix (*Plenaxis*), anastrozole (*Arimidex*), bicalutamide (*Casodex*), cyproterone (*✦Androcur, Androcur Depot*), estramustine (*Emcyt*), exemestane (*Aromasin*), flutamide (*Eulexin, ✦Euflex*), fulvestrant (*Faslodex*), goserelin (*Zoladex*), letrozole (*Femara*), leuprolide (*Eligard, Lupron, Viadur*), medroxyprogesterone (*Depo-Provera*), megestrol (*Megace*), nilutamide (*Nilandron, ✦Anandron*), tamoxifen (*Nolvadex, Tamone*), testolactone (*Teslac*), toremifene (*Fareston*), triptorelin (*Trelstar Depot*). **Immunomodulators:** aldesleukin (*Proleukin, interleukin-2*), alemtuzumab (*Campath*), BCG (*Bacillus of Calmette & Guerin, Pacis, TheraCys, TICE BCG*), bevacizumab (*Avastin*), cetuximab (*Erbitux*), denileukin (*Ontak*), gemtuzumab (*Mylotarg*), ibritumomab (*Zevalin*), imatinib (*Gleevec*), interferon alfa-2a (*Roferon-A*), interferon alfa-2b (*Intron A*), interferon alfa-n3

(*Alferon N*), rituximab (*Rituxan*), tositumomab (*Bexxar*), trastuzumab (*Herceptin*). **Mitotic Inhibitors**: docetaxel (*Taxotere*), etoposide (*VP-16, Etopophos, Toposar, VePesid*), paclitaxel (*Taxol, Onxol*), teniposide (*Vumon, VM-26*), vinblastine (*Velban, VLB*), vincristine (*Oncovin, Vincasar, VCR*), vinorelbine (*Navelbine*). **Platinum-Containing Agents**: carboplatin (*Paraplatin*), cisplatin (*Platinol-AQ*), oxaliplatin (*Eloxatin*). **Radiopharmaceuticals**: samarium 153 (*Quadramet*), strontium-89 (*Metastron*). **Miscellaneous**: arsenic trioxide (*Trisenox*), asparaginase (*Elspar*, ✤*Kidrolase*), bexarotene (*Targretin*), bortezomib (*Velcade*), gefitinib (*Iressa*), irinotecan (*Camptosar*), leucovorin (*Wellcovorin*, folinic acid), levamisole (*Ergamisol*), mitotane (*Lysodren*), pegaspargase (*Oncaspar*), porfimer (*Photofrin*), topotecan (*Hycamtin*), tretinoin (*Vesanoid*).

OPHTHALMOLOGY: Antibacterials – Aminoglycosides

gentamicin (*Garamycin, Genoptic, Gentak*, ✤*Alcomicin, Diogent*) ▶K ♀C ▶? $
ADULT - Ocular infections: 1-2 gtts q2-4h or ½ inch ribbon of ointment bid- tid.
PEDS - Not approved in children.
UNAPPROVED PEDS - Ocular infections: 1-2 gtts q4h or ½ inch ribbon of ointment bid-tid.
FORMS - Generic/Trade: solution 0.3% (5 ,15 mL), ointment 0.3% (3.5 g tube).
NOTES - For severe infections, use up to 2 gtts every hour.

tobramycin (*Tobrex*) ▶K ♀B ▶- $
ADULT - Ocular infections, mild to moderate: 1-2 gtts q4h or ½ inch ribbon of ointment bid-tid. Ocular infections, severe: 2 gtts q1h, then taper to q4h or ½ inch ribbon of ointment q3-4h, then taper to bid-tid.
PEDS - Not approved in children.
UNAPPROVED PEDS - Ocular infections: 1-2 gtts q4h or ½ inch ribbon of ointment bid-tid.
FORMS - Generic/Trade: solution 0.3% (5 mL). Trade only: ointment 0.3% (3.5 g tube).

OPHTHALMOLOGY: Antibacterials – Fluoroquinolones

ciprofloxacin (*Ciloxan*) ▶LK ♀C ▶? $$
ADULT - Corneal ulcers / keratitis: 2 gtts q15 minutes x 6 hours, then 2 gtts q30 minutes x 1 day; then, 2 gtts q1h x 1 day, and 2 gtts q4h x 3-14 days. Bacterial conjunctivitis: 1-2 gtts q2h while awake x 2 days, then 1-2 gtts q4h while awake x 5 days; or ½ inch ribbon ointment tid x 2 days, then ½ inch ribbon bid x 5 days.
PEDS - Bacterial conjunctivitis: use adult dose for age ≥1 yo (solution) and ≥2 yo (ointment). Not approved below these ages.
FORMS - Trade/generic: solution 0.3% (2.5,5,10 mL). Trade only: ointment 0.3% (3.5 g tube).
NOTES - Avoid the overuse of fluoroquinolones for conjunctivitis. May cause white precipitate of active drug at site of epithelial defect that may be confused with a worsening infection. Resolves within 2 weeks and does not necessitate discontinuation. Ocular administration has not been shown to cause arthropathy.

gatifloxacin (*Zymar*) ▶K ♀C ▶? $$
ADULT - Bacterial conjunctivitis: 1-2 gtts q2h while awake up to 8 times/day on days 1 & 2, then 1-2 gtts q4h up to 4 x /day on days 3-7.
PEDS - Age <1 yo: Not approved. >1 yo: Bacterial conjunctivitis: 1-2 gtts q2h while awake up to 8 times/day on days 1&2, then 1-2 gtts q4h up to 4 times/day on days 3-7.
FORMS - Trade only: solution 0.3%.
NOTES - Avoid the overuse of fluoroquinolones for conjunctivitis. Ocular administration has not been shown to cause arthropathy.

levofloxacin (*Iquix, Quixin*) ▶KL ♀C ▶? $$
ADULT - Bacterial conjunctivitis, Quixin: 1-2 gtts q2h while awake up to 8 times/day on days 1&2, then 1-2 gtts q4h up to 4 times/day on days 3-7. Bacterial conjunctivitis, Iquix: 1-2 gtts q30 min to 2h while awake and q4-6h overnight on days 1-3, then 1-2 gtts q1-4h while awake on days 4 to completion of therapy.
PEDS - Bacterial conjunctivitis, Quixin: =<1 yo: Not approved. >1yo: 1-2 gtts q2h while awake up to 8 times/day on days 1&2, then 1-2 gtts q4h up to 4 times/day on days 3-7. Bacterial conjunctivitis, Iquix: <6 yo: Not approved. =>6 yo: 1-2 gtts q30 min to 2h while awake and q4-6h overnight on days 1-3, then 1-2 gtts q1-4h while awake on days 4 to completion of therapy.
FORMS - Trade only: solution 0.5% (Quixin, 5 mL), 1.5% (Iquix, 5 mL).
NOTES - Avoid the overuse of fluoroquinolones for conjunctivitis. Ocular administration has not been shown to cause arthropathy.

moxifloxacin (*Vigamox*) ▶LK ♀C ▶? $$
  ADULT - Bacterial conjunctivitis: 1 gtt tid x 7 days.
  PEDS - Bacterial conjunctivitis: age <1 yo: Not approved. >1yo: 1 gtt tid x 7 days.
  FORMS - Trade only: solution 0.5%.
  NOTES - Avoid the overuse of fluoroquinolones for conjunctivitis. Ocular administration has not been shown to cause arthropathy.

norfloxacin (*Chibroxin*) ▶LK ♀C ▶? $
  ADULT - Bacterial conjunctivitis: 1-2 gtts qid x 7 days. Severe infections may require 1-2 gtts q2h x 1-2 days, then qid.
  PEDS - Bacterial conjunctivitis >1 year of age: 1-2 gtts qid x 7 days.
  FORMS - Trade only: solution 0.3% (5 mL).

NOTES - Avoid the overuse of fluoroquinolones for conjunctivitis. Ocular administration has not been shown to cause arthropathy.

ofloxacin (*Ocuflox*) ▶LK ♀C ▶? $$
  ADULT - Corneal ulcers/keratitis: 1-2 gtts q30 minutes while awake and 1-2 gtts 4-6 h after retiring x 2 days, then 1-2 gtts q1h while awake x 5 days, then 1-2 gtts qid x 3 days. Bacterial conjunctivitis: 1-2 gtts q2-4 h x 2 days, then 1-2 gtts qid x 5 days.
  PEDS - Bacterial conjunctivitis: age ≥1 yo: Use adult dose. <1 yo: Not approved.
  FORMS - Trade/generic soln 0.3% (5, 10 mL).
  NOTES - Avoid the overuse of fluoroquinolones for conjunctivitis. Ocular administration has not been shown to cause arthropathy.

OPHTHALMOLOGY: Antibacterials – Other

bacitracin (*AK Tracin*) ▶Minimal absorption ♀C ▶? $
  ADULT - Ocular infections: apply ¼-½ inch ribbon of ointment q3-4h or bid-qid.
  PEDS - Not approved in children.
  UNAPPROVED PEDS - Ocular infections: apply ½ inch ribbon of ointment q3-4h or bid-qid.
  FORMS - Generic/Trade: ointment 500 units/g (3.5g tube)

erythromycin (*Ilotycin, AK-Mycin*) ▶L ♀B ▶+ $
  ADULT - Ocular infections, corneal ulceration: ½ inch ribbon of ointment q3-4h or 2-8 times/day. For chlamydial infections: bid x 2 months or bid x 5 days/month for 6 months.
  PEDS - Ophthalmia neonatorum prophylaxis: ½ inch ribbon to both eyes within 1 hour of birth.
  FORMS - Generic: ointment 0.5% (1, 3.5 g tube).

fusidic acid (*Fucithalmic*) ▶L ♀? ▶? $
  ADULT - Canada only. Eye infections: 1 gtt in both eyes q12h x 7 days.
  PEDS - Canada only. Children ≥2 yo, eye infections: 1 gtt in both eyes q12h x 7 days.
  FORMS - Trade: Drops 1%. Multidose tubes of 3, 5 g. Single dose preservative-free tubes of 0.2 g in a box of 12.

Neosporin ointment (neomycin + bacitracin + polymyxin B) ▶K ♀C ▶? $
  ADULT - Ocular infections: ½ inch ribbon of ointment q3-4 h x 7-10 days or ½ inch ribbon 2-3 times/day for mild-moderate infection.
  PEDS - Not approved in children.
  UNAPPROVED PEDS - ½ inch ribbon of ointment q3-4h x 7-10 days.
  FORMS - Generic/Trade: ointment. (3.5 g tube).

NOTES - Contact dermatitis can occur after prolonged use.

Neosporin solution (neomycin + polymyxin + gramicidin) ▶KL ♀C ▶? $$
  ADULT - Ocular infections:1-2 gtts q1-6h x 7-10 days.
  PEDS - Not approved in children.
  UNAPPROVED PEDS - 1-2 gtts q1-6h x 7-10 days.
  FORMS - Generic/Trade: solution (10 mL)
  NOTES - Contact dermatitis can occur after prolonged use.

Polysporin (polymyxin B + bacitracin) ▶K ♀C ▶? $
  ADULT - Ocular infections: ½ inch ribbon of ointment q3-4h x 7-10 days or ½ inch ribbon bid-tid for mild-moderate infection.
  PEDS - Not approved in children.
  UNAPPROVED PEDS - Ocular infections: ½ inch ribbon of ointment q3-4h x 7-10 days.
  FORMS - Generic/Trade: ointment (3.5 g tube).

Polytrim (polymyxin B + trimethoprim) ▶KL ♀C ▶? $
  ADULT - Ocular infections: 1-2 gtts q3-6h x 7-10 days. Max 6 gtts/day.
  PEDS - Age ≥2 mo: Use adult dose. <2 mo: Not approved.
  FORMS - Generic/Trade: solution (10 mL).

sulfacetamide (*Sulamyd, Bleph-10, Sulf-10, Isopto Cetamide, AK-Sulf*) ▶K ♀C ▶- $
  ADULT - Ocular infections, corneal ulceration: 1-2 gtts q2-3h initially, then taper by decreasing frequency as condition allows x 7-10 days or ½ inch ribbon of ointment q3-4h initially, then taper x 7-10 days. Trachoma: 2 gtts q2h with systemic antibiotic such as doxycycline or

azithromycin.
PEDS - Age ≥2 mo: Use adult dose. <2 mo: Not approved.
FORMS - Generic only: solution 10%, 30% (15 mL). Generic/Trade: ointment 10% (3.5g tube).

Trade only: solution 10% (2.5,5,15 mL) 10, 15, 30% (15 mL)
NOTES - Ointment may be used as an adjunct to solution.

OPHTHALMOLOGY: Antihistamines, Ocular

azelastine (*Optivar*) ▶L ♀C ▶? $$
ADULT - Allergic conjunctivitis: 1 gtt in each eye bid.
PEDS - Age ≥3 yo: Use adult dose. <3yo: Not approved.
FORMS - Trade only: solution 0.05% (3, 6 mL).
NOTES - Wait 10 minutes after use before inserting contact lenses. Do not use contacts if red eyes.
emedastine (*Emadine*) ▶L ♀B ▶? $$
ADULT - Allergic conjunctivitis: 1 gtt in affected eye up to qid.
PEDS - Age ≥3 yo: Use adult dose. <3yo: Not approved.
FORMS - Trade only: solution 0.05% (5 mL).
NOTES - Wait 10 minutes after use before inserting contact lenses. Do not use contacts if red eyes.
epinastine (*Elestat*) ▶K ♀C ▶? $$$

ADULT - Allergic conjunctivitis: 1 gtt in each eye bid.
PEDS - Not approved in children <3 yo. Age ≥3 yo: Use adult dose.
FORMS - Trade only: solution 0.05% (5,10 mL).
NOTES - Do not administer while wearing soft contact lenses. Wait ≥10 minutes after administration before inserting lenses.
levocabastine (*Livostin*) ▶Minimal absorption ♀C ▶? $$$
ADULT - Seasonal allergic conjunctivitis: 1 gtt in each eye qid for up to 2 weeks.
PEDS - Age ≥12 yo: Use adult dose. <12 yo: Not approved.
FORMS - Trade only: suspension 0.05% (5,10 mL).
NOTES - Do not administer while wearing soft contact lenses. Wait ≥15 minutes after administration before inserting lenses.

OPHTHALMOLOGY: Antiviral Agents

fomivirsen (*Vitravene*) ▶Exonuclease ♀C ▶- $$$$$
ADULT - CMV retinitis in AIDS patients with failure/intolerance to other treatments: 330 mcg by intravitreal injection q2 weeks x 2 doses, then q 4 weeks.
PEDS - Not approved in children.
NOTES - Corticosteroid-responsive ocular inflammation, transient increase in intraocular pressure. Not for patients who have received cidofovir in past 2-4 weeks.
trifluridine (*Viroptic*) ▶Minimal absorption ♀C ▶- $$$
ADULT - HSV keratitis/keratoconjunctivitis: 1 gtt q2h to maximum 9 gtts/day. After re-epithelialization, decrease dose to 1 gtt q4h (minimum 5 gtts/day) while awake x 7-14 days. Maximum

of 21 days of treatment.
PEDS - Age ≥6 yo: Use adult dose. <6 yo: Not approved.
FORMS - Trade only: solution 1% (7.5 mL).
NOTES - Avoid continuous use >21 days; may cause keratitis and conjunctival scarring. Urge frequent use of topical lubricants (ie, tear substitutes) to minimize surface damage.
vidarabine (*Vira-A*) ▶Cornea ♀C ▶? $$$
ADULT - HSV keratitis/keratoconjunctivitis: ½ inch ribbon of ointment 5 times daily divided q3h while awake. After re-epithelialization, decrease dose to ½ inch ribbon bid x 5-7 days.
PEDS - Age ≥2 yo: Use adult dose. <2 yo: Not approved.
FORMS - Trade only: ointment 3% (3.5 g tube).

OPHTHALMOLOGY: Corticosteroid & Antibacterial Combinations

NOTE: Recommend that only ophthalmologists or optometrists prescribe due to infection and glaucoma risk. Monitor intraocular pressure.

***Blephamide* (prednisolone + sodium sulfacetamide)** ▶KL ♀C ▶? $
ADULT - Steroid-responsive inflammatory condition with bacterial infection or risk of bacterial

infection: Start 1-2 gtts q1h during the day and q2h during the night, then 1 gtt q4-8h; or ½ inch ribbon (ointment) tid-qid initially, then qd-bid thereafter.

PEDS - Not approved in children.

FORMS - Generic/Trade: solution/suspension (5,10 mL), Trade only: ointment (3.5 g tube).

NOTES - Shake well before using suspension. Gradually taper when discontinuing.

Cortisporin (neomycin + polymyxin + hydrocortisone) ▶LK ♀C ▶? $

ADULT - Steroid-responsive inflammatory condition with bacterial infection or risk of bacterial infection: 1-2 gtts or ½ inch ribbon of ointment q3-4h or more frequently prn.

PEDS - Not approved in children.

UNAPPROVED PEDS - 1-2 gtts or ½ inch ribbon of ointment q3-4h.

FORMS - Generic/Trade: suspension (7.5 mL), ointment (3.5 g tube).

NOTES - Shake well before using suspension. Gradually taper when discontinuing.

FML-S Liquifilm (prednisolone + sodium sulfacetamide) ▶KL ♀C ▶? $

ADULT - Steroid-responsive inflammatory condition with bacterial infection or risk of bacterial infection: Start 1-2 gtts q1h during the day and q2h during the night, then 1 gtt q4-8h; or ½ inch ribbon (ointment) tid-qid initially, then qd-bid thereafter.

PEDS - Not approved in children.

FORMS - Trade only: suspension (5,10 mL).

NOTES - Shake well before using suspension. Gradually taper when discontinuing.

Maxitrol (dexamethasone + neomycin + polymyxin) ▶KL ♀C ▶? $

ADULT - Steroid-responsive inflammatory condition with bacterial infection or risk of bacterial infection: Start 1-2 gtts q1h during the day and q2h during the night, then 1 gtt q4-8h; or ½ -1 inch ribbon (ointment) tid-qid initially, then qd-bid thereafter.

PEDS - Not approved in children.

FORMS - Trade/Generic: suspension (5 mL), ointment (3.5 g tube).

NOTES - Shake well before using suspension. Gradually taper when discontinuing.

Pred G (prednisolone + gentamicin) ▶KL ♀C ▶? $$

ADULT - Steroid-responsive inflammatory condition with bacterial infection or risk of bacterial infection: Start 1-2 gtts q1h during the day and q2h during the night, then 1 gtt q4-8h or ½ inch ribbon of ointment bid-qid.

PEDS - Not approved in children.

FORMS - Trade only: suspension (2,5,10 mL), ointment (3.5 g tube).

NOTES - Shake well before using suspension. Gradually taper when discontinuing.

TobraDex (tobramycin + dexamethasone) ▶L ♀C ▶? $$

ADULT - Steroid-responsive inflammatory condition with bacterial infection or risk of bacterial infection: 1-2 gtts q2h x 1-2 days, then 1-2 gtts q4-6h; or ½ inch ribbon of ointment bid-qid.

PEDS - <2 yo: not approved. ≥2 yo: 1-2 gtts q2h x 1-2 days, then 1-2 gtts q4-6h; or ½ inch ribbon of ointment bid-qid.

FORMS - Trade only: suspension (2.5,5,10 mL), ointment (3.5 g tube).

NOTES - Shake well before using suspension. Gradually taper when discontinuing.

Vasocidin (prednisolone + sodium sulfacetamide) ▶KL ♀C ▶? $

ADULT - Steroid-responsive inflammatory condition with bacterial infection or risk of bacterial infection: Start 1-2 gtts q1h during the day and q2h during the night, then 1 gtt q4-8h; or ½ inch ribbon (ointment) tid-qid initially, then qd-bid thereafter.

PEDS - Not approved in children.

FORMS - Generic/Trade: solution (5,10 mL)

NOTES - Shake well before using suspension. Gradually taper when discontinuing.

OPHTHALMOLOGY: Corticosteroids

NOTE: Recommend that only ophthalmologists or optometrists prescribe due to infection and glaucoma risk. Monitor intraocular pressure.

fluorometholone (*FML, FML Forte, Flarex, Fluor-Op*) ▶L ♀C ▶? $$

ADULT - 1-2 gtts q1-2h or ½ inch ribbon of ointment q4h x 1-2 days, then 1-2 gtts bid-qid or ½ inch of ointment qd-tid.

PEDS - Age ≥2 yo: Use adult dose. <2 yo: Not approved.

FORMS - Generic/Trade: suspension 0.1% (5, 10,15 mL). Trade only: suspension 0.25% (5, 10,15 mL), ointment 0.1% (3.5 g tube)

NOTES - Fluorometholone acetate (Flarex) is more potent that fluorometholone (FML, FML Forte). Shake well before using suspension. Gradually taper when discontinuing. Use caution in glaucoma.

loteprednol (*Alrex, Lotemax*) ▶L ♀C ▶? $$

ADULT - 1-2 gtts qid, may increase to 1 gtt q1h

during first week of therapy prn. Seasonal allergic conjunctivitis: 1 gtt in affected eye qid (0.2% suspension). Postoperative inflammation: 1-2 gtts qid.

PEDS - Not approved in children.

FORMS - Trade only: suspension 0.2% (Alrex 5,10 mL), 0.5% (Lotemax 2.5, 5,10,15 mL).

NOTES - Shake well before using suspension. Gradually taper when discontinuing.

prednisolone (*AK-Pred, Pred Forte, Pred Mild, Inflamase, Inflamase Forte, Econopred, Econopred Plus, ✚AK Tate, Diopred*) ▶L ♀C ▶? $$

ADULT - Solution: 1-2 gtts up to q1h during day and q2h at night, when response observed, then 1 gtt q4h, then 1 gtt tid-qid. Suspension: 1-2 gtts bid-qid.

PEDS - Not approved in children.

FORMS - Generic/Trade: suspension 1% (5,10, 15 mL), solution 0.125 (5 mL), 1% (5,10,15 mL). Trade only: suspension 0.12% (5,10 mL), solution 0.125% (5,10 mL)

NOTES - Prednisolone acetate (Pred Mild, Pred Forte) is more potent than prednisolone sodium phosphate (AK-Pred, Inflamase Forte). Shake well before using suspension. Gradually taper when discontinuing.

rimexolone (*Vexol*) ▶L ♀C ▶? $$

ADULT - Post-operative inflammation: 1-2 gtts qid x 2 weeks. Uveitis: 1-2 gtts q1h while awake x 1 week, then 1 gtt q2h while awake x 1 week, then taper.

PEDS - Not approved in children.

FORMS - Trade only: suspension 1% (5,10 mL).

NOTES - Shake well before using suspension. Gradually taper when discontinuing. Prolonged use associated with corneal/scleral perforation and cataracts.

OPHTHALMOLOGY: Decongestants, Ocular

naphazoline (*Albalon, AK-Con, Vasocon, Naphcon, Allerest, Clear Eyes*) ▶? ♀C ▶? $

ADULT - Ocular vasoconstrictor/decongestant: 1 gtt q3-4h prn up to qid for up to 4 days.

PEDS - <6 yo: not approved. ≥6 yo: 1 gtt q3-4h prn up to qid for up to 4 days.

FORMS - OTC Generic/Trade: solution 0.012, 0.02, 0.03% (15, 30 mL). Rx generic/Trade: 0.1% (15 mL).

NOTES - Overuse can cause rebound dilation of blood vessels. Do not administer while wearing soft contact lenses. Wait ≥15 minutes after

administration before inserting lenses.

Naphcon-A (naphazoline + pheniramine) ▶L ♀C ▶? $

ADULT - Ocular decongestant: 1-2 gtts bid-qid prn.

PEDS - Age ≥6 yo: Use adult dose. <6 yo: Not approved.

FORMS - OTC Trade only: solution 0.025% + 0.3% (15 mL).

NOTES - Overuse can cause rebound dilation of blood vessels. Do not administer while wearing soft contact lenses. Wait ≥15 minutes after administration before inserting lenses.

OPHTHALMOLOGY: Glaucoma Agents – Beta Blockers

NOTE: May be absorbed and cause effects, side effects and drug interactions associated with systemic beta-blocker therapy. Use caution in cardiac conditions and asthma. Morning only dosing of beta blocker eyedrops may be preferred, as evening dosing may be associated with nocturnal hypotension and reduced heart rate.

betaxolol (*Betoptic S*) ▶LK ♀C ▶? $$

ADULT - Chronic open angle glaucoma or ocular hypertension: 1-2 gtts bid.

PEDS - Not approved in children.

FORMS - Trade only: suspension 0.25% (2.5,5, 10,15 mL). Generic only: solution 0.5% (5,10, 15 mL).

NOTES - More selective beta1-blocking agent. Shake suspension before use.

carteolol (*Ocupress*) ▶KL ♀C ▶? $

ADULT - Chronic open angle glaucoma or ocular hypertension: 1 gtt bid.

PEDS - Not approved in children.

FORMS - Generic/Trade: solution 1% (5,10,15 mL).

NOTES - Intrinsic sympathomimetic activity.

levobetaxolol (*Betaxon*) ▶KL ♀C ▶? ?

ADULT - Approved but not yet marketed. Chronic open angle glaucoma or ocular hypertension: 1 gtt bid.

PEDS - Not approved in children.

FORMS - Trade only: solution 0.5%.

levobunolol (*Betagan*) ▶? ♀C ▶- $

ADULT - Chronic open angle glaucoma or ocular hypertension: 1-2 gtts (0.5%) qd-bid or 1-2 gtts (0.25%) bid.

PEDS - Not approved in children.

FORMS - Generic/Trade: solution 0.25% (5,10 mL) 0.5% (5,10,15 mL - Trade only 2 mL).

metipranolol (*Optipranolol*) ▶? ♀C ▶? $

ADULT - Chronic open angle glaucoma or ocular hypertension: 1 gtt bid.

PEDS - Not approved in children.

FORMS - Generic/Trade: solution 0.3% (5,10 mL).

timolol (*Timoptic, Timoptic XE, Istalol, Timoptic Ocudose*) ▶LK ♀C ▶+ $

ADULT - Chronic open angle glaucoma or ocular hypertension: 1 gtt (0.25 or 0.5%) bid or 1 gtt of gel (0.25 or 0.5% Timoptic XE) qd or 1 gtt (0.5% Istalol solution) qd.

PEDS - Not approved in children.

FORMS - Generic/Trade: solution 0.25, 0.5% (5,10,15 mL), preservative free 0.2 mL. Generic/Trade: gel forming solution 0.25, 0.5% (2.5*, 5 mL). Trade: solution 0.5% (Istalol) 10 mL. Note: * 0.25%Timoptic XE.

NOTES - Administer other eye meds ≥10 minutes before Timoptic XE.

OPHTHALMOLOGY: Glaucoma Agents – Carbonic Anhydrase Inhibitors

NOTE: Sulfonamide derivatives; verify absence of sulfa allergy before prescribing.

acetazolamide (*Diamox*) ▶LK ♀C ▶+ $$

ADULT - Glaucoma: immediate-release, 250 mg PO qd-qid, extended-release, 500 mg PO qd-bid. Max 1g/day. Acute glaucoma: 500 mg IV, followed by oral therapy.

PEDS - Not approved in children.

UNAPPROVED PEDS - Glaucoma: 8-30 mg/kg/day PO, divided tid. Acute glaucoma: 5-10 mg/kg IV every 6h .

FORMS - Generic/Trade: Tabs 125, 250 mg. Trade only: extended release Caps 500 mg.

NOTES - May cause metallic taste, anorexia, or diarrhea in >10 % of patients.

brinzolamide (*Azopt*) ▶LK ♀C ▶? $$

ADULT - Chronic open angle glaucoma or ocular hypertension: 1 gtt tid.

PEDS - Not approved in children.

FORMS - Trade only: susp 1% (5,10,15 mL).

NOTES - Do not administer while wearing soft contact lenses. Wait ≥15 minutes after administration before inserting lenses.

dorzolamide (*Trusopt*) ▶KL ♀C ▶- $$

ADULT - Chronic open angle glaucoma or ocular hypertension: 1 gtt tid.

PEDS - Chronic open angle glaucoma or ocular hypertension: 1 gtt tid.

FORMS - Trade only: solution 2% (5,10 mL).

NOTES - Do not administer while wearing soft contact lenses. Keep bottle tightly capped to avoid crystal formation . Wait ≥15 minutes after administration before inserting lenses. Use caution in sulfa allergy.

methazolamide (*Neptazane*) ▶LK ♀C ▶? $

ADULT - Glaucoma: 100-200 mg PO initially, then 100 mg PO q 12h until desired response. Maintenance dose: 25-50 mg PO qd-tid.

PEDS - Not approved in children.

FORMS - Generic only: Tabs 25, 50 mg.

OPHTHALMOLOGY: Glaucoma Agents – Prostaglandin Analogs

bimatoprost (*Lumigan*) ▶LK ♀C ▶? $$$

ADULT - Chronic open angle glaucoma or ocular hypertension: 1 gtt qhs.

PEDS - Not approved in children.

FORMS - Trade only: solution 0.03% (2.5, 5, 7.5 mL).

NOTES - May gradually change hazel eye color to brown and darken eyelids and lashes. Do not administer while wearing soft contact lenses. Wait ≥5 minutes after administration before inserting lenses. May aggravate intraocular inflammation.

latanoprost (*Xalatan*) ▶LK ♀C ▶? $$$

ADULT - Chronic open angle glaucoma or ocular hypertension: 1 gtt qhs.

PEDS - Not approved in children.

FORMS - Trade only: solution 0.005% (2.5 mL).

NOTES - May gradually change hazel eye color to brown. Do not administer while wearing soft contact lenses. Wait ≥5 minutes after administration before inserting lenses. May aggravate intraocular inflammation.

travoprost (*Travatan*) ▶L ♀C ▶? $$

ADULT - Glaucoma in patients intolerant to or not responding to other medications: 1 gtt qhs.

PEDS - Not approved in children.

FORMS - Trade only: solution 0.004% (2.5,5 mL).

NOTES - May gradually change hazel eye color to brown and darken eyelids and lashes. Do not administer while wearing soft contact lenses. Wait ≥5 minutes after administration before inserting lenses. May aggravate intraocular inflammation.

unoprostone (Rescula) ▸Plasma, K ♀C ▸? $$
ADULT - Chronic open angle glaucoma or ocular hypertension: 1 gtt bid.
PEDS - Not approved in children.
FORMS - Trade only: solution 0.15% (5 mL).

NOTES - Indicated for patients intolerant to or who have failed other glaucoma meds. May gradually change hazel eye color to brown and darken eyelids and lashes. Do not administer while wearing soft contact lenses. Wait ≥5 minutes after administration before inserting lenses. May aggravate intraocular inflammation.

OPHTHALMOLOGY: Glaucoma Agents – Sympathomimetics

apraclonidine (Iopidine) ▸KL ♀C ▸? $$$
ADULT - Adjunctive therapy for glaucoma: 1-2 gtts (0.5%) tid. Perioperative IOP elevations: 1 gtt (1%) 1h prior to surgery, then 1 gtt immediately after surgery.
PEDS - Not approved in children.
FORMS - Trade only: solution 0.5% (5,10 mL), 1% (0.1 mL).
NOTES - Rapid tachyphylaxis may occur. Do not use long-term. Do not administer while wearing soft contact lenses. Wait ≥15 minutes after administration before inserting lenses.

brimonidine (Alphagan P) ▸L ♀B ▸? $$
ADULT - Chronic open angle glaucoma or ocular hypertension: 1 gtt tid.
PEDS - Glaucoma >2 yo: 1 gtt tid.
FORMS - Trade only: solution 0.15% (5,10,15 mL).

NOTES - Contraindicated in patients receiving MAO inhibitors. Do not administer while wearing soft contact lenses. Wait ≥15 minutes after administration before inserting lenses. Local allergic reactions may occur in 10-30%. Alphagan P may be associated with fewer side effects.

dipivefrin (Propine) ▸Eye/plasma/L ♀B ▸? $
ADULT - Chronic open angle glaucoma or ocular hypertension: 1 gtt q12h.
PEDS - Glaucoma: 1 gtt q12h.
FORMS - Generic/Trade: solution 0.1% (5,10,15 mL).
NOTES - Do not administer while wearing soft contact lenses. Wait ≥15 minutes after administration before inserting lenses. Dipivefrin is a prodrug that becomes activated in eye to epinephrine.

OPHTHALMOLOGY: Glaucoma Agents – Other

Cosopt (dorzolamide + timolol) ▸LK ♀D ▸- $$
ADULT - Chronic open angle glaucoma or ocular hypertension: 1 gtt bid.
PEDS - Not approved in children.
FORMS - Trade only: solution dorzolamide 2% + timolol 0.5% (5,10 mL).
NOTES - Do not administer while wearing soft contact lenses. Wait ≥15 minutes after administration before inserting lenses. Use caution in sulfa allergy. See beta-blocker warnings. Avoid with severe renal impairment (CrCl <30 mL/min); caution in hepatic failure.

pilocarpine (Pilocar, Pilopine HS, Isopto

Carpine, Ocusert, Ocu Carpine, ✚Diocarpine) ▸Plasma ♀C ▸? $
ADULT - Glaucoma: 1-2 gtts up to tid-qid up to 6 times/day or ½ inch ribbon (4% gel) qhs.
PEDS - Glaucoma: 1-2 gtts up to tid-qid up to 6 times/day.
FORMS - Generic/Trade: solution 0.5, 1, 2, 3, 4, 6% (15mL). Trade only: 5%, 8% (15 mL), gel 4% (4 g tube).
NOTES - Do not administer while wearing soft contact lenses. Wait ≥15 minutes after administration before inserting lenses. Causes miosis. May cause blurred vision and difficulty with adaptation in dark.

OPHTHALMOLOGY: Mast Cell Stabilizers, Ocular

cromolyn sodium (Crolom, Opticrom) ▸LK ♀B ▸? $$$
ADULT - Allergic ocular disorders (vernal keratoconjunctivitis, vernal conjunctivitis, vernal keratitis): 1-2 gtts in each eye 4-6 times/day at regular intervals.

PEDS - Age ≥4 yo: Use adult dose. <4 yo: Not approved.
FORMS - Generic/Trade: solution 4% (10 mL).
NOTES - Works best as preventative agent; use continually during at risk season. Do not administer while wearing soft contact lenses. Wait

≥15 minutes after administration before inserting lenses. Response may take up to 6 weeks.

ketotifen (*Zaditor*) ▶Minimal absorption ♀C ▶? $$

ADULT - Allergic conjunctivitis: 1 gtt in each eye q8-12h.

PEDS - Allergic conjunctivitis children >3yo: 1 gtt in each eye q8-12h.

FORMS - Trade only: solution 0.025% (5 mL).

NOTES - Wait at least 10 minutes before inserting contacts.

lodoxamide (*Alomide*) ▶K ♀B ▶? $$$

ADULT - Allergic ocular disorders: 1-2 gtts in each eye qid for up to 3 months.

PEDS - Age ≥2 yo: Use adult dose. <2 yo: Not approved.

FORMS - Trade only: solution 0.1% (10 mL).

NOTES - Works best as preventative agent; use continually during at risk season. Do not administer while wearing soft contact lenses. Wait ≥15 minutes after administration before inserting lenses.

nedocromil (*Alocril*) ▶L ♀B ▶? $$

ADULT - Allergic conjunctivitis: 1-2 gtts in each eye bid.

PEDS - Children >3 yo: Allergic conjunctivitis: 1-2 gtts bid. Not approved in children <3yo.

FORMS - Trade only: solution 2% (5 mL).

NOTES - Solution normally appears slightly yellow. Works best as preventative agent; use continually during at risk season. Refrain from wearing contacts while exhibiting signs and symptoms of allergic conjunctivitis.

olopatadine (*Patanol*) ▶K ♀C ▶? $$$

ADULT - Allergic conjunctivitis: 1-2 gtts in each eye bid at an interval of 6-8h.

PEDS - Age ≥3 yo: Use adult dose. <3 yo: Not approved.

FORMS - Trade only: solution 0.1% (5 mL).

NOTES - Do not administer while wearing soft contact lenses. Wait ≥15 minutes after administration before inserting lenses.

pemirolast (*Alamast*) ▶? ♀C ▶? $$$

ADULT - Allergic conjunctivitis: 1-2 gtts in each eye qid.

PEDS - Not approved in children <3 yo. Children >3 yo: 1-2 gtts qid.

FORMS - Trade only: solution 0.1% (10 mL).

NOTES - Works best as preventative agent; use continually during at risk season. Decreased itching may be seen within a few days, but full effect may require up to four weeks. Refrain from wearing contacts while exhibiting signs and symptoms of allergic conjunctivitis. Wait 10 minutes before inserting contacts.

OPHTHALMOLOGY: Mydriatics & Cycloplegics

NOTE: Use caution in infants.

atropine (*Isopto Atropine*) ▶L ♀C ▶+ $

ADULT - Uveitis: 1-2 gtts (0.5 or 1% solution) up to qid or ¼ inch ribbon (1% ointment) up to tid. Refraction: 1-2 gtts (1% solution) 1 h before procedure or 1/8-1/4 inch ribbon qd-tid.

PEDS - Uveitis: 1-2 gtts (0.5%) up to tid or 1/8-1/4 inch ribbon up to tid. Refraction: 1-2 gtts (0.5%) bid x 1-3 days before procedure or 1/8 inch ribbon (1% ointment) x 1-3 days before procedure.

UNAPPROVED PEDS - Amblyopia: 1 gtt in good eye qd.

FORMS - Generic/Trade: solution 1% (5,15 mL) Generic only: ointment 1% (3.5 g tube).

NOTES - Cycloplegia lasts 5-10 days, mydriasis lasts 7-14 days. Each drop of a 1% solution contains 0.5 mg atropine.

cyclopentolate (*AK-Pentolate, Cyclogyl, Pentolair*) ▶? ♀C ▶? $

ADULT - Refraction: 1-2 gtts (1-2%), repeat in 5-10 minutes prn. Give 45 min before procedure.

PEDS - May cause CNS disturbances in children. Refraction: 1-2 gtts (0.5,1, or 2%), repeat in 5-10 minutes prn. Give 45 minutes before procedure.

FORMS - Generic/Trade: solution 1% (2,15 mL). Trade only: 0.5% (15 mL) and 2% (2,5,15 mL)

NOTES - Cycloplegia lasts 6-24 hours, mydriasis lasts 1 day.

homatropine (*Isopto Homatropine*) ▶? ♀C ▶? $

ADULT - Refraction: 1-2 gtts (2%) or 1 gtt (5%) in eye(s) immediately before procedure, repeat q5-10 minutes prn. Max 3 doses. Uveitis: 1-2 gtts (2-5%) bid-tid or as often as q3-4h.

PEDS - Refraction: 1 gtt (2%) in eye(s) immediately before procedure, repeat q10 minutes prn. Uveitis: 1 gtt (2%) bid-tid.

FORMS - Trade only: solution 2% (5 mL), 5% (15 mL). Generic/Trade: solution 5% (5 mL)

NOTES - Cycloplegia & mydriasis last 1-3 days.

phenylephrine (*Neo-Synephrine, Mydfrin, Relief*) ▶Plasma, L ♀C ▶? $

ADULT - Ophthalmologic exams: 1-2 gtts (2.5, 10%) before procedure. Ocular surgery: 1-2 gtts (2.5, 10%) before surgery. Uveitis: 1-2 gtts

(2.5, 10%) tid with atropine.

PEDS - Not routinely used in children.

FORMS - Generic/Trade: solution 2.5,10% (3*, 5, 15 mL) Note: * 2.5% Mydfrin.

NOTES - Overuse can cause rebound dilation of blood vessels. No cycloplegia; mydriasis lasts 5hours. Systemic absorption may be associated with sympathetic stimulation (eg, tachycardia).

tropicamide (*Mydriacyl*) ▶? ♀? ▶? $

ADULT - Fundus exam: 1-2 gtts (0.5%) in eye(s) 15- 20 minutes before exam, repeat q30 minutes prn.

PEDS - Not approved in children.

FORMS - Generic/Trade: solution 0.5% (15 mL), 1% (2, 3, 15 mL)

NOTES - Mydriasis and cycloplegia last 6 hours.

OPHTHALMOLOGY: Nonsteroidal Anti-Inflammatories

diclofenac (*Voltaren*) ▶L ♀B, D (3rd trimester) ▶? $$

ADULT - Post-op inflammation following cataract removal: 1 gtt qid x 2 weeks. Ocular photophobia and pain associated with corneal refractive surgery: 1-2 gtt to operative eye(s) 1 h prior to surgery and 1-2 gtt within 15 minutes after surgery, then 1 gtt qid prn for ≤3 days.

PEDS - Not approved in children.

FORMS - Trade: solution 0.1% (2.5,5 mL).

NOTES - Contraindicated for use with soft contact lenses.

flurbiprofen (*Ocufen*) ▶L ♀C ▶? $

ADULT - Inhibition of intraoperative miosis: 1 gtt q30 min beginning 2h prior to surgery (total of 4 gtts).

PEDS - Not approved in children.

UNAPPROVED ADULT - Treatment of cystoid macular edema, inflammation after glaucoma or cataract laser surgery, uveitis syndromes.

FORMS - Trade/generic: soln 0.03% (2.5 mL).

ketorolac (*Acular, Acular LS*) ▶L ♀C ▶? $$$

ADULT - Allergic conjunctivitis: 1 gtt (0.5%) qid. Post-op inflammation following cataract removal: 1 gtt (0.5%) qid beginning 24 h after surgery x 2 weeks. Post-op corneal refractive surgery: 1 gtt (0.4%) prn for up to 4 days.

PEDS - Age ≥3 yo: Use adult dose. <3 yo: Not approved.

FORMS - Trade only: solution (Acular LS) 0.4% (5 ml), (Acular) 0.5% (3,5,10 mL), preservative free (Acular) 0.5% unit dose (0.4 ml).

NOTES - Do not administer while wearing soft contact lenses. Wait ≥15 minutes after administration before inserting lenses. Avoid use in late pregnancy.

OPHTHALMOLOGY: Other

artificial tears (*Tears Naturale, Hypotears, Refresh Tears, Lacrilube, GenTeal*) ▶Minimal absorption ♀A ▶+ $

ADULT, PEDS - Ophthalmic lubricant: 1-2 gtts tid-qid prn.

FORMS - OTC soln (15, 30 mL among others).

cyclosporine (*Restasis*) ▶Minimal absorption ♀C ▶? $$$$

ADULT - Keratoconjunctivitis sicca (chronic dry eye disease): 1 gtt in each eye approximately q12h.

PEDS - Not approved in children.

FORMS - Trade: emulsion 0.05% (0.4 mL single-use vials).

NOTES - Wait ≥15 min before inserting contacts.

dapiprazole (*Rev-Eyes*) ▶Minimal absorption ♀B ▶? $

ADULT - Reversal of diagnostic mydriasis: 2 gtts in each eye, repeat in 5 minutes.

PEDS - Age ≥4 yo: Use adult dose. <4 yo: Not approved.

FORMS - Trade only: powder for solution 0.5% (5 mL).

NOTES - Wait 10 minutes after use before inserting contact lenses. Do not use contacts if eyes are red.

petrolatum (*Lacrilube, Dry Eyes, Refresh PM*, ✥*Duolube*) ▶Minimal absorption ♀A ▶+ $

ADULT - Ophthalmic lubricant: Apply ¼ inch ointment to inside of lower lid prn.

PEDS - Ophthalmic lubricant: Apply ¼ inch ointment to inside of lower lid prn.

FORMS - OTC ointment (3.5 g tube).

proparacaine (*Ophthetic*, ✥*Alcaine*) ▶L ♀C ▶? $

ADULT - Do not prescribe for unsupervised use. Corneal toxicity may occur with repeated use. Local anesthetic: 1-2 gtts before procedure. Repeat q5-10 minutes x 1-3 doses (suture or foreign body removal) or x 5-7 doses (cataract or glaucoma surgery).

PEDS - Not approved in children.
FORMS - Generic/Trade: solution 0.5% (15 mL).
tetracaine (*Pontocaine*) ▶Plasma ♀C ▶? $
ADULT - Do not prescribe for unsupervised use.
Corneal toxicity may occur with repeated use.
Local anesthetic: 1-2 gtts or ½-1 inch ribbon of
ointment before procedure.
PEDS - Not approved in children.

FORMS - Generic/Trade: solution 0.5% (15 mL).
verteporfin (*Visudyne*) ▶L/plasma ♀C ▶?
$$$$$
ADULT - Treatment of age-related macular degeneration: 6 mg/m^2 IV over 10 minutes; laser
light therapy 15 minutes after start of infusion.
PEDS - Not approved in children.
NOTES - Risk of photosensitivity x 5 days.

Visual Acuity Screen

96
20/800

873
20/400

2843   OXX 20/200
6 3 8 5 2   X O O   20/100
8 7 4 5 9   O X O   20/70
6 3 9 2 5   X O X   20/50
4 2 8 3 6 5   o x o   20/40
3 7 4 2 5 8   x x o   20/30
9 3 7 8 2 6   x o o   20/25

Hold card in good light 14 inches from eye. Record vision for each eye separately
with and without glasses. Presbyopic patients should read through bifocal glasses.
Myopic patients should wear glasses only.
Pupil Diameter (mm)

.2 3 4 5 6 7 8 9

JG Rosenbaum, MD. Pocket Vision Screen. Beachwood, Ohio

PSYCHIATRY: Antidepressants – Heterocyclic Compounds

NOTE: Gradually taper dose when discontinuing
cyclic antidepressants to avoid withdrawal symptoms after prolonged use.

amitriptyline (*Elavil*) ▶L ♀D ▶- $
ADULT - Depression: Start 25-100 mg PO qhs,
gradually increase to usual effective dose of

50-300 mg/day.
PEDS - Depression, adolescents: Use adult dosing. Not approved in children <12 yo.
UNAPPROVED ADULT - Chronic pain/migraine prevention: 10-100 mg/day.
UNAPPROVED PEDS - Depression, children: Start 1 mg/kg/day PO divided tid x 3 days, then increase to 1.5 mg/kg/day to max 5 mg/kg/day.
FORMS - Generic: Tabs 10, 25, 50, 75, 100, 150 mg. Elavil brand name no longer available, but retained here for name recognition.
NOTES - Tricyclic, tertiary amine - primarily serotonin. Demethylated to nortriptyline (primarily norepinephrine). Therapeutic range is 150-300 ng/ml (amitriptyline + nortriptyline). Orthostatic hypotension, arrhythmias, and anticholinergic side effects. Don't use with MAOIs.

amoxapine ▶L ♀C ▶- $$$
ADULT - Rarely used; other drugs preferred. Depression: Start 25-50 mg PO bid-tid, increase by 50- 100 mg bid- tid after 1 week. Usual effective dose is 150- 400 mg/day. Maximum dose is 600 mg/day.
PEDS - Not approved in children <16 yo.
FORMS - Generic: Tabs 25, 50, 100, 150 mg.
NOTES - Tetracyclic - primarily norepinephrine. Dose ≤300 mg/day may be given as a single bedtime dose. Don't use with MAO inhibitors.

clomipramine (Anafranil) ▶L ♀C ▶+ $$$
ADULT - OCD: Start 25 mg PO qhs, gradually increase over 2 weeks to usual effective dose of 150-250 mg/day, max 250 mg/day.
PEDS - OCD and ≥10 yo: Start 25 mg PO qhs, gradually increase over 2 weeks to 3 mg/kg/day or 100 mg/day, max 200 mg/day. <10 yo: Not approved.
UNAPPROVED ADULT - Depression: 100-250 mg/day. Panic disorder: 12.5 - 150 mg/day. Chronic pain: 100- 250 mg/day.
FORMS - Generic/Trade: Caps 25, 50, 75 mg.
NOTES - Tricyclic, tertiary amine- primarily serotonin. May cause seizures, orthostatic hypotension, arrhythmias, and anticholinergic side effects. Don't use with MAOIs.

desipramine (Norpramin) ▶L ♀C ▶+ $$
ADULT - Depression: Start 25-100 mg PO qd or in divided doses. Gradually increase to usual effective dose of 100-200 mg/day, max 300 mg/day.
PEDS - Not approved in children.
FORMS - Generic/Trade: Tabs 10, 25, 50, 75, 100, 150 mg.
NOTES - Tricyclic, secondary amine- primarily norepinephrine. Therapeutic range is 125-300 ng/ml. May cause less anticholinergic side ef-

fects than tertiary amines. Orthostatic hypotension, arrhythmias. Don't use with MAOIs.

doxepin (Sinequan) ▶L ♀C ▶- $$
ADULT - Depression and/or anxiety: Start 75 mg PO qhs, gradually increase to usual effective dose of 75-150 mg/day, max 300 mg/day.
PEDS - Adolescents : Use adult dose. Not approved in children <12 yo.
UNAPPROVED ADULT - Chronic pain: 50- 300 mg/day. Pruritus: start 10-25 mg at bedtime. Usual effective range 10-100 mg/day.
FORMS - Generic/Trade: Caps 10, 25, 50, 75, 100, 150 mg. oral concentrate 10 mg/mL.
NOTES - Tricyclic, tertiary amine - primarily norepinephrine. Do not mix oral concentrate with carbonated beverages. Orthostatic hypotension, arrhythmias, anticholinergic side effects. Don't use with MAOIs. Some patients with mild symptoms may respond to 25-50 mg/ day.

imipramine (Tofranil, Tofranil PM) ▶L ♀D ▶-$$
ADULT - Depression: Start 75-100 mg PO qhs or in divided doses, gradually increase to max 300 mg/day.
PEDS - Not approved for depression in children <12 yo. Enuresis dosing: see urology section.
UNAPPROVED ADULT - Panic disorder: Start 10 mg PO qhs, titrate to usual effective dose of 50-300 mg/day.
UNAPPROVED PEDS - Depression: Start 1.5 mg/kg/day PO divided tid, increase by 1-1.5 mg/kg/day q3-4 days to max 5 mg/kg/ day.
FORMS - Generic/Trade: Tabs 10, 25, 50 mg. Trade only: Caps 75, 100, 125, 150 mg. (as pamoate salt)
NOTES - Tricyclic, tertiary amine - mixed serotonin and norepinephrine. Demethylated to desipramine (primarily norepinephrine). Orthostatic hypotension, arrhythmias, and anticholinergic side effects. Don't use with MAOIs.

maprotiline (Ludiomil) ▶KL ♀B ▶? $$$
ADULT - Rarely used; other drugs preferred. Depression: Start 25 mg PO qd, gradually increase by 25 mg q2 weeks to a max dose of 225 mg/day. Usual effective dose is 150- 225 mg/day. Chronic use max dose is 200 mg/day.
PEDS - Not approved in children.
FORMS - Generic/Trade: Tabs 25, 50, 75 mg.
NOTES - Tetracyclic- primarily norepinephrine. May cause seizures. Don't use with MAOIs.

nortriptyline (Aventyl, Pamelor) ▶L ♀D ▶+ $$
ADULT - Depression: Start 25 mg PO qd-qid. Gradually increase to usual effective dose of 75-100 mg/day, max 150 mg/day.
PEDS - Not approved in children.
UNAPPROVED ADULT - Panic disorder: Start

25 mg PO qhs, titrate to usual effective dose of 50-150 mg/day.

UNAPPROVED PEDS - Depression 6-12 yo: 1-3 mg/kg/day PO divided tid-qid or 10-20 mg/d.

FORMS - Generic/Trade: Caps 10, 25, 50, 75 mg. Oral Solution 10 mg/5 mL.

NOTES - Tricyclic, secondary amine- primarily norepinephrine. Therapeutic range is 50-150 ng/ml. May cause less anticholinergic side effects than tertiary amines. Orthostatic hypotension, arrhythmias. Don't use with MAOIs.

protriptyline (*Vivactil*) ▶L ♀C ▶+ $$$
ADULT - Depression: 15-40 mg/day PO divided tid-qid. Maximum dose is 60 mg/day.
PEDS - Not approved in children.
FORMS - Trade: Tabs 5, 10 mg.
NOTES - Tricyclic, secondary amine - primarily norepinephrine. May cause less anticholinergic side effects than tertiary amines. Orthostatic hypotension, arrhythmias. Don't use with MAOIs. Increases in dose should be made in the morning.

PSYCHIATRY: Antidepressants – Monoamine Oxidase Inhibitors (MAOIs) – (serotonin, norepinephrine, and dopamine)

NOTE: May interfere with sleep; avoid qhs dosing. Must be on tyramine-free diet, stay on diet for 2 weeks after stopping. Risk of HTN crisis and serotonin syndrome with many medications, including OTC. Evaluate thoroughly for drug interactions. Allow ≥2 weeks wash-out when changing between MAOIs and SSRIs (6 weeks after fluoxetine), TCAs, and other antidepressants.

isocarboxazid (*Marplan*) ▶L ♀C ▶? $$$
ADULT - Depression: Start 10 mg PO bid, increase by 10 mg q2-4 days. Usual effective dose is 20- 40 mg/day. Maximum dose is 60 mg/day divided bid-qid.
PEDS - Not approved in children <16 yo.

FORMS - Trade: Tabs 10 mg.
phenelzine (*Nardil*) ▶L ♀C ▶? $$
ADULT - Depression: Start 15 mg PO tid. Usual effective dose is 60-90 mg/day in divided doses.
PEDS - Not approved in children <16 yo.
FORMS - Trade: Tabs 15 mg.
tranylcypromine (*Parnate*) ▶L ♀C ▶- $$
ADULT - Depression: Start 10 mg PO qam, increase by 10 mg/day at 1-3 week intervals to usual effective dose of 10-40 mg/day divided bid. Maximum dose is 60 mg/day.
PEDS - Not approved in children <16 yo.
FORMS - Trade: Tabs 10 mg.

PSYCHIATRY: Antidepressants – Selective Serotonin Reuptake Inhibitors (SSRIs) - (serotonin)

NOTE: Avoid sibutramine with SSRIs. Gradually taper when discontinuing SSRIs (except fluoxetine) to avoid withdrawal symptoms after prolonged use. Observe patients started on SSRIs for worsening depression or emergence of suicidal thoughts or behaviors especially early in therapy or after increases in dose. Monitor for emergence of anxiety, agitation, panic attacks, insomnia, irritability, hostility, impulsivity, akathisia, mania and hypomania. Use during third trimester of pregnancy is associated with neonatal complications including respiratory, gastrointestinal, and feeding problems, seizures and withdrawal symptoms. Balance these risks against those of withdrawal and depression for the mother.

citalopram (*Celexa*) ▶LK ♀C but - in 3rd trimester ▶- $$$
ADULT - Depression: Start 20 mg PO qd, increase by 20 mg at >1 week intervals. Usual effective dose 20-40 mg/day, max 60 mg/day.
PEDS - Not approved in children.

FORMS - Trade: Tabs 10, 20, 40 mg. Oral solution 10 mg/5 mL.
NOTES - Don't use with MAOIs or tryptophan.
escitalopram (*Lexapro*) ▶LK ♀C but - in 3rd trimester ▶- $$$
ADULT - Depression, generalized anxiety disorder: Start 10 mg PO qd, may increase to 20 mg PO qd after >1 week. Max 20 mg/day.
PEDS - Not approved in children.
FORMS - Trade: Tabs 5, 10, 20 mg, with the 10 & 20 mg scored. Oral Solution 1 mg/mL.
NOTES - Don't use with MAOIs. Doses of >20 mg qd have not been shown superior to 10 mg qd. Escitalopram is active isomer of citalopram.
fluoxetine (*Prozac, Prozac Weekly, Sarafem*) ▶L ♀C but - in 3rd trimester ▶- $$$
ADULT - Depression & OCD: Start 20 mg PO q am, increase after several weeks to usual effective dose of 20-40 mg/day. Max 80 mg/day. Depression, maintenance therapy: 20-40 mg/day OR 90 mg once weekly delayed release

(start 7 days after last dose of 20 mg/ day). Bulimia: 60 mg PO qam; may need to titrate up to 60 mg/day over several days. Panic disorder: Start 10 mg PO q am; titrate to 20 mg /day after 1 week; max dose 60 mg/day. Premenstrual Dysphoric Disorder (PMDD): Sarafem: 20 mg PO qd continuously, or 20 mg PO qd for 14 days prior to menses, max 80 mg daily. Doses >20 mg/day can be divided am and noon.

PEDS - Depression 7-17 yo: 10-20 mg PO q am (10 mg for smaller children), max 20 mg/day. OCD: Start 10 mg PO q am, max 60 mg/day (30 mg/day for smaller children).

UNAPPROVED ADULT - Hot flashes: 20 mg PO qd.

FORMS - Trade/generic: tabs 10 mg, caps 10, 20, 40 mg, oral soln 20 mg/5 mL. Trade: caps (Sarafem) 10, 20 mg, caps delayed release (Prozac Weekly) 90 mg. Generic: tabs 20 mg.

NOTES - Half-life of parent 1-3 days and for active metabolite norfluoxetine 6-14 days. Contraindicated with thioridazine. Don't use with cisapride, thioridazine, tryptophan, or MAOIs; caution with lithium, phenytoin, TCAs, warfarin. Pregnancy exposure associated with premature delivery, low birth weight, lower Apgars.

fluvoxamine ▶L ♀C but - in 3rd trimester ▶- $$$$

ADULT - OCD: Start 50 mg PO qhs, increase by 50 mg/day q4-7 days to usual effective dose of 100-300 mg/day divided bid. Maximum dose is 300 mg/day.

PEDS - OCD and ≥8 yo: 25 mg PO qhs, increase by 25 mg/day q4-7 days to usual effective dose of 50-200 mg/day divided bid. Max dose is 200 mg/day in children age 8-11 yo; max 300 mg/day in children >11 yo. Therapeutic effect may be seen with lower doses in girls.

FORMS - Generic: Tabs 25, 50, 100 mg.

NOTES - Contraindicated with thioridazine. Don't use with cisapride, diazepam, tryptophan, pimozide, or MAOIs; caution with benzodiazepines, theophylline, TCAs, and warfarin. Luvox brand not currently on market.

paroxetine (Paxil, Paxil CR, Pexeva) ▶LK ♀C but - in 3rd trimester ▶? $$$

ADULT - Depression: Start 20 mg PO qam, increase by 10 mg/day at intervals ≥1 week to usual effective dose of 20-50 mg/day. Max 50 mg/day. Controlled release: Start 25 mg PO qam, increase by 12.5 mg/day at intervals ≥1 week to usual effective dose of 25-62.5 mg/day, max 62.5 mg/day. OCD: Start 20 mg PO qam, increase by 10 mg/day at intervals ≥1 week to usual effective dose of 20-60 mg/day.

Max 60 mg/day. Panic disorder: Start 10 mg PO qam, increase by 10 mg/day at intervals ≥1 week to usual effective dose of 10-60 mg/day. Max 60 mg/day. Controlled release: start 12.5 mg/day, increase by 12.5 mg/day at intervals ≥1 week to usual effective range of 12.5-75 mg/day, max 75 mg/day. Social anxiety disorder: Start 20 mg PO qam, max 60 mg/day. Controlled-release: Start 12.5 mg PO qam, max 37.5 mg/day. Generalized anxiety disorder: Start 20 mg PO qam, max 50 mg/day. Post-traumatic stress disorder: Start 20 mg PO qam, usual effective dose 20-40 mg/day, max 50 mg/day. Premenstrual dysphoric disorder: Controlled-release: Continuous dosing: Start 12.5 mg PO qam, may increase dose after 1 wk to max 25 mg qam. Intermittent dosing: Start 12.5 mg PO qam 2 wks prior to menses, max 25 mg/day.

PEDS - Not recommended in children or adolescents due to increased risk of suicidal thinking and suicide attempts.

UNAPPROVED ADULT - Hot flashes: 20 mg PO qd, or 12.5-25 mg PO qd of controlled release.

FORMS - Trade/Generic: Tabs 10,20,30,40 mg. Trade: Extended-release tabs 12.5,25,37.5 mg. Oral suspension 10 mg/5 mL.

NOTES - Start at 10 mg/day and do not exceed 40 mg/day in elderly or debilitated patients or those with renal or hepatic impairment. Contraindicated with thioridazine. Don't use with MAOIs or tryptophan; caution with barbiturates, cimetidine, phenytoin, theophylline, TCAs, and warfarin. Taper after long-term therapy; reduce by 10 mg/day q week. Once down to 20 mg/day, continue for 1 week then stop. Reinstitute at full dose if withdrawal symptoms develop and taper more slowly. Pregnancy exposure associated with premature delivery, low birth weight, and lower Apgar scores. Pexeva is paroxetine mesylate and is a generic equivalent for paroxetine HCl.

sertraline (Zoloft) ▶LK ♀C but - in 3rd trimester ▶+ $$$

ADULT - Depression/OCD: Start 50 mg PO qd, may increase after 1 week. Usual effective dose is 50-200 mg/day. Max dose is 200 mg/day. Panic disorder/Posttraumatic stress disorder/Social anxiety disorder: 25 mg PO qd, may increase after 1 week to 50 mg PO qd. Usual effective dose is 50-200 mg/day. Max dose is 200 mg/day. Premenstrual dysphoric disorder: Start 50 mg PO qd (continuous) or 14 days prior to menses (intermittent), max 150 mg daily continuous or 100 mg daily intermittent. If used intermittently, start 50 mg PO qd x 3 days then increase to 100 mg.

PEDS - OCD and 6-12 yo: 25 mg PO qd, max 200 mg/day. OCD and ≥13 yo: Adult dosing.

UNAPPROVED PEDS - Major depressive disorder: Start 25 mg PO qd, usual range 50-200 mg/day.

FORMS - Trade: Tabs 25, 50, 100 mg. Oral concentrate 20 mg/mL.

NOTES - Don't use with cisapride, tryptophan, or MAOIs; caution with cimetidine, warfarin, pimozide, or TCAs. Must dilute oral concentrate before administration. Pregnancy exposure associated with premature delivery, low birth weight, and lower Apgar scores.

PSYCHIATRY: Antidepressants – Other

NOTE: For bupropion, duloxetine, venlafaxine, nefazodone, mirtazapine: Observe for worsening depression or emergence of suicidal thoughts or behaviors especially early in therapy or after increases in dose. Monitor for emergence of anxiety, agitation, panic attacks, insomnia, irritability, hostility, impulsivity, akathisia, mania, and hypomania.

bupropion (*Wellbutrin, Wellbutrin SR, Wellbutrin XL*) ▶LK ♀B ▶- $$$$

ADULT - Depression: Start 100 mg PO bid (immediate release) or 150 mg PO qam (sustained release), after 4-7 days may increase to 100 mg tid (immediate release) or 150 mg bid (sustained release). Extended release: Start 150 mg PO q am, after 4 days may increase to 300 mg q am, max 450 mg q am. Usual effective dose is 300-450 mg/day. Maximum dose is 150 mg/dose and 450 mg/day (immediate release) or 400 mg/day (sust'd release). Allow 6-8h between doses with last dose no later than 5 pm.

PEDS - Not approved in children.

UNAPPROVED ADULT - ADHD: 150-450 mg/day PO.

UNAPPROVED PEDS - ADHD: 1.4-5.7 mg/kg/day PO.

FORMS - Generic/Trade: Tabs 75,100 mg. Sustained release tabs 100, 150 mg. Trade only: sustained release tabs 200 mg (Wellbutrin SR). Ext'd-release tabs 150, 300 mg (Wellbutrin XL)

NOTES - Weak inhibitor of dopamine reuptake. Contraindicated in seizure disorders, bulimia, anorexia, with MAO inhibitors, or with abrupt alcohol or sedative withdrawal. Seizures in 0.4% of patients taking 300-450 mg per day. Wellbutrin SR is same drug as Zyban for smoking cessation.

duloxetine (*Cymbalta*) ▶L ♀C ▶? ?

ADULT - Depression: 40-60 mg/day PO given either qd or bid.

PEDS - Not approved in children.

FORMS - Trade: Caps 20, 30, 60 mg.

NOTES - Use during third trimester of pregnancy is associated with neonatal complications including respiratory, gastrointestinal, and feeding problems, seizures and withdrawal symptoms. Balance these risks against those of withdrawal and depression for the mother. Avoid in end-stage renal disease or hepatic insufficiency. Blood pressure increases of 2 mm Hg systolic and 0.5 mm Hg diastolic observed.

mirtazapine (*Remeron, Remeron SolTab*) ▶LK ♀C ▶? $$$

ADULT - Depression: Start 15 mg PO qhs, increase after 1-2 weeks to usual effective dose of 15-45 mg/day.

PEDS - Not approved in children.

FORMS - Trade/generic: Tabs 15, 30, 45 mg. Tabs, orally disintegrating (SolTab) 15, 30 mg. Trade: Tabs, orally disintegrating (SolTab) 45 mg.

NOTES - Enhances norepinephrine and serootnin release, inhibits 5-HT2 and 5-HT3 receptors. 0.1% risk of agranulocytosis. May cause drowsiness and increased appetite/weight gain. Don't use with MAOs.

moclobemide (❦*Manerix*) ▶L ♀C ▶- $$

ADULT - Canada only. Depression: 300-600 mg/day PO divided twice daily after meals.

PEDS - Not approved in children.

FORMS - Trade: tabs 150, 300 mg. Generic: tabs 100, 150, 300 mg.

NOTES - No special dietary restrictions.

nefazodone ▶L ♀C ▶? $$$

WARNING - Rare reports of life-threatening liver failure. Discontinue if clinical signs or symptoms of liver dysfunction develop. Brand product withdrawn from market in USA, Canada.

ADULT - Depression: Start 100 mg PO bid, increase by 100-200 mg/day at ≥1 week intervals to usual effective dose of 150-300 mg PO bid. Maximum dose is 600 mg/day. Start 50 mg PO bid in elderly or debilitated patients.

PEDS - Not approved in children.

FORMS - Generic: Tabs 50, 100, 150, 200, 250 mg.

NOTES - Inhibits 5-HT2 receptors, inhibits serotonin reuptake. Don't use with cisapride,

MAOIs, pimozide, or triazolam; caution with al-prazolam. Many other drug interactions.

trazodone (Desyrel) ▶L ♀C ▶- $$$$
ADULT - Depression: Start 50-150 mg/day PO in divided doses, increase by 50 mg/day q3-4 days. Usual effective dose is 400-600 mg/day in divided doses.
PEDS - Not approved in children.
UNAPPROVED ADULT - Insomnia: 50-100 mg PO qhs, max 150 mg.
UNAPPROVED PEDS - Depression 6-18 yo: Start 1.5-2 mg/kg/day PO divided bid-tid, may increase q3-4 days to max 6 mg/kg/day.
FORMS - Generic/Trade: Tabs 50, 100, 150, 300 mg.
NOTES - Inhibits 5-HT2 receptors, inhibits sero-tonin reuptake. May cause priapism. Rarely used as monotherapy for depression; most often used as a sleep aid and adjunct to another antidepressant. Use caution if coadministered with agents that inhibit or induce CYP3A4.

venlafaxine (Effexor, Effexor XR) ▶LK ♀C but - in 3rd trimester ▶? $$$$
ADULT - Depression: Start 37.5-75 mg PO qd (Effexor XR) or 75 mg/day PO divided bid-tid (Effexor). Increase in 75 mg increments q4 days to usual effective dose of 150-225 mg/day, max 225 mg/day (Effexor XR) or 375 mg/day (Effexor). Generalized anxiety disorder: Start 37.5-75 mg PO qd (Effexor XR), increase in 75 mg increments q4 days to max 225 mg/day. Social anxiety disorder: Start 37.5-75 mg PO qd (Effexor XR), max 225 mg/day.
PEDS - Not approved in children.
UNAPPROVED ADULT - Hot flashes: 37.5-75 mg/day of extended release form.
FORMS - Trade: Caps, extended release 37.5, 75, 150 mg. Tabs 25, 37.5, 50, 75, 100 mg.
NOTES - Non-cyclic, serotonin-norepinephrine reuptake inhibitor (SNRI). Decrease dose in renal or hepatic impairment. Monitor for increases in BP. Don't give with MAOIs; caution with cimetidine and haloperidol. Gradually taper dose when discontinuing therapy to avoid withdrawal symptoms after prolonged use. Used for hot flashes primarily in cancer patients. Hostility, suicidal ideation, and self-harm reported when used in children. Use during third trimester of pregnancy is associated with neonatal complications including respiratory, gastrointestinal, and feeding problems, seizures and withdrawal symptoms. Balance these risks against those of withdrawal and depression for the mother.

PSYCHIATRY: Antimanic (Bipolar) Agents

carbamazepine (Tegretol, Tegretol XR, Carbatrol, Epitol) ▶LK ♀D ▶+ $
WARNING - Aplastic anemia and agranulocytosis have been reported. Monitor WBC and platelets at baseline and periodically.
ADULT, PEDS - See neurology section.
UNAPPROVED ADULT - Mania: Start 200-600 mg/day divided tid-qid (bid for XR), increase by 200 mg/day q2-4 days. Mean effective dose = 1,000 mg/day. Max 1,600 mg/day.
FORMS - Trade: Tabs, PO 100, 200 mg (Tegretol, Epitol) Tabs, Chew 100 mg (Tegretol, Epitol) Susp 100 mg/5 mL (Tegretol) extended release tabs 100, 200, 400 mg (Tegretol XR) extended release caps 100, 200, 300 mg (Carbatrol). Generic: Tabs, PO 200 mg. Chew tabs 100 mg. Susp 100 mg/5 mL.
NOTES - Therapeutic range = 4-12 mcg/ml. Stevens-Johnson Syndrome and hepatitis. Monitor LFTs. Many drug interactions.

lamotrigine (Lamictal, Lamictal CD) ▶LK ♀C ▶- $$$$
WARNING - Potentially life-threatening rashes (eg, Stevens-Johnson Syndrome, toxic epidermal necrolysis) have been reported in 0.3% of adults and 0.8% of children, usually within 2-8 weeks of initiation; discontinue at first sign of rash. Drug interaction with valproate – see adjusted dosing guidelines.
ADULT - Bipolar disorder (maintenance): Start 25 mg PO qd, 50 mg PO qd if on carbamazepine or other enzyme-inducing drugs, or 25 mg PO qod if on valproate. Increase for weeks 3-4 to 50 mg/day, 50 mg bid if on enzyme-inducing drugs, or 25 mg/day if on valproate, then adjust over weeks 5-7 to target doses of 200 mg/day, 400 mg/day divided bid if on enzyme-inducing drugs, or 100 mg/day if on valproate. See neurology section for epilepsy dosing.
PEDS - Not approved in children.
FORMS - Trade: Tabs 25, 100, 150, 200 mg. Chew Tabs 5, 25 mg.
NOTES - Drug interactions with enzyme-inducing antiepileptic drugs (i.e. carbamazepine, phenobarbital, phenytoin, primidone) and valproic acid; may need to adjust dose if these drugs are added to or discontinued from therapy (see product insert).

lithium (Eskalith, Eskalith CR, Lithobid, ♣Lithane, Carbolith, Duralith) ▶K ♀D ▶- $

WARNING - Lithium toxicity can occur at therapeutic levels.

ADULT - Acute mania: Start 300-600 mg PO tid, usual effective dose is 900-1,800 mg/day.

PEDS - Adolescents: Adult dosing. Not approved in children <12 yo.

UNAPPROVED PEDS - Mania: Start 15-60 mg/kg/day PO divided tid-qid, adjust weekly based on therapeutic levels.

FORMS - Generic/Trade: caps 150, 300, 600 mg, tabs 300 mg. Extended release tabs 300, 450 mg. Syrup 300 mg/5 ml.

NOTES - 300 mg = 8 mEq or mmol. Steady state in 5 days (longer in elderly or renally impaired patients). Trough levels for acute mania 1.0-1.5 mEq/L, maintenance 0.6-1.2 mEq/L. Dose increase of 300 mg/day raises level by approx 0.2 mEq/L. Monitor renal, thyroid function. Diuretics, ACE inhibitors, and angiotensin receptor blockers may increase levels. NSAIDs may increase lithium levels (ASA & sulindac OK). Avoid dehydration, salt restriction. Monitor for thirst, fluid intake, and urine output; polyuria and polydipsia can occur. Concentration-related side effects (e.g. tremors, GI upset) may be decreased by extending the dosing interval to tid- qid or using the extended release product.

topiramate (Topamax) ▶K ♀C ▶? $$$$$

ADULT - See neurology section

PEDS - Not approved in children.

UNAPPROVED ADULT - Bipolar disorder: Start 25-50 mg/day PO, titrate prn to max 400 mg/day. Alcohol dependence: Start 25 mg/day PO, titrate weekly to max 150 mg bid.

FORMS - Trade only: tabs 25, 100, 200 mg. sprinkle caps 15, 25 mg.

NOTES - Give ½ usual adult dose to patients with renal impairment (CrCl <70 ml/ min). Confusion, renal stones, glaucoma, and weight loss may occur.

valproic acid (Depakene, Depakote, Depakote ER, divalproex, ♥Epiject, Epival, Deproic) ▶L ♀D ▶+ $$$

WARNING - Fatal hepatic failure has occurred especially in children <2 yo with multiple anticonvulsants and co-morbidities. Monitor LFTs frequently during first 6 months. Life-threatening cases of pancreatitis have been reported after initial or prolonged use. Evaluate for abdominal pain, N/V, and/or anorexia and discontinue valproate if pancreatitis is diagnosed.

ADULT - Mania: 250 mg PO tid (Depakote), titrate to therapeutic trough level of 50-125 mcg/ml or to a maximum dose of 60 mg/kg/day.

PEDS - Not approved for mania in children.

FORMS - Generic/Trade: Caps (Depakene) 250 mg. Syrup (Depakene) 250 mg/ 5 mL. Trade only: sprinkle Caps (Depakote) 125 mg. Tabs, Enteric Coated (Depakote) 125, 250, 500 mg. Tabs, extended release (Depakote ER) 250, 500 mg.

NOTES - Contraindicated in urea cycle disorders. May cause hyperammonemia. Therapeutic range = 50-125 mcg/ml. Depakote and Depakote ER are not interchangeable. Depakote releases divalproex sodium over 8-12h (qd-qid dosing) and Depakote ER releases divalproex sodium over 18-24h (qd dosing). Contraindicated in hepatic dysfunction. Many drug interactions. Reduce dose in elderly. GI irritation, thrombocytopenia may occur. Children receiving other anticonvulsants may require higher doses. Depakene (valproic acid), Depakote (divalproex sodium). Depakote ER about 10% less bioavailable than Depakote. May need to increase dose.

PSYCHIATRY: Antipsychotics - Atypical – Serotonin Dopamine Receptor Antagonists (SDAs)

NOTE: Extrapyramidal side effects including tardive dyskinesia may occur with antipsychotics. Increased risk of hyperglycemia / diabetes mellitus; monitor glucose periodically.

clozapine (Clozaril, FazaClo ODT) ▶L ♀B ▶- $$$$$

WARNING - Risk of agranulocytosis is 1-2%, monitor WBC counts q week x 6 months, then q2 weeks. Contraindicated if WBC <3,500 cells/mm3. Discontinue if WBC <3,000 cells/mm3. Risk of seizures, orthostatic hypotension, respiratory/ cardiac arrest. Risk of myocarditis; monitor especially during the first month.

ADULT - Treatment refractory schizophrenia & suicidal behavior with schizophrenia or schizoaffective disorder: Start 12.5 mg PO qd- bid, increase by 25-50 mg/day to usual effective dose of 300-450 mg/day. Maximum dose is 900 mg/day. Retitrate dose if stopped more than 3-4 days.

PEDS - Not approved in children.

FORMS - Generic/Trade: Tabs 25, 100 mg.

Trade: Orally disintegrating tab (FazaClo ODT) 25, 100 mg (scored).

NOTES - Low EPS and tardive dyskinesia risk. May be effective for treatment resistant patients who have not responded to conventional agents. Associated with significant weight gain and increased risk of developing new onset diabetes - monitor weight, fasting blood glucose, and triglycerides before initiation and at regular intervals during treatment. Excessive sedation or respiratory depression may occur when combined with CNS depressants especially benzodiazepines. If an orally disintegrating tab is split, discard the remaining portion.

olanzapine (*Zyprexa, Zyprexa Zydis*) ▶L 9C ▶- $$$$$

ADULT - Agitation in acute bipolar mania or schizophrenia: Start 10 mg IM, may repeat in ≥2h to max 30 mg/day (reduce dose to 2.5-5 mg in the elderly or debilitated). Psychotic disorders, oral therapy: Start 5-10 mg PO qd. Increase weekly to usual effective dose of 10-15 mg/day. Max 20 mg/day. Bipolar disorder, monotherapy, acute manic or mixed episodes and maintenance: Start 10-15 mg PO qd. Adjust dose at intervals ≥24 h in 5 mg/day increments to usual effective dose of 5-20 mg/day. Max 20 mg/day. Bipolar mania, adjunctive: Start 10 mg PO qd; usual effective dose 5-20 mg/day. Max 20 mg/day.

PEDS - Not approved in children.

FORMS - Trade: Tabs 2.5,5,7.5,10,15 mg. Orally disintegrating tabs (Zyprexa Zydis) 5,10, 15,20 mg.

NOTES - Use for short-term (3-4 weeks) acute manic episodes associated with bipolar disorder. Associated with significant weight gain and increased risk of developing new-onset diabetes - monitor weight, fasting blood glucose, and triglycerides before initiation and at regular intervals during treatment. Monitor for orthostatic hypotension when given IM.

quetiapine (*Seroquel*) ▶LK 9C ▶- $$$$$

ADULT - Psychotic disorders: Start 25 mg PO bid, increase by 25- 50 mg bid-tid on day 2-3, to target dose of 300-400 mg/day divided bid-tid. Usual effective dose is 150-750 mg/day. Maximum dose is 800 mg/day. Acute bipolar mania, monotherapy or adjunctive: Start 50 mg PO bid on day 1, then increase by 100 mg/day over next 3 days to reach the following maximal rate: 100 mg bid, 150 mg bid, and then 200 mg bid. If tolerated and necessary, may then increase to 300 mg bid on day 5 and 400

mg bid thereafter.

PEDS - Not approved in children.

UNAPPROVED ADULT - Bipolar disorder: 100-200 mg per day in divided doses.

FORMS - Trade: Tabs 25, 100, 200, 300 mg.

NOTES - Eye exam for cataracts recommended q 6 months. Low EPS, tardive dyskinesia risk.

risperidone (*Risperdal, Risperdal Consta*) ▶LK 9C ▶- $$$$$

ADULT - Psychotic disorders: Start 1 mg PO bid, increase by 1 mg bid on the second and third day, then at intervals ≥1 week (some patients may require slower titration). Start 0.5 mg/dose in the elderly, debilitated, renally or hepatically impaired, or hypotensive patients. Titrate by ≤0.5 mg BID. Usual effective dose is 4-8 mg/day divided qd-bid; maximum dose is 16 mg/day. Long-acting injection (Consta) for schizophrenia: Start 25 mg IM q 2 weeks while continuing oral dose x 3 weeks. May increase q 4 weeks to max 50 mg q 2 weeks. Bipolar mania: Start 2-3 mg PO qd, may adjust by 1 mg/day at 24-hr intervals to max of 6 mg/day.

PEDS - Not approved in children.

UNAPPROVED PEDS - Psychotic disorders, mania, aggression: 0.5-1.5 mg/day PO.

FORMS - Trade: Tabs 0.25, 0.5, 1, 2, 3, 4 mg. Orally disintegrating tablets (M-TAB) 0.5, 1, 2 mg. Oral solution 1 mg/ml.

NOTES - Solution is compatible with water, coffee, orange juice, and low-fat milk; is NOT compatible with cola or tea. Increased risk of stroke and transient ischemic attacks when used for dementia-related psychoses. Place orally disintegrating tablets on tongue and do not chew. Establish tolerability with oral form before starting long-acting injection. Alternate injections between buttocks.

ziprasidone (*Geodon*) ▶L 9C ▶- $$$$$

WARNING - May prolong QTc. Avoid with drugs that prolong QTc or in those with QT syndrome or cardiac arrhythmias.

ADULT - Schizophrenia: Start 20 mg PO bid with food, adjust at >2 day intervals to max 80 mg PO bid. Acute agitation in schizophrenia: 10-20 mg IM. May repeat 10 mg dose q 2 hours, 20 mg dose q 4 hours, max 40 mg per day. Bipolar mania: Start 40 mg PO bid with food, adjust to 60-80 mg bid on day 2. Usual range 40-80 mg bid.

PEDS - Not approved in children.

FORMS - Trade: Caps 20,40,60,80 mg.

NOTES – Carbamazepine, ketoconazole interactions. Low EPS and tardive dyskinesia risk.

PSYCHIATRY: Antipsychotics – D2 Antagonists – High Potency (1-5 mg = 100 mg CPZ)

NOTE: Can give in qhs doses, but may be divided initially to decrease side effects and increase daytime sedation. EPS side effects including tardive dyskinesia may occur with antipsychotics.

fluphenazine (*Prolixin*, ♥*Modecate, Moditen*) ►LK ♀C ▶? $$$
ADULT - Psychotic disorders: Start 0.5-10 mg/day PO divided q6-8h. Usual effective dose 1-20 mg/day. Max dose is 40 mg/day PO or 1.25-10 mg/day IM divided q6-8h. Max dose is 10 mg/day IM. May use long-acting formulations (enanthate/decanoate) when patients are stabilized on a fixed daily dose. Approximate conversion ratio: 12.5- 25 mg IM/ SC (depot) q3 weeks = 10- 20 mg/day PO.
PEDS - Not approved in children.
FORMS - Generic/Trade: Tabs 1, 2.5, 5, 10 mg. Elixir 2.5 mg/5 ml. Oral concentrate 5 mg/ml.
NOTES - Do not mix oral concentrate with coffee, tea, cola, or apple juice.

haloperidol (*Haldol*) ►LK ♀C ▶- $$
ADULT - Psychotic disorders/Tourette's: 0.5-5 mg PO bid-tid. Usual effective dose 6-20 mg/day, max dose 100 mg/day or 2-5 mg IM q1-8h prn. May use long-acting (depot) form when patients are stabilized on a fixed daily dose. Approx. conversion ratio: 100- 200 mg IM (depot) q4 weeks = 10 mg/day PO haloperidol.
PEDS - Psychotic disorders age 3- 12 yo: 0.05-0.15 mg/kg/day PO divided bid-tid. Tourette's or non-psychotic behavior disorders age 3- 12 yo: 0.05- 0.075 mg/kg/day PO divided bid-tid. Increase dose by 0.5 mg q week to maximum dose of 6 mg/day. Not approved for IM administration in children.
UNAPPROVED ADULT - Acute psychoses and combative behavior: 5-10 mg IV/IM, repeat prn in 10-30 min.
UNAPPROVED PEDS - Psychosis 6-12 yo: 1-3 mg/dose IM (as lactate) q4-8h, max 0.15 mg/kg/day.
FORMS - Generic/ Trade: Tabs 0.5, 1, 2, 5, 10, 20 mg. Oral concentrate 2 mg/ml.
NOTES - Therapeutic range is 2- 15 ng/ml.

perphenazine (*Trilafon*) ►LK ♀C ▶? $$$
ADULT - Psychotic disorders: Start 4-8 mg PO tid or 8-16 mg PO bid-qid (if hospitalized), maximum PO dose is 64 mg/day. Can give 5-10 mg IM q6h, max IM dose is 30 mg/day.
PEDS - Not approved for children <12 yo.
FORMS - Generic/Trade: Tabs 2, 4, 8, 16 mg. Oral concentrate 16 mg/5 ml.
NOTES - Do not mix oral concentrate with coffee, tea, cola, or apple juice.

pimozide (*Orap*) ►L ♀C ▶- $$$
ADULT - Tourette's: Start 1-2 mg/day PO in divided doses, increase q2 days to usual effective dose of 1-10 mg/day. Maximum dose is 0.2 mg/kg/day up to 10 mg/day.
PEDS - Tourette's age >12 yo: 0.05 mg/kg PO qhs, increase q3 days to maximum of 0.2 mg/kg/day up to 10 mg/day.
FORMS - Trade only: Tabs 1, 2 mg.
NOTES - QT prolongation may occur. Monitor ECG at baseline and periodically throughout therapy. Contraindicated with macrolide antibiotics, nefazodone, and sertraline. Use caution with inhibitors of CYP3A4.

thiothixene (*Navane*) ►LK ♀C ▶? $$
ADULT - Psychotic disorders: Start 2 mg PO tid. Usual effective dose is 20-30 mg/day, maximum dose is 60 mg/day PO.
PEDS - Adolescents: Adult dosing. Not approved in children <12 yo.
FORMS - Generic/Trade: Caps 2, 5, 10. Oral concentrate 5 mg/ml. Trade only: Caps 20 mg. Generic only: Caps 1 mg.

trifluoperazine (*Stelazine*) ►LK ♀C ▶- $$$
ADULT - Psychotic disorders: Start 2-5 mg PO bid. Usual effective dose is 15-20 mg/day, some patients may require ≥40 mg/day. Can give 1-2 mg IM q4-6h prn, maximum IM dose is 10 mg/day. Anxiety: 1-2 mg PO bid for up to 12 weeks. Maximum dose is 6 mg/day.
PEDS - Psychotic disorders 6-12 yo: 1 mg PO qd-bid, gradually increase to maximum dose of 15 mg/day. Can give 1 mg IM qd-bid.
FORMS - Generic/Trade: Tabs 1, 2, 5, 10 mg. Trade only: oral concentrate 10 mg/ml.
NOTES - Dilute oral concentrate before giving.

PSYCHIATRY: Antipsychotics – D2 Antagonists – Mid Potency (10 mg = 100 mg CPZ)

NOTE: Extrapyramidal side effects including tardive dyskinesia may occur with antipsychotics.

loxapine (*Loxitane*, ✚*Loxapac*) ▶LK ♀C ▶- $$$$
ADULT - Psychotic disorders: Start 10 mg PO bid, usual effective dose is 60-100 mg/day divided bid- qid. Maximum dose is 250 mg/day.
PEDS - Not approved in children.
FORMS - Generic/Trade: Caps 5,10,25,50 mg.

methotrimeprazine (✚*Nozinan*) ▶L♀? ▶? $\$-$$
ADULT - Canada only. Anxiety/analgesia: 6-25 mg PO per day given tid. Sedation: 10-25 mg hs. Psychoses/intense pain: Start 50-75 mg PO per day given in 2-3 doses, max 1000 mg/day. Postoperative pain: 20-40 mg PO or 10-25 mg IM q 8h. Anesthesia premedication: 10-25 mg IM or 20-40 mg PO q 8h with last dose of 25-50 mg IM 1h before surgery. Limit therapy to ≤30 days.
PEDS - Canada only. 0.25 mg/kg/day given in 2-3 doses, max 40 mg/day for child <12 yo.
FORMS - Trade/Generic: Tabs 2, 5, 25, 50 mg. Trade: Oral liquid 5 mg/m, drops 40 mg/mL.

molindone (*Moban*) ▶LK ♀C ▶? $$$$$
ADULT - Psychotic disorders: Start 50-75 mg/day PO divided tid-qid, usual effective dose is 50-100 mg/day. Maximum dose is 225 mg/day.
PEDS - Adolescents: Adult dosing. Not approved in children <12 yo.
FORMS - Trade: Tabs 5, 10, 25, 50 mg.

PSYCHIATRY: Antipsychotics – D2 Antagonists – Low Potency (50-100 mg = 100 mg CPZ)

NOTE: Extrapyramidal side effects including tardive dyskinesia may occur with antipsychotics.

chlorpromazine (*Thorazine*, ✚*Largactil*) ▶LK ♀C ▶- $
ADULT - Psychotic disorders: 10-50 mg PO bid-qid or 25-50 mg IM, can repeat in 1 hour. Severe cases may require 400 mg IM q4-6h up to max of 2,000 mg/day IM. Hiccups: 25-50 mg PO/IM tid-qid. Persistent hiccups may require 25-50 mg in 0.5-1 L NS by slow IV infusion.
PEDS - Severe behavioral problems/ psychotic disorders age 6 months-12 yo: 0.5 mg/kg PO q4-6h prn or 1 mg/kg PR q6-8h prn or 0.5 mg/kg IM q6-8h prn.
FORMS - Generic/Trade: Tabs 10, 25, 50, 100, 200 mg. Oral concentrate 30 mg/ml, 100 mg/ml. Trade only: sustained release Caps 30, 75, 150 mg. Syrup 10 mg/5 ml. Suppositories 25, 100 mg.
NOTES - Monitor for hypotension if IM, IV use.

thioridazine (*Mellaril*) ▶LK ♀C ▶? $
WARNING - Can cause QTc prolongation, torsade arrhythmias, and sudden death.
ADULT - Psychotic disorders: Start 50-100 mg PO tid, usual effective dose is 200-800 mg/day divided bid-qid. Maximum dose is 800 mg/day.
PEDS - Behavioral disorders 2- 12 yo: 10- 25 mg PO bid-tid, maximum dose is 3 mg/kg/day.
FORMS - Generic: Tabs 10,15,25,50,100,150, 200 mg. Oral concentrate 30,100 mg/ml.
NOTES - Not recommended as first-line therapy. Contraindicated if history of cardiac arrhythmias, congenital long QT syndrome, or if taking fluvoxamine, propranolol, pindolol, drugs that inhibit CYP 2D6 (e.g. fluoxetine, paroxetine), and other drugs that prolong the QTc interval. Only use for patients with schizophrenia who do not respond to other antipsychotics. Monitor baseline ECG and potassium. Pigmentary retinopathy with doses >800 mg/day.

PSYCHIATRY: Antipsychotics – Dopamine-2 / Serotonin-1 Partial Agonist & Serotonin-2 Antagonist

aripiprazole (*Abilify*) ▶L ♀C ▶? $$$$$
ADULT - Schizophrenia: Start 10-15 mg qd. Max 30 mg qd.
PEDS - Not approved in children.

FORMS - Trade: Tabs 5,10,15,20,30 mg.
NOTES - Low EPS and tardive dyskinesia risk. Monitor glucose periodically to assess for hyperglycemia / diabetes.

PSYCHIATRY: Anxiolytics / Hypnotics - Benzodiazepines - Long Half-Life (25-100 hours)

NOTE: To avoid withdrawal, gradually taper when discontinuing after prolonged use. Use cautiously in the elderly; may accumulate and lead to side effects, psychomotor impairment.

bromazepam (♣*Lectopam*) ▶L ♀D ▶- $
ADULT - Canada only. 6-18 mg/day PO in equally divided doses.
PEDS - Not approved in children.
FORMS - Trade/generic: Tabs 1.5, 3, 6 mg.
NOTES - Do not exceed 3 mg/day initially in the elderly or debilitated. Gradually taper when discontinuing after prolonged use. Half life ~20 hours in adults but increased in elderly. Cimetidine may prolong elimination.

chlordiazepoxide (*Librium*) ▶LK ♀D ▶- ©IV $
ADULT - Anxiety: 5-25 mg PO tid-qid or 25-50 mg IM/IV tid-qid (acute/severe anxiety). Acute alcohol withdrawal: 50-100 mg PO/IM/IV, repeat q3-4h prn up to 300 mg/day.
PEDS - Anxiety and >6 yo: 5-10 mg PO bid-qid.
FORMS - Generic/Trade: Caps 5, 10, 25 mg.
NOTES - Half-life 5-30 h.

clonazepam (*Klonopin*, ♣*Rivotril, Clonapam*) ▶LK ♀D ▶? ©IV $$
ADULT - Panic disorder: 0.25 mg PO bid, increase by 0.125- 0.25 mg q3 days to maximum dose of 4 mg/day.
PEDS - Not approved for peds panic disorder.
UNAPPROVED ADULT - Restless legs syndrome: start 0.25 mg PO qhs. Max 2 mg qhs.
FORMS - Generic/Trade: Tabs 0.5, 1, 2 mg. Trade: Orally disintegrating tabs (Klonopin Wafers) 0.125, 0.25, 0.5, 1, 2 mg.
NOTES - Half-life 18- 50 h.

clorazepate (*Tranxene, Genxene*) ▶LK ♀D ▶- ©IV $$
ADULT - Anxiety: Start 7.5-15 mg PO qhs or bid-tid, usual effective dose is 15-60 mg/day.
Acute alcohol withdrawal: 60-90 mg/day on first day divided bid-tid, gradually reduce dose to 7.5-15 mg/day over 5 days. Max dose is 90 mg/day. May transfer patients to single-dose tabs (Tranxene-SD) when dose stabilized.
PEDS - Not approved in children <9 yo.
FORMS - Generic/Trade: Tabs 3.75, 7.5, 15 mg. Trade only: extended release Tabs 11.25, 22.5 mg.
NOTES - Half-life 40-50 h.

diazepam (*Valium*, ♣*Vivol, E Pam*) ▶LK ♀D ▶- ©IV $
ADULT - Anxiety: 2-10 mg PO bid-qid or 2-20 mg IM/IV, repeat dose in 3-4h prn. Alcohol withdrawal: 10 mg PO tid-qid x 24 hr then 5 mg PO tid-qid prn.
PEDS - Not approved for anxiety in children.
UNAPPROVED ADULT - Loading dose strategy for alcohol withdrawal: 10-20 mg PO or 10 mg slow IV in closely monitored setting, then repeat similar or lower doses q1-2 hr prn until sedated. Further doses should be unnecessary due to long half-life.
FORMS - Generic/Trade: Tabs 2,5,10 mg. Oral solution 5 mg/5 ml. Oral concentrate (Intensol) 5 mg/ml.
NOTES - Half-life 20-80h. Respiratory depression may occur.

flurazepam (*Dalmane*) ▶LK ♀X ▶- ©IV $
ADULT - Insomnia: 15-30 mg PO qhs.
PEDS - Not approved in children <15 yo.
FORMS - Generic/Trade: Caps 15, 30 mg.
NOTES - Half-life 70-90h. For short term treatment of insomnia.

PSYCHIATRY: Anxiolytics / Hypnotics - Benzodiazepines - Medium Half-Life (10-15 hours)

NOTE: Gradually taper when discontinuing after prolonged use to avoid withdrawal.

estazolam (*ProSom*) ▶LK ♀X ▶- ©IV $$
ADULT - Insomnia: 1-2 mg PO qhs for up to 12 weeks. Reduce dose to 0.5 mg in elderly, small, or debilitated patients.
PEDS - Not approved in children.
FORMS - Generic/Trade: Tabs 1, 2 mg.
NOTES - For short term treatment of insomnia.

lorazepam (*Ativan*) ▶LK ♀D ▶- ©IV $$$
ADULT - Anxiety: Start 0.5-1 mg PO bid-tid, usual effective dose is 2-6 mg/day. Maximum dose is 10 mg/day PO. Anxiolytic/sedation: 0.04-0.05 mg/kg IV/IM; usual dose 2 mg, max 4 mg. Insomnia: 2-4 mg PO qhs.
PEDS - Not approved in children.

UNAPPROVED ADULT - Alcohol withdrawal: 1-2 mg PO/IM/IV q 2-4 hr prn or 2 mg PO/IM/IV q6h x 24 hr then 1 mg q6h x 8 doses.
UNAPPROVED PEDS - Anxiolytic/Sedation: 0.05 mg/kg/dose q4-8h PO/IV, max 2 mg/dose.
FORMS - Generic/Trade: Tabs 0.5, 1, 2 mg. Trade only: oral concentrate 2 mg/ml.
NOTES - Half-life 10-20h. No active metabolites. For short term treatment of insomnia.

temazepam (*Restoril*) ▶LK ♀X ▶- ©IV $
ADULT - Insomnia: 7.5- 30 mg PO qhs x 7-10 d.
PEDS - Not approved in children.
FORMS - Generic/Trade: Caps 7.5, 15, 30 mg.
NOTES - Half-life 8-25h. For short term treatment of insomnia.

PSYCHIATRY: Anxiolytics / Hypnotics - Benzodiazepines - Short Half-Life (<12 hours)

NOTE: Gradually taper when discontinuing after prolonged use to avoid withdrawal.

alprazolam (*Xanax, Xanax XR*) ▶LK ♀D ▶- ©IV $

ADULT - Anxiety: Start 0.25-0.5 mg PO tid, may increase q3-4 days to a maximum dose of 4 mg/day. Use 0.25 mg PO bid in elderly or debilitated patients. Panic disorder: Start 0.5 mg PO tid (or 0.5-1.0 mg PO qd of Xanax XR), may increase by up to 1 mg/day q3-4 days to usual effective dose of 5-6 mg/day (3-6 mg/day for Xanax XR), maximum dose is 10 mg/day.

PEDS - Not approved in children.

FORMS - Generic/Trade: Tabs 0.25, 0.5, 1, 2 mg. Generic only: Oral concentrate 1 mg/mL. Extended release tabs: 0.5, 1, 2, 3 mg.

NOTES - Half-life 12h, but need to give tid. Divide administration time evenly during waking hours to avoid interdose symptoms. Don't give with antifungals (i.e. ketoconazole, itraconazole); use caution with macrolides, propoxyphene, oral contraceptives, TCAs, cimetidine, antidepressants, anticonvulsants, paroxetine, sertraline, and others that inhibit CYP 3A4.

oxazepam (*Serax*) ▶LK ♀D ▶- ©IV $$$

ADULT - Anxiety: 10-30 mg PO tid-qid. Acute alcohol withdrawal: 15-30 mg PO tid-qid.

PEDS - Not approved in children <6 yo.

UNAPPROVED ADULT - Restless legs syndrome: start 10 mg PO qhs. Max 40 mg qhs.

FORMS - Generic/Trade: Caps 10, 15, 30 mg. Trade only: Tabs 15 mg.

NOTES - Half-life 8 hours.

triazolam (*Halcion*) ▶LK ♀X ▶- ©IV $

ADULT - Hypnotic: 0.125- 0.25 mg PO qhs x 7-10 days, maximum dose is 0.5 mg/day. Start 0.125 mg/day in elderly or debilitated patients.

PEDS - Not approved in children.

UNAPPROVED ADULT - Restless legs syndr: Start 0.125 mg PO qhs, max 0.5 mg qhs.

FORMS - Generic/Trade: Tabs 0.125, 0.25 mg.

NOTES - Half-life 2-3 hours. Anterograde amnesia may occur. Don't use with protease inhibitors, ketoconazole, itraconazole, or nefazodone; use caution with macrolides, cimetidine, and other CYP 3A4 inhibitors.

PSYCHIATRY: Anxiolytics / Hypnotics – Other

buspirone (*BuSpar, Vanspar*) ▶K ♀B ▶- $$$

ADULT - Anxiety: Start 15 mg "dividose" daily (7.5 mg PO bid), increase by 5 mg/day q2-3 days to usual effective dose of 30 mg/day, maximum dose is 60 mg/day.

PEDS - Not approved in children.

FORMS - Generic/Trade: tabs 5, 7.5,10, 15 mg. Trade only: Dividose tab 15, 30 mg (scored to be easily bisected or trisected).

NOTES - Slower onset than benzodiazepines; optimum effect requires 3-4 wks of therapy. Don't use with MAOIs; caution with itraconazole, cimetidine, nefazodone, erythromycin, and other CYP 3A4 inhibitors.

butabarbital (*Butisol*) ▶LK ♀D ▶? ©III $$

ADULT - Rarely used; other drugs preferred. Sedative: 15-30 mg PO tid-qid. Hypnotic: 50-100 mg PO qhs for up to 2 weeks.

PEDS - Pre-op sedation: 2-6 mg/kg PO before procedure, maximum 100 mg.

FORMS - Trade: Tabs 30, 50 mg. elixir 30 mg/5 ml.

chloral hydrate (*Aquachloral Supprettes*) ▶LK ♀C ▶+ ©IV $

ADULT - Sedative: 250 mg PO/PR tid after meals. Hypnotic: 500- 1,000 mg PO/PR qhs. Acute alcohol withdrawal: 500- 1,000 mg PO/PR q6h prn.

PEDS - Sedative: 25 mg/kg/day PO/PR divided tid-qid, up to 500 mg tid. Hypnotic: 50 mg/kg PO/PR qhs, up to max of 1 g. Pre-anesthetic: 25- 50 mg/kg PO/PR before procedure.

UNAPPROVED PEDS - Sedative: higher than approved doses 75-100 mg/kg PO/PR.

FORMS - Generic/Trade: Caps 500 mg. syrup 500 mg/ 5 mL. Trade only: rectal suppositories: 325, 650 mg.

NOTES - Give syrup in ½ glass of juice, water.

diphenhydramine (*Allermax, Benadryl, Diphen, Banophen, Diphenhist, Sominex, Siladryl, ✦Allerdryl, Allernix*) ▶LK ♀B ▶- $

ADULT - Insomnia: 25-50 mg PO qhs.

PEDS - Insomnia ≥12 yo: 25-50 mg PO qhs.

FORMS - OTC/Generic/Trade: Tabs/Caps 25, 50 mg. Soln 6.25 mg/5 ml, 12.5 mg/5 ml. Elixir 12.5 mg/ml. OTC only: chew Tabs 12.5 mg. OTC/Rx/Generic/Trade: Caps 25, 50 mg. Oral solution 12.5 mg/5 ml.

NOTES - Anticholinergic side effects are enhanced in the elderly, and may worsen dementia or delirium. Avoid use with donepezil, rivastigmine, galantamine, and tacrine.

zaleplon (*Sonata*, ♣ *Starnoc*) ▶L ♀C ▶- ©IV $$$
ADULT - Insomnia: 5-10 mg PO qhs prn, maximum 20 mg.
PEDS - Not approved in children.
FORMS - Trade: Caps 5, 10 mg.
NOTES - Half-life = 1 hour. Useful if problems with sleep initiation or morning grogginess. For short term treatment of insomnia. Take immediately before bedtime or after going to bed and experiencing difficulty falling asleep. Use 5 mg dose in patients with mild to moderate hepatic impairment, elderly patients, and in patients taking cimetidine. Possible drug interactions with rifampin, phenytoin, carbamazepine, and phenobarbital. Do not use for benzodiazepine or alcohol withdrawal.

zolpidem (*Ambien*) ▶L ♀B ▶+ ©IV $$$
ADULT - Hypnotic: 5- 10 mg PO qhs. Maximum dose is 10 mg.
PEDS - Not approved in children.
FORMS - Trade: Tabs 5, 10 mg.
NOTES - Half-life = 2.5 hours. Useful if problems with early morning awakening. For short term treatment of insomnia. Do not use for benzodiazepine or alcohol withdrawal.

zopiclone (♣ *Imovane*) ▶L ♀D ▶- $
ADULT - Canada only. Short-term treatment of insomnia: 5-7.5 mg PO qhs. In elderly or debilitated, use 3.75 mg qhs initially, and increase prn to 5-7.5 mg qhs. Maximum 7.5 mg qhs.
PEDS - Not approved in children.
FORMS - Trade: tabs 5, 7.5 mg. Generic: tabs 7.5 mg.
NOTES - Treatment should usually not exceed 7-10 days without re-evaluation.

PSYCHIATRY: Combination Drugs

Limbitrol (chlordiazepoxide + amitriptyline) ▶LK ♀D ▶- ©IV $$$
ADULT - Rarely used; other drugs preferred. Depression/ Anxiety: 1 tab PO tid-qid, may increase up to 6 tabs/day.
PEDS - Not approved in children <12 yo.
FORMS - Generic/Trade: Tabs, chlordiazepoxide/ amitriptyline: 5/12.5, 10/25.

Symbyax (olanzapine + fluoxetine) ▶LK ♀C ▶- ?
ADULT - Bipolar depression: Start 6/25 mg PO qhs. Max 18/75 mg/day.
PEDS - Not approved in children <12 yo.
FORMS - Trade: Caps (olanzapine/fluoxetine) 6/25, 6/50, 12/25, 12/50 mg.
NOTES - Efficacy beyond 8 weeks not established. Monitor weight, fasting glucose, and triglycerides before initiation and periodically during treatment. Contraindicated with thioridazine; don't use with cisapride, thioridazine, tryptophan, or MAOIs; caution with lithium, phenytoin, TCAs, ASA, NSAIDs and warfarin. Pregnancy exposure to fluoxetine associated with premature delivery, low birth weight, and lower Apgar scores.

Triavil (perphenazine + amitriptyline) ▶LK ♀D ▶? $$
ADULT - Rarely used; other drugs preferred. Depression/ Anxiety: 1 tab (2-25 or 4-25) PO tid-qid. Max 8 tabs/day (2-25 or 4-25).
PEDS - Not approved in children.
FORMS - Generic/Trade: Tabs, perphenazine/ amitriptyline: 2/10, 2/25, 4/10, 4/25, Generic: Tabs perphenazine/amitriptyline: 4/50.

PSYCHIATRY: Drug Dependence Therapy

acamprosate (*Campral*) ▶K ♀C ▶? ?
ADULT - Maintenance of abstinence from alcohol: 666 mg (2 tabs) PO tid. Start after alcohol withdrawal and patient is abstinent.
PEDS - Not approved in children.
FORMS - Trade: delayed-release tabs 333 mg.
NOTES - Reduce dose to 333 mg if CrCl 30-50 ml/min. Contraindicated if CrCl <30 ml/min.

buprenorphine (*Subutex*) ▶L ♀C ▶- ©III $$$$$
ADULT - Treatment of opioid dependence: Induction 8 mg SL on day 1, 16 mg SL on day 2.

Maintenance: 16 mg SL qd. Can individualize to range of 4-24 mg SL qd.
PEDS - Not approved in children.
FORMS - Trade: SL tabs 2, 8 mg
NOTES - Subutex is preferred over Suboxone for induction. Suboxone preferred for maintenance. Prescribers must complete training and apply for special DEA number. See www.suboxone.com.

bupropion (*Zyban, Buproban*) ▶LK ♀B ▶- $$$$
ADULT - Smoking cessation: Start 150 mg PO q

am x 3 days, then increase to 150 mg PO bid x 7-12 wks. Allow 8h between doses with last dose no later than 5 pm. Maximum dose is 150 mg PO bid. Target quit date should be after at least 1 wk of therapy to achieve steady state. Stop if no progress towards abstinence by 7th wk. Write "dispense behavioral modification kit" on first script.

PEDS - Not approved in children.

FORMS - Trade: Ext'd release tabs 150 mg.

NOTES - Zyban is same drug as antidepressant Wellbutrin SR. Contraindicated in seizure disorders, bulimia, anorexia, or those taking MAO inhibitors. Seizures occur in 0.4% of patients taking 300-450 mg/day. Buproban is an approved generic not yet marketed.

clonidine (*Catapres, Catapres-TTS*) ▶LK ♀C ▶? $

ADULT - See cardiovascular section

PEDS - Not approved in children <12 yo.

UNAPPROVED ADULT - Opioid withdrawal: 0.1-0.3 mg PO q 6h. Alcohol withdrawal, adjunct: 0.3-0.6 mg PO q6h. Smoking cessation: 0.15-0.4 mg/day PO divided tid-qid or 0.2 mg patch (TTS-2) q week. ADHD: 5 mcg/kg/day PO x 8 weeks.

UNAPPROVED PEDS - ADHD: 5 mcg/kg/day PO x 8 weeks.

FORMS - Generic/Trade: Tabs, non-scored 0.1, 0.2, 0.3 mg. Trade only: transdermal weekly patch 0.1 mg/day (TTS-1), 0.2 mg/day (TTS-2), 0.3 mg/day (TTS-3).

NOTES - Rebound HTN may occur with abrupt discontinuation. Transdermal Therapeutic System (TTS) is designed for seven day use so that a TTS-1 delivers 0.1 mg/day x 7 days. May supplement first dose of TTS with oral x 2-3 days until therapeutic level is achieved.

disulfiram (*Antabuse*) ▶L ♀C ▶? $$

WARNING - Never give to the intoxicated.

ADULT - Sobriety: 125-500 mg PO qd.

PEDS - Not approved in children.

FORMS - Trade only: Tabs 250 mg.

NOTES - Patient must abstain from any alcohol for ≥12 h before using. Disulfiram-alcohol reaction may occur for up to 2 weeks after discontinuing disulfiram. Metronidazole and alcohol in any form (eg, cough syrups, tonics) contraindicated. Hepatotoxicity.

methadone (*Dolophine, Methadose*, ✦*Metadol*) ▶L ♀B ▶+ ©II $$

WARNING - High doses (mean ~400 mg/day) have been inconclusively associated with arrhythmia (torsade de pointes), particularly in those with pre-existing risk factors.

ADULT - Opioid dependence: 20-100 mg PO qd.

PEDS - Not approved in children.

FORMS - Generic/Trade: Tabs 5,10,40 mg. Oral soln 5&10 mg/5 ml. Oral concentrate 10 mg/ml.

NOTES - Treatment >3 wks is maintenance and only permitted in approved treatment programs. Drug interactions leading to decreased methadone levels with enzyme-inducing HIV drugs (I.e. efavirenz, nevirapine); monitor for opiate withdrawal symptoms and increase methadone if necessary. Rapid metabolizers may require more frequent daily dosing.

naltrexone (*ReVia, Depade*) ▶LK ♀C ▶? $$$$

WARNING - Hepatotoxicity with higher than approved doses.

ADULT - Alcohol dependence: 50 mg PO qd. Opioid dependence: Start 25 mg PO qd, increase to 50 mg qd if no signs of withdrawal.

PEDS - Not approved in children.

FORMS - Generic/Trade: Tabs 50 mg.

NOTES - Avoid if recent (past 7-10 days) ingestion of opioids. Conflicting evidence of efficacy for chronic, severe alcoholism.

nicotine gum (*Nicorette, Nicorette DS*) ▶LK ♀X ▶- $$$$$

ADULT - Smoking cessation: Gradually taper 1 piece (2 mg) q1-2h x 6 weeks, 1 piece (2 mg) q2-4h x 3 weeks, then 1 piece (2 mg) q4-8h x 3 weeks. Max 30 pieces/day of 2 mg gum or 24 pieces/day of 4 mg gum. Use 4 mg pieces (Nicorette DS) for high cigarette use (>24 cigarettes/day).

PEDS - Not approved in children.

FORMS - OTC/Generic/Trade: gum 2, 4 mg.

NOTES - Chew slowly and park between cheek and gum periodically. May cause N/V, hiccups. Coffee, juices, wine, and soft drinks may reduce absorption. Avoid eating/ drinking x 15 minutes before/during gum use. Available in original, orange, or mint flavor. Do not use beyond 6 months.

nicotine inhalation system (*Nicotrol Inhaler*) ▶LK ♀D ▶- $$$$$

ADULT - Smoking cessation: 6-16 cartridges/ day x 12 weeks.

PEDS - Not approved in children.

FORMS - Trade: Oral inhaler 10 mg/cartridge (4 mg nicotine delivered), 42 cartridges/box.

nicotine lozenge (*Commit*) ▶LK ♀D ▶- $$$$$

ADULT - Smoking cessation: In those who smoke <30 min after waking use 4 mg lozenge; others use 2 mg. Take 1-2 lozenges q1-2 h x 6 weeks, then q2-4h in weeks 7-9, then q4-8h in weeks 10-12. Length of therapy 12 weeks.

PEDS - Not approved in children.

FORMS - Trade – OTC/Trade: lozenge 2 mg, 4 mg in 72- and 168-count packages

NOTES - Allow lozenge to dissolve and do not chew. Do not eat or drink within 15 minutes before use. Avoid concurrent use with other sources of nicotine.

nicotine nasal spray (Nicotrol NS) ▶LK ♀D ▶- $$$$$

ADULT - Smoking cessation: 1-2 doses each hour, with each dose = 2 sprays, one in each nostril (1 spray = 0.5 mg nicotine). Minimum recommended 8 doses/day, max 40 doses/d.

PEDS - Not approved in children.

FORMS - Trade: nasal solution 10 mg/ml (0.5 mg/inhalation); 10 ml bottles.

nicotine patches (Habitrol, Nicoderm, Nicotrol) ▶LK ♀D ▶- $$$$

ADULT - Smoking cessation: Start one patch (14- 22 mg) qd and taper after 6 weeks. Total duration of therapy is 12 weeks.

PEDS - Not approved in children.

FORMS - OTC/Rx/Generic/Trade: patches 11, 22 mg/ 24 hours. 7, 14, 21 mg/ 24 h (Habitrol & NicoDerm). OTC/Trade: 15 mg/ 16 h (Nicotrol).

NOTES - Ensure patient has stopped smoking. Dispose of patches safely; can be toxic to kids, pets.

Suboxone (buprenorphine + naloxone) ▶L ♀C ▶- ©III $$$$$

ADULT - Treatment of opioid dependence: Maintenance: 16 mg SL qd. Can individualize to range of 4-24 mg SL qd.

PEDS - Not approved in children.

FORMS - Trade: SL tabs 2/0.5 and 8/2 mg buprenorphine / naloxone

NOTES - Suboxone preferred over Subutex for unsupervised administration. Titrate in 2-4 mg increments / decrements to maintain therapy compliance and prevent withdrawal. Prescribers must complete training and apply for special DEA number. See www.suboxone.com.

BODY MASS INDEX*	Heights are in feet and inches; weights are in pounds					
BMI	*Classification*	*4'10"*	*5'0"*	*5'4"*	*5'8"*	*6'0"*	*6'4"*
<19	Underweight	<91	<97	<110	<125	<140	<156
19-24	Healthy Weight	91-119	97-127	110-144	125-163	140-183	156-204
25-29	Overweight	120-143	128-152	145-173	164-196	184-220	205-245
30-40	Obese	144-191	153-204	174-233	197-262	221-293	246-328
>40	Very Obese	>191	>204	>233	>262	>293	>328

*BMI = kg/m^2 = (weight in pounds)(703)/(height in inches)^2. Anorectants appropriate if BMI ≥30 (with comorbidities ≥27); surgery an option if BMI >40 (with comorbidities 35-40).   www.nhlbi.nih.gov

PSYCHIATRY: Stimulants / ADHD / Anorexiants

Adderall (dextroamphetamine + amphetamine) ▶L ♀C ▶- ©II $$

WARNING - Chronic overuse/abuse can lead to marked tolerance and psychic dependence; caution with prolonged use.

ADULT - Narcolepsy: Start 10 mg PO q am, increase by 10 mg q week, maximum dose is 60 mg/day divided bid-tid at 4-6h intervals. ADHD: Start 10 mg PO q am (Adderall XR), increase by 5-10 mg q week, max dose 30 mg/day.

PEDS - Narcolepsy: 6-12 yo: Start 5 mg PO qd, increase by 5 mg q week. Age >12 yo: Start 10 mg PO qam, increase by 10 mg q week, maximum dose is 60 mg/day divided bid-tid at 4-6h intervals. ADHD: 3-5 yo: Start 2.5 mg qd, increase by 2.5 mg q week. Age ≥6 yo: Start 5 mg PO qd-bid (Adderall) or 10 mg PO qd (Adderall XR), increase by 5 mg (Adderall) or 5-10 mg (Adderall XR) q week, maximum dose is 40 mg/day (Adderall) divided bid-tid at 4-6h intervals or 30 mg/day (Adderall XR). Not

recommended for children <3 yo.

FORMS - Trade/Generic: Tabs 5, 7.5, 10, 12.5, 15, 20, 30 mg. Trade: Capsules, extended release (Adderall XR) 5,10, 15, 20, 25, 30 mg.

NOTES - Capsules may be opened and the beads sprinkled on applesauce; do not chew beads. Adderall XR should be given upon awakening. Avoid evening doses. Monitor growth and use drug holidays when appropriate. May increase pulse and BP.

atomoxetine (Strattera) ▶K ♀C ▶? $$$$

ADULT - ADHD: Start 40 mg PO qd, then increase after >3 days to target of 80 mg/day divided qd-bid. Max dose 100 mg/day.

PEDS - ADHD: Children/adolescents ≤70 kg: Start 0.5 mg/kg qd, then increase after >3 days to target dose of 1.2 mg/kg/day divided qd-bid. Max dose 1.4 mg/kg or 100 mg per day. If >70 kg use adult dose.

FORMS - Trade: caps 10, 18, 25, 40, 60 mg.

NOTES - If taking strong CYP2D6 inhibitors,

use same starting dose but only increase if well-tolerated at 4 weeks and symptoms unimproved. May be stopped without tapering. Monitor growth.

benzphetamine (*Didrex*) ▶K ♀X ▶? ©III $$$

WARNING - Chronic overuse/abuse can lead to marked tolerance and psychic dependence; caution with prolonged use.

ADULT - Short-term treatment of obesity: Start with 25-50 mg once daily in the morning and increase if needed to 1-3 times daily.

PEDS - Not approved if <12 years of age.

FORMS - Trade: tabs 50 mg.

NOTES - Tolerance to anorectic effect develops within weeks and cross-tolerance to other drugs in class common.

caffeine (*NoDoz, Vivarin, Caffedrine, Stay Awake, Quick-Pep*) ▶L ♀B ▶? $

ADULT - Fatigue: 100- 200 mg PO q3-4h prn.

PEDS - Not approved in children <12 yo.

FORMS - OTC/Generic/Trade: Tabs/Caps 200 mg. OTC/Trade: Extended-release tabs 200 mg. Lozenges 75 mg.

dexmethylphenidate (*Focalin*) ▶LK ♀C ▶? ©II $$

WARNING - Chronic overuse/abuse can lead to marked tolerance and psychic dependence; caution with prolonged use.

ADULT - ADHD: Patients not taking racemic methylphenidate or who are on other stimulants start 2.5 mg PO bid, max 20 mg/24 hr. Patients taking racemic methylphenidate use conversion of 2.5 mg for each 5 mg of methylphenidate, max 20 mg/day. Doses should be ≥4h apart.

PEDS - ADHD and ≥6 yo: If not already on racemic methylphenidate or other stimulants, start 2.5 mg PO bid, max 20 mg/24 hr. If already on racemic methylphenidate, use conversion of 2.5 mg for each 5 mg of methylphenidate given bid, max 20 mg/day. Doses should be ≥4h apart.

FORMS - Trade: tabs 2.5 mg, 5 mg, 10 mg.

NOTES - Avoid evening doses. Monitor growth and use drug holidays when appropriate. May increase pulse and BP. 2.5 mg is equivalent to 5 mg racemic methylphenidate.

dextroamphetamine (*Dexedrine, Dextrostat*) ▶L ♀C ▶- ©II $$

WARNING - Chronic overuse/abuse can lead to marked tolerance and psychic dependence; caution with prolonged use.

ADULT - Narcolepsy: Start 10 mg PO qam, increase by 10 mg q week, max 60 mg/day divided qd (sustained release) or bid-tid at 4-6h in-

tervals.

PEDS - Narcolepsy: 6-12 yo: Start 5 mg PO qam, increase by 5 mg q week. Age >12 yo: Start 10 mg PO qam, increase by 10 mg q week, max 60 mg/day divided qd (sustained release) or bid-tid at 4-6h intervals. ADHD: age 3-5 yo: Start 2.5 mg PO qd, increase by 2.5 mg q week. Age ≥6 yo: Start 5 mg PO qd-bid, increase by 5 mg q week, max 40 mg/day divided qd-tid at 4-6h intervals. Not recommended for patients <3 yo.

FORMS - Trade/Generic: Tabs 5, 10 mg. Extended Release caps 5, 10, 15 mg.

NOTES - Avoid evening doses. Monitor growth and use drug holidays when appropriate. May increase pulse and BP.

diethylpropion (*Tenuate, Tenuate Dospan*) ▶K ♀B ▶? ©IV $

WARNING - Chronic overuse/abuse can lead to marked tolerance and psychic dependence; caution with prolonged use.

ADULT - Short-term treatment of obesity: 25 mg PO tid 1 hr before meals and mid evening if needed or 75 mg sustained-release daily at midmorning.

PEDS - Not approved if <12 years of age.

FORMS - Trade/generic: tabs 25 mg, sustained-release tabs 75 mg.

NOTES - Tolerance to anorectic effect develops within weeks and cross-tolerance to other drugs in class common.

methylphenidate (*Ritalin, Ritalin LA, Ritalin SR, Methylin, Methylin ER, Metadate ER, Metadate CD, Concerta*) ▶LK ♀C ▶? ©II $$$

WARNING - Chronic overuse/abuse can lead to marked tolerance and psychic dependence; caution with prolonged use.

ADULT - Narcolepsy: 10 mg PO bid-tid before meals. Usual effective dose is 20-30 mg/day, max 60 mg/day. Use sustained release Tabs when the 8-hour dosage corresponds to the titrated 8-hour dosage of the conventional Tabs.

PEDS - ADHD ≥6 yo: Start 5 mg PO bid before breakfast and lunch, increase gradually by 5-10 mg/day at weekly interval to max 60 mg/day. Sustained and extended release: start 20 mg PO qd, max 60 mg daily. Concerta (extended release) start 18 mg PO qam; titrate in 9-18 mg increments at weekly intervals to max 54 mg/day. Consult product labeling for dose conversion from other methylphenidate regimens. Discontinue after 1 month if no improvement observed.

FORMS - Trade: tabs 5, 10, 20 mg (Ritalin, Methylin, Metadate). Extended release tabs 10, 20 mg (Methylin ER, Metadate ER). Extended release tabs 18, 27, 36, 54 mg (Concerta). Extended release caps 20, 30 mg (Metadate CD) May be sprinkled on food. Sustained-release tabs 20 mg (Ritalin SR). Extended release caps 10, 20, 30, 40 mg (Ritalin LA). Generic: tabs 5, 10, 20 mg, extended release tabs 10, 20 mg, sustained-release tabs 20 mg.

NOTES - Avoid evening doses. Monitor growth and use drug holidays when appropriate. May increase pulse and BP. Ritalin LA may be opened and sprinkled on applesauce.

modafinil (*Provigil*, ✚*Alertec*) ▶L ♀C ▶? ©IV $$$$

ADULT - Narcolepsy and sleep apnea/hypopnea: 200 mg PO qam. Shift work sleep disorder: 200 mg PO one hour before shift.

PEDS - Not approved in children <16 yo.

FORMS - Trade: Tabs 100, 200 mg.

NOTES - May increase levels of diazepam, phenytoin, TCAs, warfarin, or propranolol; may decrease levels of cyclosporine, oral contraceptives, or theophylline.

pemoline (*Cylert*) ▶LK ♀B ▶? ©IV $$$

WARNING - Should not be used as first line drug therapy for ADHD due to life-threatening hepatic failure.

PEDS - ADHD age >6 yo: Start 37.5 mg PO q am, increase by 18.75 mg at 1 week intervals to usual effective dose of 56.25- 75 mg/day. Maximum dose is 112.5 mg/day.

UNAPPROVED ADULT - Narcolepsy: 50- 200 mg/day PO divided bid.

FORMS - Generic/Trade: tabs 18.75, 37.5, 75 mg. chew tabs 37.5 mg.

NOTES - Monitor ALT at baseline and q2 weeks thereafter; discontinue if >2 x normal. Avoid evening doses. Monitor growth and use drug holidays when appropriate.

phendimetrizine (*Bontril SR, Melfiat, Prelu-2*) ▶K ♀C ▶? ©III $$

WARNING - Chronic overuse/abuse can lead to marked tolerance and psychic dependence; caution with prolonged use.

ADULT - Short-term treatment of obesity: Start 35 mg 2 or 3 times daily 1 hr before meals. Sustained-release 105 mg once in the morning before breakfast.

PEDS - Not approved in children <12 yo.

FORMS - Trade/generic: tabs/caps 35 mg, sustained-release caps 105 mg.

NOTES - Tolerance to anorectic effect develops within weeks and cross-tolerance to other drugs in class common.

phentermine (*Adipex-P, Ionamin, Pro-Fast*) ▶KL ♀C ▶- ©IV $$

ADULT - Obesity: 8 mg PO tid before meals or 1-2 h after meals. May give 15-37.5 mg PO q am or 10-14 h before bedtime.

PEDS - Not approved in children <16 yo.

FORMS - Generic/Trade: Caps 15, 18.75, 30, 37.5 mg. Tabs 8, 30, 37.5 mg. Trade only: extended release Caps 15, 30 mg (Ionamin).

NOTES - Indicated for short term (8-12 weeks) use only. Contraindicated for use during or within 14 days of MAOIs (hypertensive crisis).

sibutramine (*Meridia*) ▶KL ♀C ▶- ©IV $$$

ADULT - Obesity: Start 10 mg PO q am, may titrate to 15 mg/day after one month. Maximum dose is 15 mg/day.

PEDS - Not approved in children <16 yo.

FORMS - Trade: Caps 5, 10, 15 mg.

NOTES - May increase pulse and BP. Don't use in patients with uncontrolled HTN or heart disease. Caution using with SSRIs or other antidepressants. Contraindicated for use during or within 14 days of MAOIs (hypertensive crisis).

PSYCHIATRY: Other

benztropine (*Cogentin*, ✚*Bensylate*) ▶LK ♀C ▶? $

ADULT - Drug-induced extrapyramidal disorders: 1-4 mg PO/IM/IV qd-bid.

PEDS - Not approved in children

FORMS - Generic: Tabs 0.5, 1, 2 mg.

NOTES - Anticholinergic side effects are enhanced in the elderly, and may worsen dementia or delirium. Avoid use with donepezil, rivastigmine, galantamine, or tacrine.

clonidine (*Catapres, Catapres-TTS*) ▶LK ♀C ▶? $

ADULT - See cardiovascular section.

PEDS - Not approved in children <12 yo.

UNAPPROVED ADULT - Tourette's syndrome: 3-5 mcg/kg/day PO divided bid-qid.

UNAPPROVED PEDS - ADHD: Start 0.05 mg qhs, titrate to 0.05-0.3 mg/day in 3-4 divided doses. Tourette's syndrome: 3-5 mcg/kg/day PO divided bid-qid.

FORMS - Generic/Trade: Tabs 0.1, 0.2, 0.3 mg. Trade only: transdermal weekly patch 0.1 mg/day (TTS-1), 0.2 mg/day (TTS-2), 0.3 mg/day (TTS-3).

NOTES - Rebound HTN may occur with abrupt withdrawal.

diphenhydramine (*Benadryl, Banophen, Allermax, Diphen, Diphenhist, Siladryl, Sominex, ♥Allerdryl, Allernix*) ▶LK♀B▶-$
ADULT - Drug-induced extrapyramidal disorders: 25-50 mg PO tid-qid or 10-50 mg IV/IM tid-qid.
PEDS - Drug-induced extrapyramidal disorders: 12.5-25 mg PO tid-qid or 5 mg/kg/day IV/IM divided qid, max 300 mg/day.
FORMS - OTC/Generic/Trade: Tabs 25, 50 mg. OTC/Trade only: chew tabs 12.5 mg. OTC/Rx/ Generic/Trade: Caps 25, 50 mg. Oral solution 12.5 mg/5 ml.

NOTES - Anticholinergic side effects are enhanced in the elderly, and may worsen dementia or delirium. Avoid use with donepezil, rivastigmine, galantamine, or tacrine.
guanfacine (*Tenex*) ▶K ♀B ▶? $$$
ADULT - See cardiovascular section
PEDS - Not approved in children.
UNAPPROVED PEDS - ADHD: Start 0.5 mg PO qd, titrate by 0.5 mg q3-4 days as tolerated to 0.5 mg PO tid.
FORMS - Generic/Trade: Tabs 1, 2 mg.
NOTES - Less sedation and hypotension compared to clonidine.

PULMONARY: Beta Agonists

NOTE: Palpitations, tachycardia, lightheadedness, tremor, nervousness, headache, & nausea may occur; these effects may be more pronounced with systemic administration. Decreases in potassium can occur, rarely leading to adverse cardiovascular effects; monitor accordingly.
albuterol (*Ventolin, Ventolin HFA, Proventil, Proventil HFA, Volmax, VoSpire ER, Ventodisk, ♥Airomir, Ventodisk, salbutamol*) ▶L ♀C ▶? $
ADULT - Asthma: MDI: 2 puffs q4-6h prn. Soln for inhalation: 2.5 mg nebulized tid-qid. Dilute 0.5 ml 0.5% soln with 2.5 ml NS. Deliver over ~ 5-15 min. One 3 ml unit dose (0.083%) nebulized tid-qid. Caps for inhalation: 200-400 mcg inh q4-6h via a Rotahaler device. 2-4 mg PO tid-qid or extended release 4-8 mg PO q12h up to 16 mg PO q12h.
PEDS - Asthma: MDI: ≥4 yo: 1-2 puffs q4-6 h prn. Soln for inhalation (0.5%): 2-12 yo: 0.1-0.15 mg/kg/dose not to exceed 2.5 mg tid-qid, diluted with NS to 3 ml. Caps for inhalation: ≥4 yo 200-400 mcg inhaled q4-6h via a Rotahaler device. Tabs, syrup 6-12 yo: 2-4 mg PO tid-qid, max dose 24 mg/d in divided doses or extended release 4 mg PO q12h. Syrup 2-5 yo: 0.1-0.2 mg/kg/dose PO tid up to 4 mg tid. Prevention of exercise-induced bronchospasm ≥4 yo (Proventil HFA, Ventolin HFA): 2 puffs 15 minutes before exercise.
UNAPPROVED ADULT - COPD: MDI, soln for inhalation: use asthma dose. Acute asthma: MDI, soln for inhalation: dose as above q20 min X 3 or until improvement. Continuous nebulization: 10-15 mg/h until improvement.
UNAPPROVED PEDS - Acute asthma: soln for inhalation: 0.15 mg/kg (minimum 2.5 mg) q 20 minutes x 3 doses then 0.15-0.3 mg/kg up to

10 mg q1-4 hrs as needed, or 0.5 mg/kg/hour continous nebulization. MDI: 4-8 puffs q20 minutes for 3 doses then every 1-4 hours prn. Soln for inhalation (0.5%): <2 yo: 0.05 - 0.15 mg/kg/ dose q4-6h. Syrup <2 yo: 0.3 mg/kg/24h PO divided tid, max dose 12 mg/24h. Prevention of exercise-induced bronchospasm: MDI: ≥4 yo 2 puffs 15 minutes before exercise.
FORMS - Generic/Trade: MDI 90 mcg/actuation, 200/canister. "HFA" inhalers use hydrofluoroalkane propellant instead of CFCs but are otherwise equivalent. Soln for inhalation 0.5% (5 mg/ml) in 20 ml with dropper. Nebules for inhalation 3 ml unit dose 0.083%. Extended release tabs 4 & 8 mg. Trade only:1.25 mg & 0.63 mg/3 ml unit dose. Tabs 2 & 4 mg. Syrup 2 mg/5 ml. Caps for inhalation 200 mcg microfine in packs of 24s & 96s w/ Rotahaler.
NOTES - Do not crush/chew extended release tablets. Volmax must be refrigerated.
fenoterol (*♥Berotec*) ▶L ♀C ▶? $
ADULT - Canada only. Acute asthma: MDI: 1-2 puffs tid-qid; maximum 8 puffs/day. Soln for nebulization: up to 2.5 mg q6 hours.
PEDS - Not approved in children.
FORMS - Trade: MDI 100 mcg/actuation. Soln for inhalation: Unit dose 2 ml vials of 0.625 mg/ml and 0.25 mg/ml (no preservatives), and 20 ml bottles of 1 mg/ml (with preservatives that may cause bronchoconstriction in those with hyperreactive airways).
formoterol (*Foradil, ♥Oxeze*) ▶L ♀C ▶? $$$
ADULT - Asthma maintenance, COPD: 1 puff bid. Prevention of exercise-induced bronchospasm: 1 puff 15 min prior to exercise.
PEDS - Asthma maintenance ≥5 yo: 1 puff bid. Prevention of exercise-induced bronchospasm ≥12 yo: Use adult dose.
FORMS - Trade: DPI 12 mcg, 60 blisters/pack.

NOTES - Not for use for the relief of acute bronchospasm.

levalbuterol (Xopenex) ▶L ♀C ▶? $$$$
ADULT - Asthma: Soln for inhalation: 0.63-1.25 mg nebulized q6-8h.
PEDS - Asthma: Soln for inhalation ≥12 yo: Use adult dose. 6-11 yo: 0.31 mg nebulized tid.
FORMS - Trade: soln for inhalation 0.63 & 1.25 mg in 3 ml unit-dose vials.
NOTES - R-isomer of albuterol. Dyspepsia may occur.

metaproterenol (Alupent, Metaprel, Pro-Meta, ✦orciprenaline) ▶L ♀C ▶? $$
ADULT - Asthma: MDI: 2-3 puffs q3-4h; max dose 12 puffs/day. Soln for inhalation: 0.2-0.3 ml of 5% soln in 2.5 ml NS. 20 mg PO tid-qid.
PEDS - Asthma: soln for inhalation: >6 yo 0.1-0.3 ml of the 5% soln in 2.5 ml NS. Tabs or syrup: >9 yo or >60 lbs: 20 mg PO tid-qid. 6-9 yo or <60 lbs: 10 mg PO tid-qid. 2-5 yo: 1.3-2.6 mg/kg/day PO in divided doses tid-qid.
UNAPPROVED PEDS - Asthma: MDI: >6 yo 2-3 puffs q3-4h; max dose 12 puffs/day. Soln for inhalation: 0.1-0.3 ml of the 5% soln in 2.5 ml NS q4-6h prn or q20 min until improvement. Tabs, syrup: <2 yo: 0.4 mg/kg/dose PO tid-qid.
FORMS - Trade: MDI 0.65 mg/actuation in 100 & 200/canister. Trade/Generic: Soln for inhalation 0.4, 0.6% in unit-dose vials; 5% in 10 & 30 ml with dropper. Syrup 10 mg/5 ml. Generic: Tabs 10 & 20 mg.

pirbuterol (Maxair) ▶L ♀C ▶? $$
ADULT - Asthma: MDI: 1-2 puffs q4-6h. Max dose 12 puffs/day.
PEDS - Not approved in children.
UNAPPROVED PEDS - Asthma ≥12 yo: Use adult dose.

FORMS - Trade: MDI 0.2 mg/actuation, 400/canister.
NOTES - Breath actuated autohaler.

salmeterol (Serevent Diskus) ▶L ♀C ▶? $$$
WARNING - SMART trial suggests a small but significant increase in respiratory adverse events and asthma-related deaths (?greater in African-Americans). Do not abruptly stop therapy. Avoid in significantly worsening or acute asthma. Use only with corticosteroids.
ADULT - Asthma/ COPD maintenance: 1 puff bid. Prevention of exercise-induced bronchospasm: 1 puff 30 minutes before exercise.
PEDS - Asthma maintenance ≥4 yo: 1 puff bid. Prevention of exercise-induced bronchospasm: 1 puff 30 minutes before exercise.
FORMS - Trade: DPI (Diskus): 50 mcg, 60 blisters.
NOTES - Not for use for the relief of acute bronchospasm.

terbutaline (Brethine, Bricanyl) ▶L ♀B ▶- $$
ADULT - Asthma: 2.5-5 mg PO q6h while awake. Max dose 15 mg/24h. 0.25 mg SC into lateral deltoid area; may repeat x1 within 15-30 min. Max dose 0.5 mg/4h. See entry in OB/GYN section for use as tocolytic.
PEDS - Not approved in children.
UNAPPROVED PEDS - Asthma: >12 yo: use adult dose, max 7.5 mg/24h; ≤12 yo: 0.05 mg/kg/dose tid, increase to max of 0.15 mg/kg/dose tid, max 5 mg/day. Acute asthma: 0.01 mg/kg SC q20 minutes x 3 doses then q2-6 hrs as needed.
FORMS - Generic/trade: Tabs 2.5 & 5 mg (Brethine scored).
NOTES - Give 50% normal dose in renal insufficiency; avoid in renal failure.

WHAT COLOR IS WHAT INHALER? (Body then cap - Generics may differ)

Advair	purple	Combivent	clear/orange	Proventil	yellow/ orange
Aerobid	grey/purple	Flovent	orange/ peach	Pulmicort	white/brown
Aerobid-M	grey/green	Foradil	grey/beige	QVAR 40mcg	beige/grey
Alupent	clear/blue	Intal	white/blue	QVAR 80mcg	mauve/grey
Atrovent	clear/green	Maxair	blue/white	Tilade	white/white
Azmacort	white/white	Maxair Autohaler	white/white	Ventolin	light blue/navy

PULMONARY: Combinations

Advair (fluticasone + salmeterol) ▶L ♀C ▶? $$$-$$$$
WARNING - SMART trial suggests a small but significant increase in respiratory adverse events and asthma-related deaths associated with salmeterol (? greater in African-Americans). It is not known if concurrent fluticasone decreases this risk. Do not abruptly stop therapy. Do not use for rescue in significantly worsening or acute asthma.
ADULT - Asthma: 1 puff bid (all strengths). COPD with chronic bronchitis: 1 puff bid (250/50 only).
PEDS - Asthma maintenance ≥12 yo: Use adult

dose. 4-11 yo: 1 puff bid (100/50 only).
FORMS - Trade: DPI: 100/50, 250/50, 500/50 mcg fluticasone propionate/mcg salmeterol per actuation. 60 doses per DPI.
NOTES - 1 puff of Advair is the equivalent of 2 puffs of Serevent MDI or 1 puff Serevent Diskus, PLUS 2 puffs of Flovent 44 (Advair 100/50), Flovent 110 (Advair 250/50), or Flovent 220 (Advair 500/50) mcg MDI. See individual components for additional information. Ritonavir & other CYP3A4 inhibitors such as ketoconazole significantly increase fluticasone concentrations, resulting in systemic effects, including adrenal suppression.

Combivent (albuterol + ipratropium) ▶L ♀C ▶? $$
ADULT - COPD: MDI: 2 puffs qid. Max dose 12 puffs/24 hours.
PEDS - Not approved in children.
FORMS - Trade: MDI: 90 mcg albuterol/18 mcg ipratropium per actuation, 200/canister.
NOTES - Contraindicated with soy & peanut allergy. Refer to components.

DuoNeb (albuterol + ipratropium, ♥Combivent inhalation solution) ▶L ♀C ▶? $$$$
ADULT - COPD: One unit dose nebulized qid; may add 2 doses/day prn to max of 6 doses/day.
PEDS - Not approved in children.
FORMS - Trade: Unit dose: 2.5 mg albuterol/0.5 mg ipratropium per 3 ml vial, premixed. 30 & 60 vials/carton.
NOTES - Refer to components

Symbicort (budesonide + formoterol) ▶L ♀C ▶? $$
ADULT - Canada only. Asthma maintenance: 1-2 puffs bid.
PEDS - Canada only. Asthma maintenance ≥12 yo: Use adult dose.
FORMS - Trade: DPI: 100/6 and 200/6 mcg budesonide/mcg formoterol per actuation.
NOTES - Inhibitors of CYP3A4 (eg, ketoconazole) may increase budesonide levels. See individual components for additional information.

PULMONARY: Inhaled Steroids

NOTE: See Endocrine-Corticosteroids when oral steroids necessary. Beware of adrenal suppression when changing from systemic to inhaled steroids. Inhaled steroids are not for treatment of acute asthma; higher doses may be needed for severe asthma and exacerbations. Adjust to lowest effective dose for maintenance. Use of a DPI, a spacing device, & rinsing the mouth with water after each use may decrease the incidence of thrush & dysphonia. Pharyngitis & cough may occur with all products. Use with caution in patients with active or quiescent TB, untreated systemic fungal, bacterial, viral or parasitic infections or in patients with ocular HSV. Inhaled steroids produce small, transient reductions in growth velocity in children.

beclomethasone (QVAR, ♥Vanceril) ▶L ♀C ▶? $$
ADULT - Asthma maintenance: 40 mcg 1-4 puffs bid. 80 mcg 1-2 puffs bid.
PEDS - Asthma maintenance in 5-11 yo: 40 mcg 1-2 puffs bid.
UNAPPROVED ADULT - Asthma maintenance: NHLBI dosing schedule (puffs/day divided bid): Low dose 2-6 puffs of 40 mcg or 1-3 puffs of 80 mcg. Medium dose: 6-12 puffs of 40 mcg or 3-6 puffs of 80 mcg. High dose: >12 puffs of 40 mcg or >6 puffs 80 mcg.
UNAPPROVED PEDS - Asthma maintenance: NHLBI dosing schedule (puffs/day divided bid): 2-4 puffs of 40 mcg or 1-2 puffs of 80 mcg. Medium dose: 4-8 puffs of 40 mcg or 2-4 puffs of 80 mcg. High dose: >8 puffs of 40 mcg or >4 puffs of 80 mcg.
FORMS - Trade: MDI (non-CFC): 40 mcg & 80 mcg/actuation, 100 actuations/canister.

budesonide (Pulmicort Turbuhaler, Pulmicort Respules) ▶L ♀B ▶? $$$$
ADULT - Asthma maintenance: DPI: 1-2 puffs qd-bid up to 4 puffs bid.
PEDS - Asthma maintenance 6-12 yo: DPI: 1-2 puffs qd-bid. 12 mo - 8 yo: Suspension for inhalation (Respules): 0.5 mg - 1 mg qd or divided bid.
UNAPPROVED ADULT - Asthma maintenance: NHLBI dosing schedule (puffs/day qd or divided bid) DPI: Low dose: 1-3 puffs. Medium dose: 3-6 puffs. High dose: >6 puffs.
UNAPPROVED PEDS - Asthma maintenance: (NHLBI dose in puffs/day qd or divided bid) DPI: Low dose: 1-2 puffs. Medium dose: 2-4 puffs. High dose: >4 puffs. Suspension for inhalation (qd or divided bid): Low dose: 0.5 mg. Medium dose: 1 mg. High dose: 2 mg.
FORMS - Trade: DPI: 200 mcg powder/actuation, 200/canister. Respules: 0.25 mg/2 ml & 0.5 mg/2 ml unit dose.
NOTES - Respules should be delivered via a jet nebulizer with a mouthpiece or face mask.

CYP3A4 inhibitors such as ketoconazole, erythromycin, ritonavir, etc may significantly increase systemic concentrations, possibly causing adrenal suppression.

flunisolide (*Aerobid, Aerobid-M*) ▶L ♀C ▶? $$$

ADULT - Asthma maintenance: MDI: 2 puffs bid up to 4 puffs bid.

PEDS - Asthma maintenance: 6-15 yo: MDI: 2 puffs bid.

UNAPPROVED ADULT - Asthma maintenance: NHLBI dosing schedule (puffs/day divided bid): Low dose: 2-4 puffs. Medium dose: 4-8 puffs. High dose: >8 puffs.

UNAPPROVED PEDS - Asthma maintenance: NHLBI dosing schedule (puffs/day divided bid): Low dose: 2-3 puffs. Medium dose: 4-5 puffs. High dose: >5 puffs.

FORMS - Trade: MDI: 250 mcg/actuation, 100/canister. AeroBid-M: menthol flavor.

fluticasone (*Flovent, Flovent Rotadisk*) ▶L ♀C ▶? $$$

ADULT - Asthma maintenance: MDI: 2 puffs bid up to 4 puffs bid. Max dose 880 mcg bid. DPI (Rotadisk): 1 puff bid up to 2 puffs bid. Max dose 500 mcg bid.

PEDS - Asthma maintenance 4-11 yo: DPI (Rotadisk): 1 puff bid up to max dose 100 mcg bid.

UNAPPROVED ADULT - Asthma maintenance: NHLBI dosing schedule (puffs/day divided bid): Low dose: 2-6 puffs of 44 mcg MDI or 50 mcg DPI. Medium dose: 6-15 puffs of 44 mcg MDI or 6-12 puffs 50 mcg DPI. 3-6 puffs of 110 mcg MDI or 100 mcg DPI. 2-3 puffs of 220 mcg MDI or 2 puffs 250 mcg DPI. High dose: >6 puffs 110 mcg MDI or 100 mcg DPI. >3 puffs 220 mcg DPI or >2 puffs 250 mcg DPI.

UNAPPROVED PEDS - Asthma maintenance:

NHLBI dosing schedule (puffs/day divided bid): Low dose: 2-4 puffs of 44 mcg MDI or 50 mcg DPI. Medium dose: 4-10 puffs of 44 mcg MDI or 4-8 puffs 50 mcg DPI. 1-4 puffs of 110 mcg MDI or 2-4 puffs 100 mcg DPI. 1-2 puffs of 220 mcg MDI or 1 puff 250 mcg DPI. High dose: >10 puffs 44 mcg MDI or >8 puffs 50 mcg DPI. >4 puffs 110 mcg MDI or 100 mcg DPI. >2 puffs 220 mcg DPI or >1 puff 250 mcg DPI.

FORMS - Trade: MDI: 44, 110, 220 mcg/actuation in 60 & 120/canister. DPI (Rotadisk): 50, 100, & 250 mcg/actuation, in 4 blisters containing 15 Rotadisks (total of 60 doses) with inhalation device.

NOTES - Ritonavir & other CYP3A4 inhibitors such as ketoconazole significantly increase fluticasone concentrations, resulting in systemic effects, including adrenal suppression. Rotadisk contains lactose; may cause anaphylactic reactions in patients with severe milk allergy.

triamcinolone (*Azmacort*) ▶L ♀D ▶? $$$

ADULT - Asthma maintenance: MDI: 2 puffs tid-qid or 4 puffs bid. Max dose 16 puffs/day. Severe asthma: 12-16 puffs/day and adjust downward.

PEDS - Asthma maintenance >12 yo: Use adult dose. 6-12 yo: 1-2 puffs tid-qid or 2-4 puffs bid. Max dose 12 puffs/day.

UNAPPROVED ADULT - Asthma maintenance: NHLBI dosing schedule (puffs/day divided bid): Low dose: 4-10 puffs. Medium dose: 10-20 puffs. High dose: >20 puffs.

UNAPPROVED PEDS - Asthma maintenance: NHLBI dosing schedule (puffs/day divided bid): Low dose: 4-8 puffs. Medium dose: 8-12 puffs. High dose: >12 puffs.

FORMS - Trade: MDI: 100 mcg/actuation, 240/canister. Built-in spacer.

INHALED STEROIDS: ESTIMATED COMPARATIVE DAILY DOSES*

Drug	Form	ADULT			CHILD (≤12 yo)		
		Low	Medium	High	Low	Medium	High
beclomethasone MDI	40 mcg/puff	2-6	6-12	>12	2-4	4-8	>8
	80 mcg/puff	1-3	3-6	>6	1-2	2-4	>4
budesonide DPI	200 mcg/dose	1-3	3-6	>6	1-2	2-4	>4
	Soln for nebs	-	-	-	0.5 mg	1 mg	2 mg
flunisolide MDI	250 mcg/puff	2-4	4-8	>8	2-3	4-5	>5
fluticasone MDI	44 mcg/puff	2-6	6-15	>15	2-4	4-10	>10
	110 mcg/puff	1-2	3-6	>6	1	1-4	>4
	220 mcg/puff	1	2-3	>3	n/a	1-2	>2
fluticasone DPI	50 mcg/dose	2-6	6-12	>12	2-4	4-8	>8
	100 mcg/dose	1-3	3-6	>6	1-2	2-4	>4
	250 mcg/dose	1	2-3	>2	n/a	1	>2
triamcinolone MDI	100 mcg/puff	4-10	10-20	>20	4-8	8-12	>12

*MDI=metered dose inhaler. DPI=dry powder inhaler. All doses in puffs (MDI) or inhalations (DPI).
Reference: http://www.nhlbi.nih.gov/guidelines/asthma/execsumm.pdf

PREDICTED PEAK EXPIRATORY FLOW (liters/min)   Am Rev Resp Dis 1963; 88:644

Age (yrs)	Women (height in inches)					Men (height in inches)					Child (height in inches)	
	55"	60"	65"	70"	75"	60"	65"	70"	75"	80"		
20	390	423	460	496	529	554	602	649	693	740	44"	160
30	380	413	448	483	516	532	577	622	664	710	46"	187
40	370	402	436	470	502	509	552	596	636	680	48"	214
50	360	391	424	457	488	486	527	569	607	649	50"	240
60	350	380	412	445	475	463	502	542	578	618	52"	267
70	340	369	400	432	461	440	477	515	550	587	54"	293

PULMONARY: Leukotriene Inhibitors

NOTE: Not for treatment of acute asthma. Abrupt substitution for corticosteroids may precipitate Churg-Strauss syndrome.

montelukast (*Singulair*) ▶L ♀B ▶? $$$
ADULT - Asthma maintenance, allergic rhinitis: 10 mg PO q pm.
PEDS - Asthma maintenance, allergic rhinitis: 6-14 yo: 5 mg PO q pm. 2-5 yo: 4 mg (chew tab or oral granules) PO q pm. Asthma 12-23 months: 4 mg (oral granules) PO q pm.
UNAPPROVED PEDS - Allergic rhinitis: 12-23 months: 4 mg (oral granules) PO q pm.
FORMS - Trade: Tabs 4, 5 mg (chew cherry flavored) & 10 mg. Oral granules 4 mg packet, 30/box.
NOTES - Chew tabs contain phenylalanine. Oral granules may be placed directly into the mouth or mixed with a spoonful of applesauce, carrots, rice or ice cream. If mixed with food, must be taken within 15 minutes. Do not mix with liquids. Levels decreased by phenobarbital & rifampin. Dyspepsia may occur.

zafirlukast (*Accolate*) ▶L ♀B ▶- $$$
ADULT - Asthma maintenance: 20 mg PO bid, 1h ac or 2h pc.
PEDS - Asthma maintenance ≥12 yo: use adult dose. 5-11 yo: 10 mg PO bid, 1h ac or 2h pc.
UNAPPROVED ADULT - Allergic rhinitis: 20 mg PO bid, 1h ac or 2h pc.
FORMS - Trade: Tabs 10, 20 mg.
NOTES - Potentiates warfarin & theophylline. Levels increased by erythromycin. Nausea may occur. If liver dysfunction is suspected, discontinue drug & manage accordingly.

zileuton (*Zyflo*) ▶L ♀C ▶? $$$$
WARNING - Contraindicated in active liver disease.
ADULT - Asthma maintenance: 600 mg PO qid.
PEDS - Asthma maintenance ≥12 yo: use adult dose.
FORMS - Trade: Tabs 600 mg.
NOTES - Monitor LFTs for elevation. Potentiates warfarin, theophylline, & propranolol. Dyspepsia & nausea may occur.

PULMONARY: Other

acetylcysteine (*Mucomyst, Mucosil-10, Mucosil-20, ♥Parvolex*) ▶L ♀B ▶? $$$
ADULT - Mucolytic nebulization: 3-5 ml of the 20% soln or 6-10 ml of the 10% soln tid-qid. Instillation, direct or via tracheostomy: 1-2 ml of a 10% to 20% soln q1-4h; via percutaneous intratracheal catheter: 1-2 ml of the 20% soln or 2-4 ml of the 10% soln q1-4h. See entry in the Contrast Media section for use in mitigating contrast nephropathy.
PEDS - Mucolytic nebulization: Use adult dose.
FORMS - Generic/Trade: soln 10 & 20% in 4,10, & 30 ml vials.
NOTES - Increased volume of liquefied bronchial secretions may occur; maintain an open airway. Watch for bronchospasm in asthmatics. Stomatitis, N/V, fever, & rhinorrhea may occur.

A slight disagreeable odor may occur & should soon disappear. A mask may cause stickiness on the face after nebulization; wash with water.

alpha-1 proteinase inhibitor (*alpha-1 antitrypsin, Aralast, Prolastin, Zemaira*) ▶Plasma ♀C ▶? $$$$$
WARNING - Possible transmission of viruses and Creutzfeldt-Jakob disease.
ADULT - Congenital alpha-1 proteinase inhibitor deficiency with emphysema: 60 mg/kg IV once weekly.
PEDS - Not approved in children.
NOTES - Contraindicated in selected IgA deficiencies with known antibody to IgA. Hepatitis B vaccine recommended before use.

aminophylline (♥*Phyllocontin*) ▶L ♀C ▶? $
ADULT - Asthma: loading dose if currently not

receiving theophylline: 6 mg/kg IV over 20-30 min. Maintenance IV infusion 1g in 250 ml D5W (4 mg/ml) at 0.5-0.7 mg/kg/h (70kg: 0.7 mg/kg/h = 11 ml/h). In patients with cor pulmonale, CHF, liver failure, use 0.25 mg/kg/h. If currently on theophylline, each 0.6 mg/kg aminophylline will increase the serum theophylline concentration by approximately 1 mcg/ml. Maintenance: 200 mg PO bid-qid.

PEDS - Asthma loading dose if currently not receiving theophylline: 6 mg/kg IV over 20-30 min. Maintenance >6 mo: 0.8-1 mg/kg/hr IV infusion. >1 yo: 3-4 mg/kg/dose PO q6h.

UNAPPROVED PEDS - Neonatal apnea of prematurity: loading dose 5-6 mg/kg IV/PO. Maintenance: 1-2 mg/kg/dose q6-8 h IV/PO.

FORMS - Generic: Tabs 100 & 200 mg. Oral liquid 105 mg/5 ml. Trade: Tabs controlled release (12hr) 225 mg, scored.

NOTES - Aminophylline is 79% theophylline. Administer IV infusion ≤25 mg/min. Multiple drug interactions (especially ketoconazole, rifampin, carbamazepine, isoniazid, phenytoin, macrolides, zafirlukast & cimetidine). Review meds before initiating treatment. Irritability, nausea, palpitations & tachycardia may occur. Overdose may be life-threatening.

beractant (*Survanta*) ▶Lung ♀? ▶? $$$$$
PEDS - RDS (hyaline membrane disease) in premature infants: Specialized dosing.

caffeine citrate (*Cafcit*) ▶L ♀C ▶? $$$$$
WARNING - Watch for necrotizing enterocolitis.
ADULT - Not approved in adults.
PEDS - Apnea of prematurity between 28-33 weeks gestational age: Load 20 mg/kg IV over 30 min. Maintenance 5 mg/kg PO q 24h.
FORMS - Trade: Oral solution: 20 mg/ml in 3 ml vials. Preservative-free.
NOTES - 2 mg caffeine citrate = 1 mg caffeine base. Avoid serum levels >50 mg/L; monitor periodically. Obtain baseline serum levels if on theophylline. Tachycardia, irritability, hyper/hypoglycemia. Seizures with overdose.

calfactant (*Infasurf*) ▶Lung ♀? ▶? $$$$$
PEDS - RDS (hyaline membrane disease) in premature infants: Specialized dosing.

cromolyn sodium (*Intal, Gastrocrom, Nalcrom*) ▶LK ♀B ▶? $$$
ADULT - Asthma maintenance: MDI: 2-4 puffs qid. Soln for inhalation: 20 mg inh qid. Prevention of exercise-induced bronchospasm: MDI: 2 puffs 10-15 min prior to exercise. Soln for nebulization: 20 mg 10-15 min prior. Mastocytosis: 200 mg PO qid, 30 min ac & qhs.
PEDS - Asthma maintenance >5 yo: MDI: 2 puffs qid. >2 yo: soln for nebulization: 20 mg inh qid. Prevention of exercise-induced bronchospasm >5 yo: MDI: 2 puffs 10-15 min prior to exercise. >2 yo soln for nebulization: 20 mg 10-15 min prior. Mastocytosis: 2-12 yo: 100 mg PO qid 30 min ac & qhs.
FORMS - Trade: MDI 800 mcg/actuation, 112 & 200/canister. Oral concentrate 5 ml/100 mg in 8 amps/foil pouch. Generic/Trade: Soln for nebs: 20 mg/2 ml.
NOTES - Not for treatment of acute asthma. Pharyngitis may occur. Directions for oral concentrate: 1) Break open and squeeze liquid contents of ampule(s) into a glass of water. 2) Stir soln. 3) Drink all of the liquid.

dexamethasone (*Decadron*) ▶L ♀C ▶- $
ADULT - Not approved for pulmonary use
PEDS - Not approved in children.
UNAPPROVED PEDS - Bronchopulmonary dysplasia in preterm infants: 0.5 mg/kg PO/IV divided q12h x 3 days, then taper. Croup: 0.15-0.6 mg/kg PO or IM x 1. Acute asthma: >2 yo: 0.6 mg/kg to max 16 mg PO qd x 2 days.
FORMS - Generic/Trade: Tabs 0.25,0.5,0.75,1, 1.5,2,4,6 mg, various scored. Elixir: 0.5 mg/5 ml. Oral soln: 0.5 mg/5 ml & 0.5 mg/0.5 ml.

dornase alfa (*Pulmozyme*) ▶L ♀B ▶? $$$$$
ADULT - Cystic fibrosis: 2.5 mg neb qd-bid.
PEDS - Cystic fibrosis ≥6 yo: 2.5 mg nebulized qd-bid.
UNAPPROVED PEDS - Has been used in a small number of children as young as 3 mo with similar efficacy and side effects.
FORMS - Trade: soln for inhalation: 1 mg/ml in 2.5 ml vials.
NOTES - Voice alteration, pharyngitis, laryngitis, & rash may occur.

doxapram (*Dopram*) ▶L ♀B ▶? $$
ADULT - Acute hypercapnia due to COPD: 1-2 mg/min IV, max 3 mg/min. Maximum infusion time: 2 hours.
PEDS - Not approved in children.
UNAPPROVED PEDS - Apnea of prematurity unresponsive to methylxanthines: Load 2.5-3 mg/kg over 15 min, then 1 mg/kg/h titrated to lowest effective dose. Max: 2.5 mg/kg/h. Contains benzyl alcohol; caution in neonates.
NOTES - Monitor arterial blood gases at baseline and q2h during infusion. Do not use with mechanical ventilation. Contraindicated with seizure disorder, severe hypertension, CVA, head injury, CAD and severe CHF.

epinephrine (*EpiPen, EpiPen Jr, adrenalin*) ▶Plasma ♀C ▶- $$
ADULT - Acute asthma & hypersensitivity reac-

tions: 0.1 to 0.3 mg of 1:1,000 soln SC. Hypersensitivity: 0.01 mg/kg SC autoinjector.

PEDS - Acute asthma: 0.01 ml/kg (up to 0.5 ml) of 1:1,000 soln SC; repeat q15 min x 3-4 doses prn. Sustained release: 0.005 ml/kg (up to 0.15 ml) of 1:200 soln SC; repeat q8-12h prn. Hypersensitivity reactions: 0.01 mg/kg SC autoinjector. Consider EpiPen Jr. in those <30 kg.

FORMS - Soln for inj: 1:1,000 (1 mg/ml in 1 ml amps). Sust'd formulation (Sus-Phrine): 1:200 (5 mg/ml) in 0.3 ml amps or 5 ml multi-dose vials. Injectable allergy kit: EpiPen (0.3 mg), EpiPen Jr (0.15 mg).

NOTES - Directions for injectable kit use: Remove cap. Place black tip end on thigh & push down to inject. Hold in place for 10 seconds. May be injected directly through clothing. Cardiac arrhythmias & hypertension may occur. For emergencies only.

epinephrine racemic (*AsthmaNefrin, MicroNefrin, Nephron, S-2, ♣Vaponefrin*) ▶Plasma ♀C ▶- $

ADULT - See cardiovascular section

PEDS - Severe croup: inhalation soln: 0.05 ml/kg/dose diluted to 3 ml w/NS over 15 min prn not to exceed q1-2h dosing. Max dose 0.5 ml.

FORMS - Trade: soln for inhalation: 2.25% epinephrine in 15 & 30 ml.

NOTES - Cardiac arrhythmias and hypertension may occur.

ipratropium (*Atrovent*) ▶Lung ♀B ▶? $$

ADULT - COPD maintenance: MDI: 2 puffs qid; may use additional inhalations not to exceed 12 puffs/day. Soln for inhalation: 500 mcg nebulized tid-qid.

PEDS - Not approved in children <12 yo.

UNAPPROVED PEDS - Asthma: MDI: >12 yo: use adult dose. =<12 yo: 1-2 puffs tid-qid. Soln for inhalation: >12 yo: 250-500 mcg/dose tid-qid; =<12 yo: 250 mcg/dose tid-qid. Acute asthma: 2-18yo: 500 mcg nebulized with 2nd & 3rd doses of albuterol.

FORMS - Trade: MDI: 18mcg/actuation, 200/canister. Generic/Trade: Soln for nebulization: 0.02% (500 mcg/vial) in unit dose vials.

NOTES - MDI is contraindicated with soy & peanut allergy. Caution with glaucoma, BPH, or bladder neck obstruction. Cough, dry mouth & blurred vision may occur.

ketotifen (*Zaditen*) ▶L ♀C ▶- $$

ADULT - Not approved.

PEDS - Canada only. Asthma maintenance: 6 mo to 3 yo: 0.05 mg/kg PO bid. Children >3 yo: 1 mg PO bid.

FORMS - Generic/Trade: Tabs 1 mg. Syrup

1mg/5 ml.

NOTES - Several weeks may be necessary before therapeutic effect. Full clinical effectiveness is generally reached after 10 weeks.

methacholine (*Provocholine*) ▶Plasma ♀C ▶? $$

WARNING - Life-threatening bronchoconstriction can result; have resuscitation capability available.

ADULT - Diagnosis of bronchial airway hyperreactivity in non-wheezing patients with suspected asthma: 5 breaths each of ascending serial concentrations. 0.025 mg/ml to 25 mg/ml, via nebulization. The procedure ends when there is a ≥20% reduction in the FEV1 compared with baseline.

PEDS - Diagnosis of bronchial airway hyperreactivity: use adult dose.

NOTES - Avoid with epilepsy, bradycardia, vagotonia, peptic ulcer disease, thyroid disease, urinary tract obstruction or other conditions that could be adversely affected by a cholinergic agent. Hold beta-blockers. Do not inhale powder.

nedocromil (*Tilade*) ▶L ♀B ▶? $$

ADULT - Asthma maintenance: MDI: 2 puffs qid. Reduce dose to bid-tid as tolerated.

PEDS - Asthma maintenance >6 yo: MDI: 2 puffs qid.

FORMS - Trade: MDI: 1.75 mg/actuation, 112/canister.

NOTES - Not for treatment of acute asthma. Unpleasant taste & dysphonia may occur.

nitric oxide (*INOmax*) ▶Lung, K ♀C ▶? $$$$

PEDS - Respiratory failure with pulmonary hypertension in infants >34 weeks old: Specialized dosing.

NOTES - Risk of methemoglobinemia increases with concomitant nitroprusside or nitroglycerin.

omalizumab (*Xolair*) ▶Plasma, L ♀B ▶? $$$$$

WARNING - Anaphylaxis may occur within 2 hours of administration.

ADULT - Moderate to severe asthma with perennial allergy: 150-375 mg SC q 2-4 weeks, based on pretreatment serum total IgE level & body weight.

PEDS - Moderate to severe asthma with perennial allergy: ≥12 yo: use adult dose.

NOTES - Not for treatment of acute asthma. Divide doses >150 mg over >1 injection site.

poractant (*Curosurf*) ▶Lung ♀? ▶? $$$$$

PEDS - RDS (hyaline membrane disease) in premature infants: Specialized dosing.

theophylline (*Elixophyllin, Uniphyl, Theo-24, T-Phyl, ♣Theo-Dur, Theolair*) ▶L ♀C

▶+ $

ADULT - Asthma: 5-13 mg/kg/day PO in divided doses. Max dose 900 mg/day.

PEDS - Asthma, initial: >1 yo & <45 kg: 12-14 mg/kg/day PO divided q4-6h to max of 300 mg/24h. Maintenance: 16-20 mg/kg/day PO divided q4-6h to max of 600 mg/24h. >1 yo & ≥45 kg: Initial: 300 mg/24h PO divided q6-8h. Maintenance: 400-600 mg/24h PO divided q6-8h. Infants 6-52 weeks: [(0.2 x age in weeks) + 5] x kg = 24hr dose in mg PO divided q6-8h.

UNAPPROVED ADULT - COPD: 10 mg/kg/day PO in divided doses.

UNAPPROVED PEDS - Apnea & bradycardia of prematurity: 3-6 mg/kg/day PO divided q6-8h. Maintain serum concentrations 3-5 mcg/ml.

FORMS - Trade: Elixophyllin Liquid 80 mg/15 ml. Qd sustained release tabs: Uniphyl 400. Caps: Theo-24: 100, 200, 300, 400 mg. Bid sustained release tabs: T-Phyl 200 mg. Generic: Theophylline ER tabs: 100, 200, 300, 600 mg. Caps: 125, 200, 300 mg.

NOTES - Multiple drug interactions (especially ketoconazole, rifampin, carbamazepine, isoniazid, phenytoin, macrolides, zafirlukast & cimetidine). Review meds before initiating treatment. Irritability, nausea, palpitations & tachycardia may occur. Overdose may be life-threatening.

tiotropium (*Spiriva*) ▶K ♀C ▶- $$$

ADULT - COPD maintenance: Handihaler: 18 mcg inhaled qd.

PEDS - Not approved in children.

FORMS - Trade: Capsule for oral inhalation, 18 mcg. To be used with "Handihaler" device only. Packages of 6 or 30 capsules with Handihaler device.

NOTES - Not for acute bronchospasm. Administer at the same time each day. Use with caution in narrow-angle glaucoma, BPH, or bladder-neck obstruction. Avoid touching opened capsule. Glaucoma, eye pain, or blurred vision may occur if powder enters eyes. May increase dosing interval if CrCl <50 ml/ min.

TOXICOLOGY

acetylcysteine (*Mucomyst, Acetadote, ♣Parvolex*) ▶L ♀B ▶? $$$$

ADULT - Acetaminophen toxicity: Mucomyst – loading dose 140 mg/kg PO or NG, then 70 mg/kg q4h x 17 doses. May be mixed in water or soft drink diluted to a 5% solution. Acetadote (IV) – loading dose 150 mg/kg in 200 ml of D5W infused over 15 min; maintenance dose 50 mg/kg in 500 ml of D5W infused over 4 hours followed by 100 mg/kg in 1000 ml of D5W infused over 16 hours.

PEDS - Acetaminophen toxicity: same as adult dosing.

FORMS - Generic/Trade: solution 10%, 20%. Trade: IV (Acetadote)

NOTES - May be diluted with water or soft drink to a 5% solution; use diluted solution within 1 hour. Repeat loading dose if vomited within 1 hour. Critical ingestion-treatment interval for maximal protection against severe hepatic injury is between 0-8 hours. Efficacy diminishes after 8 hours & treatment initiation between 15 & 24 hours post ingestion yields limited efficacy. However, treatment should not be withheld, since the reported time of ingestion may not be correct. Anaphylactoid reactions usually occurs 30-60 mins after initiating infusion. Stop infusion, administer antihistamine or epinephrine, restart infusion slowly. If anaphylactoid reactions return or severity increases, then stop treatment.

charcoal (activated charcoal, *Actidose-Aqua, CharcoAid, EZ-Char, ♣Charcodate*) ▶Not absorbed ♀+ ▶+ $

ADULT - Gut decontamination: 25-100 g (1-2 g/ kg or 10 times the amount of poison ingested) PO or NG as soon as possible. May repeat q1-4h prn at doses equivalent to 12.5g/hr. When sorbitol is coadministered, use only with the first dose if repeated doses are to be given.

PEDS - Gut decontamination: <1 yo - 1 g/kg; 15-30 g or 1-2 g/kg if 1-12 yo PO or NG as soon as possible. Repeat doses in children have not been established, but half the initial dose is recommended. Repeat q 2-6h prn. When sorbitol is coadministered, use only with the first dose if repeated doses are to be given.

FORMS - OTC/Generic/Trade: Powder 15,30, 40,120,240 g. Solution 12.5 g/60 ml, 15 g/75 ml, 15g/120 ml, 25 g/120 ml, 30 g/120 ml, 50 g/240 ml. Suspension 15g/120 ml, 25g/120ml, 30g/150 ml, 50g/240 ml. Granules 15g/120 ml.

NOTES - Some products may contain sorbitol to improve taste and reduce GI transit time. Chocolate milk/powder may enhance palatability for pediatric use. Not usually effective for toxic alcohols (methanol, ethylene glycol, isopropanol), heavy metals (lead, iron, bromide), arsenic, lithium, potassium, hydrocarbons, and caustic ingestions (acids, alkalis). Mix powder with 8 oz water. Greatest effect when administered <1 hour of ingestion.

deferoxamine (Desferal) ▶K ♀C ▶? $$$$$

ADULT - Chronic iron overload: 500 mg- 1000 mg IM qd and 2 g IV infusion (≤15 mg/kg/hr) with each unit of blood or 1-2 g SC qd (20-40 mg/kg/day) over 8-24 h via continuous infusion pump. Acute iron toxicity: IV infusion up to 15 mg/kg/hr (consult poison center).

PEDS - Acute iron toxicity: IV infusion up to 15 mg/kg/hr (consult poison center).

NOTES - Contraindicated in renal failure/ anuria unless undergoing dialysis.

dimercaprol (BAL in oil) ▶KL ♀C ▶? $$$$$

ADULT - Specialized dosing for arsenic, mercury, gold, and lead toxicity. Consult poison center. Mild arsenic or gold toxicity: 2.5 mg/kg IM qid x 2 days, then bid x 1 day, then qd x 10 days. Severe arsenic or gold toxicity: 3 mg/kg IM q4h x 2 days, then qid x 1 day, then bid x 10 days. Mercury toxicity: 5 mg/kg IM initially, then 2.5 mg/kg qd-bid x 10 days. Begin therapy within 1-2 h of toxicity. Acute lead encephalopathy: 4 mg/kg IM initially, then q4h in combination (separate syringe) with calcium edetate x 2-7 days. May reduce dose to 3 mg/kg IM for less severe toxicity. Deep IM injection needed.

PEDS - Not approved in children.

UNAPPROVED PEDS - Same as adult dosing. Consult poison center.

edetate (EDTA, Endrate, Meritate) ▶K ♀C ▶- $$$

WARNING - Beware of elevated intracranial pressure in lead encephalopathy.

ADULT - Consult poison center. Lead toxicity: 1000 mg/m²/day IM (divided into equal doses q8-12h) or IV (infuse total dose over 8-12h) x 5 days. Interrupt therapy for 2-4 days, then repeat same regimen. Two courses of therapy are usually necessary. Acute lead encephalopathy: edetate disodium alone or in combination with dimercaprol. Lead nephropathy: 500 mg/m²/dose q24h x 5 doses (creat 2-3 mg/dl), q48h x 3 doses (creat 3-4 mg/dl), or once weekly (creat >4 mg/dl). May repeat at one month intervals.

PEDS - Specialized dosing for lead toxicity; same as adult dosing. Consult poison center.

ethanol (alcohol) ▶L ♀D ▶+ $

PEDS - Not approved in children.

UNAPPROVED ADULT - Consult poison center. Specialized dosing for methanol, ethylene glycol toxicity if fomepizole is unavailable or delayed: 1000 mg/kg (10 ml/kg) of 10% ethanol (100 mg/ml) IV over 1-2h then 100 mg/kg/h (1 ml/kg/h) to keep ethanol level approximately 100 mg/dl.

flumazenil (Romazicon, ♣Anexate) ▶LK ♀C ▶? $$$

WARNING - Do not use in chronic benzodiazepine use or acute overdose with tricyclic antidepressants due to seizure risk.

ADULT - Benzodiazepine sedation reversal: 0.2 mg IV over 15 sec, then 0.2 mg q1 min prn up to 1 mg total dose. Usual dose is 0.6-1 mg. Benzodiazepine overdose reversal: 0.2 mg IV over 30 sec, then 0.3-0.5 mg q30 sec prn up to 3 mg total dose.

PEDS - Not approved in children.

UNAPPROVED PEDS - Benzodiazepine overdose reversal: 0.01 mg/kg IV. Benzodiazepine sedation reversal: 0.01 mg/kg IV initially (max 0.2 mg), then 0.005-0.01 mg/kg (max 0.2 mg) q1 min to max total dose 1 mg. May repeat doses in 20 min, max 3 mg in 1 hour.

NOTES - Onset of action 1-3 min, peak effect 6-10 min. For IV use only, preferably through an IV infusion line into a large vein. Local irritation may occur following extravasation.

fomepizole (Antizol) ▶L ♀C ▶? $$$$$

ADULT - Consult poison center. Ethylene glycol or methanol toxicity: 15 mg/kg IV (load), then 10 mg/kg IV q12h x 4 doses, then 15 mg/kg IV q12h until ethylene glycol or methanol level <20 mg/dl. Administer doses as slow IV infusions over 30 minutes. Increase frequency to q4h during hemodialysis.

PEDS - Not approved in children.

ipecac syrup ▶Gut ♀C ▶? $

ADULT - Emesis: 15- 30 ml, then 3- 4 glasses of water.

PEDS - AAP no longer recommends home ipecac for poisoning. Emesis, <1 yo: 5- 10 ml, then ½ - 1 glass of water (controversial in children <1 year). Emesis, 1- 12 yo: 15 ml, then 1-2 glasses of water. May repeat dose (15 ml) if vomiting does not occur within 20- 30 minutes.

FORMS - Generic/OTC: syrup.

NOTES - Many believe ipecac to be contraindicated in infants <6 months of age. Do not use if any potential for altered mental status (eg, seizure, neurotoxicity), strychnine, beta blocker, calcium channel blocker, clonidine, digitalis glycoside, corrosive, petroleum distillate ingestions, or if at risk for GI bleeding (coagulopathy).

methylene blue (Urolene blue) ▶K ♀C ▶? $$

ADULT - Methemoglobinemia: 1- 2 mg/kg IV over 5 minutes.

PEDS - Not approved in children.

UNAPPROVED PEDS - Methemoglobinemia: 1-2 mg/kg/dose IV over 5 minutes; may repeat in 1 hour prn.

NOTES - Avoid in patients with G6PD deficiency. May turn urine blue-green.

penicillamine (*Cuprimine, Depen*) ▶K ♀D ▶- $$$$

WARNING - Fatal drug-related adverse events have occurred, caution if penicillin allergy.

ADULT - Consult poison center: Specialized dosing for copper toxicity: 750 mg- 1.5 g/day PO x 3 months based on 24-hour urinary copper excretion, max 2 g/day. May start 250 mg/day PO in patients unable to tolerate.

PEDS - Specialized dosing for copper toxicity. Consult poison center.

FORMS - Trade: Caps 125, 250 mg; Tabs 250 mg.

NOTES - Patients may require supplemental pyridoxine 25-50 mg/day PO. Promotes excretion of heavy metals in urine.

physostigmine (*Antilirium*) ▶LK ♀D ▶? $

WARNING - Discontinue if excessive salivation, emesis, frequent urination, or diarrhea. Rapid administration can cause bradycardia, hypersalivation, respiratory difficulties and seizures. Atropine should be available as an antagonist.

ADULT - Life-threatening anticholinergic toxicity: 2 mg IV/IM, administer IV slowly, ≤1 mg/min. May repeat q 10-30 min for severe toxicity.

PEDS - Life-threatening anticholinergic toxicity: 0.02 mg/kg IM/IV injection, administer IV slowly, ≤0.5 mg/min. May repeat q15-30 min until a therapeutic effect or max 2 mg dose.

UNAPPROVED ADULT - Postanesthesia reversal of neuromuscular blockade: 0.5 - 1 mg IV/IM, administer IV slowly, ≤1mg/min. May repeat q 10-30 min prn.

FORMS - Generic/Trade: 1mg/ml in 2ml ampules

pralidoxime (*Protopam, 2-PAM*) ▶K ♀C ▶? $$$

ADULT - Consult poison center: Specialized dosing for organophosphate toxicity: 1-2 g IV infusion over 15-30 min or slow IV injection ≥5 min (max rate 200 mg/min). May repeat dose after 1 h if muscle weakness persists.

PEDS - Not approved in children.

UNAPPROVED ADULT - Consult poison center: 20-40 mg/kg/dose IV infusion over 15-30 min.

UNAPPROVED PEDS - Consult poison center. 25 mg/kg load then 10-20 mg/kg/hr or 25-50 mg/kg load followed by repeat dose in 1-2 hours then q10-12h.

NOTES - Administer <36h of exposure when possible. Rapid administration may worsen cholinergic symptoms. Give in conjunction with atropine. IM or SC may be used if IV access is not available.

sorbitol ▶Not absorbed ♀+ ▶+ $

ADULT - Cathartic: 1-2 ml/kg of 70% soln PO.

PEDS - Not approved in children.

UNAPPROVED PEDS - 4.3 ml/kg of 35% soln (diluted from 70% stock) PO as a single dose.

FORMS - Generic: oral solution 70%.

NOTES - Can be given with activated charcoal to improve taste and decrease gastric transit time. Acts as an osmotic cathartic. May precipitate electrolyte losses.

succimer (*Chemet*) ▶K ♀C ▶? $$$$$

PEDS - Lead toxicity ≥1 yo: Start 10 mg/kg PO or 350 mg/m² q8h x 5 days, then reduce the frequency to q12h x 2 weeks. Not approved in children <12 mo.

FORMS - Trade: Caps 100 mg.

NOTES - Manufacturer recommends doses of 100 mg (8-15 kg), 200 mg (16-23 kg), 300 mg (24-34 kg), 400 mg (35-44 kg), and 500 mg (≥45 kg). Can open cap and sprinkle medicated beads over food, or give them in a spoon and follow with fruit drink. Indicated for blood lead levels >45 mcg/dl. Allow at least 4 weeks between edetate disodium and succimer treatment.

ANTIDOTES

Toxin	Antidote/Treatment	Toxin	Antidote/Treatment
acetaminophen	N-acetylcysteine	ethylene glycol	fomepizole
antidepressants, cyclic	bicarbonate	heparin	protamine
arsenic, mercury	dimercaprol (BAL)	iron	deferoxamine
benzodiazepine	flumazenil	lead	EDTA, succimer
beta blockers	glucagon	methanol	fomepizole
calcium channel blockers	calcium chloride, glucagon	methemoglobin	methylene blue
cyanide	Lilly cyanide kit	narcotics	naloxone
digoxin	dig immune Fab	organophosphates	atropine+pralidoxime
		warfarin	vitamin K, FFP

UROLOGY: Benign Prostatic Hyperplasia

alfuzosin (*UroXatral*) ▶KL ♀B ▶- $$$
WARNING - Postural hypotension with or without symptoms may develop within a few hours after administration. Avoid in moderate or severe hepatic insufficiency. Avoid co-administration with potent CYP3A4 inhibitors.
ADULT - BPH: 10 mg PO qd after a meal.
PEDS - Not approved in children.
FORMS - Trade only: extended-release tabs 10 mg
NOTES - Caution in congenital or acquired QT prolongation & severe renal insufficiency.

doxazosin (*Cardura*) ▶L ♀C ▶? $
ADULT - BPH: Start 1 mg PO qhs, titrate by doubling the dose over at least 1-2 week intervals up to a maximum of 8 mg PO qhs.
PEDS - Not approved in children.
FORMS - Generic/Trade: Tabs 1, 2, 4, 8 mg.
NOTES - Beware of dizziness, drowsiness, lightheadedness, syncope, postural hypotension; monitor BP closely. If therapy is interrupted for several days, restart at 1 mg dose. Alpha blockers are generally considered to be first line treatment in men with more than minimal symptoms.

dutasteride (*Avodart*) ▶L ♀X ▶- $$$
ADULT - BPH: 0.5 mg PO qd.
PEDS - Not approved in children.
FORMS - Trade: Capsule 0.5 mg.
NOTES - 6 months' therapy may be needed to assess effectiveness. Pregnant or potentially pregnant women should not handle capsules due to fetal risk from absorption. Caution in hepatic insufficiency. Dutasteride will decrease PSA by 50%; new baseline PSA should be established after 3-6 months to assess potentially cancer-related PSA changes.

finasteride (*Proscar*) ▶L ♀X ▶- $$$
ADULT - 5 mg PO qd alone or in combination with doxazosin to reduce the risk of sympto-matic progression of BPH.
PEDS - Not approved in children.
FORMS - Trade: Tabs 5 mg.
NOTES - Therapy for 6-12 months may be needed to assess effectiveness. Pregnant or potentially pregnant women should not handle crushed tabs because of possible absorption and fetal risk. Use with caution in hepatic insufficiency. Monitor PSA before therapy; finasteride will decrease PSA by 50% in patients with BPH, even with prostate cancer; does not appear to alter detection of prostate cancer.

tamsulosin (*Flomax*) ▶LK ♀B ▶- $$$
ADULT - BPH: 0.4 mg PO qd 30 min after the same meal each day. If an adequate response is not seen after 2-4 wks, may increase dose to 0.8 mg PO qd. If therapy is interrupted for several days, restart at the 0.4 mg dose.
PEDS - Not approved in children.
FORMS - Trade: Caps 0.4 mg.
NOTES - Dizziness, headache, abnormal ejaculation. Less risk for postural hypotension than with other alpha blockers. Alpha blockers are generally considered to be first line treatment in men with more than minimal symptoms.

terazosin (*Hytrin*) ▶LK ♀C ▶? $
ADULT - BPH: Start 1 mg PO qhs, titrate dose in a stepwise fashion to 2, 5, or 10 mg PO qhs to desired effect. Treatment with 10 mg PO qhs for 4-6 weeks may be needed to assess benefit. Maximum 20 mg/day.
PEDS - Not approved in children.
FORMS - Generic/Trade: Caps 1, 2, 5, 10 mg.
NOTES - Beware of dizziness, drowsiness, lightheadedness, syncope, postural hypotension; monitor BP closely. If therapy is interrupted for several days, restart at 1 mg dose. Alpha blockers are generally considered to be first line treatment in men with more than minimal symptoms.

UROLOGY: Bladder Agents

B&O Supprettes (belladonna + opium) ▶L ♀C ▶? ©II $$$
ADULT - Bladder spasm: 1 suppository PR qd-bid, max 4 doses/day.
PEDS - Not approved in children <12 yo.
FORMS - Generic/Trade: suppositories 30 mg opium [15A], 60 mg opium [16A].
NOTES - Store at room temperature. Contraindicated in narrow-angle glaucoma, obstructive conditions (e.g. pyloric or duodenal obstruction, obstructive intestinal lesions or ileus, achalasia, and obstructive uropathies).

bethanechol (*Urecholine*, ✦*Duvoid*, *Myotonachol*) ▶L ♀C ▶? $
ADULT - Urinary retention: 10-50 mg PO tid-qid or 2.5-5 mg SC tid-qid. Take 1 hour before or 2 h after meals to avoid N/V. Determine the minimum effective dose by giving 5-10 mg PO

initially and repeat at hourly intervals until response or to a maximum of 50 mg.

PEDS - Not approved in children.

UNAPPROVED PEDS - Urinary retention/abdominal distention: 0.6 mg/kg/day PO divided q6-8h or 0.12-0.2 mg/kg/day SC divided q6-8h.

FORMS - Generic/Trade: Tabs 5, 10, 25, 50 mg.

NOTES - May cause drowsiness, lightheadedness, and fainting. Not for obstructive urinary retention. Avoid with cardiac disease, hyperthyroidism, parkinsonism, peptic ulcer disease, and epilepsy.

desmopressin (*DDAVP*, ✚*Minirin*) ▸LK ♀B ▸? $$$$

ADULT - Primary nocturnal enuresis: 10- 40 mcg (0.1- 0.4 ml) intranasally qhs, administer ½ of dose per nostril or 0.2- 0.6 mg PO qhs.

PEDS - Primary nocturnal enuresis ≥6 yo: 10-40 mcg (50% of the dose in each nostril) intranasally qhs or 0.2-0.6 mg PO qhs.

FORMS - Generic/Trade: Tabs 0.1, 0.2 mg; Nasal solution 0.1 mg/ml (10 mcg/ spray).

NOTES - Infants and children require careful fluid intake restrictions since hyponatremic seizures have been reported with both therapeutic and higher doses. Prime the nasal spray pump, stable for ≤3 wks at room temperature, otherwise refrigerate.

dimethyl sulfoxide (*DMSO, Rimso-50*) ▸KL ♀C ▸? $$$

ADULT - Interstitial cystitis: Instill 50 mL solution into bladder by catheter & allow to remain for 15 min; expelled by spontaneous voiding. Repeat q2 weeks until symptomatic relief is obtained; thereafter, may increase time intervals between treatments.

PEDS - Not approved in children.

NOTES - Apply analgesic lubricant gel to urethra prior to inserting the catheter to avoid spasm. May administer oral analgesics or suppositories containing belladonna & opium prior to instillation to reduce spasms. May give anesthesia in patients with severe interstitial cystitis and very sensitive bladders during the 1st, 2nd & 3rd treatment. May cause lens opacities & changes in refractive index; perform eye exams before & periodically during treatment. May cause hypersensitivity reaction by liberating histamine. Monitor liver & renal function tests & CBC q6 months. May be harmful in patients with urinary tract malignancy; can cause DMSO-induced vasodilation Peripheral neuropathy may occur when used with sulindac. Garlic-like taste may occur within a few minutes of administration; odor on breath & skin

may be present & remain for up to 72 h.

flavoxate (*Urispas*) ▸K ♀B ▸? $$$$

ADULT - Bladder spasm: 100 or 200 mg PO tid-qid. Reduce dose when improved.

PEDS - Not approved in children <12 yo.

FORMS - Trade: Tabs 100 mg.

NOTES - May cause dizziness, drowsiness, dry mouth, blurred vision, N/V, urinary retention. Contraindicated in glaucoma, obstructive conditions (eg, pyloric or duodenal obstruction, obstructive intestinal lesions or ileus, achalasia, GI hemorrhage, and obstructive uropathies).

hyoscyamine (*Anaspaz, A-spaz, Cystospaz, ED Spaz, Hyosol, Hyospaz, Levbid, Levsin, Levsinex, Medispaz, NuLev, Spacol, Spasdel, Symax*) ▸LK ♀C ▸- $

ADULT - Bladder spasm: 0.125-0.25 mg PO q4h or prn; or 0.375-0.75 mg PO q12h (extended release). Max 1.5 mg/day.

PEDS - Bladder spasm >12 yo: Adult dosing.

FORMS - Generic/Trade: Tabs 0.125. Extended release tabs 0.375 mg. Sublingual tabs 0.125 mg. Extended release caps 0.375 mg. Elixir 0.125 mg/5 ml. Drops 0.125 mg/1 ml. Trade only: Tabs 0.15 mg (Hyospaz, Cystospaz). Tabs, orally disintegrating 0.125 (NuLev).

NOTES - May cause dizziness, drowsiness, dry mouth, blurred vision, N/V, urinary retention. Contraindicated in glaucoma, obstructive conditions (eg, pyloric or duodenal obstruction, obstructive intestinal lesions or ileus, achalasia, GI hemorrhage, and obstructive uropathies), unstable cardiovascular status, and myasthenia gravis.

imipramine (*Tofranil, Tofranil-PM*) ▸L ♀B ▸? $

ADULT - See psychiatry section

PEDS - Enuresis ≥6 yo: 10- 25 mg/day PO given one hour before bedtime, then increase in increments of 10-25 mg at 1-2 week intervals not to exceed 50 mg/day in 6-12 yo children or 75 mg/day in children >12 yo. Do not exceed 2.5 mg/kg/day.

UNAPPROVED ADULT - Enuresis: 25-75 mg PO qhs.

FORMS - Generic/Trade: Tabs 10, 25, 50 mg. Trade only: Caps (Tofranil-PM) 75, 100, 125, 150 mg.

NOTES - Potential cardiac toxicity, especially with overdoses. Contraindicated with MAO inhibitors or recent MI.

methylene blue (*Methblue 65, Urolene blue*) ▸Gut/K ♀C ▸? $

ADULT - Dysuria: 65-130 mg PO tid after meals with liberal water.

PEDS - Not approved in children.

FORMS - Trade only: Tabs 65 mg.

NOTES - May turn urine, stool, skin, contact lenses, and undergarments blue-green.

oxybutynin (*Ditropan, Ditropan XL, Oxytrol*, ✚*Oxybutyn*) ▶LK ♀B ▶? $

ADULT - Bladder instability: Ditropan: 2.5-5 mg PO bid-tid, max 5 mg PO qid. Ditropan XL: 5-10 mg PO qd same time each day, increase 5 mg/day q week to 30 mg/day. Oxytrol: 1 patch twice weekly on abdomen, hips or buttocks.

PEDS - Bladder instability >5 yo: 5 mg PO bid, max dose: 5 mg PO tid. >6 yo: 5 mg PO qd, max 20 mg/day (Ditropan XL). Transdermal patch not approved in children.

UNAPPROVED PEDS - Bladder instability ≤5 yo: 0.2 mg/kg/dose PO bid-qid.

FORMS - Generic/Trade: Tabs 5 mg; syrup 5 mg/5 ml. Trade only: extended release tabs (Ditropan XL) 5, 10, 15 mg. Transdermal product (Oxytrol) 3.9 mg/day.

NOTES - May cause dizziness, drowsiness, blurred vision, dry mouth, urinary retention. Contraindicated with glaucoma, obstructive uropathy or GI disease, unstable cardiovascular status, and myasthenia gravis. Transdermal patch causes less dry mouth than oral form; avoid dose reduction by cutting.

pentosan (*Elmiron*) ▶LK ♀B ▶? $$$$

ADULT - Interstitial cystitis: 100 mg PO tid 1 hour before or 2 h after a meal.

PEDS - Not approved in children.

FORMS - Trade: Caps 100 mg.

NOTES - Pain relief usually occurs at 2-4 months and decreased urinary frequency takes 6 months. May increase risk of bleeding. Use with caution in hepatic or splenic dysfunction.

phenazopyridine (*Pyridium, Azo-Standard, Urogesic, Prodium, Pyridiate, Urodol, Baridium, UTI Relief*, ✚*Phenazo*) ▶K ♀B ▶? $

ADULT - Dysuria: 200 mg PO tid after meals x 2 days.

PEDS - Dysuria in children 6-12 yo: 12 mg/kg/day PO divided tid x 2 days.

FORMS - OTC/Generic/Trade: Tabs 95, 97.2 mg. Generic/Trade: Tabs 100, 200 mg.

NOTES - May turn urine/contact lenses orange. Contraindicated with hepatitis or renal insufficiency.

***Prosed/DS* (methenamine + phenyl salicylate + methylene blue + benzoic acid + atropine + hyoscyamine)** ▶KL ♀C ▶? $$$

ADULT - Bladder spasm: 1 tab PO qid with liberal fluids.

PEDS - Not approved in children

FORMS - Trade only: Tabs methenamine 81.6 mg + phenyl salicylate 36.2 mg + methylene blue 10.8 mg + benzoic acid 9.0 mg + atropine sulfate 0.06 mg+hyoscyamine sulfate 0.06 mg.

NOTES - May cause dizziness, drowsiness, blurred vision, dry mouth, N/V, urinary retention. May turn urine/contact lenses blue.

tolterodine (*Detrol, Detrol LA*) ▶L ♀C ▶- $$$

ADULT - Overactive bladder: 2 mg PO bid (Detrol) or 4 mg PO qd (Detrol LA). Decrease dose to 1 mg PO bid (Detrol) or 2 mg PO qd (Detrol LA) if adverse symptoms, hepatic insufficiency or specific coadministered drugs (see notes).

PEDS - Not approved in children.

FORMS - Trade: Tabs 1, 2 mg. Caps, extended release 2, 4 mg.

NOTES - Contraindicated with urinary or gastric retention, or uncontrolled glaucoma. Drug interactions with CYP3A4 inhibitors (eg, erythromycin, ketoconazole, itraconazole); decrease dose to 1 mg PO bid or 2 mg qd (Detrol LA).

trospium (*Sanctura*) ▶LK ♀C ▶? ?

ADULT - Overactive bladder with urge incontinence: 20 mg PO bid. Renal impairment (CrCl <30 ml/min): 20 mg PO qhs. If ≥75 yo may taper down to 20 mg qd.

PEDS - Not approved in children.

FORMS - Trade only: Tab 20 mg

NOTES - Contraindicated with uncontrolled narrow-angle glaucoma, urinary retention, gastroparesis. May cause heat stroke due to decreased sweating. Take on an empty stomach. Improvement in signs & symptoms may be seen in a week. Causes minimum CNS side effects. Approved but not yet available.

***Urised* (methenamine + phenyl salicylate + atropine + hyoscyamine + benzoic acid + methylene blue, *Usept*)** ▶K ♀C ▶? $$$$

ADULT - Dysuria: 2 Tabs PO qid.

PEDS - Dysuria >6 yo: reduce dose based on age and weight. Not recommended for children <6 yo.

FORMS - Trade: Tab (methenamine 40.8 mg + phenyl salicylate 18.1 mg + atropine 0.03 mg + hyoscyamine 0.03 mg + 4.5 mg benzoic acid + 5.4 mg methylene blue).

NOTES - Take with food to minimize GI upset. May precipitate urate crystals in urine. Avoid use with sulfonamides. May turn urine/contact lenses blue.

***UTA* (methenamine + sodium phosphate + phenyl salicylate + methylene blue + hyoscyamine)** ▶KL ♀C ▶? $$$

ADULT - Treatment of irritative voiding/relief of inflammation, hypermotility & pain with lower urinary tract infection/relief of urinary tract symptoms caused by diagnostic procedures: 1 cap PO qid with liberal fluids.

PEDS - <6 yo: not recommended. >6 yo: dosing must be individualized by physician.

FORMS - Trade only: Caps (methenamine 120 mg + sodium phosphate 40.8 mg + phenyl salicylate 36 mg + methylene blue 10 mg + hyoscyamine 0.12 mg).

NOTES - May turn urine/feces blue to blue-green. Take 2 hours apart from ketoconazole. May decrease absorption of thiazide diuretics. Antacids and antidiarrheals may decrease effectiveness of methenamine.

UROLOGY: Erectile Dysfunction

alprostadil (*Muse, Caverject, Caverject Impulse, Edex*) ▶L ♀- ▶- $$$$

ADULT - Erectile dysfunction: 1.25-2.5 mcg intracavernosal injection over 5-10 seconds initially using a ½ inch, 27 or 30 gauge needle. If no response, may give next higher dose after 1 hour, max 2 doses/day. May increase by 2.5 mcg and then 5-10 mcg incrementally on separate occasions. Dose range= 1-40 mcg. Alternative: 125-250 mcg intraurethral pellet (Muse). Increase or decrease dose on separate occasions until erection achieved. Maximum intraurethral dose 2 pellets/24h. The lowest possible dose to produce an acceptable erection should be used.

PEDS - Not approved in children.

UNAPPROVED ADULT - Erectile dysfunction intracorporeal injection: Specially formulated mixtures of alprostadil, papaverine and phentolamine. 0.10-0.50 ml injection.

FORMS - Trade: Syringe system (Edex) 10, 20, 40 mcg; (Caverject) 5, 10, 20 mcg; (Caverject Impulse) 10, 20 mcg. Pellet (Muse) 125, 250, 500, 1000 mcg. Intracorporeal injection of locally-compounded combination agents (many variations): "Bi-mix" can be 30 mg/ml papaverine + 0.5 to 1 mg/ml phentolamine, or 30 mg/ml papaverine + 20 mcg/ml alprostadil in 10 ml vials. "Tri-mix" can be 30 mg/ml papaverine + 1 mg/ml phentolamine + 10 mcg/ml alprostadil in 5, 10 or 20 ml vials.

NOTES - Contraindicated in patients at risk for priapism, with penile fibrosis (Peyronie's disease), with penile implants, in women or children, in men for whom sexual activity is inadvisable, and for intercourse with a pregnant woman. Onset of effect is 5-20 minutes.

sildenafil (*Viagra*) ▶LK ♀B ▶- $$$

WARNING - Contraindicated in patients taking nitrates in prior/subsequent 24 hours.

ADULT - Erectile dysfunction: 50 mg PO approximately 1h (range 0.5-4h) before sexual activity. Usual effective dose range: 25-100 mg. Maximum 1 dose/day. Use lower dose (25 mg) if >65 yo, hepatic/renal impairment, or certain coadministered drugs (see notes). Not FDA-approved in women.

PEDS - Not approved in children.

UNAPPROVED ADULT - Antidepressant-associated sexual dysfunction: Same dose as above.

FORMS - Trade: Tabs 25, 50, 100 mg. Unscored tab but can be cut in half.

NOTES - Drug interactions with cimetidine, erythromycin, ketoconazole, itraconazole, saquinavir, ritonavir and other CYP3A4 inhibitors; use 25 mg dose. Do not exceed 25 mg/48 h with ritonavir. Doses >25 mg should not be taken <4h after an alpha-blocker. Caution if stroke, MI or other cardiovascular event within last 6 months.

tadalafil (*Cialis*) ▶L ♀B ▶- $$$

WARNING - Contraindicated with nitrates & alpha-blockers (except tamsulosin 0.4 mg qd).

ADULT - Erectile dysfunction: 10 mg PO prior to sexual activity. (Optimal timing of administration unclear, but should be ≥30-45 min before sexual activity.) May increase to 20 mg or decrease to 5 mg. Max 1 dose/day. Start 5 mg (max 1 dose/day) if moderate renal impairment (CrCl 31-50 ml/min). Max 5 mg/day if severe renal impairment (CrCl <30 ml/min) on dialysis. Max 10 mg/day if mild to moderate hepatic impairment; avoid in severe hepatic impairment. Max 10 mg once in 72 hours if concurrent potent CYP3A4 inhibitors.

PEDS - Not approved in children.

FORMS - Trade: Tabs 5,10,20 mg.

NOTES - If nitrates needed give ≥48 hours after the last tadalafil dose. Improves erectile function for up to 36 hours. Not FDA-approved for women. Not recommended if MI in prior 90 days, angina during sexual activity, NYHA Class ≥II in prior 6 months, hypotension (<90/50), hypertension (>170/100) or stroke in prior 6 months. Rare reports of prolonged erections.

vardenafil (*Levitra*) ▶LK ♀B ▶- $$$

WARNING - Contraindicated with nitrates (time interval for safe administration unknown) and alpha-blockers.

ADULT - Erectile dysfunction: 10 mg PO 1 h before sexual activity. Usual effective dose range: 5-20 mg. Maximum 1 dose/day. Use lower dose (5 mg) if ≥65 yo or moderate hepatic impairment (max 10 mg); 2.5 mg when coadminister with certain drugs (see notes). Not FDA-approved in women.

PEDS - Not approved in children.

FORMS - Trade: Tabs 2.5, 5, 10, 20 mg

NOTES - See the following parenthetical vardenafil dose adjustments when taken with ritonavir (max 2.5mg/72 hr); indinavir, ketoconazole 400 mg qd, or itraconazole 400 mg qd (max 2.5mg/24 hr); ketoconazole 200 mg qd, itraconazole 200 mg qd, or erythromycin (max 5 mg/24 hr). Avoid with alpha blockers & antiarrhythmics. Caution if stroke, MI or other cardiovascular event within last 6 months, prolonged QT interval, unstable angina, severe liver impairment, end stage renal disease or retinitis pigmentosa.

yohimbine (Yocon, Yohimex) ▶L ♀- ▶- $

ADULT - No approved indications.

PEDS - No approved indications.

UNAPPROVED ADULT - Erectile dysfunction: 1 tab PO tid. If side effects (eg, tremor, tachycardia, nervousness) occur, reduce to ½ tab tid, followed by gradual increases to 1 tab tid.

FORMS - Generic/Trade: 5.4 mg tab

NOTES - Prescription yohimbine and yohimbine bark extract (see Herbal section) are not interchangeable. Contraindicated with renal disease. Avoid with antidepressant use, psychiatric disorders, the elderly, women, or ulcer history. Efficacy of therapy >10 weeks unclear. American Urological Association does not recommend as a standard treatment due to unproven efficacy.

UROLOGY: Nephrolithiasis

acetohydroxamic acid (Lithostat) ▶K ♀X ▶? $$$

ADULT - Chronic UTI, adjunctive therapy: 250 mg PO tid-qid for a total dose of 10-15 mg/kg/day. Maximum dose is 1.5 g/day. Decrease dose in patients with renal impairment to no more than 1 g/day.

PEDS - Adjunctive therapy in chronic ureasplitting UTI: 10 mg/kg/day PO divided bid-tid.

FORMS - Trade: Tabs 250 mg.

NOTES - Do not use if CrCl <20 ml/min. Administer on an empty stomach.

allopurinol (Zyloprim, ♣Purinol) ▶K ♀C▶+$

ADULT - Recurrent calcium oxalate stones : 200-300 mg PO qd-bid. Reduce dose in renal insufficiency (CrCl 10-20 ml/ min= 200 mg/day, CrCl <10 ml/min = 100 mg/day).

PEDS - Not approved for urolithiasis in children.

FORMS - Generic/Trade: Tabs 100, 300 mg.

NOTES - Incidence of rash is increased in renal impairment and with ampicillin. Discontinue if rash or allergic symptoms. Do not restart after severe rash. Drug interaction with warfarin & azathioprine.

cellulose sodium phosphate (Calcibind) ▶Fecal ♀C ▶+ $$$$

WARNING - Avoid in CHF or ascites due to high sodium content.

ADULT - Absorptive hypercalciuria Type 1 (>16 yo): Initial dose with urinary calcium >300 mg/day (on moderate calcium-restricted diet) – 5 g with each meal; decrease dose to 5 g with supper, 2.5 g with each remaining meal when calcium declines to <150 mg/day. Initial dose with urinary calcium 200-300 mg/day (controlled calcium-restricted diet) – 5 g with supper, 2.5 g with each remaining meal. Mix with water, soft drink or fruit juice; ingest within 30 min of meal.

PEDS - Do not use if <16 yo.

FORMS - Trade only: bulk powder 300 mg

NOTES - Give concomitant supplement of 1.5 g magnesium gluconate with 15 g/day; 1 g magnesium gluconate with 10 g/day. Take magnesium supplement ≥1h before or after each dose to avoid binding. May cause hyperparathyroidism; long-term use may cause hypomagnesemia, hyperoxaluria, hypomagnesuria, depletion of trace metals (copper, zinc, iron); monitor calcium, magnesium, trace metals and CBC q3-6 months; monitor parathyroid hormone once between the first 2 weeks and 3 months, then q3-6 months thereafter. Adjust or stop treatment if PTH rises above normal; stop when inadequate hypocalciuric response (urinary calcium of <30 mg/5 g of cellulose sodium phosphate) occurs while patient is on moderate calcium restriction. Avoid Vitamin C supplementation since metabolized to oxalate.

chlorthalidone (Hygroton, Thalitone) ▶L ♀D▶+ $

ADULT - See cardiovascular section

PEDS - Not approved in children.

UNAPPROVED ADULT - Nephrolithiasis: 25-50

mg PO qd.

UNAPPROVED PEDS - See CV section

FORMS - Trade only: Tabs, non-scored (Thalitone) 15 mg. Generic/Trade: Tabs, non-scored (Thalitone, Hygroton) 25,50, scored (Hygroton) 100 mg.

NOTES - Beware of azotemia, hypokalemia

citrate (Polycitra-K, Urocit-K, Bicitra, Oracit, Polycitra, Polycitra-LC) ▶K ♀C ▶? $$$

ADULT - Urinary alkalinization: 1 packet in water/juice PO tid-qid with meals. 15-30 ml PO solution tid-qid with meals. 10-20 mEq PO Tabs tid-qid with meals. Max 100 mEq/day.

PEDS - Urinary alkalinization: 5-15 ml PO qid with meals.

FORMS - Trade: Polycitra-K packet (potassium citrate): 3300 mg. Urocit-K wax (potassium citrate): Tabs 5, 10 mEq. Oracit oral solution: 5

ml = sodium citrate 490 mg. Generic: Polycitra-K oral solution (5 ml = potassium citrate 1100 mg), Bicitra oral solution (5 ml = sodium citrate 500 mg), Polycitra-LC oral solution (5 ml = potassium citrate 550 mg + sodium citrate 500 mg), Polycitra oral syrup (5 ml = potassium citrate 550 mg + sodium citrate 550 mg).

NOTES - Contraindicated in renal insufficiency, PUD, UTI, and hyperkalemia.

hydrochlorothiazide (HCTZ, Esidrix, HydroDIURIL, Oretic, Microzide, Ezide, Hydrocot, Aquazide H) ▶L ♀D ▶+ $

ADULT, PEDS - See cardiovascular section

UNAPPROVED ADULT - Nephrolithiasis: 50-100 mg PO qd.

FORMS - Generic/Trade: Tabs 25, 50, 100 mg; Solution 50 mg/ 5 mL; Caps 12.5 mg.

NOTES - Beware of azotemia, hypokalemia.

UROLOGY: Prostate Cancer

abarelix (Plenaxis) ▶KL ♀X ▶- $$$$$

WARNING - Immediate-onset of systemic allergic reactions which increases with treatment duration. Patients should be observed for ≥30 min following each injection. Physicians who have enrolled in Plenaxis PLUS Program may prescribe. Serum testosterone suppression decreases with continued dosing in some patients. Effectiveness beyond 12 months has not been established. Treatment failure can be detected by measuring serum total testosterone concentrations just prior to administration on Day 29 & every 8 weeks thereafter.

ADULT - Palliative treatment of prostate cancer, in whom LHRH agonist therapy is not appropriate & who refuse surgical castration & have ≥1 of the following: risk of neurological compromise due to metastases, ureteral or bladder outlet obstruction due to local encroachment or metastatic disease, or severe bone pain from skeletal metastases persisting on narcotic analgesia. 100 mg IM to the buttock on Day 1, 15, 29 (week 4) & every 4 weeks thereafter.

PEDS - Not approved in children.

NOTES - Monitor LFTs and PSA. Avoid use in patients with known hypersensitivity with carboxymethylcellulose. May prolong QT interval. May decrease bone mineral density. Decrease in effectiveness are seen more in patients who weigh >225 pounds.

bicalutamide (Casodex) ▶L ♀X ▶- $$$$$

ADULT - Prostate cancer: 50 mg PO qd in combination with a LHRH analog (e.g. goserelin or leuprolide). Not indicated in women.

PEDS - Not approved in children.

FORMS - Trade: Tabs 50 mg.

NOTES - Monitor LFTs and PSA. May cause increased INR with warfarin. Gynecomastia and breast pain occur.

flutamide (Eulexin, ✦Euflex) ▶KL ♀D ▶- $$$$$

ADULT - Prostate cancer: 250 mg PO q8h in combination with a LHRH analog (e.g. goserelin or leuprolide). Not indicated in women.

PEDS - Not approved in children.

FORMS - Generic/Trade: Caps 125 mg.

NOTES - Monitor LFTs and PSA. May cause increased INR with warfarin. Gynecomastia and breast pain occur.

goserelin (Zoladex) ▶L ♀X ▶- $$$$$

ADULT - Prostate cancer: 3.6 mg implant SC into upper abdominal wall every 28 days, or 10.8 mg implant SC q12 weeks.

PEDS - Not approved in children.

FORMS - Trade: Implants 3.6, 10.8 mg.

NOTES - Transient increases in testosterone and estrogen occur.

leuprolide (Eligard, Lupron, Lupron Depot, Oaklide, Viadur) ▶L ♀X ▶- $$$$$

ADULT - Advanced prostate cancer: Lupron: 1 mg SC qd. Eligard: 7.5mg SC q month, 22.5mg SC q3 months or 30 mg SC q4 months. Lupron depot: 7.5mg IM q month, 22.5mg IM q3 months or 30 mg IM q4 months. Viadur: 65 mg SC implant q12 months.

PEDS - Not approved for this indication.

NOTES - Transient increases in testosterone and estrogen occur. Periodically monitor PSA,

acid phosphatase, and testosterone levels.
nilutamide (*Nilandron*, ♥*Anandron*) ▶K ♀C
▶? $$$$$
ADULT - Prostate cancer: 300 mg PO qd for 30 days, then 150 mg PO qd. Begin therapy on same day as surgical castration.

PEDS - Not approved in children.
FORMS - Trade: Tabs 50 mg.
NOTES - Contraindicated in severe hepatic or respiratory insufficiency. Beware of delay in eyes adapting to dark, interstitial pneumonitis, hepatitis, and aplastic anemia.

UROLOGY: Other

aminohippurate (*PAH*) ▶K ♀C ▶? $$$$
ADULT - Estimation of effective renal plasma flow & measurement of functional capacity of renal tubular secretory mechanism: Specialized infusion dosing available.
PEDS - Not approved in children.

NOTES - May precipitate CHF. Patients receiving sulfonamides, procaine or thiazolsulfone may interfere with chemical color development essential for analysis. Concomitant use of probenecid my result in erroneously low effective renal plasma flow.

Index

908	53	*Abelcet*	34	Pulmonary	277	acyclovir
15-methyl-prostaglandin F2 alpha	241	*Abenol*	29	Toxicology	280	Antimicrobials 46
		Abilify	265	*Acidophilus*	209	Dermatology 128
2-PAM	282	*Abreva*		*Aciphex*	189	*Adacel* 212
3TC	50	Dermatology	128	acitretin	127	*Adalat*
5-aminosalicylic acid	193	ENT	175	*Aclovate*	129	Cardiovascular 109
		acamprosate	268	Acne	120	OB/GYN 241
5-ASA	193	acarbose	141	acrivastine	174	*Adalat CC*
5-FU		*Accolate*	277	*ActHIB*	212	Cardiovascular 109
Dermatology	123	*Accupril*	85	*Acticin*	126	OB/GYN 241
Oncology	246	*Accuretic*	99	*Actidose-Aqua*	280	*Adalat XL*
6-MP		*Accutane*	122	*Actifed Cold & Allergy*	166	Cardiovascular 109
Gastroenterology	193	ACE inhibitors	83			OB/GYN 241
Oncology	246	acebutolol	105	*Actifed Cold & Sinus*	166	adalimumab 12
8-MOP	128	*acemannan*	204			adapalene 120
		Aceon	85	*Actigall*	195	*Adderall* 270
		Acetadote	280	Actinic Keratosis	123	adefovir 56
		acetaminophen		*Actiq*	24	*Adenocard* 88
		Analgesics 17, 26-30		*Activase*		adenosine 88
A/T/S	122	ENT	166-169	Cardiovascular	117	*ADH*
A1C home testing	145	Neurology	227	Neurology	230	Cardiovascular 93
A-200	126	OB/GYN	246	*Activase rt-PA*		Gastroenterology196
abacavir	49-51	acetazolamide		Cardiovascular	117	*Adipex-P* 272
abarelix		Cardiovascular	110	Neurology	230	*Adoxa* 37, 78
Oncology	246	Ophthalmology	252	activated charcoal	280	adrenalin
Urology	288	acetic acid		*Activella*	235	Cardiovasc 91, 116
Abbokinase	118	ENT	165	*Actonel*	139	Pulmonary 278
Abbokinase Open - Cath	118	ENT	166	*Actos*	142	*Adriamycin* 246
Abbreviations	4	acetohydroxamic acid	287	*Actron*	20	*Adrucil* 246
ABC	49	*Acetoxyl*	121	*Acular*	255	Adult emerg drugs 302
abciximab	104	acetylcysteine		*Acular LS*	255	Adult immunizations 214
		Contrast Media	120	*Acutrim Natural AM*	205	*Advair* 274

Advate	202	nists	85	Cardiovascular	119	amoxicillin
Advicor	96	*Aldurazyme*	161	Urology	286	Antimicrobials 70
Advil	20	alefacept	127	*Alrex*	250	Gastroenterology 186
Aerius	162	alemtuzumab	246	*Alsoy*	152	amoxicillin-clavulanate
Aerobid	276	alendronate	138	*Altace*	85	71
Aerobid-M	276	*Alertec*	272	alteplase		*Amoxil* 70
Aesculus hippocasta-		*Alesse*	237	Cardiovascular	117	amphetamine 270
num	208	*Aleve*	21	Neurology	230	*Amphojel* 183
Aflexa	208	*Aleve Cold & Sinus*166		*Alternagel*	183	*Amphotec* 34
African plum tree	210	*Alfenta*	30	*Alterra*	210	amphotericin B deoxy-
Afrin	177	alfentanil	30	*Altocor*	97	cholate 33
agalsidase beta	158	*Alferon N*	247	*Altoprev*	97	amphotericin B lipid
Agenerase	52	alfuzosin	283	altretamine	246	formulations 34
Aggrastat	105	*Alimta*	246	*Alu-Cap*	183	ampicillin 71
Aggrenox		*Alinia*	43	aluminum acetate	165	ampicillin-sulbactam72
Cardiovascular	104	alitretinoin	133	aluminum chloride	134	amprenavir 52
Neurology	230	*Alka-Seltzer*	183	aluminum hydroxide		*Amrinone* 116
Agoral	190	*Alkeran*	246	Analgesics	16	amyl nitrite 114
Agrylin	201	*Allegra*	163	Gastroent 183, 184		*Anacin* 18
Airomir	273	*Allegra-D*	169	*Alupent*	274	*Anafranil* 257
AK Tate	251	*Aller-Chlor*	163	*Alu-Tab*	183	anagrelide 201
AK Tracin	248	*Allerdryl*		Alzheimer's disease		anakinra 12
AK-Con	251	ENT	164		219	**ANALGESICS** 12
Akineton	228	Psychiatry 273, 267		amantadine		*Anandron*
AK-Mycin	248	*Allerest*	251	Antimicrobials	55	Oncology 246
AK-Pentolate	254	*Allerfrim*	167	Neurology	229	Urology 289
AK-Pred	251	*Allermax* 267, 273		*Amaryl*	144	*Anaprox* 21
AK-Sulf	248	*Allernix*		*Amatine*	116	*Anaspaz* 284
Alamast	254	ENT	164	*Ambien*	268	anastrozole 246
Alavert	163	Psychiatry 273, 267		*AmBisome*	34	*Ancef* 59
Alavert D-12	166	*Aller-Relief*	163	amcinonide	129	*Ancobon* 35
Albalon	251	*Allium sativum*	207	*Amen*	239	*Andriol* 137
albendazole	42	allopurinol		*Amerge*	226	andro 204
Albenza	42	Endocrine	146	*Amevive*	127	*Androcur* 246
Albumarc	118	Urology	287	*Amicar*	201	*Androcur Depot* 246
albumin	118	*Alluna*	211	*Amidate*	30	*Androderm* 137
Albuminar	118	*Almora*	150	amifostine	246	*Androgel* 137
albuterol	273, 275	almotriptan	225	*Amigesic*	19	Androgens 137
Alcaine	255	*Alocril*	254	amikacin	32	*Android* 137
alclometasone dipro-		aloe vera	204	*Amikin*	32	androstenedione 204
pionate	129	*Alomide*	254	amiloride	101, 111	*Anectine* 32
alcohol	281	*Alora*	233	aminocaproic acid	201	**ANESTHESIA** 30
Alcomicin	247	alosetron	192	aminoglutethimide	159	*Anexate* 281
Aldactazide	99	*Aloxi*	180	Aminoglycosides	32	*Anexsia* 26
Aldactone		alpha-1 antitrypsin	277	aminohippurate	289	*Angelica sinensis* 206
Cardiovascular	86	alpha-1 proteinase in-		aminolevulinic acid	134	*Angiomax* 198
Endocrine	162	hibitor	277	aminophylline	277	Angiotensin Receptor
Aldara	128	alpha-galactosidase		amiodarone	89	Blockers 86
aldesleukin	246		192	amitriptyline	256, 268	anhydrous glycerins
Aldomet	88	*Alphagan P*	253	amlexanox	175	166
Aldoril	99	alprazolam	267	amlodipine	96,100,108	*Ansaid* 20
Aldosterone Antago-		alprostadil		amoxapine	257	*Antabuse* 269

Anthemis nobilis – Roman chamomile 205
Anthra-Derm 127
Anthraforte 127
anthralin 127
Anthranol 127
Anthrascalp 127
Antiadrenergic agents 87
Antibacterials, topical 123
Antibacterials, ophthalmic 247
Anticoagulants 196
Anticonvulsants 220
Antidepressants 256
Antidiarrheals 178
Antidotes 282
Antidysrhythmics 88
Antiemetics 180
Antifungals, systemic 33
Antifungals, topical 124
Antihistamines, systemic 162
Antihistamines, ophthalmic 249
Antihyperlipidemics 93
Antihypertensives 99
Antilirium 282
Antimalarials 36
Antimanic agents 261
ANTIMICROBIALS 32
Antiminth 44
Antimycobacterials 40
Antiparasitics, systemic 42
Antiparasitics, topical 126
Antiplatelet drugs 104
Antipsoriatics 127
Antipsychotics 262
antipyrine 165
Antirheumatics 12
Antispas 186
Antitussives 164
Antiulcer 183
antivenin - crotalidae immune Fab ovine polyvalent 216
antivenin - crotalidae polyvalent 216

antivenin - latrodectus mactans 216
Antivert
　Gastroenterology 181
　Neurology 231
Antivirals, systemic 45
Antivirals, topical 128
Antivirals, ophthalmic 249
Antizol 281
Anturane 147
Anusol Hemorrhoidal Ointment 133
Anusol Suppositories 133
Anusol-HC 133
Anxiolytics / Hypnotics 265
Anzemet 180
APGAR score 241
Aphthasol 175
Apidra 145
Aplisol 219
Apo-Gain 136
Apokyn 229
apomorphine 229
apraclonidine 253
aprepitant 180
Apresazide 99
Apresoline 102
Apri 237
Aprodine 167
aprotinin 201
APV 52
Aquachloral Supprettes 267
AquaMephyton 157
Aquasol A 158
Aquatensen 113
Aquazide H 288
AraC 246
Aralast 277
Aralen 37
Aramine 116
Aranesp 201
Arava 13
Aredia 139
argatroban 198
Aricept 219
Arimidex 246
aripiprazole 265
Aristocort

Dermatology 132
Endocrine 141
Aristolochia 204
aristolochic acid 204
Aristospan 141
Arixtra 197
Armour Thyroid 154
arnica 204
Arnica montana 204
Aromasin 246
arsenic trioxide 247
Artane 228
Arthrotec 19
articaine 31
artichoke leaf extract 204
artificial tears 255
ASA (aspirin)
　Analgesics
　　16-18, 26-27
　Cardiovasc 97, 104
　Gastroenterology 183
　Neurology 227, 230
Asacol 193
Asaphen
　Analgesics 18
　Cardiovascular 104
Asarum 204
ascorbic acid 154
Ascriptin 16
Aslera 206
asparaginase 247
A-spaz 284
Aspirin (ASA)
　Analgesics
　　16-18, 26-27
　Cardiovasc 97, 104
　Gastroenterology 183
　Neurology 227, 230
Astelin 176
AsthmaNefrin 279
astragalus 204
Astragalus membranaceus 204
Atacand 86
Atacand HCT 99
Atacand Plus 99
Atamet 229
Atapryl 230
Atarax 164
Atasol 29
atazanavir 52

atenolol 101, 105
Atgam 217
Ativan
　Neurology 223
　Psychiatry 266
atomoxetine 270
Atopic Dermatitis 129
atorvastatin 96
atovaquone 38, 42
atracurium 31
atropine
　Cardiovascular 89
　Gastroenterology 178, 179, 187
　Ophthalmology 254
　Urology 285
Atrovent 279
Atrovent Nasal Spray 177
ATV 52
augmented betamethasone dipropionate 129
Augmentin 71
Augmentin ES-600 71
Augmentin XR 71
Auralgan 165
auranofin 12
Aurolate 12
Avage 123
Avalide 99
Avandamet 141
Avandia 142
Avapro 86
Avastin 246
Avaxim 212
Aveeno 136
Avelox 77
Aventyl 257
Aviane 237
Avinza 25
Avirax 46
Avodart 283
Avonex 227
Axert 225
Axid 184
Axid AR 184
Aygestin 240
azacitidine 246
Azactam 79
Azasan 13
azatadine 163, 174

azathioprine	13	*BayRho-D*		benzoic acid	285	*Bicillin L-A*	68

azathioprine 13
azelaic acid 121, 134
azelastine
  ENT 176
  Ophthalmology 249
Azelex 121
azithromycin 66
Azmacort 276
Azopt 252
Azo-Standard 285
AZT 51
aztreonam 79
Azulfidine
  Analgesics 14
  Gastroenterology 195
Azulfidine EN-tabs
  Analgesics 14
  Gastroenterology 195

B

B&O Supprettes 283
B6 245
B12 245
BabyBIG 216
Bacid 209
Baciguent 123
Bacillus of Calmette &
  Guerin 246
bacitracin
  Dermatol 123, 124
  Ophthalmology 248
baclofen 14
Bacterial pathogens 60
Bactocill 70
Bactrim 78
Bactroban 124
BAL in oil 281
balsalazide 192
banana bag 151
Banophen 267, 273
Baridium 285
barium sulfate 120
basiliximab 218
Bayer
  Analgesics 18
  Cardiovascular 104
Baygam 217
BayHep B 216
BayRab 217

BayRho-D
  Immunology 218
  OB/GYN 246
BayRho-D Mini Dose
  Immunology 218
  OB/GYN 246
BayTet 218
BCG 246
BCG vaccine 211
BCNU 246
B-D Glucose 145
Beano 192
becaplermin 134
beclomethasone
  ENT 177
  Pulmonary 275
Beconase AQ 177
belladonna
  Gastroenterology 186
  Urology 283
Bellergal Spacetabs 186
Bellergal-S 186
Benadryl
  ENT 164, 176
  Psychiatry 273, 267
Benadryl Allergy &
  Cold 167
Benadryl-D Allergy &
  Sinus 167
BenaMist 177
benazepril 83, 100
bendroflumethiazide
  100, 101, 112
BeneFin 210
Benefix 202
Benicar 87
Benicar HCT 99
Benoxyl 121
Bensylate
  Neurology 228
  Psychiatry 272
Bentyl 186
Bentylol 186
Benuryl 146
Benylin 164
Benylin XL 66
BenylinDME 167
Benzac 121
BenzaClin 121
Benzamycin 121
benzathine penicillin
  68, 69
benzocaine 165

benzoic acid 285
benzonatate 164
benzoyl peroxide
  121, 122
benzphetamine 271
benztropine 272
benztropine mesylate
  228
benzylpenicilloyl poly-
  lysine 69
beractant 278
Berotec 273
Beta Agonists 273
Beta blockers 105
Betaderm 130
Betagan 251
Betaloc 107
betamethasone
  Dermatology 133
  Endocrine 139
betamethasone dipro-
  pionate 129
betamethasone so-
  dium phosphate 244
betamethasone valer-
  ate 130
Betapace 93
Betapace AF 93
Betaseron 228
betaxolol
  Cardiovascular 106
  Ophthalmology 251
Betaxon 251
bethanechol 283
Betnesol 139
Betnovate 130
Betoptic S 251
bevacizumab 246
bexarotene 247
Bextra 18
Bexxar 247
bezafibrate 98
Bezalip 98
bicalutamide
  Oncology 246
  Urology 288
bicarbonate
  Cardiovascular 89
  Gastroenterology 183
Bicillin C-R 69

Bicillin L-A 68
Bicitra 288
BiCNU 246
Bifidobacteria 209
bilberry 204
Biltricide 44
bimatoprost 252
Biolean 206
BioRab 215
biotin 156
biperiden 228
bisacodyl 189
bismuth subsalicylate
  178, 186
bisoprolol 101, 106
Bisphosphonates 138
bitter melon 204
bitter orange 205
bivalirudin 198
black cohosh 205
Bladder agents 283
Blenoxane 246
bleomycin 246
Bleph-10 248
Blephamide 249
Blocadren 108
Body mass index 270
Bonamine
  Gastroenterology 181
  Neurology 231
Bonefos 138
Bonine
  Gastroenterology 181
  Neurology 231
Boniva 139
Bontril SR 272
boric acid 242
bortezomib 247
bosentan 102
Botox 134
Botox Cosmetic 134
botulinum toxin 134
botulism immune
  globulin 216
BPH 283
Bragantia 204
Bravelle 239
Brethine
  OB/GYN 241
  Pulmonary 274
bretylium 90
Bretylol 90

Brevibloc	106	*Caelyx*	246	*Capoten*	83	*Cartrol*	106
Brevicon	237	*Cafcit*	278	*Capozide*	99	carvedilol	106
Brevital	30	*Cafergot*	226	capsaicin	134	casanthranol	191
Bricanyl		*Caffedrine*	271	captopril	83, 99	cascara	189
OB/GYN	241	caffeine		*Carac*	123	*Casodex*	
Pulmonary	274	Analgesics 17, 26, 27		Carafate		Oncology	246
brimonidine	253	Neurology 226, 227		ENT	176	Urology	288
brinzolamide	252	Psychiatry	271	Gastroenterology 188		caspofungin	34
bromazepam	266	caffeine citrate	278	carbamazepine		castor oil	189
Bromfenex	170	calamine	134	Neurology	220	*Cataflam*	19
Bromfenex PD	170	*Calan*	110	Psychiatry	261	*Catapres*	
bromocriptine		*Calcibind*	287	carbamide peroxide		Cardiovascular	87
Endocrine	159	*Calciferol*	158		165	OB/GYN	245
Neurology	229	*Calcijex*	154	*Carbapenems*	58	Psychiatry 269, 272
brompheniramine 167,		*Calcimar*	159	*Carbatrol*		*Catapres-TTS*	
168, 170, 171, 174		calcitonin	159	Neurology	220	OB/GYN	245
budesonide		calcitriol	154	Psychiatry	261	Psychiatry 269, 272
ENT	177	calcium acetate	147	*Carbex*	230	*Cathflo*	117
Gastroenterology 192		calcium carbonate		carbidopa 229, 230		*Caverject*	286
Pulmonary	275	Analgesics	16	carbidopa-levodopa		*Caverject Impulse*	286
Bufferin	16	Endocrine	147		229	CCNU	246
bumetanide	111	Gastroenter 183-185		carbinoxamine 170,174		*Ceclor*	60
Bumex	111	OB/GYN	245	*Carbocaine*	31	*Cedax*	64
Buminate	118	Calcium channel		*Carbodec DM*	170	*Cedocard SR*	114
bupivacaine	31	blockers	108	*Carbolith*	261	*CeeNu*	246
Buprenex	22	calcium chloride	147	carboplatin	247	cefaclor	60
buprenorphine		calcium citrate	148	carboprost	241	cefadroxil	59
Analgesics	22	calcium gluconate	148	*Cardene*	109	cefazolin	59
Psychiatry 268, 270		calfactant	278	*Cardene SR*	109	cefdinir	63
Buproban	268	*Calsan*	147	**CARDIAC PROTO-**		cefditoren	63
bupropion 260, 268		*Caltine*	159	**COLS**	303	cefepime	65
Burinex	111	*Caltrate*	147	Cardiac parameters		cefixime	63
burn plant	204	*Camila*	237		115	*Cefizox*	65
BuSpar	267	*Campath*	246	Cardiac protocols	303	*Cefobid*	64
buspirone	267	*Campral*	268	*Cardio-Omega 3*	99	cefoperazone	64
busulfan	246	*Camptosar*	247	**CARDIOVASCULAR**		*Cefotan*	60
Busulfex	246	*Canasa*	193		83	cefotaxime	64
butabarbital	267	*Cancenex*	210	*Cardizem*	109	cefotetan	60
butalbital	17, 26	*Candicas*	34	*Cardizem CD*	109	cefoxitin	60
butenafine	124	*Candistatin*		*Cardizem LA*	109	cefpodoxime	64
Butisol	267	Antimicrobials	36	*Cardizem SR*	109	cefprozil	61
butoconazole	242	Dermatology	125	*Cardura*		ceftazidime	64
butorphanol	22	*Canesten*		Cardiovascular	87	ceftibuten	64
		Antimicrobials	34	Urology	283	*Ceftin*	61
		Dermatology	125	carisoprodol 15, 17, 27		ceftizoxime	65
		OB/GYN	242	carmustine	246	ceftriaxone	65
		Cantil	187	*Carnitor*	152	cefuroxime	61
C.E.S.	233	capecitabine	246	carteolol		*Cefzil*	61
cabergoline	159	*Capital with Codeine*		Cardiovascular	106	*Celebrex*	18
CAD 10-year risk	95	suspension	26	Ophthalmology	251	celecoxib	18
Caduet	96	*Cartia XT*	109	*Celestoderm*	130
				Cartilade	210	*Celestone*	

Endocrine	139	ate	175
OB/GYN	244	chlorodeoxyadenosine	
Celestone Soluspan			246
	139	*Chloromycetin*	80
Celexa	258	chloroquine	37
Cellcept	218	chlorothiazide	112
cellulose sodium phos-		chlorpheniramine	
phate	287	163, 166, 168, 169,	
Celontin	223	170, 172-174	
Cena-K	151	chlorpromazine	265
Cenestin	233	chlorpropamide	143
cephalexin	59	chlorthalidone	
Cephalosporins	59	Cardiovascular	
Cephulac	190	100, 101, 113	
Ceptaz	64	Urology	287
Cerebyx	221	*Chlor-Trimeton*	163
Certain Dri	134	chlorzoxazone	15
Cerubidine	246	cholestyramine	93
Cerumenex	166	choline magnesium tri-	
Cervidil	238	salicylate	19
cetirizine	163, 175	chondroitin	205
cetrorelix acetate	234	choriogonadotropin	
Cetrotide	234	alfa	238
cetuximab	246	chorionic gonadotropin	
cevimeline	175		238
chamomile	205	*Chronovera*	110
chaparral	205	*Chronulac*	190
CharcoAid	280	Chrysanthemum pa-	
charcoal	280	rthenium	207
Charcodate	280	*Cialis*	286
chasteberry	205	ciclopirox	124
Chemet	282	*Cidecin*	80
Chemstrip bG	145	cidofovir	45
Cheracol D Cough	167	cilazapril	84, 100
Chibroxin	248	cilostazol	119
Child immunizations		*Ciloxan*	247
	214	cimetidine	184
Children's Advil Cold		*Cimicifuga racemosa*	
	167		205
Children's NasalCrom		cinacalcet	159
	177	*Cipro*	74
ChiRhoClin	195	*Cipro HC Otic*	165
Chirocaine	31	*Cipro XR*	74
Chlo-Amine	163	*Ciprodex Otic*	165
chloral hydrate	267	ciprofloxacin	
chlorambucil	246	Antimicrobials	74
chloramphenicol	80	ENT	165
chlordiazepoxide		Ophthalmology	247
Gastroenterology	193	cisapride	192
Psychiatry	266, 268	cisatracurium	31
Chlordrine SR	170	cisplatin	247
chlorhexidine glucon-		citalopram	258

Citracal	148	Psychiatry	266
citrate		clonazepam	
Gastroenterology	183	Neurology	221
Urology	288	Psychiatry	266
Citri Lean	207	clonidine	
Citrocarbonate	183	Cardiovasc	87, 100
Citro-Mag	190	OB/GYN	245
Citrucel	190	Psychiatry	269, 272
Citrus aurantium	205	clopidogrel	104
cladribine	246	clorazepate	266
Claforan	64	*Clotrimaderm*	
Clarinex	162	Antimicrobials	34
clarithromycin		Dermatology	125
Antimicrobials	66	OB/GYN	242
Gastroenterology	186	clotrimazole	
Claritin	163	Antimicrobials	34
Claritin Hives Relief	163	Dermatology	125,133
Claritin RediTabs	163	ENT	175
Claritin-D 12 hr	167	OB/GYN	242
Claritin-D 24 hr	167	cloxacillin	70
Clavulin	71	clozapine	262
Clear Eyes	251	*Clozaril*	262
Clearasil	121	coal tar	134
clemastine	163	cobalamin	155
Clenia	121	codeine	
Cleocin		Analgesics	23, 26-28
Antimicrobials	80	ENT	170-174
OB/GYN	242	*Codeprex*	170
Cleocin T	121	coenzyme Q10	205
clidinium	193	*Cogentin*	
Climara	233	Neurology	228
Climara Pro	235	Psychiatry	272
clindamycin		*Cognex*	220
Antimicrobials	80	*Colace*	
Dermatology	121,122	ENT	165
OB/GYN	242	Gastroenterology	190
Clinistix	145	*Colazal*	192
Clinitest	145	*Colbenemid*	146
Clinoril	22	colchicine	146
clobazam	220	colesevelam	94
clobetasol	130	*Colestid*	94
Clobex	130	*Colestid Flavored*	94
clocortolone pivalate		colestipol	94
	130	colistin	165
Cloderm	130	*Colyte*	191
clodronate	138	*Combantrin*	44
clofazimine	40	*CombiPatch*	235
Clomid	238	*Combipres*	100
clomiphene	238	*Combivent*	275
clomipramine	257	*Combivent inhalation*	
Clonapam		*solution*	275
Neurology	221	*Combivir*	49

comfrey 205
Commiphora mukul
  extract 208
Commit 269
Compazine 182
Comtan 228
Comvax 212
Concerta 271
Condyline 128
Condylox 128
cone flower 206
Congest 233
Conray 120
CONTRAST MEDIA
  119
Conversions 9
Copaxone 227
Copegus 58
CoQ-10 205
Cordarone 89
Cordran 130
Cordran SP 130
Coreg 106
Corgard 107
Corlopam 102
Cormax 130
Correctol 189
Cortaid 131
Cortamed 131
Cortate 131
Cortef 140
Corticaine 131
Corticosteroids 129
Corticosteroids 139
Corticosteroids 249
Corticosteroids 141
Cortifoam 131, 133
cortisone 140
Cortisporin
  Dermatology 133
  Ophthalmology 250
Cortisporin Otic 165
Cortisporin TC Otic 165
Cortizone 131
Cortoderm 131
Cortone 140
Cortrosyn 160
Corvert 91
Corynanthe yohimbe
  211
Corzide 100
Cosamin DS 208

Cosmegen 246
Cosopt 253
cosyntropin 160
Cotazym 194
cotrimoxazole 78
Coumadin 199
Covera-HS 110
Coversyl 85
Cozaar 86
Cranactin 205
cranberry 205
Crataegus laevigata
  208
creatine 206
Creon 194
creosote bush 205
Crestor 97
Crixivan 53
CroFab 216
Crolom 253
cromolyn 177
cromolyn sodium
  Ophthalmology 253
  Pulmonary 278
crotamiton 126
Cryselle 237
crystalline DMSO2 209
Cubicin 80
Culturelle 209
Cuprimine 282
Curosurf 279
Cutar 134
Cutivate 131
cyanocobalamin
  155, 156
Cyclessa 237
cyclobenzaprine 15
Cyclocort 129
Cyclogyl 254
Cyclomen 245
cyclopentolate 254
cyclophosphamide 246
cyclosporine
  Immunology 218
  Ophthalmology 255
Cydec Drops 170
Cyklokapron 203
Cylert 272
Cymbalta 260
Cynara scolymus 204
Cynara-SL 204
cyproheptadine 163

cyproterone
  Dermatology 121
  Oncology 246
Cystografin 120
Cystospaz 284
Cytadren 159
cytarabine 246
Cytomel 153
Cytosar-U 246
Cytotec
  Gastroenterology 187
  OB/GYN 238
Cytovene 46
Cytoxan 246

D

D.H.E. 45 226
D2T5 212
d4T 50
dacarbazine 246
daclizumab 218
dactinomycin 246
Dalacin 242
Dalacin C 80
Dalacin T 121
dalfopristin 82
Dalmane 266
dalteparin 196
danazol 245
Danocrine 245
Dantrium 15
dantrolene 15
dapiprazole 255
dapsone 40
Daptacel 212
daptomycin 80
Daraprim 44
darbepoetin 201
Darvocet 26
Darvon Compound
  Pulvules 26
Darvon Pulvules 26
Darvon-N 26
daunorubicin 246
DaunoXome 246
Daypro 21
Daypro Alta 21
d-biotin 155
DDAVP

Endocrine 160
  Hematology 201
  Urology 284
ddC 51
ddI 49
Debacterol 175
Debrox 165
Decadron
  Endocrine 140
  Neurology 230
  OB/GYN 245
  Pulmonary 278
Deca-Durabolin 137
Declomycin 160
Deconamine 170
Decongestants 164
Decongestants 251
Deconsal II 170
Defen-LA 170
deferoxamine 281
dehydroepiandroster-
  one 206
Delatestryl 137
delavirdine 48
Delestrogen 233
Delsym 164
Delta-Cortef 140
Deltasone 140
Demadex 111
demeclocycline 160
Demerol 24
Demser 103
Demulen 1/35 237
Demulen 1/50 237
Denavir
  Dermatology 128
  ENT 176
denileukin 246
Depacon 224
Depade 269
Depakene
  Neurology 224, 227
  Psychiatry 262
Depakote
  Neurology 224, 227
  Psychiatry 262
Depakote ER
  Neurology 224, 227
  Psychiatry 262
Depen 282
Depo-Cyt 246
DepoDur 25

Depo-Estradiol	233
Depo-Medrol	
Endocrine	140
Neurology	231
Depo-Provera	
OB/GYN	239
Oncology	246
Depotest	137
Depo-Testosterone	137
Deproic	
Neurology	224, 227
Psychiatry	262
Derma-Smooth-FS	130
Dermasone	130
DERMATOLOGY	120
Dermatomes	225
Dermatop	132
Dermazin	124
Dermolate	131
Dermovate	130
deserpidine	100
Desferal	281
desipramine	257
desloratadine	162
desmopressin	
Endocrine	160
Hematology	201
Urology	284
Desocort	130
Desogen	237
desogestrel	237
desonide	130
DesOwen	130
desoximetasone	130
Desquam	121
Desyrel	261
Detrol	285
Detrol LA	285
Detussin	171
dexamethasone	
Endocrine	140
ENT	165
Neurology	230
OB/GYN	245
Ophthalmology	250
Pulmonary	278
Dexasone	
Endocrine	140
Neurology	230
Dexatrim Natural Ephedrine Free	205
dexbrompheniramine	
	168
dexchlorpheniramine	
	163
Dexedrine	271
DexFerrum	149
Dexiron	149
dexmedetomidine	30
dexmethylphenidate	
	271
Dexone	140
dexrazoxane	246
dextran	118
dextroamphetamine	
	270, 271
dextromethorphan	
	164, 167-174
dextrose	145
Dextrostat	271
Dextrostix	145
DHEA	206
DHPG	46
DHT	155
DiaBeta	144
Diabetes numbers	143
Diabetes-Related	141
Diabinese	144
Diamicron	144
Diamicron MR	144
Diamox	
Cardiovascular	110
Ophthalmology	252
Diane-35	121
Diarr-eze	179
Diascan	145
Diastat	
Analgesics	15
Neurology	221
Diastix	145
diatrizoate	120
Diatx	155
diazepam	
Analgesics	15
Neurology	221
Psychiatry	266
diazoxide	
Cardiovascular	102
Endocrine	145
Dibenzyline	103
dibucaine	133
Dicetel	195
dichloralphenazone	227
Diclectin	180
diclofenac	
Analgesics	19
Dermatology	123
Ophthalmology	255
dicloxacillin	70
dicyclomine	186
didanosine	49
Didrex	271
Didronel	138
diethylpropion	271
difenoxin	179
Differin	120
diflorasone	130
Diflucan	
Antimicrobials	34
OB/GYN	245
diflunisal	19
Digibind	90
Digifab	90
digitalis	90
Digitek	90
digoxin	90
digoxin immune Fab	90
dihydrocodeine	27
dihydroergotamine	226
dihydrotachysterol	155
diiodohydroxyquin	43
Dilacor XR	109
Dilantin	223
Dilatrate-SR	114
Dilaudid	24
Dilaudid-5	24
Diltia XT	109
diltiazem	109
Diltiazem CD	109
dimenhydrinate	181
dimercaprol	281
Dimetane-DX Cough Syrup	171
Dimetapp Cold & Allergy	167
Dimetapp Decongestant Infant Drops	165
Dimetapp Decongestant Plus Cough Infant Drops	167
Dimetapp DM Cold & Cough	167
Dimetapp Multisymptom Cold & Allergy	168
Dimetapp Nighttime	
Flu	168
Dimetapp Non-Drowsy Flu	168
dimethyl sulfone	209
dimethyl sulfoxide	284
dinoprostone	238
Diocarpine	253
Diodoquin	43
Diogent	247
Diopred	251
Dioscorea villosa	211
Diovan	87
Diovan HCT	100
Dipentum	194
Diphen	267, 273
Diphenhist	267, 273
diphenhydramine	
ENT	164, 167
Psychiatry	267, 273
diphenoxylate	178
diphtheria tetanus & acellular pertussis vaccine	212
diphtheria-tetanus toxoid	212
dipivefrin	253
Diprivan	31
Diprolene	129
Diprolene AF	129
Diprosone	129
dipyridamole	
Cardiovascular	104
Neurology	230
dirithromycin	67
Disalcid	19
DisperMox	70
disopyramide	90
disulfiram	269
Ditropan	285
Ditropan XL	285
Diuretics	110
Diuril	112
Diutensen-R	100
divalproex	
Neurology	224
Psychiatry	262
Dixirit	245
DLV	48
DMSO	284
dobutamine	115
Dobutrex	115
docetaxel	247

docosanol
  Dermatology 128
  ENT 175
docusate 191, 192
docusate calcium 190
docusate sodium
  ENT 165
  Gastroenterology 190
dofetilide 90
dolasetron 180
Dolobid 19
Dolophine
  Analgesics 24
  Psychiatry 269
Domeboro Otic 165
domperidone 193
Dona 208
donepezil 219
dong quai 206
Donnatal 187
Donnazyme 194
dopamine 115
Dopram 278
dornase alfa 278
Doryx
  Antimicrobials 37, 78
  Dermatology 121
dorzolamide 252, 253
Dostinex 159
Dovonex 127
doxacurium 31
doxapram 278
doxazosin
  Cardiovascular 87
  Urology 283
doxepin
  Dermatology 134
  Psychiatry 257
doxercalciferol 155
Doxil 246
doxorubicin liposomal 246
doxorubicin non-lipo-
  somal 246
Doxycin
  Antimicrobials 37, 78
  Dermatology 121
doxycycline
  Antimicrobials 37, 78
  Dermatology 121
  ENT 175
doxylamine

Analgesics 27
Gastroenter 180, 181
Dramamine 181
Drisdol 158
Dristan 12 Hr Nasal 177
Drithocreme 127
Drixoral Cold & Allergy 168
Drixoral Cold & Flu 168
dronabinol 181
droperidol 181
drospirenone 237
drotrecogin 80
Droxia 246
Drug dependence 268
Drug therapy web
  sites 10
Drugs in pregnancy 235
Dry Eyes 255
Drysol 134
Dryvax 215
DT 212
DTaP 212, 213, 215
DTIC-Dome 246
Duac 122
Dulcolax 189
duloxetine 260
Duolube 255
DuoNeb 275
Duragesic 24
Duralith 261
Duratuss 171
Duratuss GP 171
Duratuss HD 171
Duricef 59
dutasteride 283
Duvoid 283
Dyazide 100
Dynabac 67
Dynacin 79
DynaCirc 109
DynaCirc CR 109
Dynapen 70
Dyrenium 112

E

E Pam
  Analgesics 15
  Neurology 221

Psychiatry 266
E. angustifolia 206
E. pallida 206
E. purpurea 206
Ear preparations 165
echinacea 206
Echinacin Madaus 206
EchinaGuard 206
EC-Naprosyn 21
econazole 125
Econopred 251
Econopred Plus 251
Ecostatin 125
Ecotrin
  Analgesics 18
  Cardiovascular 104
Ectosone 130
ED Spaz 284
Edecrin 111
edetate 281
Edex 286
edrophonium 231
EDTA 281
EES 68
efalizumab 128
efavirenz 48
Effer-K 151
Effexor 261
Effexor XR 261
Efidac/24 165
eflornithine 135
Efudex 123
EFV 48
EGb 761 207
Egozinc-HC 133
ELA-Max 135
Elavil 256
Eldepryl 230
elderberry 206
Eldopaque 135
Eldoquin 135
Eldoquin Forte 135
Electropeg 191
eletriptan 225
Elidel 129
Eligard
  Oncology 246
  Urology 288
Elimite 126
Elitek 146
Elixophyllin 279

Ellence 246
Elmiron 285
Elocom 131
Elocon 131
Eloxatin 247
Elspar 247
Eltroxin 152
Emadine 249
Emcyt 246
emedastine 249
Emend 180
Emergency contracep-
  tion 236
**EMERGENCY
DRUGS** 302
Emetrol 182
EMLA 135
Emo-Cort 131
Empirin 104
Empirin with Codeine 26
Empracet 28
Emtec 28
emtricitabine 50, 51
Emtriva 50
E-mycin 67
enalapril 84, 100, 101
enalaprilat 84
Enbrel 12
Endantadine
  Antimicrobials 55
  Neurology 229
Endocodone 25
**ENDOCRINE/META-
BOLIC** 137
Endrate 281
Enduron 113
Enduronyl 100
Enemol 192
Enfamil 152
enfuvirtide 47
Engerix-B 212
Enjuvia 234
Enlon 231
enoxacin 75
enoxaparin 196
Enpresse 237
ENT 162
ENT combinations 166
entacapone 228, 230
Entex LA 171
Entex Liquid 171

Entex PSE	171	ertapenem	58
Entocort EC	192	*Erybid*	67
Entozyme	194	*Eryc*	67
Entrophen		*Erycette*	122
Analgesics	18	*Eryderm*	122
Cardiovascular	104	*Erygel*	122
ephedra	206	*Eryped*	68
Ephedra sinica	206	*Erysol*	122
ephedrine	115	*Ery-Tab*	67
Epiject		*Erythrocin IV*	68
Neurology	224, 227	*Erythromid*	67
Psychiatry	262	erythromycin	
epinastine	249	Dermatology	121,122
epinephrine		Ophthalmology	248
Cardiovasc	91, 116	erythromycin base	67
Pulmonary	278	erythromycin estolate	
epinephrine racemic			67
	279	erythromycin ethyl	
EpiPen		succinate	68, 77
Cardiovascular	91	erythromycin lacto-	
Pulmonary	278	bionate	68
EpiPen Jr		erythropoietin	202
Cardiovascular	91	escitalopram	258
Pulmonary	278	*Esclim*	233
EpiQuin Micro	135	*Esgic Plus*	17
epirubicin	246	*Esidrix*	288
Epitol		*Eskalith*	261
Neurology	220	*Eskalith CR*	261
Psychiatry	261	esmolol	106
Epival		esomeprazole	188
Neurology	224, 227	*Esoterica*	135
Psychiatry	262	*Estalis*	235
Epivir	50	estazolam	266
Epivir-HBV	50	esterified estrogens	
eplerenone	85		232, 236
epoetin	202	*Estrace*	232, 243
Epogen	202	*Estraderm*	233
epoprostenol	102	estradiol	232, 235-237
Eprex	202	estradiol acetate vagi-	
eprosartan	86, 101	nal ring	242
eptifibatide	105	estradiol cypionate	233
Epzicom	50	estradiol gel	233
Equalactin	191	estradiol topical emul-	
Erbitux	246	sion	233
Erectile dysfunction	286	estradiol transdermal	
Ergamisol	247	system	233
ergocalciferol	158	estradiol vaginal ring	
ergotamine			243
Gastroenterology	186	estradiol vaginal tab	
Neurology	226		243
Errin	237	estradiol valerate	233
Ertaczo	126	*Estradot*	233
estramustine	246	*Excedrin Migraine*	
Estrasorb	233	Analgesics	17
Estratest	236	Neurology	227
Estratest H.S.	236	*Exelon*	220
Estring	243	exemestane	246
Estrogel	233	*Ex-Lax*	191
estrogen cream	243	*Exsel*	136
Estrogens	232	*EZ-Char*	280
estrogens conjugated		ezetimibe	98
	233, 236	*Ezetrol*	98
estrogens synthetic		*Ezide*	288
conjugated A	233		
estrogens synthetic			
conjugated B	234		
estropipate	234		
Estrostep Fe OB/GYN	237		
etanercept	12	*Fabrazyme*	158
ethacrynic acid	111	*Factive*	77
ethambutol	40	factor VIIa	202
ethanol	281	factor VIII	202
ethinyl estradiol		factor IX	202
Dermatology	121	famciclovir	47
OB/GYN	236, 237,	famotidine	184, 185
	244-246	*Famvir*	47
Ethmozine	92	*Fansidar*	38
ethosuximide	221	*Fareston*	246
ethynodiol	237	*Faslodex*	246
Ethyol	246	fat emulsion	151
etidronate	138	*FazaClo ODT*	262
etodolac	20	*Feen-a-Mint*	189
etomidate	30	felbamate	221
etonogestrel	244	*Felbatol*	221
Etopophos	247	*Feldene*	22
etoposide	247	felodipine	100, 109
Euflex		*Femapron*	205
Oncology	246	*Femara*	246
Urology	288	*FemHRT*	236
Euglucon	144	*Femizol-M*	243
Eulexin		*FemPatch*	233
Oncology	246	*Femring*	242
Urology	288	*Fenesin DM*	171
Eurax	126	fenofibrate	98
evening primrose oil		fenoldopam	102
	206	fenoprofen	20
Everone	137	fenoterol	273
Evista		fentanyl	
Endocrine	161	Analgesics	24
OB/GYN	240	Anesthesia	30
Evoxac	175	fentanyl transdermal	24
Evra	245	fenugreek	206
Exanta	199	*FeoSol Tabs*	148
		Fergon	148

F

Fer-in-Sol 148
Ferodan 148
Fero-Grad 148
Ferrlecit 151
ferrous gluconate 148
ferrous sulfate 148
Fertinex 239
feverfew 207
Fexicam 22
fexofenadine 163, 169
Fiberall 191
FiberCon 191
Fidelin 206
filgrastim 203
Finacea 121, 134
finasteride
　Dermatology 135
　Urology 283
Finevin 121
Fioricet 17
Fioricet with Codeine 26
Fiorinal 17
Fiorinal C-1/2 26
Fiorinal C-1/4 26
Fiorinal with Codeine 26
fish oil 99
FK 506 219
Flagyl
　Antimicrobials 43, 81
　OB/GYN 243
Flamazine 124
Flarex 250
flavoxate 284
Flebogamma 217
flecainide 91
Fleet enema 192
Fleet Flavored Castor Oil 189
Fleet Mineral Oil Enema 190
Fleet Pain Relief 133
Fleet Phospho-Soda 192
Fletcher's Castoria 191
Flexeril 15
Flexium 210
Flextend 208
floctafenine 20
Flolan 102
Flomax 283

Flonase 177
Florazole ER 43, 81
Florinef 140
Florone 130
Flovent 276
Flovent Rotadisk 276
Floxin 75
Floxin Otic 166
floxuridine 246
fluconazole
　Antimicrobials 34
　OB/GYN 245
flucytosine 35
Fludara 246
fludarabine 246
fludrocortisone 140
Flumadine 55
flumazenil 281
FluMist 213
flunarizine 227
flunisolide
　ENT 177
　Pulmonary 276
fluocinolone 130, 136
fluocinonide 130
Fluoderm 130
Fluor-A-Day 149
fluoride 149
Fluoride dose 149
fluorometholone 250
Fluor-Op 250
Fluoroplex 123
fluorouracil
　Dermatology 123
　Oncology 246
Fluotic 149
fluoxetine 258, 268
fluoxymesterone 137
fluphenazine 264
flurandrenolide 130
flurazepam 266
flurbiprofen
　Analgesics 20
　Ophthalmology 255
flutamide
　Oncology 246
　Urology 288
fluticasone
　ENT 177
　Pulmonary 274, 276
fluticasone propionate 131

fluvastatin 97
Fluviral 213
Fluvirin 213
fluvoxamine 259
Fluzone 213
FML 250
FML Forte 250
FML-S Liquifilm 250
Focalin 271
folate 155
folic acid
　Endocrine 155, 156
　OB/GYN 245
folinic acid 247
follintropin alpha 238
follintropin beta 239
Follistim 239
Follistim AQ 239
Follistim-Antagon Kit 234
Foltx 156
Folvite 155
fomepizole 281
fomivirsen 249
fondaparinux 197
Foradil 273
formoterol 273, 275
Formulas 10
formulas - infant 152
Fortamet 142
Fortaz 64
Forteo 162
Fortovase 54
Fosamax 138
fosamprenavir 53
foscarnet 45
Foscavir 45
fosfomycin 80
fosinopril 84, 101
fosphenytoin 221
Fragmin 196
French maritime pine tree bark 209
Frisium 220
Froben 20
Froben SR 20
Frosst 222 AF 29
Frosst 292 26
Frosst 692 26
Frova 226
frovatriptan 226
FSH 238, 239

FSH/LH 239
FTC 50
FTV 54
Fucidin 123
Fucidin H 133
Fucithalmic 248
FUDR 246
fulvestrant 246
Fungizone 33
Furadantin 82
furosemide 111
fusidic acid
　Dermatology 123,133
　Ophthalmology 248
Fuzeon 47

G

G115 207
gabapentin 222
Gabitril 224
gadodiamide 119
gadopentetate 119
galantamine 219
Gamimune 217
gamma hydroxybutyrate 232
Gammagard 217
Gammar 217
Gamunex 217
ganciclovir 46
ganirelix 234
Gani-Tuss NR 171
Gantrisin 78
Garamycin
　Antimicrobials 32
　Dermatology 123
　Ophthalmology 247
garcinia 207
Garcinia cambogia 207
garlic supplements 207
Gastrocrom 278
GASTROENTEROLOGY 178
Gastrografin 120
Gas-X 188
gatifloxacin
　Antimicrobials 76
　Ophthalmology 247
Gaviscon 183

G-CSF	203	Glucovance	142
gefitinib	247	GlucoWatch	145
Gelclair	175	Glutose	145
gemcitabine	246	glyburide	142, 144
gemfibrozil	98	glycerin	190
gemifloxacin	77	GlycoLax	191
gemtuzumab	246	glycopyrrolate	193
Gemzar	246	Glycyrrhiza glabra	209
Gengraf	218	Glycyrrhiza uralensis	209
Genisoy	211	Glynase PresTab	144
Genoptic	247	Glysennid	191
Genotropin	160	Glyset	141
Gentak	247	GM-CSF	203
gentamicin		GnRH Agonists	234
Antimicrobials	32	gold sodium thioma-	
Dermatology	123	late	12
Ophthal	247, 250	goldenseal	208
GenTeal	255	GoLytely	191
Gentran	118	gonadotropins	239
Genxene	266	Gonal-F	238
Geodon	263	Gonal-F RFF Pen	238
GHB	232	Goody's Extra	
GI cocktail	187	Strength Headache	
ginger	207	Powder	17
ginkgo biloba	207	goserelin	
Ginkgold	207	OB/GYN	234
Ginkoba	207	Oncology	246
Ginsai	207	Urology	288
Ginsana	207	Gout-Related	146
ginseng - American	207	gramicidin	248
ginseng - Asian	207	granisetron	180
Glasgow coma scale		grapeseed extract	208
	220	Gravol	181
glatiramer	227	"green goddess"	187
Glaucoma	251	Grisactin 500	35
Gleevec	246	griseofulvin	35
Gliadel	246	griseofulvin ultrami-	
gliclazide	144	crosize	35
glimepiride	144	Gris-PEG	35
glipizide	142, 144	growth hormone hu-	
GlucaGen	145	man	160
Glucometer	145	guaiacolsulfonate	172
Gluconorm	143	guaifenesin	
Glucophage	142	164, 167-173, 175	
Glucophage XR	142	Guaifenex DM	171
glucosamine	208	Guaifenex PSE	171
glucose home testing		Guaitex II SR/PSE	172
	145	guanabenz	87
Glucostix	145	guanfacine	
Glucotrol	144	Cardiovascular	88
Glucotrol XL	144	Psychiatry	273
guggul	208		215
guggulipid	208	hepatitis A vaccine	212
Guiatuss	164	hepatitis B immune	
Guiatuss AC	172	globulin	216
Guiatuss PE	168	hepatitis B recombi-	
Guiatussin DAC	172	nant vaccines	215
Gynazole	242	hepatitis B vaccine	212
Gyne-Lotrimin	242	Hepsera	56
Gynodiol	232	Heptovir	50
		HERBAL & ALTER-	
		NATIVE	204
		Herceptin	247
H		Hespan	118
		hetastarch	118
H pylori treatment	186	Hexabrix	120
Habitrol	270	Hexadrol	140
haemophilus b vaccine		Hexalen	246
	212	Hextend	118
halcinonide	131	HibTITER	212
Halcion	267	Hiprex	81
Haldol	264	Histinex HC	172
HalfLytely and Bisaco-		Histussin D	172
dyl Tablet Kit	191	Histussin HC	172
Halfprin	104	Hivid	51
halobetasol propionate	131	homatropine	
Halog	131	ENT	173
haloperidol	264	Ophthalmology	254
Halotestin	137	Hormone replacement	
Halotussin AC	172		235
Halotussin DAC	172	horse chestnut seed	
Havrix	212	extract	208
hawthorn	208	Hp-Pac	186
H-BIG	216	HTN risk stratification	
HCE50	208		112
hCG	238	huang qi	204
HCTZ		huckleberry	204
Cardiovascular	113	Humalog	145
Urology	288	Humatin	44
Healthy Woman	211	Humatrope	160
HeartCare	208	Humibid DM	172
Hectorol	155	Humibid LA	172
Helidac	186	Humira	12
Helixate	202	Humulin	145
Hemabate	241	Hyalgan	29
HEMATOLOGY	196	hyaluronate	29
Hemcort HC	133	hyaluronic acid	135
Hemofil M	202	Hycamtin	247
Hemorrhoid care	133	Hycodan	173
Hepalean	197	Hycort	131
heparin	197	Hycotuss	173
Heparin dosing	198	Hyderm	131
hepatitis A inactivated		hydralazine	

99, 101, 102
HydraSense   178
Hydrastis canadensis
208
Hydrea   246
hydrochlorothiazide
Cardiovascular
99-101, 113, 114
Urology   288
Hydrocil   191
hydrocodone
Analgesics   26-28
ENT   171-175
hydrocortisone
Dermatology
131, 133, 136
Endocrine   140
ENT   165, 166
Ophthalmology   154
hydrocortisone acetate
131
hydrocortisone buty-
rate   131
hydrocortisone probu-
tate   131
hydrocortisone valer-
ate   131
Hydrocortone   140
Hydrocot   288
HydroDIURIL   288
Hydromorph Contin   24
hydromorphone   24
hydroquinone   135, 136
Hydroval   131
hydroxychloroquine   13
hydroxyprogesterone
caproate   239
hydroxyurea   246
hydroxyzine   164
Hygroton   287
hylan GF-20   29
hyoscyamine
Gastroenterology   187
Urology   284, 285
Hyosol   284
Hyospaz   284
Hypaque   120
Hypericum perforatum
210
Hyperstat   102
Hypotears   255
Hytakerol   155

Hytrin
Cardiovascular   88
Urology   283
Hytuss   164
Hyzaar   100

I

ibandronate   139
ibritumomab   246
ibuprofen
Analgesics   20, 28
ENT   167
ibutilide   91
Idamycin   246
Idarac   20
idarubicin   246
IDV   53
Ifex   246
ifosfamide   246
Ilotycin   248
Imagent   120
imatinib   246
Imdur   114
imipenem-cilastatin   58
imipramine
Psychiatry   257
Urology   284
imiquimod   128
Imitrex   226
immune globulin - in-
tramuscular   217
immune globulin - in-
travenous   217
Immunine VH   202
IMMUNIZATIONS   211
Immunizations   211
Immunoglobulins   216
Immunosuppression
218
Imodium   179
Imodium AD   179
Imodium Advanced 178
Imogam   217
Imovane   268
Imovax Rabies   215
Imuran   13
inamrinone   116
indapamide   113

Inderal   108
Inderal LA   108
Inderide   100
INDEX   289
indinavir   53
Indocid
Analgesics   20
Cardiovascular   119
OB/GYN   240
Indocin
Analgesics   20
OB/GYN   240
Indocin IV   119
Indocin SR   20
indomethacin
Analgesics   20
Cardiovascular   119
OB/GYN   240
Infanrix   212
Infasurf   278
InFed   149
Infergen   56
Inflamase   251
Inflamase Forte   251
infliximab
Analgesics   13
Gastroenterology 193
influenza vaccine   213
Infufer   149
INH   40
Inhaled Steroids
275, 276
Inhaler colors   274
Inhibace   84
Inhibace Plus   100
Innohep   198
InnoPran XL   108
INOmax   279
Inspra   85
Insta-Glucose   145
INSTRUCTIONS   3
insulin   144, 145
Intal   278
Integrilin   105
interferon alfa-2a   246
interferon alfa-2b
Antimicrobials   56, 57
Oncology   246
interferon alfacon-1   56
interferon alfa-n3   246
interferon beta-1A   227
interferon beta-1B   228

interleukin-2   246
IntestiFlora   209
Intralipid   151
Intron A
Antimicrobials   56
Oncology   246
Intropin   115
Invanz   58
Inversine   103
Invirase   54
iodine   153
iodixanol   120
iodoquinol   43
Iodotope   153
iohexol   120
Ionamin   272
iopamidol   120
Iopidine   253
iothalamate   120
ioversol   120
ioxaglate   120
ipecac syrup   281
IPOL   214
ipratropium
ENT   177
Pulmonary   275, 279
Iquix   247
irbesartan   86, 99
Iressa   247
irinotecan   247
iron dextran   149
iron polysaccharide 149
iron sucrose   149
ISMO   114
isocarboxazid   258
isometheptene   227
Isomil   152
isoniazid   40-42
isopropyl alcohol   166
isoproterenol   91
Isoptin   110
Isopto Atropine   254
Isopto Carpine   253
Isopto Cetamide   248
Isopto Homatropine
254
Isordil   114
isosorbide dinitrate 114
isosorbide mononitrate
114
Isotamine   40
isotretinoin   122

Isotrex	122	Kemadrin	228	Ku-Zyme	194	Lectopam	266
Isovue	120	Kenalog		Ku-Zyme HP	194	leflunomide	13
isoxsuprine	119	Dermatology	132	K-vescent	151	Legalon	209
isradipine	109	Endocrine	141	Kwai	207	Lenoltec	28
Istalol	252	Kenalog in Orabase		Kwellada	126	leopard's bane	204
Isuprel	91		176	Kwellada-P	126	lepirudin	199
itraconazole	35	Keppra	223	Kyolic	207	Lescol	97
IV solutions	147	Kerlone	106	Kytril	180	Lescol XL	97
Iveegam	217	Ketalar	30			Lessina	237
ivermectin	43	ketamine	30			letrozole	246
		Ketek	66	**L**		leucovorin	247
J		ketoconazole				Leukeran	246
		Antimicrobials	36	labetalol	107	Leukine	203
		Dermatology	125	Labor induction	238	Leukotriene inhibitors	
Jantoven	199	Ketoderm	125	Lac-Hydrin	135		277
Japanese encephalitis		Ketolides	66	Lacrilube	255	leuprolide	
vaccine	213	ketoprofen	20	Lactaid	193	OB/GYN	234
JE-Vax	213	ketorolac		lactase	193	Oncology	246
Jolivette	237	Analgesics	21	lactic acid	135	Urology	288
Junel 1.5/30	237	Ophthalmology	255	Lactinex	209	Leupron	246
Junel 1.5/30 Fe	237	ketotifen		Lactobacillus	209	Leustatin	246
Junel 1/20	237	Ophthalmology	254	lactulose	190	levalbuterol	274
Junel Fe 1/20	237	Pulmonary	279	Lamictal		levamisole	247
		K-G Elixir	151	Neurology	222	Levaquin	76
K		Kidrolase	247	Psychiatry	261	Levatol	108
		Kineret	12	Lamictal CD		Levbid	284
		Kira	210	Neurology	222	levetiracetam	223
K+10	151	Klaron	122	Psychiatry	261	Levitra	286
K+8	151	Klean-Prep	191	Lamisil		Levlen	237
K+Care	151	K-Lease	151	Antimicrobials	36	Levlite	237
K+Care ET	151	Klonopin		Dermatology	126	levobetaxolol	251
Kabikinase	117	Neurology	221	Lamisil AT	126	levobunolol	251
Kadian	25	Psychiatry	266	lamivudine	49-51	levobupivacaine	31
Kala	209	K-Lor	151	lamotrigine		levocabastine	
Kaletra	54	Klor-con	151	Neurology	222	ENT	177
Kaochlor	151	Klorvess	151	Psychiatry	261	Ophthalmology	249
Kaon	151	Klorvess Effervescent		Lamprene	40	levocarnitine	152
Kaon Cl	151		151	Lanoxicaps	90	levodopa	230
Kaopectate	178	Klotrix	151	Lanoxin	90	Levo-Dromoran	24
karela	204	K-Lyte	151	lansoprazole	186, 188	levofloxacin	
Kariva	237	K-Lyte Cl	151	Lansoyl	190	Antimicrobials	76
kava	208	K-Norm	151	Lantus	145	Ophthalmology	247
Kay Ciel	151	Kolyum	151	Lanvis	246	levonorgestrel	
Kayexalate	162	kombucha tea	208	Largactil	265		235, 245, 246
Kaylixir	151	Kondremul	190	Lariam	38	levonorgestrel	237
K-Dur	151	Konsyl	191	laronidase	161	Levophed	116
Keflex	59	Konsyl Fiber	191	Larrea divaricata	205	Levora	237
Keftab	59	Korean red ginseng		Lasix	111	levorphanol	24
Kefurox	61		207	latanoprost	252	Levo-T	152
Kefzol	59	K-Phos	150	Laxatives	189	Levothroid	152
		Kristalose	190	LDL goals	94	levothyroxine	152, 154
		K-Tab	151			Levoxyl	152

Levsin	
Gastroenterology	187
Urology	284
Levsinex	284
Levulan Kerastick	134
Lexapro	258
Lexiva	53
Lexxel	100
LI-160	210
Librax	193
Librium	266
licorice	209
Lidemol	130
Lidex	130
Lidex-E	130
lidocaine	
Analgesics	29
Anesthesia	31
Cardiovascular	91
Dermatology	135
lidocaine viscous	175
Lidoderm	
Analgesics	29
Dermatology	135
Limbitrol	268
Lincocin	81
lincomycin	81
lindane	126
linezolid	81
Lioresal	14
liothyronine	153, 154
Lipidil Micro	98
Lipidil Supra	98
Lipitor	96
Liposyn	151
lisinopril	84, 101
Lithane	261
lithium	261
Lithobid	261
Lithostat	287
LiveBac	209
Livostin	249
Livostin Nasal Spray	
	177
Lo/Ovral	237
Local anesthetics	31
LoCHOLEST	93
LoCHOLEST Light	93
Locoid	131
Lodine	20
Lodine XL	20
Lodosyn	229

Iodoxamide	254
Loestrin 21 1.5/30	237
Loestrin 21 1/20	237
Loestrin Fe 1.5/30	237
Loestrin Fe 1/20	237
Lofibra	98
lomefloxacin	75
Lomotil	178
lomustine	246
Loniten	103
Loperacap	179
loperamide	178
Lopid	98
lopinavir-ritonavir	54
Lopressor	107
Lopressor HCT	100
Loprox	124
Lorabid	61
loracarbef	61
loratadine	163,166,167
lorazepam	
Neurology	223
Psychiatry	266
Lorcet	26
Lortab	27
losartan	86, 100
Losec	188
Lotemax	250
Lotensin	83
Lotensin HCT	100
loteprednol	250
Lotrel	100
Lotriderm	133
Lotrimin	125
Lotrimin Ultra	124
Lotrisone	133
Lotronex	192
lovastatin	96, 97
Lovenox	196
Low-Ogestrel	237
Loxapac	265
loxapine	265
Loxitane	265
Lozide	113
Lozol	113
LPV/r	54
L-thyroxine	152
Ludiomil	257
Lugol's Solution	153
Lumbosacral spine	219
Lumigan	252
Luminal	223

Lupron	
OB/GYN	234
Urology	288
Lupron Depot	
OB/GYN	234
Urology	288
Luride	149
Lustra	135
Luxiq foam	130
Lyderm	130
lymphocyte immune	
globulin human	217
Lysodren	247
Lyteprep	191

M

M.O.S.	25
ma huang	206
Maalox	183
Macrobid	82
Macrodantin	82
Macrodex	118
Macrolides	66
mafenide	123
Mag-200	150
magaldrate	184
Maganate	150
magic mouthwash	176
Maglucate	150
magnesium carbonate	
Analgesics	16
Gastroenterol	183
magnesium chloride	
	150
magnesium citrate	190
magnesium gluconate	
	150
magnesium hydroxide	
Analgesics	16
Gastroenterology	
	183-185, 190
magnesium oxide	
Analgesics	16
Endocrine	150
magnesium sulfate	
Endocrine	150
OB/GYN	241
Magnevist	119
Mag-Ox 400	150

Magtrate	150
Malarone	38
malathion	126
maltodextrin	175
Manchurian or Kar-	
gasok tea	208
Mandelamine	81
Manerix	260
mannitol	231
Mantoux	219
maprotiline	257
Marcaine	31
Marine Lipid Concen-	
trate	99
Marinol	181
Marplan	258
Mast cell stabilizers	253
Matricaria recutita –	
German chamomile	
	205
Matulane	246
Mavik	85
MAX EPA	
Cardiovascular	99
Endocrine	152
Maxair	274
Maxalt	226
Maxalt MLT	226
Maxaquin	75
Maxeran	181
Maxidone	27
Maxiflor	130
Maximum Strength	
Pepcid AC	184
Maxipime	65
Maxitrol	250
Maxivate	129
Maxzide	100
Maxzide-25	100
MD-Gastroview	120
measles mumps & ru-	
bella vaccine	213
mebendazole	43
mecamylamine	103
mechlorethamine	246
Meclicot	
Gastroenterol	181
Neurology	231
meclizine	
Gastroenterol	181
Neurology	231
meclofenamate	21

Medispaz	284	Oncology	246	
Medivert		Meridia		
Gastroenterol	181	Gastroenterol	195	
Neurology	231	Psychiatry	272	
Medrol		Meritate	281	
Endocrine	140	meropenem	59	
Neurology	231	Merrem IV	59	
medroxyprogesterone		Mersyndol with Co-		
OB/GYN	236, 239	deine	27	
Oncology	246	mesalamine	193	
medroxyprogesterone		Mesasal	193	
- injectable	239	M-Eslon	25	
mefloquine	38	mesna	246	
Mefoxin	60	Mesnex	246	
Megace		Mestinon	232	
OB/GYN	240	mestranol	237	
Oncology	246	Metabolife 356	206	
Megacillin	68	Metadate CD	271	
megestrol		Metadate ER	271	
OB/GYN	240	Metadol		
Oncology	246	Analgesics	24	
melaleuca oil	211	Psychiatry	269	
Melanex	135	Metaglip	142	
melatonin	209	Metamucil	191	
Melfiat	272	Metaprel	274	
Mellaril	265	metaproterenol	274	
meloxicam	21	metaraminol	116	
melphalan	246	Metastron	247	
memantine	220	metaxalone	16	
Menest	232	metformin	141, 142	
Meni-D		methacholine	279	
Gastroenterol	181	methadone		
Neurology	231	Analgesics	24	
meningococcal poly-		Psychiatry	269	
saccharide vaccine	213	Methadose		
		Analgesics	24	
Menjugate	213	Psychiatry	269	
Menofem	205	methazolamide	252	
Menomune-A/C/Y/W-		Methblue 65	284	
135	213	methenamine	285	
Menostar	233	methenamine hippu-		
menotropins	239	rate	81	
Mentax	124	methenamine mande-		
mepenzolate	187	late	81	
meperidine	24	Methergine	241	
mephentermine	116	methimazole	153	
Mephyton	157	Methitest	137	
mepivacaine	31	methocarbamol	16	
Mepron	42	methohexital	30	
mequinol	136	methotrexate		
mercaptopurine		Analgesics	14	
Gastroenterol	193	Oncology	246	
methotrimeprazine	265	Dermatology	125	
methoxsalen	128	OB/GYN	243	
methsuximide	223	Micort-HC Lipocream		
methyclothiazide			131	
	100, 113	Micozole		
methylaminolevulinate		Dermatology	125	
	135	OB/GYN	243	
methylcellulose	190	MICRhoGAM		
methyldopa	88, 99	Immunology	218	
methylene blue		OB/GYN	246	
Toxicology	281	Microgestin Fe 1.5/30		
Urology	284, 285		237	
methylergonovine	241	Microgestin Fe 1/20		
Methylin	271		237	
Methylin ER	271	Micro-K	151	
methylphenidate	271	Micro-K LS	151	
methylprednisolone		Micronase	144	
Endocrine	140	MicroNefrin	279	
Neurology	231	Micronor	237	
methylsulfomethane		Microzide		
	209	Cardiovascular	113	
methyltestosterone		Urology	288	
Endocrine	137	Midamor	111	
OB/GYN	236	midazolam	30	
Meticorten	140	midodrine	116	
metipranolol	252	Midrin	227	
metoclopramide	181	Mifeprex	245	
metolazone	113	mifepristone	245	
Metopirone	161	miglitol	141	
metoprolol	100, 107	miglustat	161	
Metrika A1CNow	145	Migraine	225	
MetroCream	124	Migra-Lief	207	
MetroGel	124	Migranal	226	
MetroGel-Vaginal	243	MigraSpray	207	
MetroLotion	124	mild & strong silver		
metronidazole		protein	211	
Antimicrobials	43, 81	Milk of Magnesia	190	
Dermatology	124	milk thistle	209	
Gastroenterol	186	milrinone	116	
OB/GYN	243	mineral oil	190	
metyrapone	161	Minerals	147	
metyrosine	103	Minipress	88	
Mevacor	97	Minirin		
mexiletine	92	Endocrine	160	
Mexitil	92	Urology	284	
Miacalcin	159	Minitran	115	
Micanol	127	Minizide	101	
Micardis	87	Minocin	79	
Micardis HCT	101	minocycline	79	
Micardis Plus	101	Minox	136	
Micatin	125	minoxidil		
miconazole		Cardiovascular	103	

Dermatology	136	Monopril HCT	101	OB/GYN	244	Narcan	29
Minoxidil for Men	136	montelukast		Mydfrin	254	Nardil	258
Mintezol	45	ENT	178	Mydriacyl	255	Nasacort	178
MiraLax	191	Pulmonary	277	Mydriatics/Cyclople-		Nasacort AQ	178
Mirapex	230	Monurol	80	gics	254	Nasacort HFA	178
Mircette	237	moricizine	92	Mylanta	176	NaSal	178
mirtazapine	260	Morinda citrifolia	209	Mylanta Children's	183	Nasal preps	176
misoprostol		morphine	25	Mylanta suspension		NasalCrom	177
Analgesics	19	Motilium	193		184	Nasalide	177
Gastroenterology	187	Motofen	179	Myleran	246	Nasarel	177
OB/GYN	238	Motrin	20	Mylicon	188	Nascobal	155
Mithracin	246	Mouth & lip preps	175	Mylotarg	246	Nasonex	177
mithramycin	246	Movana	210	Myochrysine	12	nateglinide	143
mitomycin	246	moxifloxacin		Myotonachol	283	Natrecor	119
Mitomycin-C	246	Antimicrobials	77	Mysoline	224	Natulan	246
mitotane	247	Ophthalmology	247	Mytussin DM	168	Naturetin-5	112
mitoxantrone	246	MS Contin	25	M-Zole	243	Navane	264
Mivacron	32	MSIR	25	NABI-HB	216	Navelbine	247
mivacurium	32	MSM	209			Nebcin	33
M-M-R II	213	Mucinex	164			NebuPent	44
Moban	265	Mucinex DM	173	**N**		Necon 0.5/35	237
Mobic	21	Mucomyst				Necon 1/35	237
Mobicox	21	Contrast Media	120			Necon 1/50	237
moclobemide	260	Pulmonary	277	nabumetone	21	Necon 10/11	237
modafinil	272	Toxicology	280	N-acetyl-5-methoxy-		Necon 7/7/7	237
Modecate	264	Mucosil-10	277	tryptamine	209	nedocromil	
Modicon	237	Mucosil-20	277	nadolol	100, 107	Ophthalmology	254
Moditen	264	Multiple sclerosis	227	nafarelin	234	Pulmonary	279
Modulon	195	multivitamins	156	nafcillin	70	nefazodone	260
Moduret	101	mupirocin	124	naftifine	125	NegGram	74
Moduretic	101	Murine Ear	165	Naftin	125	nelfinavir	54
moexipril	84, 101	Muscle relaxants	14	nalbuphine	22	Nembutal	30
molindone	265	Muse	286	Nalcrom	278	neomycin	
mometasone	177	Mustargen	246	Nalfon	20	Dermatol	124, 133
mometasone furoate		Mutamycin	246	nalidixic acid	74	ENT	165, 166
	131	MVI	156	Nallpen	70	Gastroenterology	194
Momordica charantia		Myambutol	40	nalmefene	28	Ophthalmol	248, 250
	204	Mycelex		naloxone		Neoral	218
Monarc-M	202	Antimicrobials	34	Analgesics	29	Neosar	246
Monazole	243	Dermatology	125	Psychiatry	270	Neosporin cream	124
Monistat	243	ENT	175	naltrexone	269	Neosporin ointment	
Monistat 1-Day	244	Mycelex 7	242	Namenda	220	Dermatology	124
Monistat-Derm	125	Mycelex-3	242	nandrolone	137	Ophthalmology	248
Monitan	105	Mycifradin	194	naphazoline	251	Neosporin solution	248
Monoclate P	202	Mycobutin	41	Naphcon	251	neostigmine	231
Monocor	106	Mycolog II	133	Naphcon-A	251	Neo-Synephrine	
Monodox	37, 78	mycophenolate mofetil		Naprelan	21	Cardiovascular	117
monogyna	208		218	Naprosyn	21	ENT	178
Monoket	114	Mycostatin		naproxen		Ophthalmology	254
MonoNessa	237	Antimicrobials	36	Analgesics	21	Neovisc	29
Mononine	202	Dermatology	125	ENT	166	Nephrocap	156
Monopril	84	ENT	176	naratriptan	226	Nephrolithiasis	286

Nephron	279	
Nephrovite	156	
Neptazane	252	
Nerve roots	219	
nesiritide	119	
NESP	201	
nettle root	209	
Neulasta	203	
Neumega	203	
Neupogen	203	
NEUROLOGY	219	
Neuromuscular block-		
ers	31	
Neurontin	222	
Neutra-Phos	150	
Neutrexin	45	
nevirapine	48	
Nexium	188	
NFV	54	
niacin		
Cardiovascular	96,98	
Endocrine	156	
niacin	156	
niacinamide	155	
Niacor		
Cardiovascular	98	
Endocrine	156	
Niaspan		
Cardiovascular	98	
Endocrine	156	
Niastase	202	
nicardipine	109	
Nicoderm	270	
Nicolar	98	
Nicorette	269	
Nicorette DS	269	
nicotine gum	269	
nicotine inhalation sys-		
tem	269	
nicotine lozenge	269	
nicotine nasal spray		
	270	
nicotine patches	270	
nicotinic acid	98	
Nicotrol	270	
Nicotrol Inhaler	269	
Nicotrol NS	270	
nifedipine		
Cardiovascular	109	
OB/GYN	241	
Niferex	149	
Niferex-150	149	

Nilandron		
Oncology	246	
Urology	289	
Nilstat		
Antimicrobials	36	
Dermatology	125	
ENT	176	
OB/GYN	244	
nilutamide		
Oncology	246	
Urology	289	
Nimbex	31	
nimodipine	232	
Nimotop	232	
Nipent	246	
Nipride	103	
nisoldipine	109	
nitazoxanide	43	
nitisinone	161	
Nitrates	113	
nitric oxide	279	
Nitro-BID	114	
Nitro-Dur	115	
nitrofurantoin	82	
nitroglycerin intrave-		
nous infusion	114	
nitroglycerin ointment		
	114	
nitroglycerin spray	114	
nitroglycerin sublingual		
	114	
nitroglycerin sustained		
release	115	
nitroglycerin transder-		
mal	115	
nitroglycerin transmu-		
cosal	115	
Nitroguard	115	
Nitrol	114	
Nitrolingual	114	
Nitropress	103	
nitroprusside	103	
NitroQuick	114	
Nitrostat	114	
Nix	126	
nizatidine	184	
Nizoral		
Antimicrobials	36	
Dermatology	125	
NoDoz	271	
Nolvadex		
Endocrine	162	

	OB/GYN	240
	Oncology	246
noni		209
Non-Opioid Combo		16
Nora-BE		237
Norco		27
Norcuron		32
Nordette		237
Norditropin		160
norelgestromin		245
norepinephrine		116
norethindrone		
	235-237, 240	
Norflex		16
norfloxacin		
	Antimicrobials	75
	Ophthalmology	248
Norgesic		17
norgestimate		237
norgestimate		237
norgestimate		236
norgestrel		237
Norinyl 1+35		237
Norinyl 1+50		237
Noritate		124
Normodyne		107
Noroxin		75
Norpace		90
Norpace CR		90
Norpramin		257
Nor-Q.D.		237
Nortrel 0.5/35		237
Nortrel 1/35		237
Nortrel 7/7/7		237
nortriptyline		257
Norvasc		108
Norvir		54
Nostril		178
Nostrilla		177
NOTICES		2
Novafed A		173
Novahistex		171
Novantrone		246
Novasen		
	Analgesics	18
	Cardiovascular	104
Novasoy		211
Novolin		145
NovoLog		145
NovoRapid		145
NovoSeven		202
Novothyrox		152

Nozinan	265	
NSAIDs	18	
NSAIDs, opthal	255	
Nubain	22	
Nu-Iron	149	
Nu-Iron 150	149	
NuLev		
Gastroenterology	187	
Urology	284	
NuLytely	191	
Numby Stuff	135	
Numorphan	25	
Nupercainal	133	
Nuprin	20	
Nuromax	31	
Nursoy	152	
Nutritionals	151	
Nutropin	160	
Nutropin AQ	160	
NuvaRing	244	
NVP	48	
Nyaderm		
Antimicrobials	36	
Dermatology	125	
OB/GYN	244	
nystatin		
Antimicrobials	36	
Dermatology	125,133	
ENT	176	
OB/GYN	244	

O

Oaklide	288	
oatmeal	136	
OB/GYN	232	
Ocean	178	
Octagam	217	
Octostim	201	
octreotide	194	
Ocu Carpine	253	
Ocufen	255	
Ocuflox	248	
Ocupress	251	
Ocusert	253	
Oenothera biennis	206	
Oesclim	233	
ofloxacin		
Antimicrobials	75	
ENT	166	

Ophthalmology 248
Ogen 234
Ogestrel 237
olanzapine 263, 268
olmesartan 87, 99
olopatadine 254
olsalazine 194
Olux 130
omalizumab 279
omega-3 fatty acid
  Cardiovascular 99
  Endocrine 152
omeprazole 188
Omnicef 63
Omnipaque 120
Omniscan 119
Oncaspar 247
ONCOLOGY 246
Oncovin 247
ondansetron 180
One-a-day Bedtime &
  Rest 208, 211
One-a-day Prostate
  Health 210
One-a-day Tension &
  Mood 210
Ontak 246
Onxol 247
OPHTHALMOLOGY
  247
Ophthetic 255
Opioid Combos 26
Opioid equivalency 23
Opioids 22
opium
  Gastroenterol 179
  Urology 283
opium tincture 179
oprelvekin 203
Opticrom 253
Optimine 163
Optipranolol 252
Optiray 120
Optivar 249
Oracit 288
Oracort 176
Oral anticoagulation
  199
Oral contraceptives
  237
Oramorph SR 25
Orap 264

Orapred 140
Oraquix 31
Orbenin 70
orciprenaline 274
Oretic
  Cardiovascular 113
  Urology 288
Orfadin 161
Orgalutran 234
Orimune 214
Orinase 143
orlistat 194
orphenadrine
  Analgesics 16
  Analgesics 17
Ortho Evra 245
Ortho Novum 10/11
  237
Ortho Tri-Cyclen 237
Ortho Tri-Cyclen Lo
  237
Ortho-Cept 237
Ortho-Cyclen 237
Ortho-Est 234
Ortho-Novum 1/35 237
Ortho-Novum 1/50 237
Ortho-Novum 7/7/7
  237
Orthovisc 29
Orudis 20
Orudis E 20
Orudis KT 20
Orudis SR 20
Oruvail 20
Os-Cal 147
oseltamivir 55
Osmitrol 231
Ostac 138
Osteoforte 158
Outpt peds drugs 6
Ovarian stimulants 234
Ovcon-35 237
Ovcon-50 237
Ovide 126
Ovidrel 238
Ovol 188
Ovral 237
Ovrette 237
oxacillin 70
oxaliplatin 247
Oxandrin 137
oxandrolone 137

oxaprozin 21
oxazepam 267
oxcarbazepine 223
Oxeze 273
oxiconazole 125
Oxistat 125
Oxizole 125
oxprenolol 107
Oxsoralen-Ultra 128
oxyacantha 208
oxybate 232
Oxybutyn 285
oxybutynin 285
Oxycocet 27
Oxycodan 27
oxycodone 25, 27, 28
OxyContin 25
Oxyderm 121
OxyFAST 25
OxyIR 25
oxymetazoline 177
oxymorphone 25
oxytocin 238, 242
Oxytrol 285

P

P450 enzymes 8
Pacerone 89
Pacis
  Immunology 211
  Oncology 246
paclitaxel 247
PAH 289
palivizumab 56
palonosetron 180
pamabrom
  Analgesics 30
  OB/GYN 246
Pamelor 257
pamidronate 139
Panadol 29
Panax ginseng 207
Panax quinquefolius L.
  207
Pancrease 194
pancreatin 194
pancrelipase 194
pancuronium 32
Pandel 131

Panglobulin 217
Panretin 133
Pantoloc 189
pantoprazole 189
pantothenic acid
  155, 156
papaverine 119
paracetamol 29
Parafon Forte DSC 15
Paraplatin 247
paregoric 179
paricalcitol 156
Pariet 189
Parkinsonian agents
  228
Parlodel
  Endocrine 159
  Neurology 229
Parnate 258
paromomycin 44
paroxetine 259
Parvolex
  Contrast Media 120
  Pulmonary 277
  Toxicology 280
Patanol 254
Pausinystalia yohimbe
  211
Pavulon 32
Paxil 259
Paxil CR 259
PCO 208
Peak flow 277
PediaCare Infants'
  Decongestant Drops
  165
Pediapred 140
Pediarix 213
Pediazole 68, 77
Pediotic 166
Peds rehydration 152
Peds vitals, IV drugs 7
PedvaxHIB 212
pegaspargase 247
Pegasys 57
pegfilgrastim 203
peginterferon alfa-2a
  57
peginterferon alfa-2b
  57
PEG-Intron 57
Peg-Lyte 191

pegvisomant	161	pethidine	24	Pilopine HS	253	Polaramine	163
pemetrexed	246	petrolatum	255	Pima Syrup	153	polio	213
pemirolast	254	Pexeva	259	pimecrolimus	129	poliovirus vaccine	214
pemoline	272	PGE1	238	pimozide	264	Polocaine	31
penbutolol	108	PGE2	238	pinaverium	195	polycarbophil	191
penciclovir		Pharmorubicin	246	pindolol	108	Polycitra	288
Dermatology	128	Phazyme	188	Pinworm	44	Polycitra-K	288
ENT	176	Phenazo	285	Pin-X	44	Polycitra-LC	288
Penetrex	75	phenazopyridine	285	pioglitazone	142	polyethylene glycol	191
penicillamine	282	phendimetrizine	272	Piper methysticum	208	polyethylene glycol	
penicillin G	69	phenelzine	258	piperacillin	73	with electrolytes	191
penicillin V	69	Phenergan		piperacillin-tazobac-		Polygam	217
Penicillins	68	ENT	164	tam	73	Polyhistine	173
Penicillins	70	Gastroenterology	182	piperonyl butoxide		poly-L-lactic acid	136
Penlac	124	Phenergan VC	173		126, 127	Polymox	70
Pentacarinat	44	Phenergan VC w/ co-		Pipracil	73	polymyxin	
Pentam	44	deine	173	pirbuterol	274	Dermatology	124,133
pentamidine	44	Phenergan/Dextro-		piroxicam	22	ENT	165, 166
Pentasa	193	methorphan	173	Pitocin	238, 242	Ophthalmol	248, 250
pentazocine	22, 28	pheniramine		Pitressin		Polysporin	
pentobarbital	30	ENT	173	Cardiovascular	93	Dermatology	124
Pentolair	254	Ophthalmology	251	Endocrine	162	Ophthalmology	248
pentosan	285	phenobarbital		Gastroenterology	196	Polytar	134
pentostatin	246	Gastroent	186, 187	pivampicillin	72	polythiazide	101, 113
Pentothal	31	Neurology	223	plague vaccine	213	Polytopic	124
pentoxifylline	119	phenoxybenzamine		Plan B	245	Polytrim	248
Pen-Vee K	69		103	Plaquenil	13	Pondocillin	72
Pepcid	184	phentermine	272	Plasbumin	118	Pontocaine	256
Pepcid AC	184	phentolamine	103	plasma protein fraction		poractant	279
Pepcid Complete	184	phenyl salicylate	285		118	porfimer	247
Pepcid RPD	184	phenylephrine		Plasmanate	118	Portia	237
Peptic Relief	185	Cardiovascular	117	Plasmatein	118	potassium	151
Pepto-Bismol	178	ENT	171-174, 178	Platinol-AQ	247	Potassium forms	151
Peptol	184	Ophthalmology	254	Plavix	104	potassium iodide	153
Percocet	27	phenyltoloxamine	173	Plenaxis		Potent V	211
Percocet-demi	27	Phenytek	223	Oncology	246	Power-Dophilus	209
Percodan	27	phenytoin	223	Urology	288	PPD	219
Percodan-demi	27	PhosLo	147	Plendil	109	pralidoxime	282
Percolone	25	phosphorated carbo-		Pletal	119	pramipexole	230
perflexane	120	hydrates	182	plicamycin	246	Pramosone	136
pergolide	230	phosphorus	150	Pneumo 23	213	pramoxine	133, 136
Pergonal	239	Photofrin	247	pneumococcal 23-		Prandase	141
Periactin	163	Phrenilin	17	valent vaccine	213	Prandin	143
Peri-Colace	191	Phrenilin Forte	17	pneumococcal 7-		Prasterone	206
Peridex	175	Phyllocontin	277	valent conjugate		Pravachol	97
perindopril	85	physostigmine	282	vaccine	214	pravastatin	97, 97
Periogard	175	phytonadione	157	Pneumovax	213	Pravigard PAC	97
Periostat	175	Phytosoya	211	Podocon-25	129	praziquantel	44
Permax	230	Pilocar	253	Podofilm	129	prazosin	88, 101
permethrin	126	pilocarpine		podofilox	128	Precedex	30
perphenazine	264,268	ENT	176	Podofin	129	Precose	141
Persantine	104	Ophthalmology	253	podophyllin	129	Pred Forte	251

Pred G	250	
Pred Mild	251	
prednicarbate	132	
prednisolone		
Endocrine	140	
Ophthalmol	249, 251	
prednisone	140	
Pred-Pak	140	
Prefest	236	
Pregnyl	238	
Prelone	140	
Prelu-2	272	
Premarin	233, 243	
Premesis-Rx	245	
Premphase	236	
PremPlus	236	
Prempro	236	
Pre-Pen	69	
Prepidil	238	
Prepulsid	192	
Pressors/Inotropes	115	
Pressyn AR		
Cardiovascular	93	
Endocrine	162	
Gastroenterol	196	
Pretz	178	
Prevacid	188	
Prevacid NapraPac		
	188	
Prevalite	93	
Preven	246	
Prevex-B	130	
Prevex-HC	131	
Previfem	237	
Prevnar	214	
PrevPac	186	
Priftin	41	
prilocaine		
Anesthesia	31	
Dermatology	135	
Prilosec	188	
Primacor	116	
Primadophilus	209	
primaquine	39	
Primaxin	58	
primidone	224	
Primsol	83	
Principen	71	
Prinivil	84	
Prinzide	101	
Priorix	213	
ProAmatine	116	

Pro-Banthine	187	
probenecid	146	
Probiotica	209	
probiotics	209	
procainamide	92	
procaine penicillin	69	
Procanbid	92	
procarbazine	246	
Procardia		
Cardiovascular	109	
OB/GYN	241	
Procardia XL		
Cardiovascular	109	
OB/GYN	241	
Prochieve	244	
prochlorperazine	182	
Procrit	202	
Proctofoam NS	133	
procyanidolic oligo-		
mers	208	
procyclidine	228	
Procytox	246	
Prodium	285	
Prodium Plain	191	
Profasi	238	
Pro-Fast	272	
progesterone gel	244	
progesterone in oil	240	
progesterone micro-		
nized	240	
Progestins	239	
Proglycem	145	
Prograf	219	
proguanil	38	
Prolastin	277	
Proleukin	246	
Prolixin	264	
Proloprim	83	
Promega		
Cardiovascular	99	
Endocrine	152	
Promensil	210	
Pro-Meta	274	
promethazine		
ENT	164, 173	
Gastroenterol	182	
Prometrium	240	
Promotion	208	
Pronestyl	92	
Propacet	27	
propafenone	92	
Propanthel	187	

propantheline	187	
proparacaine	255	
Propasi HP	239	
Propecia	135	
Propiderm	129	
Propine	253	
propofol	31	
propoxyphene	26-28	
propranolol	100, 108	
Propulsid	192	
Propyl Thyracil	153	
propylene glycol		
	166, 175	
propylthiouracil	153	
Proscar	283	
Prosed/DS	285	
Prosobee	152	
ProSom	266	
prostaglandin E1	119	
Prostata	210	
Prostate cancer	288	
Prostatonin	210	
Prostigmin	231	
Prostin E2	238	
Prostin VR Pediatric		
	119	
protamine	203	
Protenate	118	
Protonix	189	
Protopam	282	
Protopic	129	
protriptyline	258	
Protropin	160	
Proventil	273	
Proventil HFA	273	
Provera	239	
Provigil	272	
Provocholine	279	
Provol	210	
Prozac	258	
Prozac Weekly	258	
Pseudo-Chlor	173	
pseudoephedrine		
	165-175	
Psorcon	130	
Psorcon E	130	
PSYCHIATRY	256	
psyllium	191	
PTU	153	
Pulmicort Respules	275	
Pulmicort Turbuhaler		
	275	

PULMONARY	273	
Pulmozyme	278	
Purge	189	
Purinethol		
Gastroenterol	193	
Oncology	246	
Purinol	287	
PVF	69	
pycnogenol	209	
pygeum africanum	210	
pyrantel	44	
pyrazinamide	41, 42	
pyrethrins	126, 127	
Pyridiate	285	
Pyridium	285	
pyridostigmine	232	
pyridoxine		
Endocrine	155-157	
Gastroenterol	180	
pyrilamine	173, 174	
pyrimethamine	38, 44	
PZA	41	

Q

QT interval drugs	7	
Quadramet	247	
Quanterra	210	
Quanterra Mental		
Sharpness	207	
Quelicin	32	
Questran	93	
Questran Light	93	
quetiapine	263	
Quick-Pep	271	
quinapril	85, 99	
quinidine	93	
quinidine gluconate	39	
quinine	39	
quinine sulfate	16	
Quinolones	74	
quinupristin	82	
Quixin	247	
QVAR	275	

R

R&C	126	

RabAvert	215	Renografin	120	Rifadin	41, 82	Rogaine Forte	136
rabeprazole	189	Renova	123	Rifamate	41	Rogitine	103
rabies immune globu-		ReoPro	104	rifampin	41, 42, 82	Rolaids	184
lin human	217	repaglinide	143	rifapentine	41	Rolaids Calcium Rich	
rabies vaccine	215	Repronex	239	Rifater	42		183
Rabies Vaccine Ad-		Requip	230	rifaximin	82	Romazicon	281
sorbed	215	Rescriptor	48	Rilutek	232	Rondec	174
"rally pack"	152	Rescula	253	riluzole	232	Rondec DM	174
raloxifene		Resectisol	231	Rimactane	41, 82	Rondec DM Infant	
Endocrine	161	reserpine	88, 100, 101	rimantadine	55	Drops	174
OB/GYN	240	RespiGam	218	rimexolone	251	Rondec Infant Drops	
ramipril	85	Restasis	255	Rimostil	210		174
Raniclor	60	Restoril	266	Rimso-50	284	ropinirole	230
ranitidine	185	Restylane	135	Riomet	142	Rosasol	124
Rapamune	219	Retavase	117	Riopan	184	rosiglitazone	141, 142
Rapinex	188	reteplase	117	Ripped Fuel	206	Rosula	122
Raptiva	128	Retin-A	123	risedronate	139	rosuvastatin	97
rasburicase	146	Retin-A Micro	123	Risperdal	263	Rowasa	193
rauwolfia	101	Retisol-A	123	Risperdal Consta	263	Roxanol	25
Rauzide	101	Retrovir	51	risperidone	263	Roxicet	27
Reactine	163	Reversol	231	Ritalin	271	Roxicodone	25
Rebetol	58	Revex	28	Ritalin LA	271	RSV immune globulin	
Rebetron	57	Rev-Eyes	255	Ritalin SR	271		218
Rebif	227	ReVia	269	ritonavir	54	RTV	54
Recombivax HB	212	Reyataz	52	Rituxan	247	RU-486	245
red clover isoflavone		Rheomacrodex	118	rituximab	247	Rubex	246
extract	210	Rheumatrex		rivastigmine	220	Rubini	206
Redoxon	154	Analgesics	14	Rivotril		Rufen	20
Refludan	199	Oncology	246	Neurology	221	Rylosol	93
Refresh PM	255	Rhinalar	177	Psychiatry	266	Ryna-12 S	174
Refresh Tears	255	Rhinocort	177	rizatriptan	226	Rynatan	174
Regitine	103	Rhinocort Aqua	177	Robaxin	16	Rynatan Pediatric	
Reglan	181	RHO immune globulin		Robaxin-750	16	Suspension	174
Regonal	232	Immunology	218	Robinul	193	Rythmodan-LA	90
Regranex	134	OB/GYN	246	Robinul Forte	193	Rythmol	92
Relafen	21	Rhodacine	20	Robitussin	164	Rythmol SR	92
Relenza	56	Rhodis	20	Robitussin AC	173		
Relief	254	Rhodis EC	20	Robitussin CF	168		
Relpax	225	Rhodis SR	20	Robitussin DAC	173		
Remeron	260	RhoGAM		Robitussin DM	168		
Remeron SolTab	260	Immunology	218	Robitussin PE	169		
Remicade		OB/GYN	246	Rocaltrol	154	S	
Analgesics	13	Rhophylac	218	Rocephin	65	S.A.S.	14
Gastroenterol	193	Rhotral	105	rocuronium	32	S-2	279
Remifemin	205	Rhovail	20	Rofact	41, 82	s-adenosylmethionine	
remifentanil	31	ribavirin	57	rofecoxib			210
Reminyl	219	ribavirin - inhaled	58	Analgesics	18	Saint John's wort	210
Remodulin	103	ribavirin - oral	58	Neurology	227	Saizen	160
Renagel	162	riboflavin	155-157	Roferon-A	246	Salagen	176
Renedil	109	RID	127	Rogaine	136	Salazopyrin	
Renese	113	Ridaura	12	Rogaine Extra		Analgesics	14
Renese-R	101	rifabutin	41	Strength	136	Gastroenterol	195
						Salazopyrin EN	195

Salazopyrin EN-Tabs 14
salbutamol 273
Salflex 19
saline nasal spray 178
salmeterol 274
Salofalk 193
salsalate 19
samarium 153 247
Sambucas nigra 206
Sambucol 206
SAM-e 210
sammy 210
Sanctura 285
Sandimmune 218
Sandoglobulin 217
Sandostatin 194
Sandostatin LAR 194
Sans-Acne 122
saquinavir 54
Sarafem 258
sargramostim 203
Sarna-HC 131
saw palmetto 210
SBE prophylaxis 72
scopolamine 182, 187
Sculptra 136
SeaMist 178
Sea-Omega 99
SecreMax 195
secretin 195
Sectral 105
Sedapap 17
Selective Estrogen
Receptor Modulators
240
selegiline 230
selenium sulfide 136
Selpak 230
Selsun 136
Semprex-D 174
senna 191, 192
Senokot 191
Senokot-S 192
SenokotXTRA 191
Sensipar 159
Sensorcaine 31
Septocaine 31
Septra 78
Ser-Ap-Es 101
Serax 267
Serenoa repens 210

Serevent Diskus 274
Serophene 238
Seroquel 263
Serostim 160
Serpasil 88
sertaconazole 126
sertraline 259
sevelamer 162
Seville orange 205
shark cartilage 210
Sibelium 227
sibutramine
Gastroenterol 195
Psychiatry 272
Siladryl 267, 273
sildenafil 286
Silvadene 124
silver - colloidal 211
silver ion 211
silver sulfadiazine 124
Silybum marianum 209
silymarin 209
simethicone
178, 184, 188
Similac 152
Simulect 218
simvastatin 97, 98
Sinemet 229
Sinemet CR 229
Sinequan 257
Sinex 178
Singulair
ENT 178
Pulmonary 277
Sinupret 206
sirolimus 219
Skelaxin 16
Skelid 139
Sleep-Tite 208, 211
Slo-Niacin 156
Slow-Fe 148
Slow-K 151
Slow-Mag 150
Slow-Trasicor 107
smallpox vaccine 215
sodium ferric glucon-
ate complex 151
sodium iodide I-131
153
Sodium Iodide I-131
Therapeutic 153
sodium phosphate

Gastroenterol 192
Urology 285
sodium polystyrene
sulfonate 162
sodium sulfacetamide
Dermatol 121, 122
Ophthalmol 249, 250
Solag 136
Solagé 136
Solaquin 135
Solaraze 123
Solu-Cortef 140
Solugel 121
Solu-Medrol
Endocrine 140
Neurology 231
Soma 15
Soma Compound 17
Soma Compound with
Codeine 27
Somatropin 160
Somavert 161
Sominex 267, 273
Sonata 268
sorbitol
Gastroenterol 192
Toxicology 282
Soriatane 127
Sotacor 93
sotalol 93
soy 211
Soyalac 152
Spacol 284
Spasdel 284
Spectazole 125
spectinomycin 33
Spectracef 63
Spiriva 280
spironolactone
Cardiovasc 86, 99
Endocrine 162
Sporanox 35
Sprintec-28 237
SQV 54
SSKI 153
St John's wort 210
Stadol 22
Stadol NS 22
Stalevo 230
standardized extract
WS 1442 – Cratae-
gutt novo 208

stanozolol 137
starch 133
Starlix 143
Starnoc 268
Statex 25
Statins 96
stavudine 50
Stay Awake 271
STDs / Vaginitis 62
Stelazine 264
Stemetil 182
Sterapred 140
stevia 211
Stevia rebaudiana 211
Stieva-A 123
Stimate
Endocrine 160
Hematology 201
Stimulants / ADHD /
Anorexiants 270
stinging nettle 209
Strattera 270
Streptase 117
streptokinase 117
streptomycin 33
streptozocin 246
Striant 137
Stromectol 43
strontium-89 247
Sublimaze 30
Suboxone 270
Subutex 268
succimer 282
succinylcholine 32
sucralfate 188
Sudafed 165
Sudafed 12 Hour 165
Sufenta 31
sufentanil 31
Sulamyd 248
Sular 109
Sulcrate 188
Sulf-10 248
sulfacetamide 248
Sulfacet-R 122
sulfadiazine 77
sulfadoxine 38
Sulfamylon 123
sulfasalazine
Analgesics 14
Gastroenterol 195
Sulfatrim 78

sulfinpyrazone	147	tacrine	220	Psychiatry	261	lin	218
sulfisoxazole	68,77,78	tacrolimus		*Tegretol XR*		tetanus toxoid	215
Sulfonamides	77	Dermatology	129	Neurology	220	tetracaine	256
sulfonated phenolics		Immunology	219	Psychiatry	261	tetracycline	
	175	tadalafil	286	*Tegrin*	134	Antimicrobials	79
sulfur	121, 122	*Tagamet*	184	*Tegrin-HC*	131	Gastroenterol	186
sulfuric acid	175	*Tagamet HB*	184	telithromycin	65	Tetracyclines	78
sulindac	22	*Talacen*	28	telmisartan	87, 101	*Teveten*	86
sumatriptan	226	*Talwin*	22	temazepam	266	*Teveten HCT*	101
Sumycin	79	*Talwin NX*	22	*Temodal*	246	thalidomide	136
Supartz	29	*Tambocor*	91	*Temodar*	246	*Thalitone*	
SuperEPA 1200	99	*Tamiflu*	55	*Temovate*	130	Cardiovascular	113
Supeudol	25	*Tamone*		temozolomide	246	Urology	287
Supplifem	210, 211	OB/GYN	240	*Tempra*	29	*Thalomid*	136
Suprax	63	Oncology	246	tenecteplase	118	*Theo-24*	279
Supro	211	tamoxifen		*Tenex*		*Theo-Dur*	279
Surfak	190	Endocrine	162	Cardiovascular	88	*Theolair*	279
Surgam	22	OB/GYN	240	Psychiatry	273	theophylline	279
Surgam SR	22	Oncology	246	teniposide	247	*TheraCys*	246
Surpass	183	tamsulosin	283	*Ten-K*	151	Therapeutic levels	5
Survanta	278	*Tanacetum parthe-*		tenofovir	50, 51	thiabendazole	45
Sustiva	48	*nium L.*	207	*Tenoretic*	101	thiamine	155-157
Swim-Ear	166	*Tanafed*	174	*Tenormin*	105	thiethylperazine	182
Symax	284	*Tapazole*	153	*Tensilon*	231	thioguanine	246
Symbicort	275	*Tarabine*	246	*Tenuate*	271	thiopental	31
Symbyax	268	*Targretin*	247	*Tenuate Dospan*	271	*Thioplex*	246
Symmetrel		*Tarka*	101	*Tequin*	76	thioridazine	265
Antimicrobials	55	*TARO-sone*	129	*Terazol*	244	thiotepa	246
Neurology	229	*Tarsum*	134	terazosin		thiothixene	264
Symphytum officinale		*Tasmar*	228	Cardiovascular	88	*Thisylin*	209
	205	*Tavist*	163	Urology	283	thonzonium	165
Synacort	131	*Tavist ND*	163	terbinafine		*Thorazine*	265
Synacthen	160	*Taxol*	247	Antimicrobials	36	Thrombolysis in MI	117
Synagis	56	*Taxotere*	247	Dermatology	126	Thrombolytics	117
Synalar	130	tazarotene	123, 128	terbutaline		*Thyro-Block*	153
Synalgos-DC	27	*Tazicef*	64	OB/GYN	241	thyroid – dessicated	
Synamol	130	*Tazidime*	64	Pulmonary	274		154
Synarel	234	*Tazocin*	73	terconazole	244	Thyroid agents	152
Synercid	82	*Tazorac*	123, 128	teriparatide	162	*Thyroid USP*	154
Syntest D.S.	236	*Taztia XT*	109	*Teslac*	246	*Thyrolar*	154
Syntest H.S.	236	*Td*	212	*Tessalon*	164	*Thyro-Tabs*	152
Synthroid	152	*TDF*	50	*Tessalon Perles*	164	tiagabine	224
Synvisc	29	tea tree oil	211	*Tes-Tape*	145	*Tiamol*	130
		Tears Naturale	255	*Testim*	137	tiaprofenic acid	22
		Tebrazid	41	testolactone	246	*Tiazac*	109
		Tecnal	17	*Testopel*	137	*Ticar*	73
T		*Tecnal C-1/2*	26	testosterone	137	ticarcillin	73
		Tecnal C-1/4	26	*Testred*	137	ticarcillin-clavulanate	73
T3	153	tegaserod	195	*Testro AQ*	137	*Tice BCG*	
T4	152	*Tegens*	204	*Testro-L.A.*	137	Immunology	211
T-20	47	*Tegretol*		*Tetanus*	216	Oncology	246
TABLES INDEX	4	Neurology	220	tetanus immune globu-		*Ticlid*	105

ticlopidine	105	Topilene Glycol	129	Triaminic Chest Congestion	169
Tigan	182	topiramate			166, 167, 174
Tikosyn	90	Neurology	224	Triaminic Cold & Allergy	169
Tilade	279	Psychiatry	262		
tiludronate	139	Topisone	129	Triaminic Cold & Cough	169
Timentin	73	Toposar	247		
Timolide	101	topotecan	247	Triaminic Cough	169
timolol		Toprol-XL	107	Triaminic Cough & Sore Throat	169
Cardiovasc	101,108	Topsyn	130		
Ophthalmol	252, 253	Toradol	21	Triaminic Oral Infant Drops	165
Timoptic	252	Torecan	182		
Tinactin	126	toremifene	246	triamterene	100, 112
Tindamax	45	torsemide	111	Triavil	268
tinidazole	45	tositumomab	247	triazolam	267
tinzaparin	198	**TOXICOLOGY**	280	Tricor	98
tioconazole	244	t-PA		Tridesilon	130
tiotropium	280	Cardiovascular	117	Tridil	114
tirofiban	105	Neurology	230	triethanolamine	166
Titralac	183	T-Phyl	279	trifluoperazine	264
tizanidine	16	Tracleer	102	trifluridine	249
TNKase	118	Tracrium	31	Trifolium pratense	210
TOBI	33	tramadol	17, 29	Trigonelle foenum-graecum	206
TobraDex	250	Trandate	107		
tobramycin		trandolapril	85, 101	trihexyphenidyl	228
Antimicrobials	33	tranexamic acid	203	TriHibit	215
Ophthalmol	247, 250	Transderm-Scop	182	Tri-K,	151
Tobrex	247	Transderm-V	182	Trikacide	43, 81
tocainide	93	Tranxene	266	Trilafon	264
Tocolytics	240	tranylcypromine	258	Trileptal	223
tocopherol	157	Trasicor	107	Tri-Levlen	237
Tofranil		trastuzumab	247	Trilisate	19
Psychiatry	257	Trasylol	201	Tri-Luma	136
Urology	284	Travatan	252	TriLyte	191
Tofranil PM	257, 284	travoprost	252	trimebutine	195
tolazamide	143	trazodone	261	trimethobenzamide	182
tolbutamide	143	trefoil	210	trimethoprim	
tolcapone	228	Trelstar Depot	246	Antimicrobials	83
Tolectin	22	Trental	119	Ophthalmology	248
Tolinase	143	treprostinil	103	trimethoprim-sulfamethoxazole	78
tolmetin	22	tretinoin			
tolnaftate	126	Dermatology	123,136	trimetrexate	45
Tol-Tab	143	Oncology	247	Trimox	70
tolterodine	285	Trexall		Tri-Nasal	178
Tomoptic Ocudose	252	Analgesics	14	Trinessa	237
Tonocard	93	Oncology	246	Trinipatch	115
Topactin	130	Triacin-C	174	Tri-Norinyl	237
Topamax		Triaderm	132	Trinovin	210
Neurology	224	triamcinolone		Tripacel	212
Psychiatry	262	Dermatology	132,133	Tripedia	212
Topical steroids	132	Endocrine	141	Triphasil	237
Topicort	130	ENT	176, 178	Tri-Previfem	237
Topicort LP	130	Pulmonary	276	triprolidine	
triptorelin	246				
Trisenox	247				
Tri-Sprintec	237				
Trivora-28	237				
Trizivir	51				
Trobicin	33				
tropicamide	255				
trospium	285				
Trusopt	252				
Truvada	51				
tuberculin PPD	219				
Tubersol	219				
Tucks	133				
Tums					
Endocrine	147				
Gastroenterol	183				
Tuss-HC	174				
Tussionex	175				
Twinrix	215				
Tylenol	29				
Tylenol w Codeine	28				
Tylox	28				
Typhim Vi	215				
typhoid vaccine	215				

U

ubiquinone	205
Ultiva	31
Ultracet	17
Ultradol	20
Ultram	29
Ultravate	131
Unasyn	72
Uniphyl	279
Uniretic	101
Unisom Nighttime Sleep Aid	181
Unithroid	152
Univasc	84
unoprostone	253
Urecholine	283
Urex	81
Urised	285
Urispas	284
Urocit-K	288
Urodol	285
urofollintropin	239
Urogesic	285

urokinase 118
Urolene blue
    Toxicology 281
    Urology 284
UROLOGY 283
Uromitexan 246
UroXatral 283
URSO 195
ursodiol 195
Ursofalk 195
Urtica dioica radix 209
Usept 285
UTA 285
Uterotonics 241
UTI Relief 285

V

Vaccinium macrocarpon 205
Vaccinium myrtillus 204
Vagifem 243
Vaginal preps 242
Vagistat-1 244
valacyclovir 47
Valcyte 46
valdecoxib 18
valerian 211
Valeriana officinalis 211
valganciclovir 46
Valisone 130
Valium
    Analgesics 15
    Neurology 221
    Psychiatry 266
valproic acid
    Neurology 224, 227
    Psychiatry 262
valrubicin 246
valsartan 87, 100
Valstar 246
Valtaxin 246
Valtrex 47
Vancenase 177
Vancenase AQ Double Strength 177
Vanceril 275
Vancocin 83

vancomycin 83
Vaniqa 135
Vanspar 267
Vantin 64
Vaponefrin 279
Vaqta 212
vardenafil 286
varicella vaccine 216
varicella-zoster immune globulin 218
Varivax 216
Vaseretic 101
Vasocidin 250
Vasocon 251
Vasodilan 119
vasopressin
    Cardiovascular 93
    Endocrine 162
    Gastroenterology 196
Vasotec 84
VCR 247
vecuronium 32
Veetids 69
Velban 247
Velcade 247
Velivet 237
Venastat 208
venlafaxine 261
Venofer 149
Venoglobulin 217
Ventodisk 273
Ventolin 273
VePesid 247
verapamil 101, 110
Verelan 110
Verelan PM 110
Vermox 43
Versed 30
Versel 136
verteporfin 256
Vesanoid 247
vetch 204
Vexol 251
Vfend 37
Viactiv 147
Viadur
    Oncology 246
    Urology 288
Viagra 286
Vibramycin
    Antimicrobials 37, 78
    Dermatology 121

Vibra-Tabs 37
Vick's 164
Vicodin 28
Vicoprofen 28
vidarabine 249
Vidaza 246
Videx 49
Videx EC 49
Vigamox 248
vinblastine 247
Vincasar 247
vincristine 247
vinorelbine 247
Viokase 194
Vioxx
    Analgesics 18
    Neurology 227
Vira-A 249
Viracept 54
Viramune 48
Virazole 58
Viread 50
Virilon 137
Viroptic 249
Visicol 192
Visipaque 120
Vistaril 164
Vistide 45
Visual acuity screen 256
Visudyne 256
vitamin A 158
vitamin B1 157
vitamin B2 157
vitamin B3
    Cardiovascular 98
    Endocrine 156
vitamin B6 157
vitamin B12 155
vitamin C 154-155
vitamin D 155, 158
vitamin D2 158
vitamin E 157
vitamin K 157
Vitamins 154
Vitex agnus castus fruit extract 205
Vitravene 249
Vitus vinifera L. 208
Vivactil 258
Vivarin 271
Vivelle 233

Vivol
    Analgesics 15
    Neurology 221
    Psychiatry 266
Vivotif Berna 215
VLB 247
VM-26 247
VMA extract 204
Volmax 273
Voltaren
    Analgesics 19
    Ophthalmology 255
Voltaren Rapide 19
Voltaren XR 19
Volume expanders 118
voriconazole 37
VoSol otic 166
VoSpire ER 273
VP-16 247
Vumon 247
Vytorin 98

W

warfarin 199
warfarin interactions 200
Welchol 94
Wellbutrin 260
Wellbutrin SR 260
Wellbutrin XL 260
Wellcovorin 247
Westcort 131
wild yam 211
Winpred 140
WinRho SDF
    Immunology 218
    OB/GYN 246
Winstrol 137
witch hazel 133
wolf's bane 204
Women's Tylenol Menstrual Relief
    Analgesics 30
    OB/GYN 246
Wyamine 116
Wycillin 69
Wygesic 28
Wytensin 87

X

Xalatan	252
Xanax	267
Xanax XR	267
Xeloda	246
Xenadrine	206
Xenical	194
Xifaxan	82
Xigris	80
ximelagatran	199
Xolair	279
Xopenex	274
Xylocaine	
Analgesics	29
Anesthesia	31
Cardiovascular	91
Dermatology	135
ENT	175
Xylocard	91
Xyrem	232

Y

Yasmin	237
yellow fever vaccine	216
YF-Vax	216
Yocon	287
Yodoxin	43
yohimbe	211
yohimbine	287
Yohimex	287

Z

Zaditen	279
Zaditor	254
zafirlukast	277
zalcitabine	51
zaleplon	268
Zanaflex	16
zanamivir	56
Zanosar	246
Zantac	185
Zantac 25	185
Zantac 75	185
Zarontin	221
Zaroxolyn	113
Zavesca	161
ZDV	51
Zebeta	106
Zegerid	188
Zelnorm	195
Zemaira	277
Zemplar	156
Zemuron	32
Zenapax	218
Zephrex-LA	175
Zerit	50
Zestoretic	101
Zestril	84
Zetia	98
Zevalin	246
Ziac	101
Ziagen	49
zidovudine	49, 51
zileuton	277
Zinacef	61
Zinecard	246
Zingiber officinale	207
ziprasidone	263
Zithromax	66
Zocor	97
Zofran	180
Zoladex	
OB/GYN	234
Oncology	246
Urology	288
zoledronic acid	139
zolmitriptan	226
Zoloft	259
zolpidem	268
Zometa	139
Zomig	226
Zomig ZMT	226
Zonalon	134
Zonegran	225
zonisamide	225
zopiclone	268
Zorbtive	160
Zostrix	134
Zostrix-HP	134
Zosyn	73
Zovia 1/35E	237
Zovia 1/50E	237
Zovirax	
Antimicrobials	46
Dermatology	128
Zyban	268
Zydone	28
Zyflo	277
Zyloprim	
Endocrine	146
Urology	287
Zymar	247
Zyprexa	263
Zyprexa Zydis	263
Zyrtec	163
Zyrtec-D	175
Zyvox	81
Zyvoxam	81

Page left blank for notes

Page left blank for notes

Page left blank for notes

Page left blank for notes

ADULT EMERGENCY DRUGS (selected)

ALLERGY	diphenhydramine (*Benadryl*): 50 mg IV/IM. epinephrine: 0.1-0.5 mg SC (1:1000 solution), may repeat after 20 minutes. methylprednisolone (*Solu-Medrol*): 125 mg IV/IM.
HYPERTENSION	esmolol (*Brevibloc*): 500 mcg/kg IV over 1 minute, then titrate 50-200 mcg/kg/minute fenoldopam (*Corlopam*): Start 0.1 mcg/kg/min, titrate up to 1.6 mcg/kg/min labetalol (*Normodyne*): Start 20 mg slow IV, then 40-80 mg IV q10 min prn up to 300 mg total cumulative dose nitroglycerin (*Tridil*): Start 10-20 mcg/min IV infusion, then titrate prn up to 100 mcg/minute nitroprusside (*Nipride*): Start 0.3 mcg/kg/min IV infusion, then titrate prn up to 10 mcg/kg/minute
DYSRHYTHMIAS / ARREST	adenosine (*Adenocard*): SVT (not A-fib/flutter): 6 mg rapid IV & flush, preferably through a central line or proximal IV. If no response after 1-2 minutes then 12 mg. A third dose of 12 mg may be given prn. amiodarone (*Cordarone, Pacerone*): Life-threatening ventricular arrhythmia: Load 150 mg IV over 10 min, then 1 mg/min x 6h, then 0.5 mg/min x 18h. atropine: 0.5-1.0 mg IV/ET, repeat q 5 min to maximum of 0.04 mg/kg. diltiazem (*Cardizem*): Rapid atrial fibrillation: bolus 0.25 mg/kg or 20 mg IV over 2 min. May repeat 0.35 mg/kg or 25 mg IV 15 min after first dose. Infusion 5-15 mg/h. epinephrine: 1 mg IV/ET for cardiac arrest. [1:10,000 solution] lidocaine (*Xylocaine*): Load 1 mg/kg IV, then 0.5 mg/kg q8-10min prn to max 3 mg/kg. Maintenance 2g in 250ml D5W (8 mg/ml) at 1-4 mg/min drip (7-30 ml/h).
PRESSORS	dobutamine (*Dobutrex*): 250 mg in 250ml D5W (1 mg/ml) at 2.5-15 mcg/kg/min. 70 kg: 21 ml/h = 5 mcg/kg/min. dopamine (*Intropin*): 400 mg in 250ml D5W (1600 mcg/ml) at 2-20 mcg/kg/min. 70 kg: 13 ml/h = 5 mcg/kg/min. Doses in mcg/kg/min: 2-5 = dopaminergic, 5-10 = beta, >10 = alpha. norepinephrine (*Levophed*): 4 mg in 500 ml D5W (8 mcg/ml) at 2-4 mcg/min. 22.5 ml/h = 3 mcg/min. phenylephrine (*Neo-Synephrine*): 50 mcg boluses IV. Infusion for hypotension: 20 mg in 250ml D5W (80 mcg/ml) at 40-180 mcg/min (35-160ml/h).
INTUBATION	etomidate (*Amidate*): 0.3 mg/kg IV. methohexital (*Brevital*): 1-1.5 mg/kg IV. rocuronium (*Zemuron*): 0.6-1.2 mg/kg IV. succinylcholine (*Anectine*): 1 mg/kg IV. Peds (<5 yo): 2 mg/kg IV preceded by atropine 0.02 mg/kg. thiopental (*Pentothal*): 3-5 mg/kg IV.
SEIZURES	diazepam (*Valium*): 5-10 mg IV, or 0.2-0.5 mg/kg rectal gel up to 20 mg PR. fosphenytoin (*Cerebyx*): Load 15-20 "phenytoin equivalents" per kg either IM, or IV no faster than 100-150 mg/min. lorazepam (*Ativan*): 0.05-0.15 mg/kg up to 3-4 mg IV/IM. phenobarbital: 200-600 mg IV at rate ≤60 mg/min; titrate prn up to 20 mg/kg phenytoin (*Dilantin*): 15-20 mg/kg up to 1000 mg IV no faster than 50 mg/min.

CARDIAC DYSRHYTHMIA PROTOCOLS (*Circulation* 2000; 102, suppl I)
For adults and children >8 years old. Alter dosing & Joules based on child's weight.

Basic Life Support
All cases: Two initial breaths, then compressions 100 per minute
One or two rescuer: 15:2 ratio of compressions to ventilations

V-Fib, Pulseless V-Tach
CPR until defibrillator ready
Defibrillate 200 J
Defibrillate 200-300 J
Defibrillate 360 J
Intubate, IV, then *options:*
- Epinephrine 1 mg IV q3-5 minutes
- Vasopressin 40 units IV once only; IV epi if no response in 5-10 min
- Defibrillate 360 J after each drug dose

Options:
- Amiodarone 300 mg IV; repeat doses 150 mg
- Lidocaine 1.0-1.5 mg/kg IV q3-5 minutes to max 3 mg/kg
- Magnesium 1-2 g IV
- Procainamide 30-50 mg/min IV to max 17 mg/kg
- Bicarbonate 1 mEq/kg IV

Defibrillate 360 J after each drug dose

Pulseless Electrical Activity (PEA)
CPR, intubate, IV.
- Consider 5 H's: hypovolemia, hypoxia, H^+ acidosis, hyper / hypokalemia, hypothermia
- Consider 5 T's: "tablets"-drug OD, tamponade-cardiac, tension pneumothorax, thrombosis-coronary, thrombosis-pulmonary embolism

Epinephrine 1 mg IV q3-5 minutes
If bradycardia, atropine 1 mg IV q3-5 min to max 0.04 mg/kg
Consider bicarbonate 1 mEq/kg IV if hyperkalemia or tricyclic/ASA overdose

Asystole
CPR, intubate, IV, assess code status
Confirm asystole in >1 lead
Search for and treat reversible causes
Consider early transcutaneous pacing
Epinephrine 1 mg IV q3-5 minutes
Atropine 1 mg IV q3-5 min to max 0.04 mg/kg

Bradycardia (<60 bpm), symptomatic
Airway, oxygen, IV
Atropine 0.5-1 mg IV q3-5 min to max 0.04 mg/kg
Transcutaneous pacemaker
Options:
- Dopamine 5-20 mcg/kg/min
- Epinephrine 2-10 mcg/min

Unstable Tachycardia (>150 bpm)
Airway, oxygen, IV
Consider brief trial of medications
Premedicate whenever possible
Synchronized cardioversion 100 J
Synchronized cardioversion 200 J
Synchronized cardioversion 300 J
Synchronized cardioversion 360 J

Stable Monomorphic V-Tach
Airway, oxygen, IV
If no CHF, then choose just one top agent (procainamide, sotalol) or other agent (amiodarone, lidocaine)
If CHF (EF<40%), then DC cardioversion after pretreatment with either:
- Amiodarone 150 mg IV over 10 min; repeat q10-15 min prn
- Lidocaine 0.5-0.75 mg/kg IV; repeat q5-10 min prn to max 3 mg/kg

Stable Wide-Complex Tachycardia
Airway, oxygen, IV
If no CHF, then *options:*
- DC cardioversion
- Procainamide 20-30 mg/min IV to max 20 mg/kg
- Amiodarone (see stable V-tach dose)
If CHF (EF<40%), then *options:*
- DC cardioversion
- Amiodarone

Stable Narrow-Complex SVT
Airway, oxygen, IV
Vagal stimulation
Adenosine 6mg IV, then 12 mg prn.
Further treatment based on specific rhythm (junctional tachycardia, PSVT, multifocal atrial tachycardia) and presence or absence of CHF.

Ordering From Tarascon Publishing

INTERNET	FAX	PHONE	MAIL
Credit card orders at www.tarascon.com	Fax credit card orders toll free to 877.929.9926	For phone orders or customer service, call 800.929.9926	Mail order & check to: Tarascon Publishing, PO Box 517, Lompoc, CA 93438

Price/Copy by # of Copies Ordered

	1–9	10–49	50–99	≥100	# Ordered	Price
TARASCON POCKET PHARMACOPOEIA®						
Classic Shirt-Pocket Edition	$9.95	$8.95	$7.95	$6.95		$
Deluxe Labcoat Pocket Edition	$17.95	$15.25	$13.45	$12.55		$
PDA software on CD-ROM, 12-month subscription*	$29.95	$25.46	$23.96	$22.46		$
PDA software on CD-ROM, 3-month subscription*	$8.97	$7.62	$7.18	$6.73		$
OTHER POCKETBOOKS & MAGNIFIER	1–9	10–49	50–99	≥100		
Tarascon Adult Emergency Pocketbook	$14.95	$13.45	$11.94	$10.44		$
Tarascon Pocket Orthopaedica®	$14.95	$13.45	$11.94	$10.44		$
Tarascon Internal Medicine & Critical Care Pocketbook	$14.95	$13.45	$11.94	$10.44		$
Tarascon Primary Care Pocketbook	$14.95	$13.45	$11.94	$10.44		$
Tarascon Pediatric Emergency Pocketbook	$11.95	$9.90	$8.95	$8.35		$
How to be a Truly Excellent Junior Medical Student	$9.95	$8.25	$7.45	$6.95		$
Sheet magnifier – fits in any book to make reading easier!	$1.00	$0.89	$0.78	$0.66		$
					Subtotal	$
SALES TAX - California only				California Sales Tax (7.75%)		$
					Shipping	$
					TOTAL	$

Palm OS or Pocket PC; download the software directly from www.tarascon.com for an approximately 10% discount!

CHOOSE SHIPPING METHOD: cost based on subtotal →

	≤$10	$10–29	$30–75	$76–300
Standard shipping	$1.00	$2.50	$6.00	$8.00
UPS 2-day air (no post office boxes)	$12.00	$14.00	$16.00	$18.00

☐ VISA ☐ Mastercard ☐ AmEx ☐ Discover

Card number _____

Expiration date _____ CID# (if available) _____

Signature _____

Name _____

Address _____

City / State / Zip _____

E-mail and phone _____